T0295244

Toward an Integrated Science of Wellbeing

Toward an Integrated Science of Wellbeing

EDITED BY ELIZABETH RIEGER,

ROBERT COSTANZA, IDA KUBISZEWSKI,

AND

PAUL DUGDALE

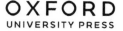

OXFORD
UNIVERSITY PRESS

Oxford University Press is a department of the University of Oxford. It furthers
the University's objective of excellence in research, scholarship, and education
by publishing worldwide. Oxford is a registered trade mark of Oxford University
Press in the UK and certain other countries.

Published in the United States of America by Oxford University Press
198 Madison Avenue, New York, NY 10016, United States of America.

© Oxford University Press 2023

All rights reserved. No part of this publication may be reproduced, stored in
a retrieval system, or transmitted, in any form or by any means, without the
prior permission in writing of Oxford University Press, or as expressly permitted
by law, by license, or under terms agreed with the appropriate reproduction
rights organization. Inquiries concerning reproduction outside the scope of the
above should be sent to the Rights Department, Oxford University Press, at the
address above.

You must not circulate this work in any other form
and you must impose this same condition on any acquirer.

Library of Congress Cataloging-in-Publication Data
Names: Rieger, Elizabeth, editor. | Costanza, Robert, editor. |
Kubiszewski, Ida, editor. | Dugdale, Paul, editor.
Title: Toward an integrated science of wellbeing / edited by Elizabeth Rieger,
Robert Costanza, Ida Kubiszewski, and Paul Dugdale.
Description: New York, NY : Oxford University Press, [2023] |
Includes bibliographical references and index. |
Identifiers: LCCN 2022058518 (print) | LCCN 2022058519 (ebook) |
ISBN 9780197567579 (hardback) | ISBN 9780197567593 (epub) |
ISBN 9780197567609
Subjects: LCSH: Happiness. | Well-being. | Conduct of life.
Classification: LCC BF575.H27 T693 2023 (print) | LCC BF575.H27 (ebook) |
DDC 158.1—dc23/eng/20230222
LC record available at https://lccn.loc.gov/2022058518
LC ebook record available at https://lccn.loc.gov/2022058519

DOI: 10.1093/med-psych/9780197567579.001.0001

Printed by Sheridan Books, Inc., United States of America

Excerpt from Mary Oliver, "The Poet with His Face in His Hands," in *New and Selected Poems,
Volume Two* (Boston: Beacon Press, 2005), reproduced with permission.

CONTENTS

LIST OF FIGURES

LIST OF TABLES

LIST OF BOXES

FOREWORD

JIGME Y. THINLEY (PRIME MINISTER OF BHUTAN, 2008–2013)

I am delighted to be writing the foreword for this book of findings and thoughts of eminent scholars and practitioners on wellbeing. Having committed much time and effort to the study and promotion of this subject, I am well aware of how far human society has strayed on a frighteningly clear self-destructive trajectory while the path to sustainable wellbeing is rapidly fading. This book will be a source of much-needed illumination.

There is no denying that sociologists, economists, neuroscientists, spiritual gurus, and experts have mined and accumulated an incredible amount of revelatory knowledge and skills on diverse aspects of human wellbeing. However, its study as a multidimensional subject has not been as central a concern as it ought to have been. With ever increasing specialisation, there is not enough acknowledgement of the interrelationships between and among the diverse conditions that are mutually dependent, vitalising, or even destructive. What is needed is a greater effort to collate this vast, dispersed wealth of knowledge so that the wisdom of a holistic, integrated approach to understanding and promoting wellbeing as a composite of constructs and scales becomes the norm. Wellbeing scholars need to work in concert.

I am reminded of my own humble appeal for an integrated approach to the august gathering of world leaders at the 63rd United Nations (UN) General Assembly in 2008. We were all shocked and dismayed by the unprecedented precipitation of a multiplicity of calamitous events in just one year. These included natural disasters; food, fuel and financial crises; failing states; deepening poverty; human trafficking and population displacement; dwindling water sources; new health hazards; and a rising incidence of terrorism, extremism, and maritime lawlessness. I was uninspired by the array of solutions put forward to meet each of the individual challenges, which the leaders seemed to think were unrelated. Nor did any appear to view the challenges from a wellbeing perspective. Instead, the focus was on how all these crises would set back economic development.

While it was perhaps inevitable that the deliberations led by industrialised nations centred on the financial crisis and the need to stimulate growth, I felt compelled to declare that "Bhutan does not look at these developments as separate, disconnected events. Rather, we see them as directly interconnected symptoms of a larger and deeper malaise that threatens our collective survival and wellbeing.

Responding to each of the challenges separately will most probably be useful in the short run, but piecemeal efforts will not lead to permanent solutions. We need to treat the disease beyond the symptoms. And the disease, we believe, has to do with our way of life that is just not rational and sustainable". I wanted the world to see these problems as pieces of one mosaic from a multidimensional perspective.

Three years later in July 2011, the 65th session of the UN General Assembly unanimously adopted the resolution, "Happiness: Toward a Holistic Approach to Development". In its preamble, the resolution states that the assembly had become "Conscious that unsustainable patterns of production and consumption can impede sustainable development", and that it recognised "the need for a more inclusive, equitable and balanced approach to economic growth that promotes sustainable development, poverty eradication, happiness and well-being of all peoples". It also welcomed "the offer of Bhutan to convene a panel discussion on the theme of happiness and well-being during its 66th session". The overwhelming response to our call led to this event being held as a 'High Level Meeting' on "Wellbeing and Happiness: Defining A New Economic Paradigm" at the UN Head Quarters on 2 April 2012.

The extraordinary constellation of great minds, nations, civil society, business and industry, spiritual leaders, and concerned citizens acknowledged human happiness and the wellbeing of all life on earth as the core goal of development. It recognised ecological sustainability, fair distribution, and the efficient use of resources as essential conditions to achieve that end. A healthy balance among natural, social, economic, and built assets was seen as being critical to the new model. This event brought to the fore the work done by my own country and the support and guidance it received from many scholars in the development of the Gross National Happiness (GNH) model. It contributed to the rapidly growing interest and practice in wellbeing around the world in both academic and policy spheres. In this regard, it is with deep appreciation that I recall how two of this book's editors—Professor Bob Costanza, with the able support of Dr. Ida Kubizweski— played a coordinating role not only at the UN but also in guiding the work of the International Group of Experts who gathered in Thimphu to deliberate further on the subject. Subsequently, the Bhutanese government submitted a report to the UN Secretary General in the run-up to the Rio+20 summit. I am very pleased that many members of this group continue to work together, and I recognise this book as a continuation of the initiative we began together.

This book suggests and explains how and why we need to study, understand, and approach the subject of wellbeing as an integrated science. The four sections examine and explain the imperative of an integrated approach to dealing with each of the four dimensions of wellbeing: namely, the psychological, physical, sociocultural, and environmental. I would humbly urge that, as integrated as the chapters are within the scope of their assigned parts of the book, the reader must remain mindful that none of the four sections is complete on its own and that each must be read as an integral part of the larger subject of human wellbeing. This is not to say that the four sections together presume to cover all facets of wellbeing.

I would go further to urge that such a holistic approach must be founded on the acceptance of reality as not being exclusive, singular, or hierarchical but rather a complex web of interdependence. Failure to appreciate this truth will distort reality and potentially create more harm than good, even with the best of intentions. Such an integrated approach is humanity's only chance for survival on the planet. Failing this, wellbeing will become an irrelevant concern.

In his book *The Wonderful Century* published in 1898, the British naturalist Alfred Russell Wallace identified "the enormous and continuous growth of wealth, without any corresponding increase in the wellbeing of the whole people" as one of the defining characteristics of the 19th century. This unconstrained pursuit of wealth, he noted, had consigned a growing proportion of the population to poverty as disparities in wealth grew and ecological degradation continued unchecked. He went on to propose that, "The final and absolute test of good government is the wellbeing and contentment of the people—not the extent of empire or the abundance of the revenue and the trade".

More than a hundred years later, this prescient call to action is at last beginning to be realised as we witness an increasing global shift from purely economic metrics of regional and national progress to frameworks that acknowledge the personal, societal, and environmental dimensions of wellbeing. The four of us (Elizabeth Rieger, Robert Costanza, Ida Kubiszewski, and Paul Dugdale) have been working on various aspects of wellbeing for many years. This book is our attempt to move toward a more integrated understanding of wellbeing that recognises the complex interconnections between these dimensions.

The prelude to the book was a forum, co-organised by Paul and attended by Elizabeth, designed to inform the development of a regional wellbeing framework. It brought together local politicians and policy executives with experts from diverse disciplines, including sociology, economics, medicine, psychology, and public administration. Despite this broad representation, as the day's discussions unfolded, some of the challenges to building a wellbeing framework that genuinely integrates across diverse perspectives became apparent. Absent, for example, was any discussion of how the proposed domains of societal wellbeing (e.g., housing, education, the economy, and so on) would yield the personal wellbeing of the population that the entire process was designed to achieve. Indeed, the construct of 'personal wellbeing' sitting at the core of the framework remained unpacked as the precise societal domains to include in the framework were discussed and debated. Moreover, linkages between societal and personal domains of wellbeing were assumed rather than properly understood. A language for integrating across levels—for simultaneously conceiving of the interplay among the individual, so-cietal, and environmental dimensions—was missing. Yet this integrated perspec-tive is required to achieve the ideals already enunciated by Wallace more than a century ago.

As Elizabeth explored these observations with her College Dean (Russell Gruen) and colleagues Robert, Ida, and Paul, the idea of an edited volume that would begin to build an integrated science of wellbeing emerged. The editorial team was created with a view to ensure comprehensive coverage in content as well as oversight of each chapter from the disciplines of psychology (Elizabeth) and medicine (Paul) and from transdisciplinary studies of society and environ-ment (Robert and Ida) to capture the full spectrum of approaches to wellbeing and ensure a 'whole systems' perspective. To join us in this endeavour, we invited both emerging and established scholars who were already making exciting con-tributions to understanding aspects of the psychological, physical, societal, or en-vironmental dimensions of wellbeing to extend their work by also examining the interconnections among each of these dimensions.

Thus began a process of learning for our editorial team as our perspectives were broadened, our ignorance was exposed, and we strove toward a shared under-standing and language. An early challenge was our realisation that the meanings and interpretation of terms can be quite different across fields. For example, from a psychological perspective, the term 'resilience' is unambiguously positive, refer-ring to the ability of individuals and communities to recover, maintain, or even enhance positive functioning in the face of adversity. However, from an ecological perspective, resilience refers to the continuation of a specific structural regime, so that even undesirable regimes can be considered resilient. For instance, coral reefs converted to less desirable algal beds are very resilient to changing into any other state. Entire societies can, likewise, be stuck in undesirable regimes, and thus, from this perspective, would be considered resilient.

We also quickly recognised that a true integration across all of the various scales, levels, and perspectives of wellbeing was not possible to achieve within this volume. Nonetheless, we believe that this book is a significant step *toward* an in-tegrated science of wellbeing. Our contributors have ably pursued the integrative venture, which we hope our readers will continue.

—Elizabeth Rieger, Robert Costanza, Ida Kubiszewski, and Paul Dugdale

Canberra and London, January 2023

DIRECTORY OF CONTRIBUTORS

EDITORS

Robert Costanza
Institute for Global Prosperity, University College London, United Kingdom

Paul Dugdale
School of Medicine and Psychology, Australian National University, Australia

Ida Kubiszewski
Institute for Global Prosperity, University College London, United Kingdom

Elizabeth Rieger
School of Medicine and Psychology, Australian National University, Australia

CONTRIBUTORS

Joanna Alexi
School of Indigenous Studies, University of Western Australia, Australia

Hilary Bambrick
School of Public Health & Social Work, Queensland University of Technology, Australia

Ee Pin Chang
School of Indigenous Studies, University of Western Australia, Australia

Bruce Chapman
College of Business and Economics, Australian National University, Australia

Michael Chapman
School of Medicine and Psychology, Australian National University, Australia

Bruce K. Christensen
School of Medicine and Psychology, Australian National University, Australia

Luca Coscieme
Hot or Cool Institute, Berlin, Germany

Robert A. Cummins
Faculty of Health, Deakin University, Australia

Kate Derry
School of Indigenous Studies, University of Western Australia, Australia

Pat Dudgeon
School of Indigenous Studies, University of Western Australia, Australia

Robert Dyball
The Fenner School of Environment and Society, Australian National University, Australia

Lorenzo Fioramonti
Centre for the Study of Governance Innovation and the Department of Political Sciences, University of Pretoria, South Africa; Member of the Italian National Parliament

Paul Gilbert
Centre for Compassion Research and Training, College of Health and Social Care Research Centre, University of Derby, United Kingdom

John Goss
Health Research Institute, Faculty of Health, University of Canberra, Australia

Carol Graham
The Brookings Institution/College Park, University of Maryland, United States

Russell L. Gruen
College of Health and Medicine, Australian National University, Australia

Amit Gupta
J. P. N. Apex Trauma Center, All India Institute of Medical Sciences, Delhi, India

Diane Jarvis
Centre for Tropical Environmental and Sustainability Science, James Cook University, Australia

Shraddha Kashyap
School of Indigenous Studies, University of Western Australia, Australia

Rebecca E. Kennedy
University of Alabama at Birmingham, United States

Julia C. Kim
GNH Centre, Bhutan

Paul Komesaroff
Faculty of Medicine, Nursing and Health Sciences, Monash University, Australia

Jenny D. V. Le
Department of Psychology, University of Rochester, United States

Margarette Leite
School of Architecture, Portland State University, United States

Phil Lignier
Centre for Tropical Environmental and Sustainability Science, James Cook University, Australia

Helen Milroy
UWA Medical School, University of Western Australia, Australia

Nancy A. Pachana
School of Psychology, University of Queensland, Australia

Sergio Palleroni
School of Architecture, Portland State University, United States

Jennifer Philip
Division of Medicine, Dentistry and Health Sciences, University of Melbourne, Australia

Kate Pickett
Department of Health Sciences, University of York, United Kingdom

Monique Platell
School of Population and Global Health, University of Western Australia, Australia

Harry T. Reis
Department of Psychology, University of Rochester, United States

Julie A. Richardson
University of Plymouth, United Kingdom

Nobhojit Roy
WHO Collaboration Centre for Research in Surgical Care Delivery in Low and Middle Income Countries, Mumbai, India

Carol D. Ryff
Institute on Aging/Department of Psychology, University of Wisconsin-Madison, United States

Jacki Schirmer
Health Research Institute, University of Canberra, Australia; Centre for Change Governance, University of Canberra, Australia

Barbara Sestak
School of Architecture, Portland State University, United States

Kane Solly
School of Psychology, University of Queensland, Australia

Robert Tanton
National Centre for Social and Economic Modelling, University of Canberra, Australia

Tsoki Tenzin
GNH Centre, Bhutan

Sotiris Vardoulakis
National Centre for Epidemiology and Population Health, Australian National University, Australia

Christian Waugh
Department of Psychology, Wake Forest University, United States

Richard Wilkinson
Division of Epidemiology and Public Health, University of Nottingham, United Kingdom

Nabeeh Zakariyya
College of Business and Economics, Australian National University, Australia

Jigme Y. Thinley
Prime Minister of Bhutan 2008–2013

Introduction

Toward an Integrated Science of Wellbeing

**ELIZABETH RIEGER, ROBERT COSTANZA,
IDA KUBISZEWSKI, AND PAUL DUGDALE ■**

BACKGROUND

There has always been interest in understanding what constitutes the good life. Starting with early philosophical writings, sustainable wellbeing at multiple scales—from physical and psychological health, through to the societal and environmental—has been a fundamental goal. Much has been written at each of these scales from the perspectives of psychology, medicine, economics, social science, ecology, and political science. However, their interconnections have received far less attention even though the identification of these interdependencies is critical to the comprehensive understanding and advancement of wellbeing.

In this book, we aim toward creating an integrated science of wellbeing that connects these scales and perspectives to better guide research and public policy. We have done this by engaging leading and emerging experts in wellbeing science from diverse fields, studying various scales and perspectives. They have all attempted to link their areas with the rest of the system. This integrated approach offers a first step toward a more complete understanding of wellbeing that we hope can propel wellbeing research and initiatives in novel and fruitful directions.

Over the past two decades the science of wellbeing has witnessed exponential growth within the individual, societal, and environmental domains. Focus on the wellbeing of the individual was greatly encouraged with the emergence of the field of positive psychology at the turn of the 21st century (Compton, 2005; Seligman & Csikszentmihalyi, 2000). Since then, there has been a burgeoning of both scientific and popular discourse identifying the elements of individual wellbeing and how these can be effectively enhanced. Yet a recurring criticism of this work has been its relative neglect of the societal and environmental factors impacting psychological and physical wellbeing. Likewise, the work undertaken on societal and environmental wellbeing can be criticised for its limited conceptualisation of what constitutes individual wellbeing and how the social and natural environment influence individual wellbeing and are influenced by the wellbeing of individuals.

Restricted conceptualisations not only limit the scope of research but also necessarily hinder the development of effective public policy. The enhancement of wellbeing is increasingly being recognised as the 'core business' of policy makers across the globe in terms of cultural and economic prosperity and is supplanting the prevailing single-minded focus on Gross Domestic Product (GDP) as the path to societal wellbeing (Costanza et al., 2014). The current overreliance on GDP as the primary national policy goal is eroding sustainable wellbeing worldwide. The UN Sustainable Development Goals (SDGs) represent an international recognition that broader shared goals are necessary (United Nations, 2015). An integrated science of wellbeing is essential to guide public policy toward these broader SDGs and the overarching goal of sustainable wellbeing. The integrated approach offered here will provide a step toward a more complete understanding of wellbeing that we hope will help to propel wellbeing research and initiatives in novel and fruitful directions.

We cannot claim to have gone far in our quest for integration. Academia and government are still siloed in disciplines and departments that do not communicate especially well. But we have hopefully taken some significant steps toward our goal of building an integrated science of wellbeing.

STRUCTURE OF THE BOOK

Our title *Toward an Integrated Science of Wellbeing* is carefully crafted. All of our authors are distinguished contributors to the science of wellbeing in their particular fields, and we have asked them to summarise some of that work in their chapters. However, most importantly for this collection, we have also asked them to consider the role of and interconnections between four different domains or scales of wellbeing research: the psychological, human biological, societal, and environmental. Hence the book is divided into four parts representing each of these domains, but throughout our authors have sought integration across levels. The Part headings, 'An Integrated Approach Includes Psychological Wellbeing . . .', 'And Physical Health and Wellbeing . . .', 'And Societal Wellbeing . . .', 'And the Wellbeing of the Built and Natural Environment', emphasise the interconnections ('And') while acknowledging the distinctions among the various levels.

In this Introduction, we first summarise the contents of each part before offering some concluding thoughts on the path forward that includes recognition of some of the challenges in developing an integrated science of wellbeing.

Part A An Integrated Approach Includes Psychological Wellbeing . . .

The task of connecting psychological wellbeing to the human biological, societal, and environmental dimensions is predicated on understanding its own dimensions. Our opening three chapters provide some clarification in this regard by addressing the long-standing distinction between two facets of psychological wellbeing, namely, the *eudaimonic* ('functioning well' in terms of realising one's full potential) and *hedonic* ('feeling well' in terms of subjective feelings of happiness and the attainment of pleasure and avoidance of pain; Ryan & Deci, 2001).

In "The Integrative Science of Eudaimonic Wellbeing: Past Progress and the Road Ahead", Carol Ryff summarises her pioneering work in defining the components of a eudaimonic conceptualisation of wellbeing (i.e., purpose in life, environmental mastery, positive relationships, autonomy, personal growth, and self-acceptance) and understanding how these connect with other dimensions such as our physical health. She goes on to offer new integrative directions by exploring the attainment of eudaimonic wellbeing through engagement with the arts and the natural world. This inspirational work is juxtaposed with the sobering message that the eudaimonic pursuit of realising our potential remains—and is increasingly—beyond the reach of many as socioeconomic disadvantage and inequality intensify (a point later elaborated on by Carol Graham in her discussion of the 'crisis of despair' and by Richard Wilkinson and Kate Pickett in their chapter on inequality and wellbeing). We are left with a clear imperative to work across scales so that societal and environmental supports and impediments to the various components of individual wellbeing can be addressed.

The next two chapters focus on the hedonic aspects of psychological wellbeing. In "Understanding the Role of Positive Emotions in Wellbeing Through Psychological, Biological, Sociocultural, and Environmental Lenses", Christian Waugh offers an integrated perspective on each stage of emotional experience (i.e., the perception of a salient stimulus, appraisal of the stimulus, production of action tendencies, and regulating our emotional states). Robert Cummins, in "Subjective Wellbeing and Resilience at the Individual Level: A Synthesis Through Homeostasis", draws a distinction between transient emotions and more stable mood states, proposing that the wellbeing mood states are comprised of happy, content, and alert and that these are under homeostatic control akin to other human biological systems. The notion that these positive mood states are unchanging within a narrow range around a setpoint for each person speaks to the broader question of which components of psychological wellbeing are changeable and to what degree (Lykken & Tellegen, 1996; Lyubomirsky, Sheldon, & Schkade, 2005). Moreover, in focusing on the role of positive affect in psychological wellbeing, these two chapters implicitly question the common practice of indexing wellbeing in terms of low levels of negative affect such as depression and anxiety. Instead, hedonic wellbeing is more than the absence of negative affect, with positive emotion a key component of several models of psychological wellbeing (e.g., Huppert & So, 2011; Seligman, 2011).

A remaining question is the role of negative emotion in wellbeing. Since the pursuit of eudaimonic wellbeing can require a degree of effort and tolerating discomfort or distress, it may at times be contrary to the experience of positive affect. As just one example of how negative emotions can be linked with facets of eudaimonic wellbeing such as mastery and sense of purpose, individuals who experience higher levels of anger (but not anxiety) regarding climate change are more likely to engage in individual and collective actions to mitigate against climate change (Stanley, Hogg, Leviston, & Walker, 2021). Thus, individual action driven by anger and dissatisfaction is necessary to improve societal and environmental wellbeing, which can create greater individual wellbeing for a larger number of people (more on this later). The assumption that positive emotions are necessarily desirable over negative ones that pervades much of the wellbeing literature has been challenged and even labelled as "toxic wellbeing" by some (Atkinson, 2021, p. 4). Nevertheless, the interest in positive emotions that was greatly propelled by the emergence of the field of positive psychology has been critical in broadening the almost singular previous focus on negative emotions, with further work now needed on the role of both positive *and* negative affect in wellbeing. For instance, Christian Waugh's own research on emotional flexibility is relevant here, in finding that people with greater resilience are more able than those with lower levels of resilience to flexibly shift between positive and negative affect in response to changing environmental circumstances (Waugh, Thompson, & Gotlib, 2011).

All models of psychological wellbeing concur in acknowledging the pivotal role of positive interpersonal relationships. Accordingly, the next three chapters in Part A, "Psychology," have a relational focus. What makes for a positive relationship, and how is it that these relationships have beneficial impacts on our wellbeing? Remarkably, given their quite distinct orientations, these chapters have considerable overlap in addressing questions of this kind. In "Evolution, Compassion, and Wellbeing", Paul Gilbert describes his innovative work offering a thoroughly biopsychosocial model of compassion grounded in an evolutionary framework. In this model, compassion (defined as a sensitivity to suffering in self and others, with a commitment to try to alleviate and prevent it) is a key element in understanding what it means to relate to ourselves and others in a manner that promotes wellbeing at the individual, societal, and environmental levels.

The role of compassion is not limited to building positive relationships, but also has implications for other dimensions of psychological wellbeing. Self-esteem, for example, features in some models of psychological wellbeing (e.g., Huppert & So, 2011) and has long been found to be strongly related to measures of happiness, wellbeing, or life satisfaction (see Diener & Diener, 1995, for cross-cultural comparisons). But the limitations of self-esteem have also been highlighted: the pursuit of self-esteem can leave us vulnerable to engaging in self-serving biases (e.g., people overestimating their intelligence) that distort reality (Leary, 2004), and it can make us want to be superior to others so that "life becomes a zero-sum game, and other people become competitors and enemies rather than supports and resources" (Crocker & Park, 2004, p. 401). Moreover, self-esteem acts as "a fair-weather friend, there for us when we succeed but deserting us precisely when we need it most—when we fail or make a fool of ourselves" (Neff & Germer, 2018, p. 22). In contrast to self-esteem, self-compassion provides a means of maintaining a positive relationship to ourselves even in the face of our inevitable failures, challenges, and personal limitations. In this sense, self-compassion provides a means of gaining self-acceptance (defined in Carol Ryff's eudaimonic wellbeing model as being able to accept both our positive and negative qualities). Understanding the role of compassion across the dimensions of psychological wellbeing, as well as across the individual, societal, and environmental scales of wellbeing, will continue to be a crucial direction of research.

In their chapter, Harry Reis and Jenny Le focus on "Perceived Partner Responsiveness and Wellbeing", with the construct of perceived partner responsiveness embodying the degree to which we view our partners as understanding, respecting, and appreciating who we are and providing us with care and support as needed. It thus shares some of the components of compassion, especially in terms of understanding the other person's needs and providing necessary support. In a novel extension of their work, the authors go beyond considering partner responsiveness in terms of dyadic personal relationships to propose broader settings where this mechanism might be at play to enhance the wellbeing of students in educational settings, groups, organisations, the operation of a society's legal and political processes, and even the environment as our planetary partner.

The final chapter focusing on relationships is that by Bruce Chapman and Nabeeh Zakariyya on "Life Satisfaction, Marital Status, and Partnership Quality: Modelling From Australia". The authors draw on a unique dataset tracking aspects of relationship quality (i.e., a person's happiness with their partner and a partner's happiness with them) and life satisfaction. Among the many interesting results emerging from this study was the finding that higher happiness with one's partner was strongly associated with higher life satisfaction, with the magnitude of this association approximately three times greater than the higher life satisfaction of the employed compared to the unemployed. This finding underscores the importance of positive relationships for wellbeing. It was similarly found that a person's happiness with their partner was positively associated with the partner's own life satisfaction, and this association was especially strong for women. The fact that women's wellbeing was found to be more contingent on the approval of their partners is consistent with the broader literature on gender differences in the importance of approval from others (Zeigler-Hill & Myers, 2012). Returning to the construct of perceived partner responsiveness, this finding also suggests that the skills of demonstrating appreciation for our partners might be especially important in the ability of men to positively impact the wellbeing of their female partners. Overall, the gendered dimensions of wellbeing require much greater attention in future integrated approaches to wellbeing.

A more concerted research focus is also required to thoroughly capture cultural diversity. As a discipline, psychology has drawn heavily from Western frameworks and samples. The subdiscipline of positive psychology has fared somewhat better in this regard (Kim, Doiron, Warren, & Donaldson, 2018), although much remains to be done in terms of informing conceptualisations of wellbeing from non-Western perspectives. This is particularly the case for Indigenous cultures subjected to the disruptive and destructive processes ensuing from colonisation. Our next chapter can be seen as part of a growing discipline of Indigenous psychology where Indigenous people themselves define the issues and promote paradigms that reflect their realities. In this chapter, Helen Milroy, Kate Derry, Shraddha Kashyap, Monique Platell, Joanna Alexi, Ee Pin Chang, and Pat Dudgeon present pioneering work by Indigenous mental health clinicians and researchers in reclaiming "Indigenous Australian Understandings of Holistic Health and Social and Emotional Wellbeing". The chapter provides an overview of the major steps in the last 30 years of consulting and embarking on the path from colonisation toward effective wellbeing interventions for Aboriginal and Torres Strait Islander peoples based on Aboriginal and Torres Strait Islander understandings of selfhood. Here, the self is inextricably linked with kinship systems, community, culture, country and land, and spirituality. Accordingly, culturally informed wellbeing interventions acknowledge this fundamentally integrated ontology of the self. The authors also describe a unique epistemology: namely, the use of artwork (Helen Milroy's evocative images) to elicit narratives to support Aboriginal and Torres Strait Islander peoples and communities in understanding and enhancing their wellbeing in a culturally responsive way. It is noteworthy that the holistic conceptualisations of Indigenous Australians, who are the most ancient continuous population on Earth (Malaspinas et al., 2016), are now leading the development of an integrated science of wellbeing.

The final chapter in Part A bridges the individual and societal sections by focusing on the psychological wellbeing of people in a particular organisational setting. In their chapter on "Wellbeing in Higher Education: Evidence- and Policy-based Strategies to Enhance the Wellbeing of People, Place, and Planet", Bruce Christensen and Rebecca Kennedy focus on the wellbeing of students in institutions of higher education in light of this population's elevated levels of psychological distress. In a sweeping yet succinct treatment of the subject matter, they begin with an overview of the evidence supporting various person-level interventions before presenting promising, albeit less extensively researched, strategies at the place and planet levels. While focused on higher education and acknowledging what can be uniquely offered by these scholarly communities in building an integrated approach to wellbeing, the chapter provides an exemplar of the range of multilevel approaches that could enhance the wellbeing of people in diverse organisational settings. As the authors note, future work is also needed to provide a similarly integrated perspective focused on the wellbeing of staff in institutions of higher education, who have been described as "pressure vessels" in light of their occupational stressors (Morrish, 2019).

Part B AND Physical Health and Wellbeing . . .

The great advances of medical science in the 20th century were based in considerable part on the adoption of 19th-century systems thinking—perhaps best exemplified by the work of Herbert Spencer—to understand the principles of physiology, disease causation, and therapeutics. Where other disciplines used the idea of the interconnected system to connect areas of investigation outward to related things, medicine pursued elaboration of the inner systems of the human body and split centrifugally—flying apart into the reductionist investigation of what we now know as the cardiovascular system, the respiratory system, the musculoskeletal system, and so on.

The limitations of this approach become apparent, at some point, to all of us who work with it. However, in clinical medical practice, it has always been necessary to do the work of drawing together knowledge from the various biological systems into a holistic therapeutic plan for the patient. Extending this, systems thinking can be a useful approach for work on integration between disciplines and between scales.

This approach is demonstrated in the chapter by Paul Dugdale, Elizabeth Rieger, and Robert Dyball on "Integrating Across Diverse Perspectives to Improve Health and Wellbeing: Obesity as an Illustrative Case". Biopsychosocial models of medical and psychological conditions have long been proposed (Engel, 1977) to understand their multidimensional aetiology but have tended to neglect the *interconnections* among the biological, psychological, and social dimensions that more recent frameworks emphasise (e.g., Tsai, Mendenhall, Trostle, & Kawachi, 2017). In this chapter, the authors focus on obesity in offering a more thoroughgoing integrated perspective. They place emphasis on the obesogenic environment while connecting these environmental conditions with examples of genetic, physiological, psychological, and social vulnerabilities in understanding the causes and potential sources of intervention and support for overweight people. Obesity illustrates several of the paradoxes that come to light when we work across scales. Between the psychological and biological scales, the profound social stigma associated with obesity works against the clear need for healthcare by people with higher levels of obesity. Looking between the environmental and human community levels, we see that the impoverishment of the environment through monocropping to support energy-dense processed food production is ironically reflected in the overnutrition of some of the human population. The chapter concludes by suggesting the sort of policy approaches that can be used to tackle obesity across scales and systems.

Our next chapter situates health and wellbeing specifically within the urban environment. In "Wellbeing and Personal Safety: Lessons from Population-Based Strategies to Reduce the Burden of Injury", Russell L. Gruen, Amit Gupta, and Nobhojit Roy describe how cities that integrate road safety, ambulance, emergency, and hospital services into city-wide trauma systems can greatly reduce death and disability arising from the accidents and injuries that accompany life in the city. The authors then reflect on how these systems can be built into the broader development of cities in the developing world. In particular, they describe how this approach has been adopted in India, starting in a few cities, but working toward a national trauma system that may show just how much this approach can reduce the global burden of injury.

The theme of integrating care across settings continues in the chapter by Kane Solly and Nancy A. Pachana, "An Integrative Perspective on Positive Ageing in Later Life". This chapter celebrates the increasing normality of people living into old age but calls out the ageist stigma that they often face. Drawing on the emergence of positive psychology, the authors outline an approach to positive ageing (while also acknowledging the potential pitfalls of a positive psychology approach). The integrated perspective provided by the authors goes beyond psychology and healthcare to show how a society that enables an ongoing contribution by people as they age, including culturally important and artistic contributions, becomes a society that is richer. Environmental considerations also feature prominently in the health and wellbeing of older adults. The innate feelings of wanting to connect to the natural world—biophilia—increase with age, while actual physical access to the natural world often decreases with age. Thoughtful, simple measures to improve access, such as parks with easily negotiable pathways, and pet ownership, can significantly improve wellbeing in this rapidly expanding population group.

There is an obvious sense in which healthcare and wellbeing relate: the purpose of healthcare is to improve the wellbeing of the individual. The chapters discussed above show that the relations go considerably further than this and sometimes in unexpected directions. But what about when the purpose of healthcare is to facilitate a good death? Michael Chapman, Jennifer Philip, and Paul Komesaroff tackle this question in "Systems of Care and Experience for Dying Well". Recognising the finitude of the human lifespan and the obvious limitations of medicine to prolong it, they examine our ideas about death, the fear and certainty of it, but also the bonding and comfort that many of our cultural practices around death bring. This more social view of death and dying is clearly related to the wellbeing of those involved and, indeed, of the broader society where meaningful reflection goes hand in hand with the practices that accompany dying and death. In an important sense, this is the chapter that shows us most clearly that wellbeing is a field worthy of reflection and study separate from the health of the individual and cannot be reduced to this or its simple aggregates in the population.

Taken together, the chapters on physical health and wellbeing show the importance of working toward an integrated science of wellbeing to improve the great projects of medical care and public health. Furthermore, they identify fruitful questions at the points of overlap between scales for further research. They also show us something about the economy of research: findings at one scale may be interesting and important for scientific inquiry at another scale, and, unless we do the thinking to relate work at one scale to another, we will miss it.

Part C AND Societal Wellbeing . . .

There are a growing number of societal wellbeing frameworks being developed and used in regions and nations around the world. These go well beyond GDP as a measure of progress and attempt to include the full range of factors that need to be considered in an integrated approach to wellbeing. Jacki Schirmer, Robert Tanton, and John Goss, in "Wellbeing Frameworks: Emerging Practice, Challenges, and Opportunities", provide a comprehensive history of the development of these frameworks and their common challenges. Increasingly, both objective and subjective measures are being included in these frameworks, which is an initial step toward integration. However, the ongoing development of an integrated science of wellbeing, as this book encourages, is much needed to evaluate the validity and utility of these frameworks. For instance, further research is required that seeks to connect the individual and societal levels of wellbeing frameworks. That is, while 'subjective wellbeing' is included in the majority of societal wellbeing frameworks, how does this relate to a more complete understanding of psychological wellbeing, such as Ryff's eudaimonic model, and how do the distinct components of models of psychological wellbeing relate to the distinct components of models of societal wellbeing?

Our next chapter provides an in-depth description of a particularly interesting and relevant example of a societal wellbeing framework: namely, the pioneering work undertaken in Bhutan. In "Weaving Wellbeing into the Fabric of the Economy: Lessons from Bhutan's Journey Toward Gross National Happiness", Julia C. Kim, Julie A. Richardson, and Tsoki Tenzin tell the amazing story of the Gross National Happiness (GNH) index and how it offers a holistic framework for wellbeing measurement and policy that integrates the individual, social, and environmental elements. In the GNH, these are defined as the four integrated pillars of sustainable wellbeing: (1) environmental conservation, (2) cultural promotion, (3) sustainable and equitable socioeconomic development, and (4) good governance.

Bhutan has been an important example of a country devoted to finding a better way to measure and use integrated wellbeing to drive policy, both locally and globally. For example, on 2 April 2012, Bhutan hosted a meeting at UN headquarters in New York City of more than 800 diverse participants from government, business, nongovernmental organisations (NGOs), and academia (including two of the authors, RC and IK). The meeting was designed to lay the ground work for a new development paradigm based on the sustainable wellbeing of all life on Earth. The Prime Minister at the time, Jigme Y. Thinley—who graciously provided the Foreword to this volume—opened the meeting with a rousing challenge.

> We desperately need an economy that serves and nurtures the wellbeing of all sentient beings on earth and human happiness that comes from living life in harmony with the natural world, with our communities, and with our inner selves. We need an economy that will serve humanity, not enslave it.

It must prevent the imminent reversal of civilisation and flourish within the natural bounds of our planet while ensuring the sustainable, equitable, and meaningful use of precious resources. (quoted in Colman, 2021, p. 241)

The UN meeting was followed up in 2013 with an International Expert Working Group (IEWG) workshop in Thimphu, Bhutan. The workshop included a group of more than 60 international experts (again including RC and IK) tasked with creating a 'new development paradigm' incorporating the ideas of GNH and other approaches to integrated wellbeing. Colman (2021) provides a detailed description of this workshop and its aftermath. There was much enthusiasm for the project and its potential impact during the workshop. Subsequently, however, under the influence of the government of India, the World Bank, and others, the entire work of the IEWG was sidelined and, under a new Prime Minister, Bhutan backed off from its original bold initiative.

But the tide has now turned as countries begin to seriously take on the challenge laid out by Jigme Thinley and Bhutan. One of the spin-offs of the 2013 workshop was the eventual creation of the Wellbeing Economy Alliance (WEAll) and the Wellbeing Economy Governments (WEGo). WEAll is a broad 'network of networks' aimed at bringing together the many organisations, governments, networks, academics, businesses, NGOs, and individuals that are already working on elements of the new economy and sustainable wellbeing. WEAll was designed to coordinate, facilitate, amplify, and catalyse the wide range of ongoing efforts around the shared goal of creating a sustainable wellbeing economy.

At a meeting in Glasgow, Scotland, in October 2017, initiated by WEAll members and hosted by Nicola Sturgeon, first Minister of Scotland, a group of governments including Scotland, Costa Rica, Slovenia, and New Zealand committed to creating a partnership to share good practice in wellbeing economy policymaking and to champion holistic and collective wellbeing as the goal of development. WEGo now includes Scotland, New Zealand, Iceland, Finland, and Wales, with several other countries and state governments close to joining. Sustainable wellbeing is gradually being accepted as the primary policy goal of at least some vanguard governments, as Jigme Thinley hoped. This volume provides additional academic support for this policy agenda.

However, in many countries, despair rather than happiness and wellbeing is prevalent, and these have been exacerbated during the COVID-19 pandemic. In Carol Graham's "America's Crisis of Despair: The Case for a Wellbeing-Based Recovery with Lessons from and for Other Countries", she chronicles this crisis and recommends tracking trends in wellbeing as part of national statistics, as is done in the United Kingdom, New Zealand, Bhutan, and other countries, as a way of solving the crisis of despair.

A key part of the problem is the rapidly increasing inequality in many countries brought about in part by the misplaced focus on GDP growth at all costs and the loss of social capital this produces. Richard Wilkinson and Kate Pickett summarise their pathbreaking work on the relationship between inequality and wellbeing in their chapter "Inequality and the Transition from GDP to Wellbeing". They show how we need to address the powerful political forces that prevent the reduction in things that we already know reduce societal wellbeing, such as homelessness, poverty, and food and job insecurity. Major reductions in inequality are necessary to transition away from government policies focused on GDP growth and to those focused on sustainable wellbeing, as the governments comprising WEGo have begun to do.

In the last chapter in this section, "An Economy Centred on Human and Ecological Wellbeing", Lorenzo Fioramonti and Luca Coscieme envision what a Wellbeing Economy (WE) that prioritises human and ecological wellbeing instead of GDP growth would look like. As mentioned earlier, several governments have recently formed the WEGo alliance to begin to implement some of these ideas. They recognise the need for an integrated approach to understanding and measuring societal wellbeing that this chapter and the rest of this volume are providing.

Part D AND the Wellbeing of the Built and Natural Environment

Although nature provides Earth's life support system, the importance of nature's direct and indirect contributions to wellbeing have only become evident within the public's awareness as the global environment has begun to visibly degrade (Bowler, Buyung-Ali, Knight, & Pullin, 2010). With increasing air and water pollution, climate disruption, loss of biodiversity, degradation of land, and an increase in natural disasters, both individuals and societies are noticing the impacts on our physical and mental health and wellbeing (Kubiszewski, Mulder, Jarvis, & Costanza, 2021; Manning & Clayton, 2018). This has become even more evident with COVID-19, as access to nature has been restricted (Grima et al., 2020; Talmage et al., 2022).

In "Natural Capital, Ecosystem Services, and Subjective Wellbeing: A Systematic Review", Diane Jarvis, Phil Lignier, Ida Kubiszewski, and Robert Costanza analyse the research that has been done on the relationship between natural capital and wellbeing over the past 20 years. They divide their analysis into four themes: (1) the degree of human intervention on the environment (e.g., urbanisation and deforestation), (2) enjoyment of specific environmental goods and services (e.g., urban greenspaces), (3) proximity to adverse consequences that result from environmental problems (e.g., pollution), and (4) overarching measures of the impact of the environment on wellbeing. From this analysis, they report that, unsurprisingly, the relationship between natural capital and wellbeing is complex and requires understanding interactions with the other types of capital (built, social, and human). However, they also report that natural capital has a significant positive impact on our physical and mental wellbeing, and its degradation is having significant negative impacts on wellbeing at all scales from individual humans, to communities, and to the entire planet.

These negative impacts are being amplified by climate change, which decreases the resilience of ecological and human systems (Doppelt, 2016; Simpson, Weissbecker, & Sephton, 2011). The chapter by Sotiris Vardoulakis and Hilary Bambrick, entitled "An Integrated Approach to Health and Wellbeing in Response to Climate Change", focuses specifically on the impacts of climate change on our wellbeing. They discuss the three types of impact that climate change has on wellbeing: (1) primary, direct impacts such as heatwaves making people sick; (2) secondary impacts, such as heatwaves causing crops to fail, which causes a food shortage; and (3) tertiary impacts, referring to more diffuse consequences such as population displacement due to conflict over natural resources or the degradation of mental wellbeing. They also note that these impacts are not equally distributed in that wealthier countries, or wealthier populations within countries, have the financial resources to buffer themselves from the worst of the climate change impacts. Women and children have also been found to be more vulnerable to climate change (Wenden, 2011). It is the poorer, more vulnerable portions of the global population that will suffer the bulk of the climate change impacts.

Some of these inequalities in the resilience to climate change stem from access to properly built infrastructure. We spend so much of our lives in the built environment that it is an obviously critical component to our wellbeing and our ability to maintain that wellbeing in response to changing conditions (Hiscock et al., 2017; Thatcher & Milner, 2014). In "Wellbeing and the Built Environment: A Case Study in the Application of Broad-Based Participatory Design," Margarette Leite, Sergio Palleroni, and Barbara Sestak look at how wellbeing depends on how we plan, design, and build the environment around us. One of the best ways to ensure that our built environment maximises wellbeing is by creating it through a participatory process with the community to guarantee that their social, environmental, and economic goals are met. To show how this can work in practice, they use a case study of eco-friendly, modular classrooms. These classrooms were built in deliberation with the community to ensure a better learning environment, one that addresses the physical, mental, intellectual, and emotional health of the students and the community as a whole.

To tie it all together, Robert Costanza, Ida Kubiszewski, and Lorenzo Fioramonti in "Sustainable Wellbeing and the United Nations Sustainable Development Goals (SDGs)" look at the relationship between the UN SDGs and wellbeing. They show that, in their current structure, the SDGs lack an overarching goal with clear metrics of progress. They propose an aggregate Sustainable Wellbeing Index (SWI) that includes the dimensions of the individual, the economy, society, and the rest of nature and that incorporates both objective and subjective indicators. This index needs to work in collaboration with a dynamic, nonlinear, systems model of the entire system of the economy-in-society-in-nature as well as the individual scale (psychological and physical). Such a model can incorporate many of the ideas in the chapters of this volume.

TOWARD INTEGRATION: AN APPROACH THAT CONNECTS PSYCHOLOGICAL, PHYSICAL, SOCIETAL, AND ENVIRONMENTAL WELLBEING

To conclude, we offer some brief observations regarding the process of developing an integrated science of wellbeing, including those factors that can facilitate this process or, conversely, render it more challenging. In thinking about our contemporary collective challenges, Yeatman (2021) has commented, "We cannot do this work if we do not rethink our place in relation to the whole. We are not outside the whole, we are within it and as dependent on its integral functioning as any other creaturely being" (p. 134). This requires us to give up the traditional scientific comfort of separating, of dis-integrating constructs such as subjectivity and objectivity. At a broader level, it involves striving against the inherent tendency in much scientific work to reduce the field of view and pursue subspeciality research interests. However, the practice of science is performed by a community of scholars that values not just dissection and specialisation, but openness, curiosity, respectfulness, and imagination, each of which aids in the creation of integrated perspectives.

Rethinking the relations between scales, or domains of research, is precisely what we had in mind in the phrase 'toward an integrated' in our title. While the development of a reductionist framework across scales is one way of integrating science, it is rarely successful. Where it is successful, it is because of a narrow scope of inquiry. More realistically, the process of 'working toward integration' by thinking through known or possible relations between fields, and doing this in dialogue with other researchers expert in a field different to one's own, will yield a wide variety of such relations. Some of these may be highly productive, some may result in useful methodological or conceptual advances, and some may be uselessly esoteric. Our hope is that framing this collection as 'toward an integrated science of wellbeing' by a community of scholars, with the expertise and commitments of our authors, would shed light on how we can achieve better and more productive integration for this critically important research.

In asking our contributors to write outside their customary scale or domain, we have implicitly suggested that they do this by listening to their own doubtful thoughts on things they are unaccustomed to writing about and sharing something of their imaginative selves with the readers. Whatever the scientific merit of what this has produced, each of their efforts has been a move toward integrating the sciences of wellbeing. We believe they have expanded the horizons of integrated explorations of wellbeing and helped to support policies to improve attainable and sustainable wellbeing for all life on earth.

REFERENCES

Atkinson, S. (2021). The toxic effects of subjective wellbeing and potential tonics. *Social Science & Medicine, 288*, 1–8. doi:10.1016/j.soccimed.2020.113098

Bowler, D. E., Buyung-Ali, L. M., Knight, T. M., & Pullin, A. S. (2010). A systematic review of evidence for the added benefits to health of exposure to natural environments. *BMC Public Health, 10*(1), 456. doi:10.1186/1471-2458-10-456

Colman, R. (2021). *What really counts: The case for a sustainable and equitable economy.* Columbia University Press.

Compton, W. C. (2005). *Introduction to positive psychology.* Thomson Wadsworth.

Costanza, R., Kubiszewski, I., Giovannini, E., Lovins, H., McGlade, J., Pickett, K. E., . . . Wilkinson, R. (2014). Development: Time to leave GDP behind. *Nature, 505*, 283–285. doi:10.1038/505283a

Crocker, J., & Park, L. E. (2004). The costly pursuit of self-esteem. *Psychological Bulletin, 130*(3), 392–414. https://doi.org/10.1037/0033-2909.130.3.392

Diener, E., & Diener, M. (1995). Cross-cultural correlates of life satisfaction and self-esteem. *Journal of Personality and Social Psychology, 68*, 653–6w63. doi:10.1037/0022-3514.68.4.653

Doppelt, B. (2016). *Transformational resilience: How building human resilience to climate disruption can safeguard society and increase wellbeing.* Routledge.

Engel, G. L. (1977). The need for a new medical model: A challenge for biomedicine. *Science, 196*, 129–136. doi:10.1126/science.847460

Grima, N., Corcoran, W., Hill-James, C., Langton, B., Sommer, H., & Fisher, B. (2020). The importance of urban natural areas and urban ecosystem services during the COVID-19 pandemic. *PLoS ONE, 15*(12), e0243344. doi:10.1371/journal.pone.0243344

Hiscock, R., Asikainen, A., Tuomisto, J., Jantunen, M., Pärjälä, E., & Sabel, C. E. (2017). City scale climate change policies: Do they matter for wellbeing? *Preventive Medicine Reports, 6*, 265–270. doi:10.1016/j.pmedr.2017.03.019

Huppert, F. A., & So, T. T. C. (2011). Flourishing across Europe: Application of a new conceptual framework for defining wellbeing. *Social Indicators Research, 110*, 837–861. doi:10.1007/s11205-011-9966-7

Leary, M. R. (2004). *The curse of the self: Self-awareness, egotism, and the quality of human life.* Oxford University Press.

Lykken, D., & Tellegen, A. (1996). Happiness is a stochastic phenomenon. *Psychological Science, 7*, 186–189.

Lyubomirsky, S., Sheldon, K. M., & Schkade, D. (2005). Pursuing happiness: The architecture of sustainable change. *Review of General Psychology, 9*, 111–131. doi:10.1037/1089-2680.9.2.111

Kim, H., Doiron, K., Warren, M. A., & Donaldson, S. I. (2018). The international landscape of positive psychology research: A systematic review. *International Journal of Wellbeing, 8*, 50–70. doi:10.5502/ijw.v8i1.651

Kubiszewski, I., Mulder, K., Jarvis, D., & Costanza, R. (2021). Toward better measurement of sustainable development and wellbeing: A small number of SDG indicators reliably predict life satisfaction. *Sustainable Development*, 1–10. doi:10.1002/sd.2234

Malaspinas, A-S., Westaway, M. C., Muller, C., Sousa, V. C., Lao, O., Alves, I., . . . Willerslev, E. (2016). A genomic history of Aboriginal Australia. *Nature, 538*, 207–214. doi:10.1038/nature18299

Manning, C., & Clayton, S. (2018). Threats to mental health and wellbeing associated with climate change. In S. Clayton & C. Manning (Eds.), *Psychology and climate change: Human perceptions, impacts, and responses* (pp. 217–244). Elsevier Academic Press.

Morrish, L. (2019). *Pressure vessels: The epidemic of poor mental health among higher education staff.* Higher Education Policy Institute.

Neff, K., & Germer, C. (2018). *The mindful self-compassion workbook: A proven way to accept yourself, build inner strength, and thrive.* Guilford Press.

Ryan, R. M., & Deci, E. L. (2001). On happiness and human potentials: A review of research on hedonic and eudaimonic well-being. *Annual Review of Psychology, 52,* 141–166. doi:10.1146/annurev.psych.52.1.141

Seligman, M. (2011). *Flourish: A new understanding of happiness and wellbeing—and how to achieve them.* Nicholas Brealey Publishing.

Seligman, M. E. P., & Csikszentmihalyi, M. (2000). Positive psychology: An introduction. *American Psychologist, 55,* 5–14. doi:1037//0003-066X.55.1.5

Simpson, D. M., Weissbecker, I., & Sephton, S. E. (2011). Extreme weather-related events: Implications for mental health and well-being. In I. Weissbecker (Ed.), *Climate change and human well-being: Global challenges and opportunities* (pp. 57–78). Springer.

Stanley, S., Hogg, T. L., Leviston, Z., & Walker, I. (2021). From anger to action: Differential impacts of eco-anxiety, eco-depression, and eco-anger on climate action and wellbeing. *Journal of Climate Change and Health, 1,* 100003. doi:10.1016/j.joclim.2021.100003

Talmage, C. A., Allgood, B., Ashdown, B. K., Brennan, A., Hill, S., Trevan, E., & Waugh, J. (2022). Tethering natural capital and cultural capital for a more sustainable post-COVID-19 world. *International Journal of Community Well-Being.* doi:10.1007/s42413-021-00151-5

Thatcher, A., & Milner, K. (2014). Changes in productivity, psychological wellbeing and physical wellbeing from working in a 'green' building. *Work, 49,* 381–393. doi:10.3233/WOR-141876

Tsai, A. C., Mendenhall, E., Trostle, J. A., & Kawachi, I. (2017). Co-occurring epidemics, syndemics, and population health. *Lancet, 389,* 978–982. doi:10.1016/S0140-6736(17)30403-8

United Nations. (2015). *Transforming our world: The 2030 agenda for sustainable development.* https://sustainabledevelopment.un.org/post2015/transformingourworld/publication

Waugh, C. E., Thompson, R. J., & Gotlib, I. H. (2011). Flexible emotional responsiveness in trait resilience. *Emotion, 11,* 1059–1067. doi:10.1037/a0021786

Wenden, A. L. (2011). Women and climate change: Vulnerabilities and challenges. In I. Weissbecker (Ed.), *Climate change and human well-being: Global challenges and opportunities* (pp. 119–33). Springer.

Yeatman, A. (2021). Restoring wholeness: Listening to country. *Griffith Review, 73,* 129–139. https://www.griffithreview.com/articles/restoring-wholeness/

Zeigler-Hill, V., & Myers, E. M. (2012). A review of gender differences in self-esteem. In S. P. McGeown (Ed.), *Psychology of gender differences* (pp. 131–143). Nova Science Publishers.

An Integrated Approach Includes
Psychological Wellbeing . . .

1

The Integrative Science
of Eudaimonic Wellbeing

Past Progress and the Road Ahead

CAROL D. RYFF ■

INTRODUCTION

The integrative science of wellbeing is covered in this chapter from the vantage point of a eudaimonic model developed more than three decades ago. In contrast to hedonic approaches that emphasise happiness and life satisfaction, eudaimonia is concerned with the realisation of personal potential and living meaningful and purposeful lives. The conceptual underpinnings of this approach are first described, followed by a brief look at its empirical measurement. Multiple topics have grown up around this model over time, such as how eudaimonia varies by age, gender, race, and educational status. Other studies have linked aspects of eudiamonic wellbeing to experiences in work and family life. Growing work has connected components of eudaimonia to health, defined not only as morbidity and mortality, but also in terms of biological risk factors. Further inquiries have linked eudaimonia to neuroscience and genetics. Lastly, whether eudaimonic wellbeing is modifiable has been the focus of numerous intervention studies. A selective look at these domains of inquiry is provided to reveal the varieties of progress made to date on the integrative science of eudaimonic wellbeing.

The remainder of the chapter then shifts to targeted directions for future research. The first topic showcases increasingly widening inequalities that have been unfolding over recent decades, especially in the United States. These socioeconomic disparities have notable implications for wellbeing and health (see also Chapters 9 and 16, this volume). The urgency of this problem has been exacerbated by the worldwide COVID-19 pandemic and its economic sequelae (see also Chapter 15, this volume). These historical changes bring into high relief a critical issue: namely, whether the realisation of human potential, arguably the essence of eudaimonia, is increasingly *not available* to large segments of contemporary societies. Continued scientific tracking of this matter is profoundly important as a window on the success or failure of the social order in our times.

The second topic brings a more hopeful future direction by seeking to build bridges to the arts and humanities as domains that may nourish wellbeing, including in the face of adversity. Scientific advances are now unfolding on these topics, though less work has examined implications for leading purposeful and meaningful lives as well as for realising personal talents and capacities. In addition, the relevance of the arts and humanities in bringing attention to human suffering greatly needs attention.

The third topic addresses environmental inputs on wellbeing, giving targeted emphasis to the natural environment as experienced in direct encounters with nature. These ideas are illustrated through poetry, literature, the visual arts, and music. The field of environmental psychology has become more prominent in recent decades with growing evidence that natural environments are linked with better mental and physical wellbeing. But again, little work has emphasised eudaimonic wellbeing and even less has focused on the role of the arts in capturing the inspirational power of nature.

Taken as a whole, the intent is to demonstrate that eudaimonic wellbeing constitutes a theoretically and philosophically rich formulation of positive functioning, which has now been empirically linked with (1) people's position in the social structure, thereby implicating differential access to power and resources; (2) proximal life experiences (stress exposures, life events, and transitions in work and family life); and (3) multiple aspects of health (disease, disability, and death) through regulation of diverse physiological systems (stress hormones, inflammatory markers, and cardiovascular risk factors), brain structures and function, and genetics. This wide panorama is nonetheless incomplete, with future work needed to showcase the import of major historical events that possibly compromise the eudaimonic potential of disadvantaged segments of contemporary societies. Alongside these distressing concerns are new inquiries on the potential of the arts to nourish wellbeing and health even during times of widespread suffering. A final new frontier brings in the natural environment and its relevance for eudaimonia and health, not only in individuals, but also in communities and societies, and importantly, for the sustainability of planet. The integrative agenda is deep and wide.

WHAT IS EUDAIMONIC WELLBEING?

This section describes a model of psychological wellbeing (Ryff, 1989) that I developed built on theories of positive psychological functioning from clinical, development, existential, and humanistic perspectives while also drawing on Aristotle's view of *eudaimonia* as the highest of all human goods (Ryff & Singer, 2008). It stands in contrast to hedonic indicators of wellbeing that are largely atheoretical in nature and focus on simple questions about happiness and life satisfaction.

This model of euadaimonic wellbeing was informed by detailed depictions of the upside of the human condition coming from the Jungian formulation of individuation (Jung, 1933), Bühler's writings about basic life tendencies that work toward the fulfillment of life (Bühler, 1935), Jahoda's perspective on positive mental health (Jahoda, 1958), Frankl's writings about the life-saving features of purpose in life (Frankl, 1959), Erikson's life-span model of ego development (Erikson, 1959), Rogers's perspective on the fully functioning person (Rogers, 1961), Allport's conception of maturity (Allport, 1961), Maslow's conception of self-actualisation (Maslow, 1968), and Neugarten's writings about the executive processes of personality in adulthood (Neugarten, 1973). These enticing perspectives had been largely missing in the empirical arena due to a lack of sound assessment procedures.

My contribution was to integrate these ideas into a model built around points of convergence among them (Ryff, 1989). This integration resulted in six core dimensions of wellbeing (see Figure 1.1). Distant philosophical input came from Aristotle's *Nichomachean Ethics* (1925), which opens with a profound query: What is the highest of all goods achievable by human action? Aristotle believed the answer was happiness but underscored notable differences in what

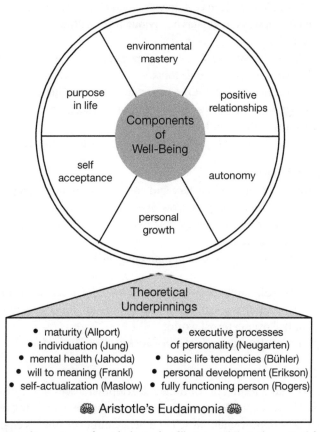

Figure 1.1 Core dimensions of psychological wellbeing and their theoretical foundations.

is meant by happiness. In his view, happiness is not about pleasure or wealth or satisfying appetites—things more aligned with hedonia, also of interest to the ancient Greeks. Instead, Aristotle defined the highest good as *activity of the soul in accord with virtue*, thereby distilling the core meaning of eudaimonia as achieving the best that is within us. It is thus a kind of personal excellence, captured by the two great Greek imperatives inscribed on the Temple of Apollo at Delphi: namely, to "know thyself" and "become who you are" (Ryff & Singer, 2008).

Translation of the identified six different aspects of wellbeing to quality assessment tools was imperative. Such operationalisation required a comprehensive approach that has been described in multiple prior publications (Ryff, 1989, 2014; Ryff & Singer, 2008). Of critical importance at the outset were clear and coherent definitions of each proposed dimension. Box 1.1 provides these definitions,

---

Box 1.1

DEFINITIONS OF THEORY-GUIDED DIMENSIONS OF EUDAIMONIC WELLBEING

Autonomy

High scorer: Is self-determining and independent; able to resist social pressures to think and act in certain ways; regulates social pressures to think and act in certain ways; regulates behaviour from within; evaluates self by personal standards.

Sample item: *"I have confidence in my own opinions, even if they are different from the way most other people think."*

Low scorer: Is concerned about the expectations and evaluations of others; relies on judgements of others to make important decisions; conforms to social pressures to think and act in certain ways.

Sample item: *"I tend to be influenced by people with strong opinions."*

Environmental Mastery

High scorer: Has a sense of mastery and competence in managing the environment; controls complex array of external activities; makes effective use of surrounding opportunities; able to choose or create contexts suitable to personal needs and values.

Sample item: *"I am quite good at managing the many responsibilities of my daily life."*

Low scorer: Has difficulty managing everyday affairs; feels unable to change or improve surrounding context; is unaware of surrounding opportunities; lacks sense of control over external world.

Sample item: *"The demands of everyday life often get me down."*

Personal Growth

High scorer: Has a feeling of continued development; sees self as growing and expanding; is open to new experiences; has sense of realising his or her potential; sees improvement in self and behaviour over time; is changing in ways that reflect more self-knowledge and effectiveness.

Sample item: "For me, life has been a continuous process of learning, changing, and growth."

Low scorer: Has a sense of personal stagnation; lacks sense of improvement or expansion over time; feels bored and uninterested with life; feels unable to develop new attitudes or behaviours.

Sample item: "When I think about it, I haven't really improved much over the years."

Positive Relations with Others

High scorer: Has warm, satisfying, trusting relationships with others; is concerned about the welfare of other others; capable of strong empathy, affection, and intimacy; understands give-and-take of human relationships.

Sample item: "I enjoy personal and mutual conversations with family and friends."

Low scorer: Has few close, trusting relationships with others; finds it difficult to be warm, open, and concerned about others; is isolated and frustrated in interpersonal relationships; not willing to make compromises to sustain important ties with others.

Sample item: "I have not experienced many warm and trusting relationships with others."

Purpose in Life

High scorer: Has goals in life and a sense of directedness; feels there is meaning to present and past life; holds beliefs that give life purpose; has aims and objectives for living.

Sample item: "I have a sense of direction and purpose in life."

Low scorer: Lacks a sense of meaning in life; has few goals or aims; lacks sense of direction; does not see purpose of past life; has no outlook or beliefs that give life meaning.

Sample item: "I don't have a good sense of what it is I'm trying to accomplish in life."

Self-Acceptance

High scorer: Possesses a positive attitude toward the self; acknowledges and accepts multiple aspects of self, including good and bad qualities; feels positive about past life.

Sample item: "When I look at the story of my life, I'm pleased with how things have turned out."

Low Scorer: Feels dissatisfied with self; is disappointed with what has occurred in past life; is troubled about certain personal qualities; wishes to be different from what he or she is.

Sample item: "My attitude about myself is probably not as positive as most people feel about themselves."

Note. Response options for all above items: 1 (*strongly disagree*) to 7 (*strongly agree*) including descriptions of both high and low scorers. These definitions, *which came from the underlying theories*, served as the basis for generating self-descriptive items intended to operationalise each dimension. Both positively and negatively worded items (drawn from the definition of both high and low scorers) were included to assess the presence or absence of each aspect of wellbeing while also guarding against response sets (e.g., the tendency to agree with all items). Detailed psychometric analyses were then conducted to refine the item pools via assessment of face and content validity, item-to-scale correlations (to ensure that each item correlated more highly with its own rather than another scale), and internal consistency (alpha) coefficients. Confirmatory factor analyses then examined whether the data supported the proposed six factor model and how the dimensions related to other constructs (convergent and discriminant validity) (Keyes, Shmotkin, & Ryff, 2002; Ryff & Keyes, 1995). In the main, these psychometric analyses, including those conducted with samples from diverse countries, have supported the proposed model. Of importance in evaluating the model's empirical structure is the need to employ scales of sufficient length (Gallagher, Lopez, & Preacher, 2009), with approaches using shortened scales showing problematic factor structures.

This detail on measurement construction is emphasised for two reasons. First, as the above progression reveals, a comprehensive approach is required to develop the high-quality measures needed to advance the field of wellbeing. Indeed, a problem with proliferating approaches to wellbeing is the lack of theoretically informed and clearly defined constructs that are accompanied by rigorous procedures to establish the validity and reliability of the relevant measures. Second, there are encouraging signs that measurement issues are receiving attention, as illustrated by the volume on *Measuring Wellbeing* (Lee, Kubzansky, & VanderWeele, 2021). This collection ends with measurement recommendations put forth by the editors and others (VanderWeele, Trudel-Fitzgerald, Allin et al., 2021) as well as a dissenting view (Ryff, Boylan, & Kirsch, 2021a) followed by a rebuttal on both sides (VanderWeele, Trudel-Fitzgerald, & Kubzansky, 2021; Ryff, Boylan, & Kirsch, 2021b). This exchange offers a useful debate on critical issues for advancing the field of wellbeing. These matters are particularly pertinent in the growing number of government surveys of wellbeing, which have been notably disconnected from the measures and findings from unfolding cohort studies (see also Chapter 13, this volume). Put another way, quality control issues in measurement of wellbeing need to be recognised because they are of no less consequence than quality control issues in assessing health or wealth.

PAST ADVANCES ON EUDAIMONIC WELLBEING: WHAT HAVE WE LEARNED?

The above model of wellbeing has had widespread impact across diverse scientific fields, with the measures translated to more than 40 languages and more than 1,200 publications generated on the antecedents, consequents, and correlates of wellbeing (Ryff, 2014, 2018). Such extensive use likely reflects, in the spirit of Aristotle, a commitment to reach for essential meanings of what constitutes the best within us. That is, the guiding model was founded on intellectually vital ideas and ideals which are seen to have relevance across multiple life domains, fields of scientific inquiry, and cultural contexts.

Many emergent findings are from the Midlife in the US (MIDUS) national longitudinal study (www.midus.wisc.edu), which has collected comprehensive biopsychosocial data on large, population-based samples of Americans. MIDUS includes measures of both eudaimonic and hedonic wellbeing and is deeply multidisciplinary in scope. Thus, the publicly available data have allowed investigators to link wellbeing to numerous domains (e.g., adult life experiences and aging, health, biology, and neuroscience). The overview below draws on previous summaries of key advances (Ryff, 2014, 2018), which include numerous findings prior to MIDUS as well as more recent reviews, with one covering sociodemographic and health correlates of both eudaimonic and hedonic wellbeing (Ryff, Boylan, & Kirsch, 2021c) and another examining the emerging science that has grown up around a specific aspect of wellbeing: namely, purposeful life engagement (Ryff & Kim, 2020).

Sociodemographic Factors and Eudaimonic Wellbeing

Initial studies based on single-point-in-time data from smaller convenience samples showed age differences in aspects of eudaimonic wellbeing (Ryff, 1989, 1991; Ryff & Keyes, 1995). Some dimensions showed increments with age (autonomy and environmental mastery), decrements with age (personal growth and purpose in life), no age differences (self-acceptance), or inconsistent patterns (positive relations with others). Subsequent longitudinal findings based on national samples offered reliable evidence of a decline from midlife to old age in personal growth and purpose in life (Springer, Pudrovska, & Hauser, 2011). Such decline may reflect structural lag—that is, the notion that social institutions have not kept up with the added years of life that many older adults now experience (Riley, Kahn, Foner, & Mack, 1994). Thus, insufficient opportunities may be available for older individuals to contribute, thereby limiting opportunities for personal growth and purposeful engagement. These hypotheses are worthy of future study, particularly given emerging links between purpose in life and numerous indicators of health, as detailed in a separate section below.

Regarding gender differences, early evidence from the Wisconsin Longitudinal Study showed that women scored higher on positive relations with others and personal growth (Marks, 1996), findings also seen in other small-sample studies (Ryff, 1995; Ryff & Heidrich, 1997). Other dimensions of eudaimonic wellbeing have not shown gender differences, and longitudinal evidence on whether life course changes in wellbeing vary for men and women have not been reported. Socioeconomic status has been linked to eudaimonic wellbeing, mostly in terms of educational attainment. Data from multiple studies (the National Survey of Families and Households, MIDUS, Whitehall, and Wisconsin Longitudinal

Study) have shown that those with higher levels of education report higher levels on all six dimensions of eudaimonic wellbeing (Marmot et al., 1998; Marmot et al., 1997). Thus, greater educational opportunities, which implicate not only access to knowledge but also to good jobs, higher incomes, and greater wealth, likely enhance all that eudaimonia entails (autonomy, mastery, personal growth, purpose in life, positive relations, and self-acceptance). Causal directionality is unclear, although there are credible reasons to believe the influences are bidirectional.

With regard to race, an early and unexpected finding from MIDUS was that African American adults reported higher levels of eudaimonic wellbeing (Ryff, Keyes, & Hughes, 2003) compared to their White counterparts. At the time, we speculated that the challenges of minority life, including unfair and unjust treatments, may hone a sense of purpose as well as inner perceptions of personal growth, autonomy, and mastery. Victor Frankl (1959) long ago put forth a powerful case that purpose and meaning are critical and life-sustaining in the face of major adversity. Subsequent work from MIDUS showed that the minority advantage in wellbeing would be even greater were it not for experiences of discrimination (Keyes, 2009). These findings point to important future hypotheses regarding the role of eudaimonic wellbeing and its consequences for health and longevity among racial/ethnic minorities.

Importantly, evidence is growing showing that sociodemographic factors often work together in shaping wellbeing. This knowledge calls for greater emphasis on intersectionality going forward—namely, how age, gender, socioeconomic status, and race/ethnicity *interact* in accounting for levels of eudaimonic wellbeing and their links to health (see Ryff, Boylan, & Kirsch, 2021a).

Experiences in Work and Family Life

Eudaimonia needs to be understood in terms of the actual experiences of people's lives, which can be examined in multiple ways. Numerous studies have shown that greater involvement in multiple life roles (e.g., worker, spouse, or parent) appears to promote higher wellbeing (e.g., Ahrens & Ryff, 2006), although the actual activities in these roles matter (e.g., helping others seems to enhance purpose and self-acceptance) (Greenfield, 2009). Those who are married have a wellbeing advantage compared to the divorced, widowed, or never married, although single women score higher on autonomy and personal growth compared to married women (Marks & Lambert, 1998). Parenting seems to enhance adult wellbeing, particularly if one's children are doing well (An & Cooney, 2006; Schmutte & Ryff, 1994), whereas the loss of a child predicts impaired wellbeing even decades later (Rogers, Floyd, Seltzer et al., 2008). Similarly, loss of a parent in childhood predicts lower levels of multiple dimensions of adult wellbeing (Maier & Lachman, 2000). Experiencing psychological or physical violence from a parent in childhood compromises adult wellbeing (Greenfield & Marks, 2010), as does caring for an ageing parent, although less so for daughters with high environmental mastery (Li, Seltzer, & Greenberg, 1999).

With regard to work, wellbeing appears to contribute to and be influenced by career pursuits, with findings varying depending on the types of work pursued (e.g., paid or unpaid) and differences between men and women (Lindfors, Berntsson, & Lundberg, 2006). The interplay between work and family life has been extensively linked to wellbeing, with findings showing both negative and positive spillover between these domains (Grzywacz, 2000; Marks, 1998). Cohort differences have been observed in how young men and women manage work and family roles, with related differences for wellbeing (Carr, 2002). For example, older women and younger men who adjusted their work schedules to meet family demands had higher self-acceptance, whereas older men and younger women had lower self-acceptance if they cut back on paid employment to accommodate family demands.

Life experiences have also been studied as stress exposures that accumulate over time. Such topics have been of interest in MIDUS (Ryff, 2019) and linked with diverse health outcomes. For example, Gruenewald et al. (2012) found links between socioeconomic adversity in childhood (i.e., parental education and welfare status) and adulthood (i.e., education, income, and difficulty paying bills) to a multisystem biological risk (i.e., allostatic load). Another example focused on the lives of African Americans, where Slopen et al. (2012, 2013) linked cumulative stress across multiple life domains (i.e., neighborhood, financial, relationship, work, perceived inequality, discrimination, and childhood adversity) to smoking behaviour. Numerous other such studies exist in MIDUS (see www.midus.wisc. edu), although few have investigated potential associations between cumulative stress exposures and eudaimonic wellbeing. An interesting hypothesis is whether the aforementioned eudaimonic advantage observed for Blacks compared to Whites constitutes a buffer (protective resource) against the adverse effects of cumulative stress.

Eudaimonia and Physical Health

Growing research has linked eudaimonic wellbeing to diagnosed disease or disability. For example, purpose in life, after adjusting for multiple covariates, has been associated with a reduced incidence of Alzheimer's disease and mild cognitive impairment (Boyle, Buchman, & Bennett, 2010) and reduced risk of stroke (Kim, Delaney, & Kubzansky, 2019; Kim, Sun, Park, & Peterson, 2013) and myocardial infarction among those with coronary heart disease (Kim, Sun, Park, Kubzansky, & Peterson, 2013). Indicators of poor health or the presence of disease have also been associated with compromised eudaimonic wellbeing (Costanzo, Ryff, & Singer, 2009; Schleicher et al., 2005), underscoring the need for longitudinal research to investigate possible bidirectional relationships.

Longitudinal community samples of older adults have shown that those with high purpose in life had reduced rates of mortality 7 years later (Boyle, Barnes, Buchman, & Bennett, 2009). Findings from MIDUS (Hill & Turiano, 2014) replicated and extended these findings, showing greater survival 14 years later among those with higher purpose in life at baseline after adjusting for numerous covari-ates. Findings from the Health and Retirement Study (HRS) showed lowest risk of all-cause mortality among those with highest levels of purpose in life as well as reduced risk of mortality from heart, circulatory, and blood conditions (Alimujiang et al., 2019). A meta-analysis of 10 prospective studies reported significant associ-ations between purpose in life and reduced all-cause mortality and reduced car-diovascular events (Cohen, Bavishi, & Rozanski, 2016). What makes these results noteworthy are the previously discussed findings that many older adults experience a decline in their sense of purpose in life as they age, with such declines having po-tentially serious consequences for health and longevity. What the mortality findings also underscore, however, is within age group variability among the aged. That is, some maintain high levels of purposeful engagement, which could inform strategies for enhancing sense of purpose in older adults (see also chapter 11, this volume). Also relevant for profiles of morbidity and mortality are findings showing that those with higher eudaimonic wellbeing are more likely to use preventive healthcare ser-vices and to practice better health behaviours (e.g., diet and exercise) (Chen, Kim, Koh, Frazier, & VanderWeele, 2019; Hill & Weston, 2019; Hooker & Masters, 2016; Kim, Kawachi, Chen, & Kubzansky, 2017; Kim, Strecher, & Ryff, 2014; Steptoe & Fancourt, 2019). Taken together, these results underscore notable benefits asso-ciated with purpose in life. The larger literature also provides evidence for other aspects of eudaimonia, some of which are covered in the next section.

Biological and Neurological Underpinnings of Eudaimonia

Researchers have been interested in possible mechanisms and processes through which eudaimonic wellbeing has its salubrious effects. Early findings showed that higher wellbeing (particularly personal growth, positive relations with others, and purpose in life) was linked with better neuroendocrine regulation, better inflam-matory profiles, lower cardiovascular risk factors, and better sleep profiles (e.g., Friedman et al., 2005; Ryff, Singer, & Love, 2004). More recent findings with na-tional samples show that aspects of eudaimonia are also associated with better glycaemic regulation (Boylan, Tsenkova, Miyamoto, & Ryff, 2017; Hafez et al., 2018), better inflammatory profiles (Friedman & Ryff, 2012; Morozink, Friedman, Coe, & Ryff, 2010), better lipid profiles (Radler, Rigotti, & Ryff, 2017), lower risk of metabolic syndrome (Boylan & Ryff, 2015), and lower allostatic load (Zilioli, Slatcher, Ong, & Gruenewald, 2015a). However, not all studies have found sig-nificant associations between eudaimonic wellbeing and biological risk factors (Feldman & Steptoe, 2003; Sloan et al., 2017), with the differences possibly linked to use of measures that were not explicitly constructed to measure eudaimonia.

Underscoring protective effects in the face of adversity, eudaimonic wellbeing may buffer against the adverse health effects of inequality. Multiple studies have shown evidence of the mitigating effects of eudaimonic wellbeing for self-rated health (Ryff, Radler, & Friedman, 2015), chronic conditions (O'Brien, 2012), in-flammatory markers (Elliot & Chapman, 2016; Morozink et al., 2010), diurnal cortisol (Zilioli, Imami, & Slatcher, 2015b), glycosylated haemoglobin (HbA1c, which is relevant for diabetes; Tsenkova, Love, Singer, & Ryff, 2007), and cardiovascular recovery following an acute stressor (Boylan, Jennings, & Matthews, 2016). The general pattern in these outcomes is that, among those with lower educational standing, having higher eudaimonic wellbeing predicts health outcomes comparable to that observed for higher educational groups.

With regard to neuroscience, an initial study using electrophysiological measures showed that higher eudaimonic wellbeing was linked with greater left than right superior frontal activation in response to emotional stimuli (Urry et al., 2004) after adjusting for hedonic indicators. Another study (van Reekum et al., 2007) used functional magnetic resonance imaging (fMRI) techniques to show that those with higher eudaimonic wellbeing had less amygdala activation in response to negative stimuli as well as more activation of regions (ventral anterior cingulate cortex) that help regulate emotion. Heller et al. (2013) used fMRI techniques to show sustained activation of reward circuitry (striatal activity) in response to positive stimuli among those with higher eudaimonic wellbeing, a pattern that was further linked with lower cortisol output over the course of the day. Schaefer et al. (2013) showed that higher purpose in life predicted less reactivity (eye-blink startle response) to negative stimuli. Finally, eudaimonic wellbeing has been linked with greater insular cortex volume, which is involved in an array of higher-order cognitive functions (Lewis, Kanai, Rees, & Bates, 2014).

Recent studies of gene expression show differential linkages to eudaimonic versus hedonic wellbeing. Specifically, eudaimonic wellbeing predicted downregulation of the conserved transcriptional response to adversity (CTRA; Cole, 2013), marked by a healthy pattern of lower expression of pro-inflammatory genes and higher expression of antibody synthesis genes. Hedonic wellbeing, in contrast, was associated with the opposite pattern (i.e., up-regulation of CTRA; i.e., the unhealthy pattern). Further studies have replicated these findings (Cole et al., 2015; Fredrickson et al., 2013, 2015). These inquiries are at the forefront of the science illuminating the mechanisms through which eudaimonia may be beneficial for health.

Taken together, notable scientific strides have occurred in linking higher eudaimonic wellbeing to reduced disease and disability, greater longevity, better regulation of multiple biological systems, brain-based assessments of adaptive emotion regulation, and healthy gene expression related to inflammatory processes. Although more research is needed, such work exemplifies an important shift in empirical research away from the long-standing focus on physiological and neurological underpinnings of psychological distress and toward the beneficial health sequelae of eudaimonic wellbeing.

Intervention Studies to Promote Wellbeing

Conceptualised as the striving to realise personal potential, eudaimonic wellbeing is not something achieved once and for all, but instead represents a life-long challenge wherein incremental improvements are always possible (Ruini, 2017). Accordingly, the main therapeutic goals of eudaimonic interventions have centred on identifying opportunities for continued personal growth and purpose, even in difficult contexts, such as dealing with the diminished health and functional capacities that accompany aging (see also Chapter 11, this volume). A recent meta-analysis (Weiss, Westerhof, & Bohlmeijer, 2016) showed that interventions can, in fact, improve wellbeing, with some targeted specifically on eudaimonia (Cantarella, Borella, Marigo, & De Beni, 2017). These endeavours build on prior work in clinical settings, such as wellbeing therapy (Fava et al., 2004; Ruini & Fava, 2009), which was designed to treat depression, mood, and anxiety disorder through the promotion of eudaimonic wellbeing. Several community-based interventions have shown gains in multiple aspects of eudaimonia among patients dealing with various health challenges (e.g., multiple sclerosis and rheumatoid arthritis) (Hart, Fonareva, Merluzzi, & Mohr, 2005; Pradhan et al., 2007). Interventions with nonclinical samples have been conducted with adolescents to prevent the emergence of psychological disorders (e.g., depression) as well as with adults to promote resilience in the workplace (Millear. Liossis, Schochet, Biggs, & Donald, 2008; Ruini et al., 2009). A program for older adults living in community settings showed enhancement of multiple aspects of eudaimonic wellbeing along with declining profiles of psychological distress (Friedman et al., 2019). Taken together, growing evidence supports the idea that eudaimonic wellbeing is modifiable and can be promoted, including in the face of significant life challenges.

TERRITORIES AHEAD IN EUDAIMONIC SCIENCE

Building on the progress described above, this section targets key directions for future, integrative research. Although socioeconomic inequality has been part of previous work, this topic now takes on great urgency due to recent historical events, including the Great Recession that began in 2008 and, more recently, the COVID-19 pandemic. Both have deepened already existing problems of inequality. The first section below frames these historical happenings as powerful forces that work against the realisation of personal potential (eudaimonia) among disadvantaged segments of society. Scientific research is essential to both document the scope of these problems and seek to address them.

The second topic below considers the interface of wellbeing with realms of life that until recently were largely absent in extant research—namely, the role of the arts and humanities in nourishing eudaimonia and thereby possibly impacting health. These lines of inquiry are about the power of art, music, and literature in uplifting the human spirit, but also encompass powerful portrayals in art of suffering and injustice that may activate needed compassion and caring among the privileged (see also Chapter 4, this volume). Such work brings to the fore problems of complacency and indifference among advantaged segments of society, topics also largely absent in prior research on health inequalities.

A final section attends to a central pillar of this edited collection: namely, environmental influences on wellbeing. These have been largely missing in prior research on eudaimonia. To consider such possibilities, focus is primarily on the natural environment, as directly experienced in nature or as taken in via multiple art forms (i.e., paintings, poetry, literature, and film). The central question is whether nature contributes to diverse aspects of eudaimonic wellbeing, and, if so, how and why. Also of interest is whether higher eudaimonia predicts greater concern about and commitment to issues of climate change, sustainability, and protecting the wellbeing of the planet. Numerous exciting hypotheses await scientific study regarding the interplay between the wellbeing of individuals and their participation in and commitment to natural environments.

Eudaimonia in Turbulent Times

As described above, considerable work has documented educational gradients in levels of eudaimonic wellbeing (Marmot et al., 1997, 1998; Ryff, 1989, 1995; Ryff & Keyes, 1995). That said, there is marked heterogeneity within educational groups (Markus, Ryff, Curhan, & Palmersheim, 2004; Ryff, 2016), which has led to important findings that document the role of eudaimonic wellbeing as a protective buffer against adverse health among less-educated adults who nonetheless report high levels of purpose, mastery, growth, positive relations, and so on.

Numerous indicators show that inequality is worsening over time (Cohen; 2018; Piketty & Saez, 2014) particularly in the United States. Referred to as the 'hoarding' of the American Dream (Reeves, 2017), the top 20% of income earners have privileged access to better educations, jobs, income, and wealth along with a greater likelihood of stable marriages to successful partners, thriving neighbourhoods, and healthier lifestyles. Such discrepancies in life opportunities and income have been linked with compromised levels of optimism, life satisfaction, and happiness among those who are disadvantaged (Graham, 2017). The Great Recession that began in 2008 exacerbated these problems, fueling dramatic increases in poverty rates (Bishaw, 2013) and accompanying health costs due to job loss, unemployment, and financial strain (Burgard & Kalousova, 2015; Kirsch & Ryff, 2016).

A unique feature of MIDUS was recruitment of two national samples situated on either side of the Great Recession. The baseline sample (aged 25–74) was recruited in 1995, followed by recruitment of a new national sample (same ages) in 2012. Over the period covered by these two samples, educational attainment in the United States improved: college-educated adults increased from 24.8% to 33.2%, and those with less than a high school level of education decreased from 15.3% to 11.3%. Despite such gains, the post-Recession sample reported less household income (after adjusting for inflation) and lower financial stability than the pre-Recession sample (Kirsch, Love, Radler, & Ryff, 2019). Similarly, the post-Recession sample had worse general health, more chronic conditions, higher body mass index (BMI), more functional limitations, and more physical health symptoms than the pre-Recession sample. With regard to psychological health, the post-Recession sample had significantly lower levels of multiple aspects of eudaimonia (i.e., autonomy, self-acceptance, and personal growth) and hedonia (i.e., positive affect and life satisfaction) than the pre-Recession sample. Further analyses revealed a steeper educational gradient in the post-Recession compared to the pre-Recession sample for BMI, functional limitations, and physical symptoms (Kirsch et al., 2019).

Other MIDUS findings (Goldman, Glei, & Weinstein, 2018) compared these two national samples on a wide array of mental health measures (positive and negative) and found that mental health was more compromised in the post-Recession sample compared to the pre-Recession sample among those with a lower socioeconomic position (measured as a composite of education, occupation, income, and wealth). This worsening of mental health among disadvantaged Americans was framed in the context of the opioid epidemic, growing alcoholism, and increased death rates, including suicide, among middle-aged White persons of low socioeconomic status (SES) (Case & Deaton, 2015; Grant et al., 2017; Kolodny et al., 2015; Schuchat, Houry, & Guy, 2017). The nomenclature increasingly used to describe these trends is *deaths of despair* (Case & Deaton, 2020; see also Chapter 15, this volume).

These findings underscore historical change in opportunities to experience eudaimonia. The central message is that the realisation of personal potential now exceeds the reach of many. Sadly, the COVID-19 pandemic exacerbated these inequities. A recent report (Pew Research Center, 2020) shows that the economic fallout from COVID-19 hit lower-income Americans the hardest, 46% of whom had trouble paying their bills compared to 16% of upper-income adults. Similarly, 35% of lower-income adults received help from a foodbank compared to 1% of upper-income adults, and 32% of lower-income adults had problems paying rent or mortgage compared to 3% of upper-income adults. Overall, 25% of US adults said they or someone in their household lost their job because of the coronavirus outbreak. Lower-income adults who were laid off due to the coronavirus were less like to return to work compared to middle- and upper-income adults who lost their jobs. Similarly, those whose ability to save money was curtailed by the recent economic upheaval were mostly lower-income adults. Another trauma has been eviction—loss of home due to inability to pay rent. Desmond (2016) brought attention to this problem in the city of Milwaukee, Wisconsin, and now runs the Eviction Lab (www.evictionlab.com) at Princeton University, where data from 25 cities are being tracked. Since the pandemic, landlords in these locations have filed about 2,500–3,000 evictions per week. Dire consequences follow for families forced out of their homes.

What is the relevance of these happenings for those interested in human wellbeing? A major point is that meaningful, happy, and fulfilled lives are increasingly not available to many individuals due to gaping discrepancies in life opportunities and resources. This renders the preoccupations with the upbeat phenomena that characterise the positive psychology movement (Seligman, 2011) strikingly out of touch with the suffering now experienced by many. Such trumpeting of the positive, alongside with negativity about the negative, was recognised well before the pandemic (e.g., Held, 2004). A voice from France depicted the problem as *Perpetual Euphoria: On the Duty to be Happy* (Bruckner, 2010), which likened pre-occupations with the positive as signaling the advent of banality akin to Voltaire's *Candide*, wherein felicity and vacuity went hand in hand.

In sum, the *intersecting catastrophes* of widening inequality subsequently compounded by the health and economic consequences of the coronavirus pandemic, demand scientific attention around the globe. On the one hand, these happenings raise the troubling possibility that wellbeing, however defined, will increasingly become the purview of privileged segments of societies. This is cause for concern: human history is replete with dire consequences that followed when blind eyes were turned toward dramatic disparities in human opportunities to lead meaningful and fulfilling lives. It is worth remembering that the ancient Greeks were also concerned about problems of greed and injustice (Balot, 2001), which they saw as violating virtues of fairness and contributing to civic strife. In turn, Dante (1308/2006) placed the sins of greed and gluttony prominently in his nine circles of hell. Will these be forces that undermine the wellbeing of many in our era? Or, alternatively, might rampant inequality carried to even greater heights by the pandemic be seen for what it is: stark evidence of societal dysfunction at structural levels that demands social change toward more equitable opportunities to realise human potential?

Nurturing Eudaimonia Through the Arts

Paradoxically, as inequality has worsened, other encouraging advances have pointed to beneficent impacts of the arts and humanities on wellbeing and health (Crawford, Brown, Baker, Tischler, & Abrams, 2015; Lomas, 2016; Royal Society for Public Health, 2013; Stuckey & Nobel, 2010; Tay, Pawelski, & Keith, 2017). A report from the World Health Organization (Fancourt & Finn, 2019) summarised evidence on the role of the arts in improving health and wellbeing in many countries. It thus appears that creating and consuming literature, poetry, the visual arts, music, dance, and film may nourish good lives even though the larger field of subjective wellbeing (eudaimonic and hedonic) has largely neglected such topics. Instead, the lion's share of inputs on wellbeing and health has focused on stress exposures and negative experience (detailed in Ryff, 2019).

An important future question is 'What cultivates sensibilities to partake of the arts'? I have argued that a broad liberal education may be important (Ryff, 2016) and have illustrated these ideas via the teaching of great literature and poetry in higher education as venues for strengthening the self and nourishing inner vitality. What we know is that the best sociodemographic predictor of attendance at arts events (e.g., music concerts, theatre, museum, and gallery exhibitions) is years of schooling (DiMaggio & Mukhtar, 2004), although less is known about whether participation rates vary depending on fields of study pursued at college or university. Such research would illuminate other questions, such as whether liberal arts training—and learning in the humanities (e.g., art, philosophy, and history) more generally—produces the capable and competent citizens needed by democratic societies (Nussbaum, 1997, 2010). Others have framed college as critical in building a defensible self that is guided by more than the bromides exchanged every day on Facebook (Deresiewicz, 2014).

Embedded within these queries is the thorny problem of elitism in higher education—something perceived long ago by Benjamin Franklin as the problematic cementing of privilege that occurs at private institutions (see Roth, 2014). In recent times, Bourdieu and Passeron (1977, 1990) have argued that elite institutions in France are the primary mechanisms through which class hierarchies are maintained across time. The miseducation of the American elite has been described as nurturing a false sense of self-worth, compromising capacities to relate to non-elites, and promoting a view of intelligence narrowly anchored in academic achievement, especially courses needed for success in law, medicine, science, and business (Deresiewicz, 2014).

These problems of elitism likely play a role in fueling the rampant inequality described above. Mendelberg, McCabe, and Thal (2016) used a large sample of US students to show that norms for financial gain are more prominent at affluent colleges compared to public universities. In addition, psychologists have shown that those from higher- compared to lower-class backgrounds have a greater sense of entitlement and higher levels of narcissism (Piff, 2014; Piff, Stancato, Côté, Mendoza-Denton, & Keltner, 2012). Those motivated by primarily extrinsic factors (e.g., financial success) also have lower wellbeing and adjustment compared to those motivated by less materialistic values (Kasser & Ryan, 1993).

Bringing these observations back to the arts and humanities, it is important to remember that much of the world's great literature has been about the suffering of the disadvantaged (e.g., Dickens, Hugo, Steinbeck, and Tolstoy). These themes are evident in contemporary fiction as well, such as *Call Me Zebra* (Van der Vliet Oloomi, 2018) and *Exit West* (Hamid, 2017), both of which tell tales of the refugee experience. Contemporary film (e.g., *The Florida Project, American Honey, Paterson, Parasite,* and *Nomadland)* also reveals the lived experiences of inequality, including homelessness, having parents with substance use problems, finding poetry in working-class lives, and the cleverness of those at the bottom vis-à-vis insensitive elites. The relevance of these domains for contemporary research on eudaimonic wellbeing is the call to investigate the role that the arts play in depicting and perhaps overcoming contemporary societal challenges. For example, do encounters with such art forms increase national quotients of caring and compassion? Do they challenge complacency and indifference among those who are not suffering? Such questions elevate themes of social justice in ongoing scholarship on wellbeing and health while pointing to the arts as venues to inform and mobilise individual and societal action about such issues.

The Natural Environment and Eudaimonic Wellbeing

Environmental psychology has come into its own as a scientific field with wide-ranging objectives (De Young, 2013; Gifford, 2014; Proshansky, 1987), such as how to address contemporary environmental problems as well as design environments to promote human capacities. Prominent distinctions are made between natural and built environments. For this chapter, I focus exclusively on natural environments (green spaces) that implicate growing concerns about urbanisation, loss of biodiversity, and environmental degradation. Substantial science now links natural environments to improved functioning, including diverse mental health outcomes, cognition, stress physiology, and sensory systems. A review by Mantler and Logan (2015) described theoretical orientations emphasising the role of nature in stress recovery processes and restoration of cognitive attention while also summarising empirical findings between 'nature connectedness' and reported vitality, positive affect, and life satisfaction as well as lower levels of anxiety and anger (see also Chapter 2, this volume). In contrast, the health correlates of 'grey space' (e.g., high in industrial activity, traffic, and noise) showed adverse links with mental health. Triguero-Mas et al. (2015) also summarised emerging links between natural outdoor environments and mental and physical health and considered intervening mechanisms (e.g., increased physical activity, social contacts, and stress reduction). Cross-sectional data from a large sample of adults in the Catalonia Health Survey did not provide evidence of these as mediators (possibly due to measurement issues), although green spaces were associated with better self-perceived health (physical and mental) across different degrees of urbanisation, levels of SES, and gender.

The above literature is interesting and important, although assessments of eudaimonic wellbeing are largely missing throughout. Most work has focused on negative indicators of mental health or limited indicators of hedonic wellbeing. Thus, questions worthy of future inquiry are whether and how encounters with nature might enhance people's knowledge of themselves (self-acceptance), their capacities to find meaning and direction in their lives (purpose in life), their sense of self-realisation (personal growth) and self-directedness (autonomy), whether they feel capable of managing their own situations (environmental mastery), and how they see the quality of their ties with others (positive relations). Collectively, these queries bring to the fore the role of nature as a source of solace and inspiration for leading well-lived lives, broadly defined. To consider how this might work, I return to the arts and humanities (including philosophy and history) as they offer long-standing evidence that nature is a profound influence on what it means to be fully alive and well.

A powerful example is the life of Alexander von Humboldt (1769–1859), beautifully written about in *The Invention of Nature* (Wulf, 2016). Primarily a scientist, naturalist, and explorer (of South America and Siberia), Humboldt influenced many of the great thinkers of his day, including Jefferson, Darwin, Wordsworth, Coleridge, Thoreau, and Goethe. Humboldt was notably ahead of his time in thinking about the degradation and exploitation of nature, warning that humankind had the power to destroy the natural environment, and he believed the consequences would be catastrophic. Humboldt had a sense of wonder about nature and believed our response to it should be based on the senses and emotion: he wanted to excite a 'love of nature' and thereby revolutionised how the natural world was seen. He believed that nature speaks to humanity in a voice 'familiar to our soul' (p. 61), thereby aligning himself with the Romantic poets of his time who believed nature could only be understood by turning inward.

Mountains, in particular, held a spell over Humboldt in a transcendental way: 'When he stood on a summit or a high ridge, he felt so moved by the scenery that his imagination carried him even higher. This imagination, he said, soothed the "deep wounds" that pure "reason" sometimes created' (p. 97). Thus, drawing on Goethe's inner circle representing German Idealism and Romanticism, Humboldt saw no irreconcilable chasm between the internal and the external world. He embraced the rationality and methods of the Enlightenment thinkers while seeing nature, not as an external mechanical system, but as a living organism that required subjectivity. This constituted a revolution in science because it required turning away from the 'dry compilation of facts' and 'crude empiricism' (p. 151). Both Goethe and Humboldt advocated for the marriage of art and science rather than seeing them as great antagonists.

An essential feature of eudaimonic wellbeing is its emphasis on inner, subjective experience, partitioned into different perceptions about the self, relationships, and life pursuits. How might nature, as expressed in poetry, nurture these subjective parts of who we are and hope to become? Mark Edmundson, Professor of English at the University of Virginia shows the way. He draws on great literature and poetry to nurture wellbeing, including ideals (values) needed by the human soul such as courage, contemplation, and compassion (Edmundson, 2015). In *Why Read* (2004), Edmundson elaborates what a liberal, humanistic education can contribute to personal becoming. Inundated with input from the internet, television, journalism, and advertising, he sees no better medium for helping young people learn how to live their lives than poetry and literature. When teaching about these works, he repeatedly asks his students 'Can you live it?', that is, does the work offer a new or better way of understanding the self and others, or point to alternative paths for living a better life?

Apropos of Humboldt and his contemporaries, Edmondson examines Wordsworth's famous poem, 'Lines Composed a Few Miles from Tintern Abbey', written in 1798. The context is that Wordsworth's life had become flat—'he lived in a din-filled city, among unfeeling people, and sensed that he is becoming one of them . . . there is a dull ache settling in his spirit' (p. 57). Returning to a scene from his childhood, he remembered himself as a young boy, free and reveling in nature. The return to nature, which is the heart of the poem, reminds him of its role in nurturing his own vitality. 'Wordsworth's poem enjoins us to feel that it (the answer to one's despondency) lies somewhere within our reach—we are creatures who have the capacity to make ourselves sick, but also the power to heal ourselves' (p. 49).

Not emphasised by Edmundson but of note is that Wordsworth's poetry served the same vital function in the life of John Stuart Mill (1893/1989) who, in his early adulthood, realised something deeply troubling: that he lacked the happiness central to the utilitarian philosophy in which he was immersed. Reflecting on his life, Mill described an early educational experience that was unquestionably exceptional but also profoundly deficient. His father began teaching him Greek and Latin at a young age and then expanded the pedagogy to fields of philosophy, science, and mathematics. However, his father was deeply opposed to anything connected to sentiment or emotion. To escape the logic machine he had become, Mill began a quest to feel, and it was the poetry of Wordsworth, mostly about nature, that ministered deeply to the longings in his soul. He credited it for helping him recover from the crisis in his mental history.

Nature is powerfully present in other art forms as well. On the heels of the Romantic era in literature was a dramatic happening—namely, the French impressionist movement (1860–1910). After centuries of religious art, mostly dark and dreary in content, the impressionists embraced a revolutionary idea: to paint outside (*en plein air*). Thus, their subject matter was suffused with light—the sun shining down on all manner of nature's beauty. This new vision gave us Monet's famed *Waterlilies*, his magnificent *Poppies*, and his *Garden at Giverny*. Cezanne captured the *Forest*, Sisley the *Fog*, and Pissarro the French countryside (*Paysage aux Patis*). Van Gogh dazzled the world with his *Starry Night* and *Sunflowers*, while Klimt, known for figurative art, created breathtaking scenes from nature (*Beech Forest* and *Fruit Trees*). From Spain, Sorolla captured seascapes (*Biarritz Beach*) and children frolicking in waves (*Ninos en el Mar*). Taken as a whole, the world came to love this art for its magnificent celebration of nature that brought joy and inspiration to all.

While the impressionists were immersed in outside adventures, others drew on nature to inspire musical creativity. From the same era were Debussy's three symphonic sketches (*La Mer*) that captured the changing moods, rhythm, and power of the sea. Other nature-inspired music included Beethoven's *Pastorale* symphony, Chopin's *Raindrop* prelude, Rimsky-Korsakov's *Flight of the Bumblebee*, and Smetana's symphonic poem about a beloved river, *The Moldau*. Important to underscore is that these works continue to evoke rich emotions in others more than a century later. That is, the glory of nature inspires enormous creativity, the products of which enrich the human experience again and again through time.

Contemporary art forms do the same, though justice cannot be done to such topics here. Of note is that the 2019 Pulitzer Prize in Literature was awarded to Richard Powers (2018) for *The Overstory*, a novel about the impact of giant, memorable trees on the lives of several distinctive people. Indeed, it is a tale about how trees changed their lives. Similarly, the 2013 Pulitzer Prize in Music was awarded to John Luther Adams for his orchestral work *Become Ocean*, which 'immerses the listener in a sonic churn, ebb and roar that conjures a world inundated by rising sea levels' (Fonseca-Wollheim, 2020). Adams thus combines musical composition with environmental activism, a theme also evident in Powers's book. On a journalistic level is *The Nature Fix* (Williams, 2017) that reports on investigations (e.g., forest-healing programs and ecotherapy) from around the world showing how nature is critical for health, happiness, and creativity. Speaking personally, great literature, art, music, and contemporary poetry about nature (e.g., Berry, 2012; Oliver, 2017) have been huge in ministering to my soul. To illustrate, I conclude with Mary Oliver's poem 'The Poet with His Face in His Hands'. It is about wanting to cry aloud for our mistakes. She admonishes us to cross forty fields and forty dark inclines to get to the place where the falls are flinging out their white sheets. In the cave behind all, you can stand there

> . . . and roar all you want
> and nothing will be disturbed, you can
> drip with despair all afternoon and still,
> on a green branch, its wings just lightly touched
> by the passing foil of the water, the thrush,
> puffing out its spotted breast, will sing
> of the perfect, stone-hard beauty of everything.

What, then, is the import of such nature poetry and other art forms about nature on the theme of this chapter—namely, the integrative science of eudaimonic wellbeing? It is simply this: alongside extant research examining people's proximity to green or grey spaces and how it matters for their mental and physical health, we need studies of how often (frequency) and how deeply (intensity) they are out in nature and, importantly, are taking it in via great literature, poetry, art, music, and film. This is not outlandish thinking: we routinely study what people eat (nutrition surveys) and drink (alcohol intake), whether they smoke, and how much physical activity they get. Varieties of participation with nature thus constitute new frontiers for what people take in as they journey through life. The central hypothesis needing careful scrutiny is whether those with higher levels of nature consumption are better able to make the most of themselves and their capacities while attending to the needs of others and the planet.

SUMMARY

This chapter revisited a model of eudaimonic wellbeing that has had widespread scientific impact. Past advances were highlighted, including how wellbeing is contoured by demographic factors, how it is linked with work and family life, and how it matters for health, including risk for disease and length of life as well as biological risk factors, neuroscience, and genetics. Whether eudaimonic wellbeing is modifiable via intervention studies was also considered. Building on these advances, three directions for future research were put forth. The first topic emphasised growing inequality and its exacerbation by the COVID-19 pandemic and its economic sequelae. Such historical change elevates the troublesome possibility that eudaimonia may increasingly be out of reach for many, a matter of grave concern. The second direction examined the role of the arts and humanities, broadly defined, as domains that may nourish eudaimonic wellbeing, including in contexts of adversity. The third topic addressed environmental inputs on wellbeing, with specific emphasis on natural environments. Although the field of environmental psychology increasingly investigates links to mental and physical health, little prior work has focused on eudaimonic wellbeing. Extending the preceding future direction, emphasis was given to depictions of nature in poetry, literature, the visual arts, and music. These constitute inputs that provide solace and inspiration, thereby likely enhancing people's capacities to make the most of their lives while also being caring and responsible citizens. Numerous future venues to investigate these hypotheses were put forth. Taken together, the overall objective has been to make the case that the pursuit of human potential (eudaimonic wellbeing) is beautifully suited for integrative science.

REFERENCES

Ahrens, C. J., & Ryff, C. D. (2006). Multiple roles and wellbeing: Sociodemographic and psychological moderators. *Sex Roles, 55*, 801–815. https://doi.org/10.1007/s11199-006-9134-8

Alimujiang, A., Wiensch, A., Bos, J., Fleischer, N. L., Mondul, A. M., McLean, K., Mukherjee, B., & Pearce, C. L. (2019). Association between life purpose and mortality among US adults older than 50 years. *JAMA Network Open, 2*(5), e194270. doi.org/10.1001/jamnetworkopen.2019.4270

Allport, G. W. (1961). *Pattern and growth in personality*. Holt, Rinehart, & Winston.

An, J. S., & Cooney, T. M. (2006). Psychological wellbeing in mid to late life: The role of generativity development and parent-child relationships across the lifespan. *International Journal of Behavioral Development, 30*, 410–421. https://doi.org/10.1177/0165025406071489

Aristotle (1925). *The Nicomachean ethnics*. Oxford University Press.

Balot, R. K. (2001). *Greed and injustice in classical Athens*. Princeton University Press.

Berry, W. (2012). *New collected poems*. Counterpoint.

Bishaw, A. (2013). *Poverty: 2000 to 2012*. www.census.gov/library/publications/2013/acs/acsbr12-01.html

Bourdieu, P., & Passeron, J. (1977). *Reproduction in education, society, and culture*. Sage.

Bourdieu, P., & Passeron, J. (1990). *Reproduction in education, society, and culture* (2nd ed.) Sage.

Boylan, J. M., Jennings, J. R., & Matthews, K. A. (2016). Childhood socioeconomic status and cardiovascular reactivity and recovery among black and white men: Mitigating effects of psychological resources. *Health Psychology, 35*(9), 957–966. https://doi.org/10.1037/hea0000355

Boylan, J. M., & Ryff, C. D. (2015). Psychological wellbeing and metabolic syndrome: Findings from the Midlife in the United States national sample. *Psychosomatic Medicine, 77*(5), 548–558. https://doi.org/10.1097/psy.0000000000000192

Boylan, J. M., Tsenkova, V. K., Miyamoto, Y., & Ryff, C. D. (2017). Psychological resources and glucoregulation in Japanese adults: Findings from MIDJA. *Health Psychology, 36*(5), 449–457. https://doi.org/10.1037/hea0000455

Boyle, P. A., Barnes, L. L., Buchman, A. S., & Bennett, D. A. (2009). Purpose in life Is associated with mortality among community-dwelling older persons. *Psychosomatic Medicine, 71*(5), 574–579. https://doi.org/10.1097/PSY.0b013e3181a5a7c0

Boyle, P. A., Buchman, A. S., & Bennett, D. A. (2010). Purpose in life is associated with a reduced risk of incident disability among community-dwelling older persons. *American Journal of Geriatric Psychiatry, 18*(12), 1093–1102. https://doi.org/10.1097/JGP.0b013e3181d6c259

Bruckner, P. (2010). *Perpetual euphoria: On the duty to be happy*. Princeton University Press.

Bühler, C. (1935). The curve of life as studied in biographies. *Journal of Applied Psychology, 43*, 653–673. https://doi.org/10.1037/h0054778

Burgard, S. A., & Kalousova, L. (2015). Effects of the Great Recession: Health and wellbeing. *Annual Review of Sociology, 41*, 181–201. doi.org/10.1146/annurev.soc-073014-112204.

Cantarella, A., Borella, E., Marigo, C., & De Beni, R. (2017). Benefits of wellbeing in training in healthy older adults. *Applied Psychology: Health and Wellbeing, 9*(3), 261–284. doi.10.1111/a0hw.12091

Carr, D. (2002). The psychological consequences of work-family tradeoffs for three cohorts of men and women. *Social Psychology Quarterly, 65*, 103–124. https://doi.org/10.2307/3090096

Case, A., & Deaton, A. (2015). Rising morbidity and mortality in midlife among white non-Hispanic Americans in the 21st century. *Proceedings of the National Academy of Sciences, 112*, 15078–15083. https://doi.org/10.1073/pnas.1518393112

Case, A., & Deaton, A. (2020). *Deaths of despair and the future of capitalism*. Princeton University Press.

Chen, Y., Kim, E. S., Koh, H. K., Frazier, A. L., & VanderWeele, T. J. (2019). Sense of mission and subsequent health and wellbeing among young adults: An outcome-wide analysis. *American Journal of Epidemiology, 188*(4), 664–673. doi.org/10.1093/ajekwz009

Cohen, P. (2018). Paychecks lag as profits soar, and prices erode wage gains. *The New York Times*, July 13. https://www.nytimes.com/2018/07/13/business/economy/wages-workers-profits.html

Cohen, R., Bavishi, C., & Rozanski, A. (2016). Purpose in life and and its relationship to all-cause mortality and cardiovascular events: A meta-analysis. *Psychosomatic Medicine, 78*, 122–133. doi.org/10.1097/PSY.0000000000000274

Cole, S. W. (2013). Social regulation of human gene expression: Mechanisms and implications for public health. *American Journal of Public Health, 103*(Suppl 1), S84–92. http://doi.org/10.2105/ajph.2012.301183

Cole, S. W., Levine, M. E., Arevalo, J. M. G., Ma, J., Weir, D. R., & Crimmins, E. M. (2015). Loneliness, eudaimonia, and the human conserved transcriptional response to adversity. *Psychoneuroendocrinology, 62*, 11–17. https://doi.org/10.1016/j.psyneuen.2015.07.001

Costanzo, E. S., Ryff, C. D., & Singer, B. H. (2009). Psychosocial adjustment among cancer survivors: Findings from a national survey of health and wellbeing. *Health Psychology, 28*(2), 147–156. https://doi.org/10.1037/a0013221

Crawford, P., Brown, B., Baker, C., Tischler, V., & Abrams, B. (2015). *Health humanities*. Palgrave Macmillan.

Dante Alighieri (1308/2006). *The divine comedy*. (A. Amari-Parker, Ed., & H. W. Longfellow, Trans.). Chartwell Books.

Desmond, M. (2016). *Evicted: Poverty and profit in the American city*. Crown Publishers.

Deresiewicz, W. (2014). *Excellent sheep: The miseducation of the American elite*. Simon & Schuster, Inc.

De Young, R. (2013). Environmental psychology overview. In A. H. Huffman & S. Klein (Eds.), *Green organizations: Driving change with IO psychology* (pp. 17–33). Routledge.

DiMaggio, P., & Mukhtar, T. (2004). Arts participation as cultural capital in the United States, 1982–2002: Signs of decline? *Poetics, 32,* 169–194.

Edmondson, M. (2004). *Why read?* Bloomsbury.

Edmondson, M. (2015). *Self and soul: A defense of ideals.* Harvard University Press.

Elliot, A. J., & Chapman, B. P. (2016). Socioeconomic status, psychological resources, and inflammatory markers: Results from the MIDUS study. *Health Psychology, 35*(11), 1205–1213. https://doi.org/10.1037/hea0000392

Erikson, E. H. (1959). Identity and the life cycle. *Psychological Issues, 1,* 1–171.

Fava, G. A., Ruini, C., Rafanelli, C., Finos, L., Conti, S., & Grandi, S. (2004). Six-year outcome of cognitive behavior therapy for prevention of recurrent depression. *American Journal of Psychiatry, 161*(10), 1872–1876. doi:10.1176/ajp/161.10.1872

Fancourt, D., & Finn, S. (2019). *What is the evidence on the role of the arts in improving health and wellbeing? A scoping review.* WHO Regional Office for Europe, Health Evidence Network (HEN) synthesis report 67.

Feldman, P. J., & Steptoe, A. (2003). Psychosocial and socioeconomic factors associated with glycated hemoglobin in nondiabetic middle-aged men and women. *Health Psychology, 22*(4), 398–405. https://doi.org/10.1037/0278-6133.22.4.398

Fonseca-Wollheim, C. (2020). Tapping forces of nature to feed the spirit. *New York Times,* November 29, AR5.

Frankl, V. E. (1959). *Man's search for meaning: An introduction to logotherapy.* Beacon Press.

Fredrickson, B. L., Grewen, K. M., Algoe, S. B., Firestine, A. M., Arevalo, J. M. G., Ma, J., & Cole, S. W. (2015). Psychological wellbeing and the human conserved transcriptional response to adversity. *PLoS One, 10*(3), e0121839. https://doi.org/10.1371/journal.pone.0121839

Fredrickson, B. L., Grewen, K. M., Coffey, K. A., Algoe, S. B., Firestine, A. M., Arevalo, J. M. G., . . . Cole, S. W. (2013). A functional genomic perspective on human wellbeing. *Proceedings of the National Academy of Sciences of the United States of America, 110*(33), 13684–13689. https://doi.org/10.1073/pnas.1305419110

Friedman, E. M., Hayney, M. S., Love, G. D., Urry, H. L., Rosenkranz, M. A., Davidson, R. J., . . . Ryff, C. D. (2005). Social relationships, sleep quality, and interleukin-6 in aging women. *Proceedings of the National Academy of Sciences, 102*(51), 18757–18762. https://doi.org/10.1073/pnas.0509281102

Friedman, E. M., Ruini, C., Foy, R., Jaros, L., Love, G., & Ryff, C. D. (2019). Lighten UP! A community-based intervention to promote eudaimonic wellbeing in older adults: A multi-site replication with 6-month follow-up. *Clinical Gerontologist, 42,* 387–397. https://doi.org/10.1080/07317115.2019.1574944

Friedman, E. M., & Ryff, C. D. (2012). Living well with medical comorbidities: A biopsychosocial perspective. *Journals of Gerontology, Series B: Psychological Sciences and Social Sciences,* 1–10. https://doi.org/10.1093/geronb/gbr152

Gallagher, M. W., Lopez, S. J., & Preacher, K. J. (2009). The hierarchical structure of wellbeing. *Journal of Personality, 77,* 1025–1050. https://doi.org/10.1111/j.1467-6494.2009.00573.x

Gifford, R. (2014). *Environmental psychology: Principles and practices* (5th ed.). Optimal Books.

Goldman, N., Glei, D. A., & Weinstein, M. (2018). Declining mental health among disadvantaged Americans. *Proceedings of the National Academy of Sciences, 115,* 7290–7295 https://doi.org/10.1073/pnas.1722023115

Graham, C. (2017). *Happiness for all? Unequal hopes and lives in pursuit of the American dream*. Princeton University Press.

Grant, B. F., Chou, S. P., Saha, T. D., Pickering, R. P., Kerridge, B. T., Ruan, W. J., . . . Hasin, D. (2017). Prevalence of 12-month alcohol use, high-risk drinking, and DMS-IV alcohol use disorder in the United States, 2001–2002 to 2012–2013: Results from the National Epidemiological Survey on Alcohol and Related Conditions. *JAMA Psychiatry, 74*, 911–923. https://doi.org/10.1001/jamapsychiatry.2017.2161

Greenfield, E. A. (2009). Felt obligation to help others as a protective factor against losses in psychological wellbeing in middle and later life. *Journal of Gerontology B: Psychological and Social Sciences, 64*, 723–732. https://doi.org/10.1093/geronb/gbp074

Greenfield, E. A., & Marks, N. F. (2010). Identifying experiences of physical and psychological violence in childhood that jeopardize mental health in adulthood. *Child Abuse and Neglect, 34*, 161–171. https://doi.org/10.1016/j.chiabu.2009.08.012

Gruenewald, T. L., Karlamangla, A. S., Hu, P., Stein-Merkin, S., Crandall, C., Koretz, B., & Seeman, T. E. (2012). History of socioeconomic disadvantage and allostatic load in later life. *Social Science and Medicine, 74*(1), 75–83. https://doi.org/10.1016/j.socscimed.2011.09.037

Grzywacz, J. D. (2000). Work-family spillover and health during midlife: Is managing conflict everything? *American Journal of Health Promotion, 14*, 236–243. https://doi.org/10.4278/0890-1171-14.4.236

Hafez, D., Heisler, M., Choi, H., Ankuda, C. K., Winkelman, T., & Kullgren, J. T. (2018). Association between purpose in life and glucose control among older adults. *Annals of Behavioral Medicine, 52*(4), 309–318. https://doi.org/10.1093/abm/kax012

Hamid, M. (2017). *Exit west*. Riverhead Books.

Hart, S., Fonareva, I., Merluzzi, N., & Mohr, D. C. (2005). Treatment for depression and its relationship to improvement in quality of life and psychological wellbeing in multiple sclerosis patients. *Quality of Life Research, 14*, 695–703. https://doi.org/10.1007/s11136-004-1364-z

Held, B. S. (2004). The negative side of positive psychology. *Journal of Humanistic Psychology, 44*, 9–46. https://doi.org/10.1177/0022167803259645

Heller, A. S., van Reekum, C. M., Schaefer, S. M., Lapate, R. C., Radler, B. T., Ryff, C. D., & Davidson, R. J. (2013). Sustained ventral striatal activity predicts eudaimonic wellbeing and cortisol output. *Psychological Science, 24*, 2191–200. https://doi.org/10.1177/0956797613490744

Hill, P. L., & Turiano, N. A. (2014). Purpose in life as a predictor of mortality across adulthood. *Psychological Science, 25*, 1482–1486. https://doi.org/10.1177/0956797614531799

Hill, P. L., & Weston, S. J. (92019). Evaluating eight-year trajectories for sense of purpose in the Health and Retirement Study. *Aging and Mental Health, 23*(2), 233–237. doi.org/10.1080/13607863.2017.1399344

Hooker, S. A., & Masters, K. S. (2016). Purpose in life is associated with physical activity measured by accelerometer. *Journal of Health Psychology, 21*(6), 962–971. doi.org/10.1177/1359105314542822

Jahoda, M. (1958). *Current concepts of positive mental health*. Basic Books.

Jung, C. G. (1933). *Modern man in search of a soul*. Harcourt Brace & World.

Kasser, T., & Ryan, R. M. (1993). A dark side of the American dream: Correlates of financial success as a central life aspiration. *Journal of Personality and Social Psychology, 65*, 410–422.

Keyes, C. L. M. (2009). The Black-White paradox in health: Flourishing in the face of social inequality and discrimination. *Journal of Personality, 77*(6), 1677–1706. https://doi.org/10.1111/j.1467-6494.2009.00597.x

Keyes, C. L. M., Shmotkin, D., & Ryff, C. D. (2002). Optimizing wellbeing: The empirical encounter of two traditions. *Journal of Personality and Social Psychology, 82,* 1007–1022. https://doi.org/10.1037/0022-3514.82.6.1007

Kim, E. S., Delaney, S. W., & Kubzansky, L. D. (2019). Sense of purpose in life and cardiovascular disease: Underlying mechanisms and future directions. *Current Cardiology Reports, 21,* 135. https://doi.org.10.1007/s11886-019-1222-9

Kim, E. S., Kawachi, I., Chen, Y., & Kubzansky, L. D. (2017). Association between purpose in life and objective measures of physical function in older adults. *JAMA Psychiatry, 74*(10), 1039. https://doi.org/10.1001/jamapsychiatry.2017.2145

Kim, E. S., Strecher, V. J., & Ryff, C. D. (2014). Purpose in life and use of preventive health care services. *Proceedings of the National Academy of Sciences of the United States of America, 111*(46), 16331–16336. https://doi.org/10.1073/pnas.1414826111

Kim, E. S., Sun, J. K., Park, N., Kubzansky, L. D., & Peterson, C. (2013). Purpose in life and reduced risk of myocardial infarction among older U.S. adults with coronary heart disease: A two-year follow-up. *Journal of Behavioral Medicine, 36*(2), 124–133. https://doi.org/10.1007/s10865-012-9406-4

Kim, E. S., Sun, J. K., Park, N., & Peterson, C. (2013). Purpose in life and reduced incidence of stroke in older adults: "The Health and Retirement Study." *Journal of Psychosomatic Research, 74*(5), 427–432. https://doi.org/10.1016/j.jpsychores.2013.01.013

Kirsch, J. A., Love, G. D., Radler, B. T., & Ryff, C. D. (2019). Scientific imperatives vis-à-vis growing inequality in America. *American Psychologist, 74,* 764–777. https://doi.org/10.1037/amp0000481

Kirsch, J. A., & Ryff, C. D. (2016). Hardships of the Great Recession and health: Understanding varieties of vulnerability. *Health Psychology Open, Jan-June,* 1-15. https://doi.org/10.1177/2055102916652390

Kolodny A., Coutwright, D. T., Hwang, C. S., Kriener, P., Eadie, J. L., Clark, T. W., & Alexander, G. C. (2015). The prescription opioid and heroin crisis: A public health approach to an epidemic of addiction. *Annual Review of Public Health, 36,* 559–574. https://doi.org/10.1146/annurev-publhealth-031914-122957

Lee, M. T., Kubzansky, L. D., & VanderWeele, T. J. (Eds.). (2021). *Measuring wellbeing: Interdisciplinary perspectives from the social sciences and humanities.* Oxford University Press. https://doi.org/10.1093/oso/9780197512531.001.0001

Lewis, G. J., Kanai, R., Rees, G., & Bates, T. C. (2014). Neural correlates of the 'good life': Eudaimonic wellbeing is associated with insular cortex volume. *Social Cognitive and Affective Neuroscience, 9,* 615–618. https://doi.org/10.1093/scan/nst032

Li, L. W., Seltzer, M. M., Greenberg, J. S. (1999). Change in depressive symptoms among daughter caregivers: An 18-month longitudinal study. *Psychology of Aging, 14,* 206–219. https://doi.org/10.1037/0882-7974.14.2.206

Lindfors, P., Berntsson, L., & Lundberg, U. (2006). Total workload as related to psychological wellbeing and symptoms of full-time employed female and male white-collar workers. *International Journal of Behavioral Medicine, 13,* 131–137. https://doi.org/10.1207/s15327558ijbm1302_4

Lomas, T. (2016). Positive art: Artistic expression and appreciation as an exemplary vehicle for flourishing. *Review of General Psychology, 20,* 171–182. https://doi.org/10.1037/gpr0000073

Maier, E. H., & Lachman, M. E. (2000). Consequences of early parental loss and separation for health and wellbeing in midlife. *International Journal of Behavioral Development, 24*, 183–189. https://doi.org/10.1080/016502500383304

Mantler, A., & Logan, A. C. (2015). Natural environments and mental health. *Advances in Integrative Medicine, 2*, 5–12. https://doi.org/10.1016/j.aimed.2015.03.002

Marks, N. F. (1996). Flying solo at midlife: Gender, marital status, and psychological wellbeing. *Journal of Marriage and the Family, 58*, 917–932. https://doi.org/10.2307/353980

Marks, N. F. (1998). Does it hurt to care? Caregiving, work-family conflict, and midlife wellbeing. *Journal of Marriage and Family, 60*, 951–966. https://doi.org/10.2307/353637

Marks, N. F., & Lambert, J. D. (1998). Marital status continuity and change among young and midlife adults: Longitudinal effects on psychological wellbeing. *Journal of Family Issues, 19*, 652–686. https://doi.org/10.1177/019251398019006001

Markus, H. R., Ryff, C. D., Curhan, K. B., & Palmersheim, K. A. (2004). In their own words: Wellbeing at midlife among high school and college educated adults. In O. G. Brim, C. D. Ryff, & R. C. Kessler (Eds.), *How healthy are we? A national study of wellbeing at midlife* (pp. 273–319). University of Chicago Press.

Marmot, M., Ryff, C. D., Bumpass, L. L., Shipley, M., & Marks, N. F. (1997). Social inequalities in health: Converging evidence and next questions. *Social Science and Medicine, 44*, 901–910. https://doi.org/10.1016/S0277-9536(96)00194-3

Marmot, M. G., Fuhrer, R., Ettner, S. L., Marks, N. F., Bumpass, L. L., & Ryff, C. D. (1998). Contribution of psychosocial factors to socioeconomic differences in health. *Milbank Quarterly, 76*, 403–448. https://doi.org/10.1111/1468-0009.00097

Maslow, A. H. (1968). *Toward a psychology of being* (2nd ed.). Van Nostrand.

Mendelberg, T., McCabe, K. T., & Thal, A. (2016). College socialization and the economic views of affluent Americans. *American Journal of Political Science, 61*, 606–623. https://doi.org/10.1111/ajps.12265

Mill, J. S. (1893/1989). *Autobiography*. Penguin.

Millear, P., Liossis, P., Shochet, I. M., Biggs, H., & Donald, M. (2008). Being on PAR: Outcomes of a pilot trial to improve mental health and wellbeing in the workplace with the Promoting Adult Resilience (PAR) program. *Behavior Change, 25*, 215–228. https://doi.org/10.1375/bech.25.4.215

Morozink, J. A., Friedman, E. M., Coe, C. L., & Ryff, C. D. (2010). Socioeconomic and psychosocial predictors of interleukin-6 in the MIDUS national sample. *Health Psychology, 29*(6), 626–635. https://doi.org/10.1037/a0021360

Neugarten, B. L. (1973). Personality change in late life: A developmental perspective. In C. Eisdorfer & M. P. Lawton (Eds.), *The psychology of adult development and aging* (pp. 311–335). American Psychological Association.

Nussbaum, M. C. (2010). *Not for profit: Why democracy needs the humanities*. Princeton University Press.

Nussbaum, M. D. (1997). *Cultivating humanity: A classical defense of reform in liberal education*. Cambridge University Press.

O'Brien, K. M. (2012). Healthy, wealthy, wise? Psychosocial factors influencing the socioeconomic status-health gradient. *Journal of Health Psychology, 17*(8), 1142–1151. https://doi.org/10.1177/1359105311433345

Oliver, M. (2017). *Devotions: The selected poems of Mary Oliver*. Penguin.

Pew Research Center. (2020). Unemployment rose higher in three months of COVID-19 than it did in two years of the Great Recession. June 11, 1–9. www.pewresearch.org/fact-tank/2020/06/11/unemployment-rose-higher-in-three-months-of-covid-19-than-it-did-in-two-years-of-the-great-recession/

Piff, P. K. (2014). Wealth and the inflated self: Class, entitlement, and narcissism. *Personality and Social Psychology Bulletin, 40*, 34–43. doi:10.11770/0146167213501699.

Piff, P. K., Stancato, D. M., Côté, S., Mendoza-Denton, R., & Keltner, D. (2012). Higher social class predicted increased unethical behavior. *Proceedings of the National Academy of Science, 109*, 4086–4091. doi.10.1073/pnas.1118373109.

Piketty, T., & Saez, E. (2014). Inequality in the long run. *Science, 344*, 838–843. https://doi.org/10.1126/science.1251936

Powers, R. (2018). *The overstory*. W. W. Norton and Co.

Pradhan, E. K., Baumgarten, M. Langenberg, P., Handwerger, B., Gilpin, A. K., Magyari, T., Hockberg, M. D., & Berman, B. M. (2007). Effect of mindfulness-based stress reduction in rheumatoid arthritis patients. *Arthiritis Care Research, 57*, 1134–1142. https://doi.org/10.1002/art.23010

Proshansky, H. M. (1987). The field of environmental psychology: Securing its future. In D. Stokols & I. Altman (Eds.), *Handbook of environmental psychology* (vol. 2, pp. 1467–1488). John Wiley & Sons.

Radler, B. T., Rigotti, A., & Ryff, C. D. (2017). Persistently high psychological wellbeing predicts better HDL cholesterol and triglyceride levels: Findings from the midlife in the U.S. (MIDUS) longitudinal study. *Lipids in Health and Disease, 17*(1), 1–9. doi.10.1186/s12944-017-0646-8

Reeves, R. V. (2017). *Dream hoarders: How the American upper middle class is leaving everyone else in the dust, why that is a problem, and what to do about it*. The Brookings Institution.

Riley, M. W., Kahn, R. L., Foner, A., & Mack, K. A. (1994). *Age and structural lag: Society's failure to provide meaningful opportunities in work, family, and leisure*. John Wiley & Sons.

Rogers, C. H., Floyd, F. J., Seltzer, M. M., Greenberg, J., & Hong, J. (2008). Long-term effects of the death of a child on parent's adjustment in midlife. *Journal of Family Psychology, 22*, 203–211. https://doi.org/10.1037/0893-3200.22.2.203

Rogers, C. R. (1961). *On becoming a person*. Houghton Mifflin.

Roth, M. S. (2014). *Beyond the university: Why liberal education matters*. Yale University Press.

Royal Society and Public Health Working Group. (2013). *Arts, health, and wellbeing beyond the Millennium: How far have we come and where do we want to go?* Royal Society for Public Health.

Ruini, C. (2017). *Positive psychology in the clinical domain: Research and practice*. Springer.

Ruini, C., & Fava, G. A. (2009). Wellbeing therapy for generalized anxiety disorder. *Journal of Clinical Psychology, 65*(5), 510–519. https://doi.org/10.1002/jclp.20592

Ruini, C., Ottolini, F., Tomba, E. Belaise, C., Albieri, E., Visani, D. Offidani, E., Caffo, E., & Fava, G. A. (2009). School intervention for promoting psychological wellbeing in adolescence. *Behavior Therapy and Experimental Psychiatry, 40*, 522–532. https://doi.org/10.1016/j.jbtep.2009.07.002

Ryff, C. D. (1989). Happiness is everything, or is it? Explorations on the meaning of psychological wellbeing. *Journal of Personality and Social Psychology, 57*, 1069–1081. doi:10.1037/0011-3514.57.6.1069.

Ryff, C. D. (1991 Jun). Possible selves in adulthood and old age: A tale of shifting horizons. *Psychology of Aging, 6*(2), 286–295. doi:10.1037//0882-7974.6.2.286.

Ryff, C. D. (1995). Psychological wellbeing in adult life. *Current Directions in Psychological Science, 4*, 99–104. https://doi.org/10.1111/1467-8721.ep10772395

Ryff, C. D. (2014). Psychological wellbeing revisited: Advances in the science and practice of eudaimonia. *Psychotherapy and Psychosomatics, 83*, 10–28. https://doi.org/10.1159/000353263

Ryff, C. D. (2016). Eudaimonic wellbeing and education: Probing the connections. In D. W. Harward (Ed.), *Wellbeing and higher education: A strategy for change and the realization of education's greater purposes* (pp. 37–48). Bringing Theory to Practice.

Ryff, C. D. (2018). Wellbeing with soul: Science in pursuit of human potential. *Perspectives in Psychological Science, 13*, 242–248. doi.10.1177/1745691617699836.

Ryff, C. D. (2019). Linking education in the arts and humanities to life-long wellbeing and health. Andrew W. Mellon Foundation. https://mellong.org/resources/articles/linking-education-arts-and-humanities-life-long-wellbeing-and-health/

Ryff, C. D., Boylan, J. M., & Kirsch, J. A. (2021a). Advancing the science of wellbeing: A dissenting view on measurement recommendations. In M. T. Lee, L. D. Kubzansky, & T. J. VanderWeele (Eds.), *Measuring wellbeing: Interdisciplinary perspectives from the social sciences and humanities* (pp. 521–535). Oxford University Press.

Ryff, C. D., Boylan, J. M., & Kirsch, J. A. (2021b). Response to response: Growing the field of wellbeing. In M. T. Lee, L. D. Kubzansky, & T. J. VanderWeele (Eds.), *Measuring wellbeing: Interdisciplinary perspectives from the social sciences and humanities* (pp. 546–554). Oxford University Press.

Ryff, C. D., Boylan, J. M., & Kirsch, J. A. (2021c). Eudaimonic and hedonic wellbeing: An integrative perspective with linkages to sociodemographic factors and health. In M. T. Lee, L. D. Kubzansky, & T. J. VanderWeele (Eds.), *Measuring wellbeing: Interdisciplinary perspectives from the social sciences and humanities* (pp. 92–135). Oxford University Press.

Ryff, C. D., & Heidrich, S. M. (1997). Experience and wellbeing: Explorations on domains of life and how they matter. *International Journal of Behavioral Development, 20*(2), 193–206. https://doi.org/10.1080/016502597385289

Ryff, C. D., & Keyes, C. L. M. (1995). The structure of psychologial wellbeing revisited. *Journal of Personality and Social Psychology, 69*(4), 719–727. https://doi.org/10.1037/0022-3514.69.4.719

Ryff, C. D., Keyes, C. L. M., & Hughes, D. L. (2003). Status inequalities, perceived discrimination, and eudaimonic wellbeing: Do the challenges of minority life Hone purpose and growth? *Journal of Health and Social Behavior, 44*(3), 275. https://doi.org/10.2307/1519779

Ryff, C. D., & Kim, E. S. (2020). Extending research linking purpose in life to health: The challenges of inequality, the potential of the arts, and the imperative of virtue. In A. L. Burrow & P. Hill (Eds.), *The ecology of purposeful living across the lifespan* (pp. 29–58). Springer Nature Switzerland AG. https://doi.org/10.1007/978-3-030-52078-6_3

Ryff, C. D., Radler, B. T., & Friedman, E. M. (2015). Persistent psychological wellbeing predicts improved self-rated health over 9–10 years: Longitudinal evidence from MIDUS. *Health Psychology Open, 2*(2). https://doi.org/10.1177/2055102915601582

Ryff, C. D., & Singer, B. H. (2008). Know thyself and become what you are: A eudaimonic approach to psychological wellbeing. *Journal of Happiness Studies, 9*, 13–39.
https://doi.org/10.1007/s10902-006-9019-0

Ryff, C. D., Singer, B. H., & Love, G. D. (2004). Positive health: Connecting wellbeing
with biology. *Philosophical Transactions: Biological Sciences, 359*(1449), 1383–1394.
https://doi.org/10.1098/rstb.2004.1521

Schaefer, S. M., Boylan, J. M., van Reekum, C. M., Lapate, R. C., Norris, C. J., Ryff, C. D.,
& Davidson, R. J. (2013). Purpose in life predicts better emotional recovery from
negative stimuli. *PLoS One, 8*, e80329. https://doi.org/10.1371/journal.pone.0080329

Schleicher, H., Alonso, C., Shirtcliff, E. A., Muller, D., Loevinger, B. L., & Coe, C. L.
(2005). In the face of pain: The relationship between psychological wellbeing and
disability in women with fibromyalgia. *Psychotherapy and Psychosomatics, 74*(4),
231–239. https://doi.org/10.1159/000085147

Schmutte, P. S., & Ryff, C. D. (1994). Success, social comparison, and self-
assessment: Parents' midlife evaluations of sons, daughters, and self. *Journal of Adult
Development, 1*, 109–126. https://doi.org/10.1007/BF02259677

Schuchat, A., Houry, D., Guy, G. P. Jr. (2017). New data on opioid use and prescribing
in the United States. *JAMA, 318*, 425–426. https://doi.org/10.1001/jama.2017.
8913

Seligman, M. E. P. (2011). *Flourish: A visionary new understanding of happiness and wellbeing*. Free Press.

Sloan, R. P., Schwarz, E., McKinley, P. S., Weinstein, M., Love, G., Ryff, C., . . . Seeman,
T. (2017). Vagally-mediated heart rate variability and indices of wellbeing: Results
of a nationally representative study. *Health Psychology, 36*(1), 73–81. https://doi.org/
10.1037/hea0000397

Slopen, N., Dutra, L. M., Williams, D. R., Mujahid, M. S., Lewis, T. T., Bennett, G.
G., . . . Albert, M. A. (2012). Psychosocial stressors and cigarette smoking among
African American adults in midlife. *Nicotine and Tobacco Research, 14*(10), 1161–
1169. https://doi.org/10.1093/ntr/nts011

Slopen, N., Kontos, E. Z., Ryff, C. D., Ayanian, J. Z., Albert, M. A., & Williams, D. R.
(2013). Psychosocial stress and cigarette smoking persistence, cessation, and re-
lapse over 9–10 years: A prospective study of middle-aged adults in the United
States. *Cancer Causes & Control, 24*(10), 1849–1863. https://doi.org/10.1007/s10
552-013-0262-5

Springer, K. W., Pudrovska, T., & Hauser, R. M. (2011). Does psychological wellbeing
change with age? Longitudinal tests of age variations and further explorations of
the multidimensionality of Ryff's model of psychological wellbeing. *Social Science
Research, 40*(1), 392–398. doi.org.10.1016/j.ssresearch.2010.05.008

Steptoe, A., & Fancourt, D. (2019). Leading a meaningful life at older ages and its relationship with social engagement, prosperity, health, biology, and time use.
Proceedings of the National Academy of Sciences, 116(4), 1207–1212. doi.org/
10.1073/pnas.1814723116

Stuckey, H. L., & Nobel, J. (2010). The connection between art, healing, and public
health: A review of current literature. *American Journal of Public Health, 100*,
254–263.

Tay, L., Pawelski, J. O., & Keith, M. G. (2017). The role of the arts and humanities in
human flourishing: A conceptual model. *Journal of Positive Psychology, 13*(3), 215–
225. doi.org/10.1080/17439760.2017.1279207.

Triguero-Mas, M., Dadvand, P., Cirach, M., Martinez, D., Medina, A., Mompart, A., Basagaña, X., Grazuleviciene, R., & Nieuwenhuijsen, M. J. (2015). Natural outdoor environments and mental and physical health: Relationships and mechanisms. *Environment International, 77*, 35–41. https://doi.org/10.1016/j.envint.2015.01.012

Tsenkova, V. K., Love, G. D., Singer, B. H., & Ryff, C. D. (2007). Socioeconomic status and psychological wellbeing predict cross-time change in glycosylated hemoglobin in older women without diabetes. *Psychosomatic Medicine, 69*(8), 777–784. https://doi.org/10.1097/PSY.0b013e318157466f

Urry, H. L., Nitschke, J. B., Dolski, I., Jackson, D. C., Dalton, K. M., Mueller, C. J., . . . Davidson, R. J. (2004). Making a life worth living: Neural correlates of wellbeing. *Psychological Science, 15*(6), 367–372. doi:10.1111/j.0956-7976.2004.00686.x

Van der Vliet Oloomi, A. (2018). *Call me zebra*. Houghton Mifflin Harcourt.

VanderWeele, T. J., Trudel-Fitzgerald, C., Allin, P., Farrelly, C., Fletcher, G., Frederick, D. E., . . . Kubzansky, L. (2021). Current recommendations on the selection of measures for wellbeing. In M. T. Lee, L. D. Kubzansky, & T. J. VanderWeele (Eds.), *Measuring wellbeing: Interdisciplinary perspectives from the social sciences and humanities* (pp. 501–520). Oxford University Press.

VanderWeele, T. J., Trudel-Fitzgeral, C., & Kubzansky, L. D. (2021). Response to "Advancing the science of wellbeing: A dissenting view on measurement recommendations." In M. T. Lee, L. D. Kubzansky, & T. J. VanderWeele (Eds.), *Measuring wellbeing: Interdisciplinary perspectives from the social sciences and humanities* (pp. 536–545). Oxford University Press.

Van Reekum, C. M., Urry, H. I., Johnstone, T., Thurow, M. E., Frye, C. J., Jackson, C. A., . . . Davidson, R. J. (2007). Individual differences in amygdala and ventromedial prefrontal cortex activity are associated with evaluation speed and psychological wellbeing. *Journal of Cognitive Neuroscience, 19*, 237–248. https://doi.org/10.1162/jocn.2007.19.2.237

Weiss, L. A., Westerhof, G. J., & Bohlmeijer, E. T. (2016). Can we increase psychological wellbeing? The effects of interventions on psychology wellbeing: A meta-analysis of randomized controlled trials. *PLoS One, 11*(6), e0158092. https://doi.org/10.1371/journal.pone.0158092

Williams, F. (2017). *The nature fix: Why nature makes us happier, healthier, and more creative*. W. W. Norton and Co.

Wulf, A. (2016). *The invention of nature: Alexander von Humboldt's new world*. Penguin Random House.

Zilioli, S., Imami, L., & Slatcher, R. B. (2015b). Life satisfaction moderates the impact of socioeconomic status on diurnal cortisol slope. *Psychoneuroendocrinology, 60*, 91–95. https://doi.org/10.1016/j.psyneuen.2015.06.010

Zilioli, S., Slatcher, R. B., Ong, A. D., & Gruenewald, T. L. (2015a). Purpose in life predicts allostatic load ten years later. *Journal of Psychosomatic Research, 79*(5), 451–457. https://doi.org/10.1016/j.jpsychores.2015.09.013

2

Understanding the Role of Positive Emotions in Wellbeing Through Psychological, Biological, Sociocultural, and Environmental Lenses

CHRISTIAN WAUGH ∎

INTRODUCTION

The central theme of this volume is that to understand an integrated science of wellbeing requires understanding the psychological, biological, sociocultural, and environmental causes and correlates of wellbeing at the individual level. The theme of this chapter is that to understand wellbeing requires understanding the integrative science of positive emotions, the most reliable source of emotion-based, hedonic wellbeing (Diener, Suh, Lucas, & Smith, 1999), as well as an occasional source and/or outcome of meaning-based, eudaimonic wellbeing (Kashdan, Biswas-Diener, & King, 2008; King, Hicks, Krull, & Del Gaiso, 2006). In this chapter, I begin by briefly defining positive emotions and describing the importance of positive emotions to the hedonic and eudaimonic dimensions of wellbeing (see also Chapters 1 and 3, this volume). This will lead to an exploration of the integrative science of positive emotions through psychological, biological, sociocultural, and environmental lenses that can in turn inform an integrative understanding of wellbeing at other scales.

POSITIVE EMOTIONS AND HEDONIC/
EUDAIMONIC WELLBEING

An emotion is a set of systems (neural, physiological, and behavioural) that co-ordinate a response to a potentially important stimulus (Tooby & Cosmides, 1990), which can be either external (e.g., a snake) or internal (e.g., the thought of a snake) to the person. Emotions are not static entities, but are dynamic processes (Scherer & Moors, 2019) that consist of (1) the perception of an important/salient stimulus, which is then (2) appraised along a number of dimensions, (3) produces action tendencies that are supported by physiological changes, and (4) can be regulated if the person's emotional goals are different from their current emotional state. Furthermore, emotions can be differentiated from each other at each of these process steps. For example, conscious and unconscious emotions may be induced by the conscious or unconscious perception of stimuli in the environment, respectively (LeDoux, 1996), and high and low arousal emotions may be differentiated by the level of physiological changes that occur during the emotion process (Russell, Weiss, & Mendelsohn, 1989).

Perhaps the most granular differentiation of emotion occurs from the appraisals people make about stimuli (Smith & Ellsworth, 1985). Appraisals are evaluations of changes in the internal (i.e., in one's mind) or external environment that are deemed relevant to one's wellbeing (Smith & Ellsworth, 1985). In other words, appraisals occur when people make personal meaning of something happening in the environment. There are many different dimensions of appraisals, but the one most relevant to this chapter is the *valence dimension*, which consists of the degree to which a stimulus is evaluated as positive and/or negative (Smith & Ellsworth, 1985). Loosely speaking, positive appraisals tend to give rise to positive emotions and negative appraisals tend to give rise to negative emotions. Importantly, positive and negative emotions are not opposite sides of the same coin but instead are independent emotional states even though they are often related to each other. Indeed, the neural structures responsible for positive and negative emotions are overlapping but distinct (Tobia, Hayashi, Ballard, Gotlib, & Waugh, 2017): positive and negative moods are sometimes negatively correlated, but not always (Zautra, Reich, Davis, Potter, & Nicolson, 2000), and there are distinct emotional states like nostalgia that are characterised by a mix of positive and negative emotions (Larsen, McGraw, & Cacioppo 2001).

This independence of positive and negative emotions is especially important for understanding the relation of each to different forms of wellbeing. Whereas positive emotions are integral to forms of wellbeing such as life satisfaction (Diener, Sandvik, & Pavot, 2009), resilience (Fredrickson, Tugade, Waugh, & Larkin, 2003), and having meaning (King et al., 2006), negative emotions are integral to forms of 'ill-being' like depression and anxiety (Watson & Clark, 1992). Positive emotions are clearly integral to wellbeing, so to understand wellbeing, it is imperative to also understand positive emotions.

Individual wellbeing can be characterised into two forms: hedonic and eudaimonic. Hedonic wellbeing refers to those forms that are most directly about feeling good about one's life; it is characterised by subjective wellbeing and, more importantly, positive emotions (Ryan & Deci, 2001; see also Chapter 3, this volume). Indeed, research suggests that one of the most reliable predictors of hedonic wellbeing is the frequency with which people feel positive emotions in their daily lives (Diener et al., 2009). On the other hand, eudaimonic wellbeing stems from Aristotle's view that not all wellbeing should be about how one feels, but rather that one form of wellbeing should be about self-actualisation and living a meaningful life (Ryan & Deci, 2001). The differentiation (or not) of hedonic and eudaimonic wellbeing is beyond the scope of this particular chapter (but see Kashdan et al., 2008; see also Chapter 1, this volume). However, it appears that although positive emotions are typically posited to be more important to hedonic than to eudaimonic wellbeing, evidence suggests that positive emotions are important to both. For example, in a series of studies, researchers found that both experimentally induced and daily forms of positive emotions were highly predictive of the degree to which people felt that they had meaning in their life—a primary component of eudaimonic wellbeing (King et al., 2006).

PERCEPTION OF AN IMPORTANT/SALIENT STIMULUS

The framing of most of the remainder of this chapter is based on the aforementioned basic process model of emotions (Scherer & Moors, 2019) in which emotions consist of (1) the perception of an important/salient stimulus, (2) which is then appraised along a number of dimensions, (3) produces action tendencies that are supported by physiological changes, and (4) can be regulated if the person's emotional goals are different from their current emotional state. In this section, I focus on the perception of a salient stimulus with respect to key psychological, biological, sociocultural, and environmental dimensions.

Psychological Lens

Emotions evolved as responses to evolutionarily important stimuli that motivated organisms to behave in a way (action tendency) to increase or maintain their evolutionary fitness (ability to survive, mate, and care for offspring). The types of stimuli that aided the evolution of negative emotions included immediate threats to one's survival or the survival of offspring/loved ones stemming from, for example, predators (Mobbs, Hagan, Dalgleish, Silston, & Prévost, 2015), other non-kin human groups (Mifune, Simunovic, & Yamagishi, 2017), and poisonous foods (Rozin, Haidt, & McCauley, 2008). Thus, this class of stimuli included threats to one's access to social (e.g., ostracism; Williams, 2006), physical (illness/injury), or material (e.g., food/shelter) resources.

The types of stimuli that aided in the evolution of positive emotions, on the other hand, included opportunities to gain or maintain resources critical for improving the organism's evolutionary fitness (Berridge & Kringelbach, 2015; Fredrickson,

1998). Therefore, positive emotions often occur in response to stimuli/situations that represent opportunities for gaining or maintaining social resources, such as making friends (Waugh & Fredrickson, 2006), which were critical for protecting against threats and for sharing other resources, including material resources, such as food (Berridge & Kringelbach, 2015) and engagement in active play (e.g., wrestling and chasing), which supported the development of muscles and skills necessary for hunting and avoiding predators (Smith, 1982).

Biological Lens

The perception of stimuli in general involves sensory neurons that receive information from the environment (e.g., optic and cochlear nerves), which then send that information to the nucleus in the thalamus associated with that sensory modality, from where information is sent to the brain's sensory regions (e.g., auditory/visual cortex). Because of their heightened biological relevance, the brain biases the perception of emotional stimuli. For example, in addition to this slower sensory organ → thalamus → sensory cortex route, some biologically relevant information takes a faster route in which it is sent directly from the thalamus to the amygdala (LeDoux, 1996). This allows the amygdala to quickly detect biologically relevant stimuli like threats, and, through reciprocal neural connections, the amygdala can bias information processing in the sensory and attention regions to better attend to and detect further threats in the environment (Sabatinelli et al., 2005).

This biologically relevant biased sensory processing also occurs for positive stimuli. Rewards are biologically relevant positive stimuli that animals are motivated to work for to obtain, presumably because these stimuli represent the potential gain or maintenance of resources as noted above. When an animal senses a potential reward or a cue that predicts a potential reward, their mesolimbic dopaminergic system (including the ventral striatum, substantia nigra, ventral tegmental area, midline cortical regions, and other regions) responds with an increase in dopamine, which represents the 'incentive salience' of that reward; that is, the degree to which the animal is motivated to try to obtain it (Berridge & Robinson, 2003). Importantly, through its role in promoting motivation, dopamine helps bias attention to these rewarding stimuli and the cues in the environment that predict them (Wickelgren, 1997). For example, this is the system that responds when new mothers see their babies (relative to seeing other babies) because their babies represent highly biologically relevant positive stimuli (Nitschke et al., 2004).

Sociocultural Lens

Humans are an inherently social species, so many of the most important biologically relevant stimuli that give rise to positive emotions represent possible gains in and/or the maintenance of social relationships. This is why, when we are born, we are already primed and ready to respond to stimuli that represent our social relationships. For example, infants are able to recognise and categorise facial expressions as early as 5 months (Bornstein & Arterberry, 2003).

Culture, as a social institution, dictates which stimuli in the environment are important and the appropriate responses to those stimuli. Throughout development, people are not only equipped with some biological preparedness to respond to important stimuli, but this preparedness is also shaped and changed when certain culturally valued emotional responses are rewarded and/or modelled (Mesquita & Boiger, 2014). Evidence from studies suggests that although different cultures often experience similar emotional responses to certain positive stimuli (e.g., those reflecting achievement and successful relationships), cultures may still differ in how they perceive these stimuli (Mesquita & Frijda, 1992). For example, both Japanese and American people perceive smiles as indicative of happiness when the smiler is surrounded by others who are also smiling; however, relative to Americans, Japanese people perceive smiles as reflecting less happiness when the smiler is surrounded by others who are expressing negative emotions (Masuda et al., 2008). Thus when perceiving facial expressions, Japanese people incorporate the surrounding context of the expression more so than do American people.

Environmental Lens

Of course, the environment contains within it the stimuli to which people emotionally respond. When discussing the environmental lens, however, I focus more on the surroundings, conditions, or world that people live in. Pertaining specifically to the natural environment, the *biophilia hypothesis* states that humans have an innate need to connect with nature because it was a source of resources critical to our evolution (Kellert & Wilson, 1993). Furthermore, this need to connect with nature goes beyond just reaping the environment for its natural resources, but also arises from the natural environment's impact on our cognition and emotion. Indeed, even brief contact with nature reliably induces positive emotions, and extended contact can produce increases in wellbeing more generally (Capaldi, Passmore, Nisbet, Zelenski, & Dopko, 2015).

One relevant theory as to why the natural environment promotes positive emotions is through its effect on attention (Kaplan & Kaplan, 1989). In this *attention restoration theory*, theorists posit that effortful attention directed to our environment can become fatiguing and make people irritable. For example, think of all the stimuli one needs to pay attention to in an office—the current project, potential emails from colleagues, the time, to mention just a few. This induces a desire to 'get away' to environments that offer a reprieve from this effortful, directed attention by promoting effortless, involuntary attention (Kaplan, 1995). Nature is a prime example of such an environment because it offers a chance to get away from complex environments requiring extended directed attention (e.g., the office) to an environment that does not require such high levels of directed attention (e.g., a park). Importantly, though, nature promotes this redirected attention because it is also fascinating and rich enough to command people's involuntary attention (Kaplan, 1995).

APPRAISALS

Psychological Lens

After perceiving a stimulus in the environment, the degree to which this stimulus induces an emotional response depends on the appraisals that people make of it. As mentioned previously, appraisals are evaluations of changes in the environment that are deemed relevant to one's wellbeing (Smith & Ellsworth, 1985). So, appraisals are dynamic transactions between the self and the environment (Lazarus & Folkman, 1984) that rely not only on properties of the environment and the stimuli being responded to but also on properties of the person, such as their values, goals, and temperament. This latter point is why different people can have different reactions to the same environmental stimulus. For example, whereas an extraverted person who values social contact might appraise a party invitation as highly positive, a socially anxious person might appraise that same party invitation as negative.

Typically, positive appraisals have been defined as those appraisals in which people evaluate the environment in terms of being high on the 'pleasantness' or 'positive valence' appraisal dimension (Smith & Ellsworth, 1985). We have recently proposed a definition of positive appraisal that incorporates its effect on people's wellbeing. Specifically, we argue that positive appraisals are those in which people make evaluations of the environment in relation to the self that leads to an increase in expected wellbeing (Waugh & McRae, unpublished manuscript). We chose to focus on increases in expected wellbeing instead of actual wellbeing based on the idea that the brain is an expectation machine, constantly forming expectations of the near and far future and comparing actual outcomes to those expectations (Wilson, Lisle, Kraft, & Wetzel, 1989). For example, if someone you like asks you out on a date, then you form a positive appraisal because your expected wellbeing in the near and far future has increased to include a possible relationship. Sometimes these increases in expected wellbeing become realised, but sometimes they do not (perhaps the date does not go as planned). Research in *affective forecasting*—estimating how one would feel in the future if a particular event occurred—has shown that people are often overly optimistic about how positive they would feel if something positive occurred (Wilson & Gilbert, 2003). However, evidence suggests that even these optimistic 'illusions' contribute positively to people's wellbeing because they help people care about others and engage in creative work (Taylor & Brown, 1988).

Biological Lens

Subcortical regions of the brain tend to be responsible for fast, primary appraisals of stimuli. For example, the amygdala processes simple forms of unpredictability, as when hearing arrhythmic tones (Herry et al., 2007), and biologically relevant representations of possible threat, such as facial expressions of fear (Morris et al., 1996). Cortical regions tend to be responsible for slower, more complex secondary appraisals of stimuli. For example, the medial prefrontal cortex processes the degree to which stimuli are relevant to one's perceived traits (Chavez, Heatherton, & Wagner, 2017).

We have argued that positive appraisals are particularly formed in the nucleus accumbens (NacC) and ventromedial prefrontal cortex (vmPFC; Waugh & McRae, unpublished manuscript). The NaCC and vmPFC are both part of the mesolimbic dopamine system responsible for identifying rewarding stimuli that organisms are motivated to work for to obtain. There is some evidence that the NaCC generates positive appraisals of primary rewards such as food and sex (Sescousse, Caldú, Segura, & Dreher, 2013). Consistent with our view of positive appraisal indicating increases in expected wellbeing, the NaCC is particularly responsive to cues that predict these primary rewards (Knutson, Adams, Fong, & Hommer, 2001). The vmPFC generates positive appraisals based on more complex associations between the self and the environment. For example, the vmPFC is involved when people think about themselves positively (Chavez et al., 2017), think about their future optimistically (Kuzmanovic, Rigoux, & Tittgemeyer, 2018), and receive positive feedback from others (Somerville, Kelley, & Heatherton, 2010). The vmPFC also seems to process increases in expected wellbeing, as studies have shown it to be responsive to food rewards that people expect to consume later (Hare, O'Doherty, Camerer, Schultz, & Rangel, 2008) and when simulating future positive events (Benoit, Szpunar, & Schacter, 2014).

Sociocultural Lens

Appraisals are evaluations of the environment in relation to the self, and this referenced self includes both one's independent sense of self as well as one's socially constructed self. People have social identities in which their sense of self is, in part, based on their membership and identification with social groups (defined, for example, in terms of our gender, ethnicity, age, and profession, and referred to as our 'in-groups'; Turner, Hogg, Oakes, Reicher, & Wetherell, 1987). When identification with an in-group is high and salient, our perception of our unique characteristics can become subordinate to the characteristics of a typical member of the group. When this occurs, people may have different emotional responses to stimuli than when they are thinking of themselves as a unique individual (Mackie, Maitner, & Smith, 2016) because their appraisal of the environment in terms of the self as individual is different from that of the self as a member of a group. For example, people may feel more pride when thinking of themselves as American than they do when thinking of themselves as an individual (Smith, Seger, & Mackie, 2007).

Culture can impact people's emotional appraisals by shaping their self-construals and by transmitting and reinforcing cultural values. People from cultures that emphasise interdependence tend to construe themselves in terms of their relationships to others, whereas people from cultures that emphasise independence tend to construe themselves in terms of their unique characteristics (Markus & Kitayama, 1991), and these different self-construals can impact emotional appraisals. For example, one study found that American participants, who tend to have more independent self-construals, tended to appraise successes as due to their own agency, whereas Japanese participants, who tend to have more interdependent construals, tended to appraise successes as due to aspects of the situation (Imada & Ellsworth, 2011). Emotional appraisals reflect what people value, and values are also shaped and reinforced by culture. For example, people from interdependent cultures tend to value low arousal positive emotions such as contentment more than they value high arousal positive emotions such as excitement (Tsai, 2007).

Environmental Lens

Appraisals of the natural environment, for the most part, follow the same rules as do appraisals of other stimuli mentioned above; however, there are particular forms of appraisal that seem to be sparked most consistently by nature. Part of the reason that people enjoy being in nature is to appreciate and immerse themselves in its 'natural beauty'. There are several sociological and philosophical theories about how people judge beauty. A fairly simple psychological theory suggests that people judge objects, others, or scenes as beautiful when they can process those stimuli fluently and easily (Reber, Schwarz, & Winkielman, 2004). For example, this is why we tend to like symmetry in objects and faces. This aesthetic preference for easily processed stimuli may stem from the fact that this processing fluency leads to a positive affective response, which is then applied to the stimulus. In short, fluency can induce positive appraisals of a stimulus stemming from the fact that this fluency induces positive emotional responses. Altogether, this suggests that people enjoy natural beauty because they can easily and fluently process the scene (perhaps due to evolved mechanisms described above), with this fluency producing positive emotional responses to nature.

Processing fluency is not the only way we can appraise nature, however, and, conversely sometimes it is a certain type of processing nonfluency that also shapes people's positive responses to nature. To illustrate, people will sometimes feel the positive emotion of awe when they encounter particular natural scenes like thunderstorms, mountains, and the desert. When faced with such scenes, people may appraise them in terms of their vastness in such a way as to diminish themselves in comparison (e.g., 'I feel so small compared to this canyon'; Shiota, Keltner, & Mossman, 2007). When this appraisal of vastness leads to a need to accommodate this new experience into one's own existing schemas of the world, it can lead to the positive emotion of awe (Shiota et al., 2007).

ACTION TENDENCIES AND BODILY RESPONSES

Psychological Lens

Emotions evolved because they motivated sets of behaviours that served to improve/protect evolutionary fitness. Thus, when people are in a heightened emotional state, they tend to have a greater likelihood of doing these evolutionarily relevant behaviours than others. These behaviours are called *action tendencies* (Frijda, 2007). For a long time, theories of emotion were largely based on investigations of negative emotions like fear and anger. It was clear that in these types of heightened negative emotional states, people's possible repertoire of action tendencies in that moment were narrowed to those that were most evolutionarily relevant. For example, if being chased by a bear, one's action tendency repertoire should hopefully only consist of run, hide, fight, and/or scream while not including irrelevant behaviours like knitting and socialising. A couple of decades ago, however, Fredrickson (1998) posed the idea that this narrowing of possible behaviours in an emotionally charged situation was mostly the providence of negative emotions and not necessarily of positive emotions. In her *broaden-and-build theory*, she proposed that, in positive emotional situations, people's behavioural repertoire is sometimes broadened, instead of narrowed, due to the evolutionary relevance of building and supporting resources rather than of protecting them. For example, when feeling positive emotions, one's social behavioural repertoire may be broadened beyond just interacting with close friends to include interacting with strangers, presumably because of the potential for gaining future relationship resources (Quoidbach, Taquet, Desseilles, de Montjoye, & Gross, 2019).

Importantly, however, this broadened behavioural repertoire stemming from positive emotions appears to apply to some types of positive emotions more so than to others. A series of studies has shown that positive emotions that are characterised by high approach tendencies, like desire/lust/craving, tend to actually narrow action tendency repertoires because the motivational force behind those emotional states is to acquire and consume something, whether it is food, sex, or other rewards (Gable & Harmon-Jones, 2008). Although these high approach positive emotions still promote the acquisition of resources, when highly motivated to acquire something, people's behavioural repertoires narrow to only those behaviours that will acquire that thing, sometimes at the expense of seizing other possible opportunities in the environment. For example, if a person is sitting on the beach and feeling content, a low approach emotion, they might feel as if there are many possible behaviours that they could do next—read, surf, reflect on life; however, if they start feeling excited (a high approach emotion) about eating a juicy apple they have in their bag, then for those next moments they will just focus on getting the apple into their mouths.

Biological Lens

In the brain, the motivated behaviour induced by high approach positive emotions is driven by the basal ganglia system (Ikemoto, Yang, & Tan, 2015). Motivated behaviours are those that are enacted to gain or avoid an expected outcome (Yin & Knowlton, 2006), which dovetails with our conception of positive appraisals as evaluations that lead to increases in expected wellbeing. The basal ganglia receive projections from all over the brain that consist of sensory (e.g., seeing ice cream) and representational inputs (e.g., thinking about ice cream). The basal ganglia then selects and amplifies some of those inputs according to the goals of the organism (Yin & Knowlton, 2006), which are partially driven by the positive appraisals of expected outcomes (e.g., the value of eating the ice cream) communicated to the basal ganglia by the vmPFC and NaCC (Haber, Kunishio, Mizobuchi, & Lynd-Balta, 1995). The basal ganglia then produces motivated motor programmes that get passed along to the regions (e.g., motor cortex and superior colliculus) responsible for the implementation of the behaviour (e.g., grabbing a spoon and eating the ice cream). That the basal ganglia are key to wellbeing is supported by findings showing that there is basal ganglia dysregulation in some disorders characterised by problems with motivated behaviour such as depression (Gunaydin & Kreitzer, 2016).

This basal ganglia system is most relevant to those positive emotional states with approach-related action tendencies. Berridge and Robinson (2003) call this the 'wanting' system in that it involves motivated behaviour when one *wants to consume* or have something. They contrast this to the 'liking' system, which is more related to the *actual consumption* of rewards, thus generating positive emotions that are lower in arousal because there is no need for arousal-supported motivated behaviour to obtain the reward. Contentment, then, is a positive emotion related to this liking system in that it is related to the consumption (i.e., savouring) of one's life circumstances. These types of low arousal positive emotions are generated, in part, by the mu-opioidergic pain-relief system. Consumption of rewards like food and social acceptance has been shown to be related to mu-opioid release (Hsu et al., 2013; Zhang & Kelley, 2000) and, although mu-opiod neurotransmitters are found all over the brain and are involved in a myriad of emotional responses, their distribution in the brain seems to be most highly correlated with brain regions involved in positive emotions (Nummenmaa et al., 2018).

Sociocultural Lens

Much like how cultural values and norms can shape appraisals of what is important and relevant, they can also shape action tendencies. The function of an action tendency is to motivate behaviour to solve problems or to gain or maintain resources, and culture can shape how those behaviours accomplish those goals by rewarding culturally normative behaviour (Mesquita & Boiger, 2014). For example, shame is an emotion that represents a threat to the self and a possible loss of social resources through one's actions. When shamed, however, people from different cultures employ different action tendencies. Those from a culture that prioritises the value of independence tend to withdraw from the situation to prevent further loss of social resources and mitigate the threat to the self, while those from an interdependent culture tend to engage in behaviours designed to restore social relationships as a way to regain social resources (Bagozzi, Verbeke, & Gavino, 2003).

As stated in the appraisal section, culture can also influence what types of positive emotions people value, with people from independent cultures more likely to value high arousal positive emotions (e.g., excitement) than those from interdependent cultures (Tsai, 2007). These valued emotions, in turn, can drive the motivated behaviours that people might expect to lead to these desired emotional states. For example, European Americans are more likely to want to listen to highly arousing music than are Chinese people (Tsai, Miao, Seppala, Fung, & Yeung, 2007), and the more people value high arousal positive emotions the more likely they are to choose stimulating versus relaxing products (Tsai, Chim, & Sims, 2015).

Environmental Lens

Generally speaking, the degree to which the environment influences motivated behaviours should be tied to whether that environment consists of threats that would lead to protective motivated behaviours (e.g., fighting or escaping) or consists of the resources that would lead to positively motivated behaviours (e.g., hunting and socialising). One way of assessing whether an environment promotes motivated behaviour is through its effect on physiological arousal, which is needed to support such behaviour. Many studies find that being in nature leads to decreases in arousal (e.g., Laumann, Gärling, & Stormark, 2003; Ulrich et al., 1991), however, suggesting that when there's no particular threat nor a particular resource to be gained, nature can undo the motivated arousal that would otherwise be directed elsewhere (Laumann et al., 2003). This relaxation of motivated arousal can then be critical for promoting physiological recovery, regeneration, and, ultimately, mental and physical health (Kaplan, 1995).

The environment can also affect the degree to which people have the action tendency of self-reflection. In the aforementioned attention restoration theory, natural environments are fascinating enough to be pleasurable but not particularly attentionally demanding, so they promote both attentional recovery and self-reflection, with the latter referring to opportunities to think about one's life and goals, for instance (Herzog, Black, Fountaine, & Knotts, 1997). Other environments, such as sports stadiums, can provide some attentional recovery because they are high in fascination, but because they are also high in attentional focus, there is not as much opportunity for reflection (Herzog et al., 1997). Taken together, these findings dovetail with the typical emotions experienced in these disparate environments, with nature being associated with low arousal, high self-reflection emotions like contentment (Richardson, McEwan, Maratos, & Sheffield, 2016) and sports stadiums (as an example) being associated with high arousal positive emotions that are low in self-reflection (Uhrich & Benkenstein, 2010).

REGULATION

Psychological Lens

When people have the goal of changing their emotion, they can employ emotion regulation techniques to do so (McRae & Gross, 2020). Because happiness can be such a valued state (Catalino, Algoe, & Fredrickson, 2014), people often have the goal of improving their positive emotions whether just for their own sake (Quoidbach, Berry, Hansenne, & Mikolajczak, 2010) or as a way to regulate stress (Waugh, 2020).

Beginning with the former, there are a myriad of ways that people can improve their positive emotions for their own sake, and empirically supported positivity interventions offer insight into what the most robust ways may be. To give just one example of the plethora of such approaches, in the Life Enhancing Activities for Family Caregivers (LEAF) positivity intervention (Moskowitz et al., 2019), participants are trained to increase their positive emotions by (1) noticing positive events, (2) capitalising on those positive events, (3) practicing gratitude, (4) practicing mindfulness, (5) aligning personal strengths with goals, and (6) engaging in acts of kindness. The LEAF intervention has been shown to successfully increase positive emotions and physical health as well as decrease depression and anxiety in caregivers of people with dementia (Moskowitz et al., 2019).

When people have the goal to regulate their positive emotions in order to improve their stress responses, I have proposed that they can do so in at least three ways (Waugh, 2020). First, positive emotions can be the targets of regulation, in which case the person's regulation goal is to increase positive emotions to feel better about the stressor. For example, someone might regulate their stress response to being in a pandemic by thinking about the positive aspects of quarantine, such as being able to spend more time with their family. Importantly, when positive emotions are the target, this leaves open the possibility that people do not necessarily feel lower levels of negative emotions about the stressor after regulation but that these negative emotions now co-exist with more positive emotions.

Second, people may increase positive emotions as a way to decrease negative emotions. In this case, successful stress regulation would be reflected by decreased negative emotions. For example, after going through a traumatic event someone might think about all the ways they have grown as a way to feel less anxious and depressed about having had to go through the event (e.g., 'I wouldn't be the person I am today if I hadn't gone through this' [Joseph, Murphy, & Regel, 2012, p. 323]), a process captured by the term *posttraumatic growth*. Last, incidental positive emotions (i.e., those that do not have to do with the regulatory process itself) may facilitate people's ability to use regulatory techniques. For example, we have shown that anticipating a future positive event can help people better regulate their responses to a current stressor (Leslie-Miller, Waugh, & Cole, 2021; Monfort, Stroup, & Waugh, 2015).

Biological Lens

As noted above, people can regulate their positive emotions by either behaving in a certain way (e.g., expressing gratitude) and/or by changing the way they appraise the environment. When changing behaviour, people employ regions of the brain that are involved in cognitive control including the ventro- and dorsolateral prefrontal cortex, dorsomedial prefrontal cortex, and anterior cingulate. These regions are crucial for maintaining regulatory goals, inhibiting nondesired behaviours, promoting desired regulatory behaviours, and monitoring regulatory progress (Buhle et al., 2014; Ochsner & Gross, 2005).

When people regulate their emotions by changing the way they appraise the environment, we have suggested that they can do so in two ways (Waugh & McRae, unpublished manuscript). First, they can positively appraise some aspects of the environment, such as noticing and savouring positive events. As noted above, these positive appraisals are generated by the vmPFC and NaCC. Second, people can reappraise some negative aspects of the environment in order to feel more positive, which is the strategy of *positive reappraisal*. Positive reappraisal involves the vmPFC and NaCC because of their role in generating positive appraisals. Unlike simply appraisal, however, positive reappraisal also recruits cognitive control regions because it involves maintaining regulatory goals, inhibiting negative appraisals, generating new semantic representations, and monitoring regulatory progress (Ochsner & Gross, 2005).

Sociocultural Lens

The sociocultural environment is a critical player in shaping people's ability or propensity to regulate their emotions. One study, for example, found that women were better at regulating their emotional responses to pain when they were with their partners than when they were by themselves (Coan, Schaefer, & Davidson, 2006). Findings like these have led theorists to propose that being in a social environment is actually the default state of being, such that our brains expect to be in such an environment and that not being in such a social environment—either through rejection or loneliness—can impair our ability to regulate our emotions (Beckes & Coan, 2011).

These social environments are constructed by cultures, and, besides shaping what emotions people value and therefore what emotions they target when regulating, culture can also shape the strategies that people use to regulate their emotions (Mesquita, De Leersnyder, & Albert, 2014). One study found that cultures that value interdependence, hierarchy, and embeddedness valued emotional suppression (i.e., regulating one's emotion by trying to suppress outward expressions of that emotion) because these cultures tend to value social cohesion that can be potentially disrupted by the outward expression of certain emotions (Matsumoto, Yoo, & Nakagawa, 2008). On the other hand, cultures that value egalitarianism and individualism were found to value reappraisal because these cultures tend to value the free expression (including emotional expression) of the individual.

Although most research on cultural differences in emotion regulation focuses on when people regulate negative emotions (Butler, Lee, & Gross, 2007), these differences also exist in how people regulate their positive emotions. In one study, researchers surveyed European American and Asian students after they had succeeded on an exam. They found that, after this success, European American students were much more likely to then plan activities involving increasing and/or maintaining their positive emotions (e.g., going to a party) than were Asian students (Miyamoto & Ma, 2011). This research indicates that people from Western cultures tend to endorse and exhibit more pro-hedonic emotion regulation in the form of savouring positive emotions than do people from Eastern cultures who are more willing to dampen positive emotions (Miyamoto & Ma, 2011).

Environmental Lens

In Gross's (2015) process model of emotion regulation, he identifies various phases of the emotional process as potential targets for regulation. Two of the earliest phases of this process model include situation selection and situation modification in which people attempt to regulate their emotions by changing the situation they are in. Put simply, changing one's environment is a primary and effective emotion regulation strategy. For example, in this chapter, I have extolled the virtues of being in a natural environment for positive emotions and wellbeing, and evidence suggests that some people understand this and hence intentionally choose to be in natural environments as a way of boosting their positive emotion (Johnsen, 2011).

The environment may also indirectly influence how people regulate their positive emotions. As mentioned above, incidental positive emotions may influence emotion regulation, so being in an environment that promotes positive emotions may also aid in the regulation of emotions. Indeed, some evidence suggests that being in a natural environment is not only a source of positive emotion but can also help facilitate emotion regulation more broadly (Richardson, 2019). One way in which this occurs is through the facilitation of cognitive functioning. Natural environments promote cognitive restoration (Kaplan, 1995), which is the rejuvenation and energising of cognitive processes like attention and cognitive control. These cognitive processes are, in turn, important for some forms of emotion regulation like cognitive reappraisal (Sheppes & Meiran, 2008). Therefore, the restorative nature of being in a natural environment may indirectly promote effective emotion regulation via the restoration and rejuvenation of cognitive processes.

LINKING POSITIVE EMOTIONS AND WELLBEING AT THE INDIVIDUAL AND COMMUNITY LEVELS

In this chapter, I focus primarily on how positive emotions contribute to an individual's wellbeing, which is distinct from the wellbeing of the community that the individual belongs to (Lee & Kim, 2015). Community wellbeing includes assessments of its members' positive emotions or happiness, but also includes other factors that transcend individuals, such as productivity, economic health, and overall health (Lee & Kim, 2015). There are, however, important links between individual levels of positive emotions and community wellbeing (Cloutier & Pfeiffer, 2017).

First, individuals' positive emotions are quite reliably influenced by the community's wellbeing (Cloutier & Pfeiffer, 2017). Being satisfied with one's community/ nation predicts one's individual wellbeing, especially for those people in countries that do not have as many material sources of wellbeing (Morrison, Tay, & Diener, 2011). In addition, I have spent much of this chapter outlining how positive emotions can be influenced by social factors such as one's culture and interactions with others. So, an individual's wellbeing will be impacted by the extent to which a community's cultural values (such as free expression of positive emotions; Miyamoto & Ma, 2011) and social structure (its closeness and promotion of social support and sharing; Cloutier & Pfeiffer, 2017) allow for the experience of positive emotions. In addition, I have reviewed how aspects of the environment, such as the presence of natural beauty, can impact positive emotions. So, an individual's wellbeing will also be impacted by the extent to which the physical manifestation of that community consists of environmental features that cultivate positive emotions (such as having greater green space; Pfeiffer & Cloutier, 2016).

Second, aspects of a community's wellbeing can be, in turn, influenced by the positive emotional wellbeing of its members (Lyubomirsky, King, & Diener, 2005). For example, increasing the wellbeing of employees can improve their organisation's productivity (Fredrickson, 2000). In addition, when people are happier, they also tend to be physically healthier (Pressman & Cohen, 2005), which can decrease the financial strain of illness on a community (Lopez-Casasnovas, Rivera, & Currais, 2005). In sum, although I have focused mostly on how positive emotions contribute to the wellbeing of individuals, it is clear that there are strong bidirectional links between these emotions and the wellbeing of the community as whole.

SUMMARY

Positive emotions are a vital aspect of emotional/hedonic and eudaimonic individual wellbeing. In this chapter, I provided an integrative perspective on the positive emotional process across psychological, biological, sociocultural, and environmental perspectives. Key aspects of this process include the following:

- The stimuli that induce positive emotions tend to be those that have been associated in our evolutionary history with the gain or maintenance of resources. Furthermore, the perception of these stimuli is directed by the mesolimbic dopaminergic system and shaped by one's cultural upbringing.
- Once perceived, the brain (vmPFC, NaCC) positively appraises the stimuli. Appraisal is the evaluation of the environment in relation to the self, and because culture and social identities directly shape our self-conception they can also shape how we positively appraise stimuli.
- These appraisals lead to motivated behaviours that have evolved to obtain or maintain resources. These motivated behaviours are generated by the vmPFC/NaCC through the basal ganglia and are shaped by cultural norms that dictate what behaviours are likely to produce positive emotions. Being in a natural environment can generally reduce the arousal associated with motivated behaviour and instead induce low arousal positive emotions such as contentment.
- Last, emotion regulation is critical to improving positive emotions and wellbeing either for their own sake or in response to a stressor. Importantly, one's culture can shape what positive emotions are targeted and what emotion regulation strategies are preferred and most successful. The brain regions responsible for positive appraisal are recruited for positive emotion regulation as well as additional regions associated with cognitive control.

In sum, fully understanding wellbeing and the role of positive emotion in it will require a comprehensive framework that integrates findings and theory across lenses and scales. Although there are now several decades of research on emotion linking the psychological with the biological, it is only in the past decade or so that researchers have begun to also identify crucial sociocultural and environmental contributors to this complex interplay. Discovering these links will firm up the foundation of wellbeing theory and knowledge to more completely understand what makes a life good.

REFERENCES

Bagozzi, R. P., Verbeke, W., & Gavino Jr, J. C. (2003). Culture moderates the self-regulation of shame and its effects on performance: The case of salespersons in the Netherlands and the Philippines. *Journal of Applied Psychology, 88*(2), 219. https://doi.org/10.1037/0021-9010.88.2.219

Beckes, L., & Coan, J. A. (2011). Social baseline theory: The role of social proximity in emotion and economy of action. *Social and Personality Psychology Compass, 5*(12), 976–988. https://doi.org/10.1111/j.1751-9004.2011.00400.x

Benoit, R. G., Szpunar, K. K., & Schacter, D. L. (2014). Ventromedial prefrontal cortex supports affective future simulation by integrating distributed knowledge. *Proceedings of the National Academy of Sciences of the United States of America, 111*(46), 16550–16555. https://doi.org/10.1073/pnas.1419274111

Berridge, K. C., & Kringelbach, M. L. (2015). Pleasure Systems in the Brain. *Neuron, 86*(3), 646–664. https://doi.org/10.1016/j.neuron.2015.02.018

Berridge, K. C., & Robinson, T. E. (2003). Parsing reward. *Trends in Neurosciences, 26*(9), 507–513. https://doi.org/10.1016/S0166-2236(03)00233-9

Bornstein, M. H., & Arterberry, M. E. (2003). Recognition, discrimination and categorization of smiling by 5-month-old infants. *Developmental Science, 6*(5), 585–599. https://doi.org/10.1111/1467-7687.00314

Buhle, J. T., Silvers, J. A., Wager, T. D., Lopez, R., Onyemekwu, C., Kober, H., Weber, J., & Ochsner, K. N. (2014). Cognitive reappraisal of emotion: A meta-analysis of human neuroimaging studies. *Cerebral Cortex, 24*(11), 2981–2990. https://doi.org/10.1093/cercor/bht154

Butler, E. A., Lee, T. L., & Gross, J. J. (2007). Emotion regulation and culture: Are the social consequences of emotion suppression culture-specific? *Emotion, 7*(1), 30.

Capaldi, C. A., Passmore, H.-A., Nisbet, E. K., Zelenski, J. M., & Dopko, R. L. (2015). Flourishing in nature: A review of the benefits of connecting with nature and its application as a wellbeing intervention. *International Journal of Wellbeing, 5*(4), 1–16. https://doi.org/do i:10.5502/ijw.v5i4.449

Catalino, L. I., Algoe, S. B., & Fredrickson, B. L. (2014). Prioritizing positivity: An effective approach to pursuing happiness? *Emotion, 14*(6), 1155–1161. https://doi.org/10.1037/a0038029

Chavez, R. S., Heatherton, T. F., & Wagner, D. D. (2017). Neural population decoding reveals the intrinsic positivity of the self. *Cerebral Cortex, 27*(11), 5222–5229. https://doi.org/10.1093/cercor/bhw302

Cloutier, S., & Pfeiffer, D. (2017). Happiness: An alternative objective for sustainable community development. In R. Phillips & C. Wong (Eds.), *Handbook of community well-being research* (pp. 85–96). Springer.

Coan, J. A., Schaefer, H. S., & Davidson, R. J. (2006). Lending a hand: Social regulation of the neural response to threat. *Psychological Science, 17*(12), 1032–1039. https://doi.org/10.1111/j.1467-9280.2006.01832.x

Diener, E., Sandvik, E., & Pavot, W. (2009). Happiness is the frequency, not the intensity, of positive versus negative affect. In E. Diener (Ed.), *Assessing well-being* (pp. 213–231). Springer.

Diener, E., Suh, E. M., Lucas, R. E., & Smith, H. L. (1999). Subjective well-being: Three decades of progress. *Psychological Bulletin, 125*(2), 276–302. https://doi.org/10.1037/0033-2909.125.2.276

Fredrickson, B. L. (1998). What good are positive emotions? *Review of General Psychology, 2*(3), 300–319. https://doi.org/10.1037/1089-2680.2.3.300

Fredrickson, B. L. (2000). Why positive emotions matter in organizations: Lessons from the broaden-and-build model. *Psychologist-Manager Journal, 4*(2), 131–142. https://doi.org/10.1037/h0095887

Fredrickson, B. L., Tugade, M. M., Waugh, C. E., & Larkin, G. R. (2003). What good are positive emotions in crisis? A prospective study of resilience and emotions following the terrorist attacks on the United States on September 11th, 2001. *Journal of Personality and Social Psychology, 84*(2), 365–376. https://doi.org/10.1037/0022-3514.84.2.365

Frijda, N. H. (2007). *The laws of emotion.* Erlbaum.

Gable, P. A., & Harmon-Jones, E. (2008). Approach-motivated positive affect reduces breadth of attention. *Psychological Science, 19*(5), 476–482. https://doi.org/10.1111/j.1467-9280.2008.02112.x

Gross, J. J. (2015). The Extended Process Model of Emotion Regulation: Elaborations, applications, and future directions. *Psychological Inquiry, 26*(1), 130–137. https://doi.org/10.1080/1047840X.2015.989751

Gunaydin, L. A., & Kreitzer, A. C. (2016). Cortico–basal ganglia circuit function in psychiatric disease. *Annual Review of Physiology, 78*(1), 327–350. https://doi.org/10.1146/annurev-physiol-021115-105355

Haber, S. N., Kunishio, K., Mizobuchi, M., & Lynd-Balta, E. (1995). The orbital and medial prefrontal circuit through the primate basal ganglia. *Journal of Neuroscience, 15*(7), 4851–4867. https://doi.org/10.1523/JNEUROSCI.15-07-04851.1995

Hare, T. A., O'Doherty, J., Camerer, C. F., Schultz, W., & Rangel, A. (2008). Dissociating the role of the orbitofrontal cortex and the striatum in the computation of goal values and prediction errors. *Journal of Neuroscience, 28*(22), 5623–5630. https://doi.org/10.1523/JNEUROSCI.1309-08.2008

Herry, C., Bach, D. R., Esposito, F., Di Salle, F., Perrig, W. J., Scheffler, K., Luthi, A., & Seifritz, E. (2007). Processing of temporal unpredictability in human and animal amygdala. *Journal of Neuroscience, 27*(22), 5958–5966. https://doi.org/10.1523/JNEUROSCI.5218-06.2007

Herzog, T. R., Black, A. M., Fountaine, K. A., & Knotts, D. J. (1997). Reflection and attentional recovery as distinctive benefits of restorative environments. *Journal of Environmental Psychology, 17*(2), 165–170. https://doi.org/10.1006/jevp.1997.0051

Hsu, D. T., Sanford, B. J., Meyers, K. K., Love, T. M., Hazlett, K. E., Wang, H., Ni, L., Walker, S. J., Mickey, B. J., & Korycinski, S. T. (2013). Response of the μ-opioid system to social rejection and acceptance. *Molecular Psychiatry, 18*(11), 1211–1217. https://doi.org/10.1038/mp.2013.96

Ikemoto, S., Yang, C., & Tan, A. (2015). Basal ganglia circuit loops, dopamine and motivation: A review and enquiry. *Behavioural Brain Research, 290,* 17–31. https://doi.org/10.1016/j.bbr.2015.04.018

Imada, T., & Ellsworth, P. C. (2011). Proud Americans and lucky Japanese: Cultural differences in appraisal and corresponding emotion. *Emotion, 11*(2), 329. https://doi.org/10.1037/a0022855

Johnsen, S. Å. K. (2011). The use of nature for emotion regulation: Toward a conceptual framework. *Ecopsychology*, *3*(3), 175–185. https://doi.org/10.1089/eco.2011.0006

Joseph, S., Murphy, D., & Regel, S. (2012). An affective-cognitive processing model of post-traumatic growth. *Clinical Psychology & Psychotherapy*, *19*(4), 316–325. https://doi.org/10.1002/cpp.1798

Kaplan, R., & Kaplan, S. (1989). *The experience of nature: A psychological perspective.* Cambridge University Press.

Kaplan, S. (1995). The restorative benefits of nature: Toward an integrative framework. *Journal of Environmental Psychology*, *15*(3), 169–182. https://doi.org/10.1016/0272-4944(95)90001-2

Kashdan, T. B., Biswas-Diener, R., & King, L. A. (2008). Reconsidering happiness: The costs of distinguishing between hedonics and eudaimonia. *Journal of Positive Psychology*, *3*(4), 219–233. https://doi.org/10.1080/17439760802303044

Kellert, S. R., & Wilson, E. O. (1993). *The biophilia hypothesis*. Island Press.

King, L. A., Hicks, J. A., Krull, J. L., & Del Gaiso, A. K. (2006). Positive affect and the experience of meaning in life. *Journal of Personality and Social Psychology*, *90*(1), 179–196. https://doi.org/10.1037/0022-3514.90.1.179

Knutson, B., Adams, C. M., Fong, G. W., & Hommer, D. (2001). Anticipation of increasing monetary reward selectively recruits nucleus accumbens. *Journal of Neuroscience*, *21*(16), RC159. https://doi.org/10.1523/JNEUROSCI.21-16-j0002.2001

Kuzmanovic, B., Rigoux, L., & Tittgemeyer, M. (2018). Influence of vmPFC on dmPFC predicts valence-guided belief formation. *Journal of Neuroscience*, *38*(37), 7996–8010. https://doi.org/10.1523/JNEUROSCI.0266-18.2018

Larsen, J. T., McGraw, A. P., & Cacioppo, J. T. (2001). Can people feel happy and sad at the same time? *Journal of Personality and Social Psychology*, *81*, 684–696. https://doi.org/10.1037/0022-3514.81.4.684

Laumann, K., Gärling, T., & Stormark, K. M. (2003). Selective attention and heart rate responses to natural and urban environments. *Journal of Environmental Psychology*, *23*(2), 125–134. https://doi.org/10.1016/S0272-4944(02)00110-X

Lazarus, R. S., & Folkman, S. (1984). *Stress, appraisal, and coping*. Springer.

LeDoux, J. E. (1996). *The emotional brain: The mysterious underpinnings of emotional life* (1996-98824-000). Simon & Schuster.

Lee, S. J., & Kim, Y. (2015). Searching for the meaning of community well-Being. In S. J. Lee, Y. Kim, & R. Phillips (Eds.), *Community well-being and community development* (pp. 9–23). Springer.

Leslie-Miller, C. J., Waugh, C. E., & Cole, V. T. (2021). Coping with COVID-19: The benefits of anticipating future positive events and maintaining optimism. *Frontiers in Psychology*, *12*(646047), 1–9. https://doi.org/10.3389/fpsyg.2021.646047

Lopez-Casasnovas, G., Rivera, B., & Currais, L. (Eds.). (2005). *Health and Economic Growth: Findings and Policy Implications*. MIT Press.

Lyubomirsky, S., King, L., & Diener, E. (2005). The benefits of frequent positive affect: Does happiness lead to success? *Psychological Bulletin*, *131*(6), 803–855.

Mackie, D. M., Maitner, A. T., & Smith, E. R. (2016). Intergroup emotions theory. In T. D. Nelson (Ed.), *Handbook of Prejudice, Stereotyping, and Discrimination* (pp. 149–174). Psychology Press.

Markus, H. R., & Kitayama, S. (1991). Culture and the self: Implications for cognition, emotion, and motivation. *Psychological Review, 98*(2), 224. https://doi.org/10.1037/0033-295X.98.2.224

Masuda, T., Ellsworth, P. C., Mesquita, B., Leu, J., Tanida, S., & Van de Veerdonk, E. (2008). Placing the face in context: Cultural differences in the perception of facial emotion. *Journal of Personality and Social Psychology, 94*(3), 365–381. https://doi.org/10.1037/0022-3514.94.3.365

Matsumoto, D., Yoo, S. H., & Nakagawa, S. (2008). Culture, emotion regulation, and adjustment. *Journal of Personality and Social Psychology, 94*(6), 925–937. https://doi.org/10.1037/0022-3514.94.6.925

McRae, K., & Gross, J. J. (2020). Emotion regulation. *Emotion, 20*(1), 1–9. https://doi.org/10.1037/emo0000703

Mesquita, B., & Boiger, M. (2014). Emotions in context: A sociodynamic model of emotions. *Emotion Review, 6*(4), 298–302. https://doi.org/10.1177/1754073914534480

Mesquita, B., De Leersnyder, J., & Albert, D. (2014). The cultural regulation of emotions. In J. J. Gross, D. Albert, A. K., Anderson, A. Appleton, & O. Ayduk (Eds.), *Handbook of emotion regulation* (2nd ed., pp. 284–301). Guilford Press.

Mesquita, B., & Frijda, N. H. (1992). Cultural variations in emotions: A review. *Psychological Bulletin, 112*(2), 179–204. https://doi.org/10.1037/0033-2909.112.2.179

Mifune, N., Simunovic, D., & Yamagishi, T. (2017). Intergroup biases in fear-induced aggression. *Frontiers in Psychology, 8*, 49. https://doi.org/10.3389/fpsyg.2017.00049

Miyamoto, Y., & Ma, X. (2011). Dampening or savoring positive emotions: A dialectical cultural script guides emotion regulation. *Emotion, 11*(6), 1346. https://doi.org/10.1037/a0025135

Mobbs, D., Hagan, C. C., Dalgleish, T., Silston, B., & Prévost, C. (2015). The ecology of human fear: Survival optimization and the nervous system. *Frontiers in Neuroscience, 9*, 55. https://doi.org/10.3389/fnins.2015.00055

Monfort, S. S., Stroup, H. E., & Waugh, C. E. (2015). The impact of anticipating positive events on responses to stress. *Journal of Experimental Social Psychology, 58*, 11–22. https://doi.org/10.1016/j.jesp.2014.12.003

Morris, J. S., Frith, C. D., Perrett, D. I., Rowland, D., Young, A. W., Calder, A. J., & Dolan, R. (1996). A differential neural response in the human amygdala to fearful and happy facial expressions. *Nature, 6603*, 812–815. https://doi.org/10.1038/383812a0

Morrison, M., Tay, L., & Diener, E. (2011). Subjective well-being and national satisfaction: Findings from a worldwide survey. *Psychological Science, 22*(2), 166–171. https://doi.org/10.1177/0956797610396224

Moskowitz, J. T., Cheung, E. O., Snowberg, K., Verstaen, A., Merrilees, J., Salsman, J. M., & Dowling, G. A. (2019). Randomized control trial of a facilitated online positive emotion regulation intervention for dementia caregivers. *Health Psychology, 38*(5), 391–402. https://doi.org/10.1037/hea0000680

Nitschke, J. B., Nelson, E. E., Rusch, B. D., Fox, A. S., Oakes, T. R., & Davidson, R. J. (2004). Orbitofrontal cortex tracks positive mood in mothers viewing pictures of their newborn infants. *Neuroimage, 21*(2), 583–592. https://doi.org/10.1016/j.neuroimage.2003.10.005

Nummenmaa, L., Saanijoki, T., Tuominen, L., Hirvonen, J., Tuulari, J. J., Nuutila, P., & Kalliokoski, K. (2018). μ-Opioid receptor system mediates reward processing

in humans. *Nature Communications*, *9*(1), 1–7. https://doi.org/10.1038/s41
467-018-03848-y

Ochsner, K. N., & Gross, J. J. (2005). The cognitive control of emotion. *Trends in Cognitive Sciences*, *9*(5), 242–249. https://doi.org/10.1016/j.tics.2005.03.010

Pfeiffer, D., & Cloutier, S. (2016). Planning for happy neighborhoods. *Journal of the American Planning Association*, *82*(3), 267–279. https://doi.org/10.1080/01944 363.2016.1166347

Pressman, S. D., & Cohen, S. (2005). Does positive affect influence health. *Psychological Bulletin*, *131*(6), 925–971.

Quoidbach, J., Berry, E. V., Hansenne, M., & Mikolajczak, M. (2010). Positive emotion regulation and well-being: Comparing the impact of eight savoring and dampening strategies. *Personality and Individual Differences*, *49*(5), 368–373. https://doi.org/10.1016/j.paid.2010.03.048

Quoidbach, J., Taquet, M., Desseilles, M., de Montjoye, Y.-A., & Gross, J. J. (2019). Happiness and social behavior. *Psychological Science*, *30*(8), 1111–1122. https://doi.org/10.1177/0956797619849666

Reber, R., Schwarz, N., & Winkielman, P. (2004). Processing fluency and aesthetic pleasure: Is beauty in the perceiver's processing experience? *Personality and Social Psychology Review*, *8*(4), 364–382. https://doi.org/10.1207/s15327957pspr0804_3

Richardson, M. (2019). Beyond restoration: Considering emotion regulation in natural well-being. *Ecopsychology*, *11*(2), 123–129. https://doi.org/10.1089/eco.2019.0012

Richardson, M., McEwan, K., Maratos, F., & Sheffield, D. (2016). Joy and calm: How an evolutionary functional model of affect regulation informs positive emotions in nature. *Evolutionary Psychological Science*, *2*(4), 308–320. https://doi.org/10.1007/s40 806-016-0065-5

Rozin, P., Haidt, J., & McCauley, C. R. (2008). Disgust. In M. Lewis, J. M. Haviland-Jones, & L. F. Barrett (Eds.), *Handbook of Emotions* (3rd ed; pp. 757–776). Guilford Press.

Russell, J. A., Weiss, A., & Mendelsohn, G. A. (1989). The affect grid: A single-item scale of pleasure and arousal. *Journal of Personality and Social Psychology*, *57*, 493–502. https://doi.org/10.1037/0022-3514.57.3.493

Ryan, R. M., & Deci, E. L. (2001). On happiness and human potentials: A review of research on hedonic and eudaimonic well-being. *Annual Review of Psychology*, *52*, 141–166. https://doi.org/10.1146/annurev.psych.52.1.141

Sabatinelli, D., Bradley, M. M., Fitzsimmons, J. R., & Lang, P. J. (2005). Parallel amygdala and inferotemporal activation reflect emotional intensity and fear relevance. *NeuroImage*, *24*(4), 1265–1270. https://doi.org/10.1016/j.neuroimage.2004.12.015

Scherer, K. R., & Moors, A. (2019). The emotion process: Event appraisal and component differentiation. *Annual Review of Psychology*, *70*, 719–745. https://doi.org/10.1146/annurev-psych-122216-011854

Sescousse, G., Caldù, X., Segura, B., & Dreher, J.-C. (2013). Processing of primary and secondary rewards: A quantitative meta-analysis and review of human functional neuroimaging studies. *Neuroscience & Biobehavioral Reviews*, *37*, 681–696. https://doi.org/10.1016/j.neubiorev.2013.02.002

Sheppes, G., & Meiran, N. (2008). Divergent cognitive costs for online forms of reappraisal and distraction. *Emotion*, *8*(6), 870–874. https://doi.org/10.1037/a0013711

Shiota, M. N., Keltner, D., & Mossman, A. (2007). The nature of awe: Elicitors, appraisals, and effects on self-concept. *Cognition and Emotion, 21*(5), 944–963. https://doi.org/10.1080/02699930600923668

Smith, C. A., & Ellsworth, P. C. (1985). Patterns of cognitive appraisal in emotion. *Journal of Personality and Social Psychology, 48*(4), 813–838. https://doi.org/10.1037/0022-3514.48.4.813

Smith, E. R., Seger, C. R., & Mackie, D. M. (2007). Can emotions be truly group level? Evidence regarding four conceptual criteria. *Journal of Personality and Social Psychology, 93*(3), 431–446. https://doi.org/10.1037/0022-3514.93.3.431

Smith, P. K. (1982). Does play matter? Functional and evolutionary aspects of animal and human play. *Behavioral and Brain Sciences, 5*(1), 139–155. https://doi.org/10.1017/S0140525X0001092X

Somerville, L. H., Kelley, W. M., & Heatherton, T. F. (2010). Self-esteem modulates medial prefrontal cortical responses to evaluative social feedback. *Cerebral Cortex, 20*(12), 3005–3013. https://doi.org/10.1093/cercor/bhq049

Taylor, S. E., & Brown, J. D. (1988). Illusion and well-being: A social psychological perspective on mental health. *Psychological Bulletin, 103*(2), 193–210. https://doi.org/10.1037/0033-2909.103.2.193

Tobia, M. J., Hayashi, K., Ballard, G., Gotlib, I. H., & Waugh, C. E. (2017). Dynamic functional connectivity and individual differences in emotions during social stress. *Human Brain Mapping, 38*, 6185–6205. https://doi.org/10.1002/hbm.23821

Tooby, J., & Cosmides, L. (1990). The past explains the present: Emotional adaptations and the structure of ancestral environments. *Ethology and Sociobiology, 11*(4–5), 375–424. https://doi.org/10.1016/0162-3095(90)90017-Z

Tsai, J. L. (2007). Ideal affect: Cultural causes and behavioral consequences. *Perspectives on Psychological Science, 2*(3), 242–259. https://doi.org/10.1111/j.1745-6916.2007.00043.x

Tsai, J. L., Chim, L., & Sims, T. (2015). *Consumer behavior, culture, and emotion.* https://doi.org/10.1093/acprof:oso/9780199388516.003.0004

Tsai, J. L., Miao, F. F., Seppala, E., Fung, H. H., & Yeung, D. Y. (2007). Influence and adjustment goals: Sources of cultural differences in ideal affect. *Journal of Personality and Social Psychology, 92*(6), 1102. https://doi.org/10.1037/0022-3514.92.6.1102

Turner, J. C., Hogg, M. A., Oakes, P. J., Reicher, S. D., & Wetherell, M. S. (1987). *Rediscovering the social group: A self-categorization theory.* Basil Blackwell.

Uhrich, S., & Benkenstein, M. (2010). Sport stadium atmosphere: Formative and reflective indicators for operationalizing the construct. *Journal of Sport Management, 24*(2), 211–237. https://doi.org/10.1123/jsm.24.2.211

Ulrich, R. S., Simons, R. F., Losito, B. D., Fiorito, E., Miles, M. A., & Zelson, M. (1991). Stress recovery during exposure to natural and urban environments. *Journal of Environmental Psychology, 11*(3), 201–230. https://doi.org/10.1016/S0272-4944(05)80184-7

Watson, D., & Clark, L. A. (1992). On traits and temperament: General and specific factors of emotional experience and their relation to the five-factor model. *Journal of Personality, 60*, 441–476. https://doi.org/10.1111/j.1467-6494.1992.tb00980.x

Waugh, C. E. (2020). The roles of positive emotion in the regulation of emotional responses to negative events. *Emotion, 20*(1), 54–58. https://doi.org/10.1037/emo0000625

Waugh, C. E., & Fredrickson, B. L. (2006). Nice to know you: Positive emotions, self-other overlap, and complex understanding in the formation of a new relationship. *Journal of Positive Psychology, 1*(2), 93–106. https://doi.org/10.1080/17439760500510569

Waugh, C. E., & McRae, K. (unpublished manuscript). *The Positive Appraisal in the Regulation of Stress (PARS) model.*

Wickelgren, I. (1997). Getting the brain's attention. *Science, 278*(5335), 35–37. https://doi.org/10.1126/science.278.5335.35

Williams, K. D. (2006). Ostracism. *Annual Review of Psychology, 58*(1), 425–452. https://doi.org/10.1146/annurev.psych.58.110405.085641

Wilson, T. D., & Gilbert, D. T. (2003). Affective forecasting. In M. P. Zanna (Ed.), *Advances in Experimental Social Psychology* (vol. 35, pp. 345–411). Academic Press. https://doi.org/10.1016/S0065-2601(03)01006-2

Wilson, T. D., Lisle, D. J., Kraft, D., & Wetzel, C. G. (1989). Preferences as expectation-driven inferences: Effects of affective expectations on affective experience. *Journal of Personality and Social Psychology, 56*(4), 519–530. https://doi.org/10.1037/0022-3514.56.4.519

Yin, H. H., & Knowlton, B. J. (2006). The role of the basal ganglia in habit formation. *Nature Reviews Neuroscience, 7*(6), 464–476. https://doi.org/10.1038/nrn1919

Zautra, A. J., Reich, J. W., Davis, M. C., Potter, P. T., & Nicolson, N. A. (2000). The role of stressful events in the relationship between positive and negative affect: Evidence from field and experimental studies. *Journal of Personality, 68*, 927–951. https://doi.org/10.1111/1467-6494.00121

Zhang, M., & Kelley, A. (2000). Enhanced intake of high-fat food following striatal mu-opioid stimulation: Microinjection mapping and fos expression. *Neuroscience, 99*(2), 267–277. https://doi.org/10.1016/S0306-4522(00)00198-6

Subjective Wellbeing and Resilience at the Individual Level

A Synthesis Through Homeostasis

ROBERT A. CUMMINS ∎

INTRODUCTION

The construct of resilience has been the focus of research efforts for the past 40 years. It has become especially topical in recent years given the various phases of the COVID-19 pandemic chronicled across the world, whereby both individuals and whole populations have been severely tested on their ability to survive multiple sources of challenge to their normal life routines. While the level of threat caused by the disease is highly variable, depending especially on geographic location and personal affluence, the societal influence of the pandemic is felt by everyone. National economies have been in tatters, international travel curtailed, unemployment rampant, and civil liberties overridden by restrictions of movement outside homes (for a harrowing account in the United States, see Chapter 15, this volume). So, what tools from scientific psychology can assist the understanding of human resilience under such conditions?

The most obvious tool is the judicious deployment of resources. At the level of government, these include effective management of the economy, maintenance of public health, and the continuation of public services. However, even rich governments have limited resources for this purpose and sometimes limited willingness to distribute their resources as well (see also Chapter 16, this volume). So, even in the most favourable national circumstances, the survival of pre-COVID societies has been jeopardised. Indeed, fundamental changes in societies appeared quite early in the pandemic. These include changed (and, for many, dramatically altered) working conditions, stresses on family life, and the chronic threat of infection.

The effects of these changes on individual people depend on many factors. Most fundamentally, it depends on the balance between personal resource availability and needs. But it is the individual's perception of these resources and needs that is so crucial to positive and negative attitude formation (see also Chapter 2, this volume). And maintaining a positive attitude under challenging conditions is the hallmark of *resilience*, a common English word meaning the power to deal effectively with challenge. An excellent definition of resilience is provided by Merriam-Webster (2021) as 'an ability to recover from, or adjust easily to, misfortune or change'.

What, then is the science of resilience? While there is a massive psychological literature on the topic, it is generally disappointing and unenlightening. There are so many ways of operationalising the Merriam-Webster definition and so many alternative definitions that the scientific community appears overwhelmed. It has produced a plethora of complex models for resilience, but they are susceptible to being variously overly complex or missing a sound theoretical foundation (see also Chapter 1, this volume). A recent example is the model of 'quantified systemic resilience' offered by Scheffer et al. (2018). However, their model is seriously flawed (for a critique, see Cummins, 2020a).

In considering how to rectify this situation, a worthy thought is that the beginnings of understanding must always be based on the most certain knowledge. And that most certain knowledge is always the simplest. In the case of resilience, the most certain knowledge comes from biology, where resilience is intimately linked to homeostatic systems. Such systems have been intensively studied over the past century and do much of the heavy lifting concerning recovery and adaptation within physiology. In this chapter, biological homeostasis will provide the starting point for developing further understanding.

This narrative proceeds as follows. Following a description of biological homeostasis, discussion moves to psychological science and the overlap of concepts which have led to understanding psychological homeostasis. Within this psychological/biological context, resilience will be examined in terms of its measurement, its control systems, and its relationship with subjective wellbeing.

BIOLOGICAL HOMEOSTASIS AND RESILIENCE

Biological resilience reflects an animal's physiological capacity to recover from or adjust easily to misfortune or change. There are really two arms to this capacity. One concerns the long-term survival of species, referred to as the animal's 'fitness'. This is a measure of an animal's reproductive success, most especially in challenging conditions as are currently being imposed on divers species through climate change (Balmford, 1996). The other arm to biological resilience is the animal's capacity to adapt its physiology to seasonal and diurnal changes in its environment. Most essential in this regard are a special set of hard-wired management systems designed to maintain key variables within a limited range of values required for normal physiological functioning. Such systems are called 'homeostatic,' as first recognised and named almost a hundred years ago (Cannon, 1929, 1932).

Biological Homeostasis

In close sympathy with the definition of resilience, *homeostasis* is the ability to restore biological control following a perturbation of a managed variable outside its normal range. The most familiar of these variables is body temperature, which is allowed only a single degree of variation under normal operating conditions in humans. Such management requires not just the genetic machinery to organise the physiological components, but also the availability of necessary resources. Thus, for example, hypothermia can come about through a lack of energy in the diet (starvation) or in any situation where body heat loss exceeds heat gain (e.g., inadequate clothing). There are many biological homeostatic systems, each managing a single variable and interacting with one another. For example, the ability of the temperature control system to instruct an increase in heat production by increasing the metabolic rate depends on an adequate supply of fuel (glucose) in the blood, which is itself under the active management of glucose homeostasis.

Essentially, all life depends on homeostasis (see Damasio, 2018), and each homeostatic system has the following characteristics:

1. It concerns the management of a single variable type (e.g., core body temperature) by a complex, multipart system. The first such system was detailed by Cannon (1932) in relation to blood glucose and core body temperature.
2. Each homeostatically managed variable has a 'setpoint'. The level of this setpoint defines the average of its normal operating level. For example, core body temperature for humans is 'set' at 36°C.
3. Each managed variable is not held rigidly at its setpoint. Rather, it can vary within a narrow range (36.5–37.5°C in the case of human body temperature), referred to as its 'setpoint range', while remaining under homeostatic control.
4. Strong forces can wrest control of the managed variable away from homeostasis, such as exposure to an overly hot or cold environment. When the level of the variable moves outside its setpoint range, this is a signal that the variable is no longer under homeostatic control. If this occurs on a chronic basis, it signals pathology. For body temperature, a value higher than 37.5°C signals fever, while a value less than 35.0°C signals hypothermia.
5. Each variable being managed (e.g., temperature) has a specific receptor which interfaces that variable with the nervous system. For example, in mammals, the temperature receptor is located in the preoptic area of the anterior hypothalamus (Romanovsky, 2007). These receptors record the momentary level of the managed variable (core body

temperature) and interface with higher-level processors concerned with homeostatic management. These processors match receptor information against the setpoint for that variable. If the level is different from the setpoint, then disparity information is sent to 'effectors'. These devices activate physiological and behavioural systems in ways to correct for the difference and so restore the level of the variable to lie closer to its setpoint.

6. Each effector system comprises a complex network of devices which, in cooperation with one another, act in ways to raise or lower the level of the variable being managed. For example, if the person is too hot, blood flow is increased to the skin to facilitate heat loss; if the person is too cold, blood flow to the skin is reduced, thereby conserving heat. Other devices to manage body temperature include adjusting metabolic rate, moving into or out of the sun, and so on.

As indicated by the complexity of such management strategies, homeostatic systems are expensive to maintain, both in terms of energy expenditure and the space they occupy in the nervous system. Thus, relatively few physiological variables are under direct homeostatic control. Direct homeostatic management is restricted to those variables which must be maintained within a narrow range of values for normal physiological functioning.

Resilience Versus Homeostasis

The above account of physiological homeostasis makes it clear that each homeostatic system is a separate entity even though they are all functionally dependent on one another. In this model, any measure of systemic (whole-body) resilience will reflect the weakest homeostatic system. If homeostatic control over blood glucose fails then, in the absence of treatment, the whole body will die. Within this perspective, an understanding of physiological resilience can be described as having the following characteristics:

1. At the level of individual homeostatic systems, resilience is a measure of capacity to manage a particular variable when its physiological subsystem is compromised. For example, if pathology involving the pancreas reduces its ability to produce insulin, the resilience of the body to manage blood glucose is compromised.

2. In this situation, the fact of diminished resilience can be applied to both glucose homeostasis and to the whole body because the whole body depends on glucose management.

3. Following this logical trail, the notion of physiological 'systemic resilience' makes little sense. Rather, systemic resilience is driven by the single most fragile homeostatic system. And the corollary of this is that the most informative measures of systemic resilience will concern

assessments of individual homeostatic systems, such as core body temperature, blood glucose, and blood oxygenation. How, then, does this logical conclusion relate to psychology?

THE TRANSITION FROM BIOLOGICAL TO PSYCHOLOGICAL HOMEOSTASIS

Perhaps the best starting point for the transition from biological to psychological homeostasis is a reminder of *evolutionary parsimony* (see phylogenetics: Wikipedia). Basically, rather than engaging in much *de novo* creation, evolution usually takes the path of modifying successfully operating systems. This understanding fits with the basic idea of conservation of energy. All biological systems are limited by the energy they can acquire, so the respecification of existing systems is more energy-efficient than experimenting with new ones. Moreover, currently operating systems are already known to interact successfully within the whole-body complex.

It follows from this parsimony theme that any psychological homeostatic system is certain to share basic characteristics with its biological counterparts and that any psychological homeostatic theory should reflect this common lineage. Moreover, any proposed theory for psychology should be simple, using a minimum number of concepts and linkages (Achenbaum & Bengtson, 1994), while keeping novel concepts as an unavoidable rarity.

In the spirit of such developmental guidelines, the successful approach to theory formation in psychology has been fundamentally reductionist, aimed at understanding the basic structure and operational character of the *simplest* psychological variables that display reliable *stability*. This line of enquiry commenced with Watson's (1930) study using data from a sample of 388 graduate students who completed multiple measures of self-happiness ratings devised by the author. His validity assumption in creating these measures was that 'the individual is called happy if he believes himself happier than most others of like age and sex, if he believes his prevailing moods cheerful, his spirits high, his satisfactions lasting, his days full of interesting and amusing things, his prevalent attitudes described by such words as "enthusiastic", "jolly", "tranquil", "joyful", "fortunate" or "well-integrated"' (p. 79).

His measurement instrument comprised six items, each with several parts representing the above aspects, and could be likely completed in 5–10 minutes. 'Each graphic rating scale was scored by a scale of units ranging from 0 at the most unhappy extreme to 100 at the happiest extreme with 50 in the middle' (Watson, 1930, p. 82). It is notable that this form of end-defined, numerical scale preceded the five-choice scale of Likert (1932), and the numerical form has only recently come back into favour with the realisation that 11-choice (0 to 10), unipolar response scales yield superior measurement sensitivity with no loss of reliability (Cummins, 2021).

In addition to the rating scales, other measures required various forms of response, including one open-ended qualitative item. So, assembling the data from each person into a single scale to produce their 'happiness rating' proved challenging. Various means were employed, which included seeking the opinion of a committee to determine comparative adjectival ratings, item weightings, subtracting negative item scores from positive item scores, and so on.

Watson then checked the internal reliability of his instrument by creating two subscale scores, each derived from a different set of items. Application of the Spearman-Brown formula, which provides a correlation corrected for test-length, yielded evidence of the scale's reliability of .83 and .85. Given the heterogeneous construction of the scale items, this level of reliability is, actually, extraordinary, and Watson needs to be credited with developing the first reflective measurement scale (i.e., where the construct to be measured determines the nature of the items that reflect its character; Diamantopoulos & Winklhofer 2001) for happiness.

But this was not his most remarkable result. Watson's table 2 presents a distribution of individual happiness scores, derived from the whole scale, on a range that extends from 100 to 380 units. The median value is 273 units. Using the formula provided in the Personal Wellbeing Index Manual (PWI; International Wellbeing Group, 2013), this value converts to a score of 71.84 percentage points (pp) on a 0 to 100 percentage point scale. This median score is just below the normative range for the PWI using Australian data (mean 75.43 pp, normative range 74.13 to 76.73 pp) and very close to the level generally reported for graduate students (e.g., 72.0 pp reported by Renn et al., 2009). It might seem incredible that the cumbersome, mixed-method instrument used by Watson some 80 years ago in the United States to measure 'happiness' produced such comparable results to the Australian normative data for the PWI (Khor, Fuller-Tysziewicz, & Hutchinson, 2020), which measures 'satisfaction'. But this result is no coincidence. It is caused by the domination of each 'happiness' or 'satisfaction' response by *homeostatically protected mood* (HPM), which is an individual difference variable, as explained later in this account.

Following Watson's lead, it was soon discovered that measures of mood happiness are both reliable and surprisingly stable over time. Just 4 years later, Hartmann (1934) obtained a test–retest reliability of .70 with two testings of happiness a month apart, while Wessman and Ricks (1966) reported that happiness-related measures taken 2 years apart correlated at .67. Similar results were reported by Bradburn (1969) in a four-wave US study. Using a three-choice response scale and follow-up measures at 3-month intervals, he measured the consistency with which people reported being 'very happy' from one wave to the next. The correlations (gamma coefficients) ranged from .65 to .84.

By the 1970s, it was clear that there was considerable stability in measures of mood happiness and that similar levels of stability were also exhibited by a new measure called Global Life Satisfaction (GLS). This measurement scale, similar in construction to Watson's single-item, graphic rating scale for happiness, asked 'How satisfied are you with your life overall?', and the measured variable became known as subjective wellbeing (SWB). Key figures in this early research were Andrews and Withey (1976), who reported test-retest reliabilities of around .68 between two administrations of their GLS measure.

The Standardisation of the SWB Metric

These results triggered mounting interest in GLS and, encouraged by the fact the scale was just a single item, GLS started to be commonly included in national surveys. Cummins (1995) identified 16 surveys which had reported a population mean score for 'life satisfaction', with a view to determining whether these means reflected the same level of stability as reported by Andrews and Withey. Hindering this approach was the discovery that, even though these surveys were restricted to Western populations, there was a great deal of variation in the response scales researchers had employed. Of particular concern was that the number of response choices in such scales were highly variable (e.g., 1–5, 0–7, 1–11, etc.). This meant that the scale mean scores could not be directly compared with one another. So Cummins devised an arithmetic conversion formula that standardised the results from different response scales into a single common metric. The resulting units were called *percentage of scale maximum* (%SM), now renamed as 'percentage points' (pp). The conversion formula continues to be used by the International Wellbeing Group (2013; section 5.2).

Using this conversion, Cummins (1995) summarised the results of the 16 surveys and found that, using the survey mean scores as data, the grand mean (and standard deviation [SD]) could be expressed as 75.0 ± 2.5pp. Cummins speculated that 'One explanation for this result could be the existence of a psychological, homeostatic mechanism' (p. 193).

Some 3 years later Cummins (1998) confirmed the population-level SWB stability and further speculated that 'It is proposed that life satisfaction is a variable under homeostatic control and with a homeostatic set-point ensuring that populations have, on average, a positive view of their lives. However, the factors that influence this set-point to lie between 80 to 60 [pp] cannot yet be specified' (p. 330).

SWB Stability and Personality

Over the following years, research attention started to shift from simple replication to the mechanism causing such SWB stability. The best guess was personality. It seemed an obvious choice. Optimism was considered as largely genetically determined (Tiger, 1979) and therefore stable. Moreover, personality in the form of extraversion and neuroticism was known to have strong links to levels of SWB (Costa & McCrae, 1980), and there was a conventional view that personality was largely genetically determined (for reviews, see Block, 1981; Brim & Kagan, 1980; Jackson & Paunonen, 1980).

Up to this point all the theorising rested on correlational data. A different methodology, using longitudinal data, yielded a new conceptual step toward understanding stability. Headey and Wearing (1989) reported that, when the level of SWB changed following some major event, it tended to return to its previous level over time. This caused the authors to propose that each person has an 'equilibrium level' of SWB and that personality has the role of restoring equilibrium after change by making certain kinds of events more likely. For example, people with strong extraversion have a higher than normal probability of experiencing positive events. So, if their SWB went down due to a negative challenge, their experience of positive events would soon restore SWB to equilibrium. Through this means, personality, life events, and SWB are in dynamic equilibrium with one another, they claimed.

Their model is, however, incomplete. Headey and Wearing never really explain how, following a deviation from equilibrium caused by an event, SWB returns to its previous level. The reasoning that someone high on extraversion will recover from low SWB because of their personality does not work for someone who is also high on neuroticism.

Breaking Away from Personality

The next step in understanding came from the doctoral thesis of Melanie Davern. In a series of studies, she demonstrated that the major correlate of SWB was not personality, as had been so long prescribed (Diener, Sandvik, Pavot, & Fujita, 1992), but rather was affect in the form of a mood (Davern, Cummins, & Stokes, 2007). While the precise composition of this mood was uncertain, it appeared to contain mildly positive affects of 'content' and 'happy', together with an activated affect, such as 'excited', 'aroused', or 'alert'. Moreover, these affects naturally cluster together on the affective circumplex (Russell, 1980), giving credence to the possibility of a simple genetic linkage.

Following Russell (1980), Davern initially referred to this mood as 'core affect'. However, when Russell (2009) started to use core affect to refer to both mood and emotion, that term was no longer appropriate. Moreover, the 'homeostatic model of SWB' was starting to take shape (Cummins, 2003). So 'core affect' was replaced by 'homeostatically protected mood (HPMood)' (Cummins, 2010). This new term not only referred exclusively to mood, thereby excluding emotion, but also linked HPMood to homeostatic management. HPMood also represented the variable that homeostasis was hypothesised to be managing.

At this point the necessary components required to claim discovery of a psychological homeostatic system were taking shape. The general stability of SWB was well established, the psychological mechanisms that could be responsible for managing levels of SWB around a 'setpoint' were being described (Cummins & Nistico 2002), and an important new variable, HPMood, had been identified. However, several key aspects of a hypothetical homeostatic system were missing. Especially, the variable that was being 'homeostatically managed' remained to be identified, as did the hypothetical setpoint for that variable. The next step in theory development involves an understanding of affect.

Affect: Mood and Emotion

The term 'affect' refers to feelings in general (Buchanan, 2007; Russell & Feldman Barrett, 1999). Affects may be further categorised into 'mood' and 'emotion', and each of these into positive and negative affect. Moods and emotions are distinguished by several features. Specifically, moods are primitive, genetic in origin, object-free, and chronic (Bower & Forgas, 2000; Oatley & Johnson-Laird 1987). Emotions are complex, acute, affective-cognitive-somatic responses to percepts or ideas (Russell, 2003; Scherer 2000). Moods and emotions also differ in that moods are low-intensity, background affects (Buchanan, 2007; Ekkekakis, 2013), while emotions may be high or low intensity (Forgas, 1995).

From this description, at a theoretical conceptual level, it makes logical sense that SWB comprises both mood and emotion. HPMood would represent the stable, genetically determined, individual difference factor which is unchanging. It is the phenotype of each person's setpoint genotype, and its level is their HPMood setpoint. The role of HPMood is to provide a low-level, background positive affect to consciousness. This proposal would account for both the chronic stability of SWB, as an individual difference, and its normal positivity due to its content (i.e., content, happy, alert).

Emotion, on the other hand, is the variable component of SWB. It is the product of information processing by sensory receptors (percepts) informing about the environment combined with information processing concerning thoughts about the self. This stream of emotion, comprising cognitive/affective information, constitutes a level of affect that is normally stronger than HPMood. Because of this, the changing information contained in the emotion can be recognised above the constant positivity of HPMood. The role of this emotion is to direct attention to new information by influencing the overall level and valence of affect in consciousness.

While this scenario has a logical appeal, the crucial evidence for HPMood setpoints was missing. While the issue of 'setpoints for SWB' had been the topic of speculation and inference for many years prior (Diener, Lucas, & Scollon; 2006; Lykken & Tellegen, 1996; McGue, Bacon, & Lykken, 1993), no direct empirical evidence for their existence had been produced. This changed with the publication of two papers, those by Cummins, Li, Wooden, and Stokes (2014) and by Capic, Li, and Cummins (2018). The first paper demonstrated the existence of setpoints for HPMood and the second paper provided confirmation.

The methodology used for both papers is much the same. Both papers employ longitudinal SWB data and engage a process called 'data-stripping'. The assumption underpinning this method is that variations in SWB are due to the emotion component, while the HPMood content remains stable. Thus, the iterative elimination of raw data from individual respondents, based on over-time confidence limits, selectively removes data that have been strongly influenced by emotion, leaving HPMood as the dominant component of the residue. A complete description of this methodology is provided by Capic and Cummins (2023). A crucial point to note, which is the source of misunderstanding for some authors (Headey, 2010), is that homeostasis theory does not claim a setpoint for SWB. The setpoint that has been demonstrated is for the HPMood component of SWB alone.

Resilience and Homeostasis

From the above description it is evident that the concepts of 'resilience' and 'SWB homeostasis' share a common theoretical base such that normal psychological functioning is stabilised and protected by a suite of devices that have evolved for that purpose. As an example of this commonality, Kunicki and Harlow (2020) note that 'resilience is commonly defined as positive adaption in the face of adversity' (p. 330). This observation is followed by a referentially intense text that concludes 'up to 20 different constructs may underlie resilience' (p. 331), listing most of the major constructs employed in SWB research. They then state that, 'for the purpose of this study, resilience was viewed from a trait perspective and defined as a higher-order construct comprised of the eight underlying constructs mentioned above' (p. 331).

In general agreement with these authors, their description is valid as far as it goes, but it fails to provide a coherent theoretical entity and platform for subsequent research. In accordance with the precepts of psychological science, such platforms provide the opportunity of disproof by critical results, rather than simply providing the basis for endless confirmatory analyses using correlational data. Homeostasis theory offers the opportunity for disproof through the following aspects:

1. Homeostasis theory goes beyond a general statement of 'positive adaptation' by proposing specific mechanisms of adaptation (Cummins, 2017).
2. Resilience theory has no single point of reference for the logic of why and how SWB recovers. Homeostasis theory does this through the reference level of HPMood, for each person, in the form of their setpoint. These setpoints have been calculated to exist as a normal distribution in population samples between 70 and 90 pp on a 0 to 100 pp scale (Capic et al., 2018; Cummins et al., 2014).
3. Unlike resilience, homeostasis theory explains why SWB is so stable. Stability is caused by the vigorous control over SWB levels such that they lie close to HPMood setpoints. Using Bayesian hierarchical modelling and longitudinal data, Anglim, Weinberg, and Cummins (2015) reported that the SWB of individuals generally fluctuated between about 2 and 3 pp either side of 75 pp.
4. Unlike resilience, the application of homeostasis theory allows us to understand why it is possible to create normative ranges for SWB. These ranges are presented for Australian data by Khor et al. (2020).

5. Unlike resilience, homeostasis theory promotes the creation of new kinds of understanding. For example, it proposes that HPMood is present not just in SWB but also within other self-report variables, such as those listed by Kunicki and Harlow (2020). Because HPMood is an individual difference variable, it is held at the same level within all such variables (e.g., optimism, self-esteem, etc.) for each person. Then, because this level of HPMood is a constant, at a different level for each individual, when data are grouped as a population sample, the HPMood content causes the self-report variables to correlate with one another. This phenomenon was noted more than 30 years ago by Meehl (1990), who dubbed such correlations the 'crud factor'.

The causal attribution of 'crud' caused by HPMood has been demonstrated by statistically removing the HPMood variance (see Cummins, 2020b). This publication shows the results from four separate studies, confirming that at least half of the variance responsible for the correlations between 10 different self-evaluative variables is HPMood. Moreover, in about half of these, the reduction is so severe after excising HPMood variance that the initially significant raw score correlation becomes nonsignificant.

Impersonal Resilience

In closing this account, it is notable that the description of homeostatic management has been restricted to the domain of psychological science and biology. The reason for omitting discussion related to community, economic, and environmental/ecological perspectives is that while these disciplines include considerations of resilience, their relationship to homeostasis is indirect. That is, while each of these areas supplies resources of relevance to homeostasis and discussion involving these areas has addressed the topic of stability in terms of open and closed systems (Cannon, 1932), ecological systems (Holling, 1973), and social systems in terms of dynamic systems theory (Carver, 1998; Vallacher & Nowak, 1997), none of them describes a homeostatic system. The essential components of homeostasis require a measurable setpoint variable, which is used as a reference point for a system of management, which normally maintains the managed variable within a narrow operating range. In sum, homeostasis is a system of management peculiar to the biological and psychological processes of organisms.

SUMMARY

Psychological homeostasis, as applied to SWB meets all the requirements for a defined, validated, and testable homeostatic system. In essence, as described within this chapter, SWB is a composite variable containing both emotion and mood. The emotion serves to inform the brain about relevant changes in the internal and external environment. The mood component is characterised as a composite of the three affects: happy, content, and alert. These combine to form HPMood, which is the phenotype of a genetically determined individual difference. HPMood exists as a weak, background affect that is present in all thoughts about the self, including SWB. Its purpose is to maintain a positive outlook in consciousness, and its level is unchanging within a narrow range, around a setpoint for each person. These setpoints are normally distributed within population samples between 70 and 90 pp, on a 0–100 scale of satisfaction (Capic et al., 2018). In summary, homeostasis theory includes units of measurement as well as ample opportunity for disproof.

There are many ways that the homeostasis proposition can be tested. One central proposition is that HPMood is present in all responses concerning general self-evaluations, such as self-esteem or SWB. This has substantial implications for interpreting results from publications involving multivariate, correlational statistics based on self-report variables. If the basis for such correlations is substantially due to HPMood, then the reported interactions using raw data are being misinterpreted (e.g., with self-esteem being highly correlated with extraversion). Rather, the true level of *substantive shared variance* between such variables can only be revealed after the shared variance of HPMood has been removed. For a detailed description of the methodology, see Capic and Cummins (2023).

This understanding has serious implications for interventions based on correlational data from self-report variables. For example, a substantial proportion of the positive psychology interventionist literature rests on self-determination theory (SDT; Deci & Ryan, 2000; Ryan & Deci, 2000; see also Cummins, 2016, for a critique). The central claim of SDT is that competence, autonomy, and relatedness are 'three basic psychological needs' which are postulated to be 'innate, essential, and universal' (Ryan & Deci, 2000, p. 74). Moreover, they state that 'a basic need . . . is an energizing state that, if satisfied, conduces toward health and well-being but, if not satisfied, contributes to pathology and ill-being'. Almost the entire evidential edifice of SDT is based on multivariate, correlational statistics based around the three 'basic needs' measured through self-report data. An interesting stress test for SDT would be to repeat key analyses supporting this proposition after removing the shared variance of HPMood.

In conclusion, the theory of subjective wellbeing homeostasis as an overarching, superordinate construct offers a simplified understanding of resilience. The core of psychological homeostasis is HPMood and the setpoint for each person that HPMood represents. An understanding of HPMood also has the potential to simplify psychology by greatly reducing the levels of automatic correlation between variables measured through self-report. After the variance contributed by HPMood has been removed, the residual strength of correlations will more closely represent the true nature of the common variance between such variables.

REFERENCES

Achenbaum, W. A., & Bengtson, V. L. (1994). Re-engaging the disengagement theory of aging: On the history and assessment of theory development in gerontology. *Gerontologist, 34*(6), 756–763.

Andrews, F. M., & Withey, S. B. (1976). *Social indicators of well-being: Americans' perceptions of life quality.* Plenum Press.

Anglim, J., Weinberg, M. K., & Cummins, R. A. (2015). Bayesian hierarchical modeling of the temporal dynamics of subjective well-being: A 10-year longitudinal analysis. *Journal of Research in Personality, 59*(3), 1–14.

Balmford, A. (1996). Extinction filters and current resilience: The significance of past selection pressures for conservation biology. *Trends in Ecology & Evolution, 11*(5), 193–196.

Block, J. (1981). Some enduring and consequential structures of personality. In A. I. Rabin (Ed.), *Further explorations in personality* (pp. 27–43). Wiley.

Bower, G. H., & Forgas, J. P. (2000). Affect, memory, and social cognition. In E. Eich, J. F. Kihlstrom, G. H. Bower, J. P. Forgas, & P. M. Niedenthal (Eds.), *Cognition and emotion* (pp. 87–168). Oxford University Press.

Bradburn, N. M. (1969). *The structure of psychological well-being.* Aldine.

Brim, O. G., & Kagan, J. (Eds.) (1980). *Constancy and change in human development.* Harvard University Press.

Buchanan, T. W. (2007). Retrieval of emotional memories. *Psychological Bulletin, 133*(5), 761–779.

Cannon, W. B. (1929). Organization for physiological homeostasis. *Physiological Reviews, 9*(3), 399–431.

Cannon, W. B. (1932). *The wisdom of the body.* Norton.

Capic, T., & Cummins, R. A. (2023). Discovering and confirming setpoints for homeostatically protected mood: An explanation of the methodology. In R. A. Cummins (Ed.), *Personal wellbeing index manual* (6th ed.) [Manuscript in preparation]. Australian Centre on Quality of Life, Deakin University.

Capic, T., Li, N., & Cummins, R. A. (2018). Confirmation of subjective wellbeing setpoints: Foundational for subjective social indicators. *Social Indicators Research, 137*(1), 1–28.

Carver, C. S. (1998). Resilience and thriving: Issues, models, and linkages. *Journal of Social Issues, 54,* 245–266.

Costa Jr P. T., & McCrae, R. R. (1980). Influence of extraversion and neuroticism on subjective well-being: Happy and unhappy people. *Journal of Personality and Social Psychology, 38*(4), 668–678. https://doi.org/10.1037/0022-3514.38.4.668

Cummins, R. A. (1995). On the trail of the gold standard for life satisfaction. *Social Indicators Research, 35*(2), 179–200.

Cummins, R. A. (1998). The second approximation to an international standard of life satisfaction. *Social Indicators Research, 43*(3), 307–334.

Cummins, R. A. (2003). Normative life satisfaction: Measurement issues and a homeostatic model. *Social Indicators Research, 64,* 225–256. https://doi.org/10.1023/A:1024712527648

Cummins, R. A. (2010). Subjective wellbeing, homeostatically protected mood and depression: A synthesis. *Journal of Happiness Studies, 11*(1), 1–17. https://doi.org/10.1007/s10902-009-9167-0

Cummins, R. A. (2016). *Self-determination theory and the theory of subjective wellbeing homeostasis: An examination of congruence.* Australian Centre on Quality of Life, Deakin University.

Cummins, R. A. (2017). Subjective wellbeing homeostasis. *Oxford Bibliographies Online.* https://www.oxfordbibliographies.com/view/document/obo-9780199828340/obo-9780199828340-0167.xml

Cummins, R. A. (2020a). Homeostasis and tipping points. *Australian Centre on Quality of Life Bulletin, 4*(40). http://www.acqol.com.au/publicationsbulletins

Cummins, R. A. (2020b). Unrealistic optimism. *Australian Centre on Quality of Life Bulletin, 4*(31). http://www.acqol.com.au/publicationsbulletins

Cummins, R. A. (2021). Likert scale developments. *Australian Centre on Quality of Life Bulletin, 5*(26). http://www.acqol.com.au/publicationsbulletins

Cummins, R. A., Li, L., Wooden, M., & Stokes, M. (2014). A demonstration of set-points for subjective wellbeing. *Journal of Happiness Studies, 15,* 183–206.

Cummins, R. A., & Nistico, H. (2002). Maintaining life satisfaction: The role of positive cognitive bias. *Journal of Happiness Studies, 3*(1), 37–69.

Damasio, A. (2018). *The strange order of things: Life, feeling, and the making of culture.* Pantheon Books.

Davern, M. T., Cummins, R. A., & Stokes, M. A. (2007). Subjective wellbeing as an affective-cognitive construct. *Journal of Happiness Studies, 8*(4), 429–449. https://doi.org/10.1007/s10902-007-9066-1

Deci, E. L., & Ryan, R. M. (2000). The "what" and "why" of goal pursuits: Human needs and the self-determination of behavior. *Psychological Inquiry, 11*(4), 227–268.

Diamantopoulos, A., & Winklhofer, H. M. (2001). Index construction with formative indicators: An alternative to scale development. *Journal of Marketing Research, 38*(2), 269–277.

Diener, E., Lucas, R. E., & Scollon, C. N. (2006). Beyond the hedonic treadmill: Revising the adaptation theory of well-being. *American Psychologist, 61*(4), 305–314.

Diener, E., Sandvik, E., Pavot, W., & Fujita, F. (1992). Extraversion and subjective well-being in a U.S. national probability sample. *Journal of Research in Personality, 26*(3), 205–215. https:doi.org/10.1016/0092-6566(92)90039-7

Ekkekakis, P. (2013). *The measurement of affect, mood, and emotion: A guide for health-behavioral research.* Cambridge University Press.

Forgas, J. P. (1995). Mood and judgment: The affect infusion model (AIM). *Psychological Bulletin, 117*(1), 39–66.

Hartmann, G. W. (1934). Personality traits associated with variations in happiness. *Journal of Abnormal and Social Psychology, 29,* 202–212.

Headey, B. (2010). The set point theory of well-being has serious flaws: On the eve of a scientific revolution. *Social Indicators Research, 97*(1), 7–21.

Headey, B., & Wearing, A. (1989). Personality, life events, and subjective well-being: Toward a dynamic equilibrium model. *Journal of Personality and Social Psychology, 57,* 731–739.

Holling, C. S. (1973). Resilience and stability of ecological systems. *Annual Review of Ecological Systems, 4,* 1–23.

International Wellbeing Group. (2013). *Personal wellbeing index manual* (5th ed.). Australian Centre on Quality of Life, School of Psychology, Deakin University.

Jackson, D. N., & Paunonen, S. V. (1980). Personality structure and assessment. *Annual Review of Psychology, 31,* 503–551. https://doi.org/10.1146/annurev.ps.31.020 180.002443

Khor, S., Fuller-Tysziewicz, M., & Hutchinson, D. (2020). Australian normative data for subjective wellbeing. In R. A. Cummins (Ed.), *Personal wellbeing index manual* (6th ed.). Australian Centre on Quality of Life, School of Psychology, Deakin University.

Kunicki, Z. J., & Harlow, L. L. (2020). Towards a higher-order model of resilience. *Social Indicators Research, 151,* 329–344.

Likert, R. (1932). A technique for the measurement of attitudes. *Archives in Psychology, 140,* 1–55.

Lykken, D. T., & Tellegen, A. (1996). Happiness is a stochastic phenomenon. *Psychological Science, 7*(3), 186–189.

McGue, M., Bacon, S., & Lykken, D. T. (1993). Personality stability and change in early adulthood: A behavioral genetic analysis. *Developmental Psychology, 29,* 96–109.

Meehl, P. E. (1990). Why summaries of research on psychological theories are often uninterpretable. *Psychological Reports, 66,* 195–244.

Merriam-Webster. (2021). *Online dictionary.* http://www.merriam-webster.com

Oatley, K., & Johnson-Laird, P. N. (1987). Towards a cognitive theory of emotions. *Cognition and Emotion, 1,* 29–50.

Renn, D., Pfaffenberger, N., Platter, M., Mitmansgruber, H., Höfer, S., & Cummins, R. A. (2009). International Well-being Index: The Austrian version. *Social Indicators Research, 90,* 243–256.

Romanovsky, A. A. (2007). Thermoregulation: Some concepts have changed. Functional architecture of the thermoregulatory system. *American Journal of Physiology-Regulatory, Integrative and Comparative Physiology, 292,* R37–R46.

Russell, J. A. (1980). A circumplex model of affect. *Journal of Personality and Social Psychology, 39,* 1161–1178.

Russell, J. A. (2003). Core affect and the psychological construction of emotion. *Psychological Review, 110,* 145–172.

Russell, J. A. (2009). Emotion, core affect, and psychological construction. *Cognition and Emotion, 23*(7), 1259–1283. https://doi.org/10.1080/02699930902809375

Russell, J. A., & Feldman Barrett, L. F. (1999). Core affect, prototypical emotional episodes, and other things called emotion: Dissecting the elephant. *Journal of Personality and Social Psychology, 76*(5), 805–819.

Ryan, R. M., & Deci, E. L. (2000). Self-determination theory and the facilitation of intrinsic motivation, social development, and well-being. *American Psychologist, 55*(1), 68–78.

Scheffer, M., Bolhuis, J. E., Borsboom, D., Buchman, T. G., Gijzel, S. M., Goulson, D., Kammenga, J. E., Kemp, B., van de Leemput, I. A., & Levin, S. (2018). Quantifying resilience of humans and other animals. *Proceedings of the National Academy of Sciences, 115*(47), 11883–11890.

Scherer, K. R. (2000). Psychological models of emotion. In J. C. Borod (Ed.), *The neuropsychology of emotion* (pp. 137–162). Oxford University Press.

Tiger, L. (1979). *Optimism: The biology of hope.* Simon & Schuster, Inc.

Vallacher, R. R., & Nowak, A. (1997). The emergence of dynamical social psychology. *Psychological Inquiry, 8,* 73–99.

Watson, G. B. (1930). Happiness among adult students of education. *Journal of Educational Psychology, 21,* 79–109.

Wessman, A. E., & Ricks, D. F. (1966). *Mood and personality.* Holt, Rinehart & Winston.

4

Evolution, Compassion, and Wellbeing

PAUL GILBERT ■

INTRODUCTION

Wellbeing is not easy to conceptualise or define (Dodge, Daly, Huyton, & Sanders, 2012). In their meta-analysis, Zessin, Dickhäuser, and Garbade (2015) referred to the distinction between subjective wellbeing, which is linked to positive affective states such as happiness and a sense of life satisfaction, and psychological wellbeing, which entails living a meaningful and purposeful life. These processes can diverge. For example, risking one's life to save others is unlikely to elicit feelings of happiness at the time but is a source of deep meaning that resonates with the person's values. Moreover, negative affect and psychopathology need to be studied separately because flourishing is not just the absence of pathology, and, indeed, individuals can flourish despite having mental health problems (Lamers, Westerhof, Glas, & Bohlmeijer, 2015).

While diverse, each of the aforementioned definitions places wellbeing very much 'within' the experience of an individual mind, but wellbeing can be extended to dyadic relationships, families, peer groups, and communities. Moreover, beyond the psychosocial, there are physical, societal, and environmental levels of wellbeing. Once again, it is quite possible for people to have one without the other. For example, one may be in a very positive frame of mind and not know one is actually dying of cancer, or even accept it as part of life; similarly, forms of head injury can be associated with denial of difficulties. Conversely, one may have positive physical wellbeing but not mental wellbeing.

In this chapter, I argue that all of these different experiences and processes, across the different domains, are influenced by caring motivation and connections. To feel cared for by others, to be caring of others, and to be caring of oneself are the foundations of wellbeing across its diverse conceptualisations.

Importantly, central to caring is compassion, which arises when we use our competencies for reasoning, empathy, and knowing awareness to intentionally try to alleviate and prevent suffering and distress and be helpful (Gilbert, 2019, 2020; Gilbert & Choden, 2013).

I begin this chapter by describing an evolutionary framework for understanding the biopsychosocial underpinnings of the emergence of compassion before making more explicit links between compassion and wellbeing, again using an integrative perspective. I then briefly describe some of the diverse approaches that can be utilised to build compassionate motivation in individuals. In the final section, I consider compassion at the societal level, contrasting 'controlling and holding' and 'caring and sharing' evolved social structures, and offer some suggestions on how we can move from the former to the latter.

AN EVOLUTIONARY FRAMEWORK OF COMPASSION: INTEGRATING BIOLOGICAL, PSYCHOLOGICAL, AND SOCIAL PROCESSES

The Evolution of Caring

Evolutionary processes provide the framework for understanding the biological underpinnings of caring, compassion, and wellbeing. The evolutionary process is driven by challenges to survival and reproduction (Workman, Reader, & Barkow, 2020). The earliest forms of reproduction were primarily to produce high numbers of offspring with high mortality. In the case of fish and turtles, for example, few will make it to adulthood to reproduce. A major change to reproductive strategies evolved with producing fewer offspring and greater parental investment, with consequent higher chances of survival to adulthood to reproduce (Geary, 2000). The central motivational system that facilitated this was *caring*. This produced organisms that were capable of *being caring* and were also *responsive to being cared for* (Cassidy & Shaver 2016; Gilbert, 1989/2016, 2005; Mayseless, 2016). Like all motivations, caring evolves as an algorithm. An algorithm is an *if* A *then* do B. At its simplest, the caring algorithm is a straightforward stimulus response algorithm of *if* signal/stimulus is one of distress or need, *then* take appropriate actions. For example, crocodiles can hear the sounds of their hatchlings, which trigger behaviours to pick them up and carry them to the water. Thereafter, no further caring behaviour emerges. In avian species, the open mouths of chicks trigger feeding behaviour. Hence, the evolution of caregiving required the evolution of feature detectors for specific signals of distress and need. In mammals, caregivers (mostly, but not always, the mother) evolved competencies to be sensitive to the signals of needs and distress (calls) of their infant(s) and to behave accordingly, such as to feed if hungry, keep warm if cold, and rescue/protect if in danger. For the infant's part, they need feature detectors for recognising and responding to parental behaviour and to be physiologically regulated as a result of these provisions. In other words, infants are able to detect, recognise, and be regulated through the interactions between themselves and the caregiver. In fact, there is now good evidence that the relationship between infants and their caregivers regulates a range of physiological systems (Hofer, 1984, 1994) and creates forms of synchrony in the physiological systems between caregivers and their children (Lunkenheimer, Tiberio, Skoranski, Buss, & Cole, 2018).

Gilbert (1989/2016, 2017a,b) refers to the caring motivational systems as a *social mentality* because the processes for giving and receiving have to co-evolve. Evolving ways of responding to an infant's distress but that the infant is nonresponsive to would not be adaptive. Equally, evolving ways of signalling distress and need, but where there is no response from another, or the signalling of distress only attracts predator attention, would not be adaptive. This is what is meant by co-evolution and co-regulation between caregiver and infant processes; they evolve together like lock and key. This also means that the caregiver and the care receiver basically engage in dynamic, reciprocal, interpersonal dances, exchanging signals that are mutually physiologically and behaviourally regulating. When these 'dances' go well—such that the caregiver experiences effectiveness and helpfulness from their behaviour, while the care receiver experiences relief from suffering and the meeting of one's needs—states of wellbeing arise that indicate this relationship is going well. Misattuned or more problematic interactions will conversely diminish wellbeing. In other words, the wellbeing of each depends on the interaction between them.

Integral to effective caring is compassion, which has been explored and defined in various ways (Gilbert, 2017a; Mascaro et al., 2020), including trying to identify clusters of phenomena (e.g., empathy and concern) associated with it (Strauss et al., 2016). The root of compassion is in caring behaviour (Gilbert, 2020). As previously stated, we can define caring, based on its evolved algorithm, as a sensitivity to distress and need that triggers appropriate behaviours to address them. From here we can define the algorithm of care-compassion as *a sensitivity to suffering in self and others with a commitment to try to alleviate and prevent it.* Although most definitions do not include the concept of prevention, it is implicit in the concept, which is why Gilbert and Choden (2013) made it explicit in their definition. Clearly, pursuing wellbeing at any moment is only part of the issue because one also wants to create the conditions for wellbeing in the future. Therefore, the prevention of suffering will be crucial to that endeavour.

From Caring to Compassion: The Evolution of a New Mind

While caring and compassion are linked, they vary in terms of their cognitive competencies and focus. Many animals who express and enact caring algorithms would not be described as compassionate. Mammals care for their offspring because of the activation of basic algorithms. So how do care and compassion vary? About a million years ago, en route to *Homo sapiens*, our ancestors quite rapidly evolved an extraordinary set of cognitive competencies that were to fundamentally affect the way all motivational systems are recruited and enacted. Gilbert

(2019, 2020, 2022) highlighted three types of cognitive competency identified by cognitive researchers from different fields, comprised of (1) reasoning, (2) empathy/mentalisation, and (3) consciousness of consciousness (mind awareness and mindfulness). These cognitive competencies are crucial to compassion.

First, humans have competencies for very complex forms of reasoning, including problem-solving, metacognition, and thinking in time (Baron-Cohen, 2020; Suddendorf, 2018). We use language and symbols to represent the world and to reason and think about the relationships in it. This is the basis of the 'scientific mind' that can not only understand the world but also change it by inventing technologies, from inventing wheels, bows, and arrows to building cities and discovering vaccines. We can also use our reasoning abilities to consider the impact that our behaviours will have. If I plant my potatoes, they will grow; if I study and practice guitar, I will get better. We can be aware that what we do today can impact our lives and those of others possibly years later (e.g., studying to pass exams to pursue a career). Clearly, our ability to reason about what is helpful versus harmful is essential for the compassionate creation of wellbeing.

A second crucial cognitive competency is mentalising (Kim, 2015; Luyten, Campbell, Allison, & Fonagy, 2020). 'Mentalisation' is an umbrella term that takes in empathy, theory of mind, and perspective-taking. It relates to the abilities to have insight into the processes occurring in one's own and other people's minds; it includes the awareness that we have motives, emotions, and beliefs that guide our (and other people's) actions. Many different species show clear indications that they can be sensitive to nonverbal signals of intention from their conspecifics (de Waal & Preston, 2017). For instance, subordinates can detect threat cues from those more dominant and back off, while, conversely, a dominant can read a submissive behaviour and reduce attacks. In the domain of caring, a mother can pick up on distress cues from her infant and provide care. More than this, however, rats have been shown to not pull a lever for food if, at the same time, a cage mate is given an electric shock, suggesting that seeing one's behaviour causing harm is aversive and can even override other motivational systems such as feeding (de Waal & Preston, 2017).

Whatever the degree of overlap in the capacities for empathy and mentalising between humans and those of other animals, ours is different because we have capacities for reasoning about the minds of others, with one aspect being able to imagine ourselves in their position (Kim, 2015; Luyten et al., 2020). This means that we are able to recognise that people do, feel, and think things because of motivation and history; that people can have intentions; and that people can deliberately deceive. With these competencies we can reason about relationships so that, for example, we are aware that if we care for our friends, this will build our relationship, but if we cheat or neglect them, our relationship will suffer.

Mentalisation enables insights into the nature of our own and others' minds (Kim, 2015; Luyten et al., 2020). While it is a competency, a bit like language, it has to be developed. It begins first with the child experiencing him- or herself as being accurately mentalised by another, usually the mother (Kim, 2015;

Luyten et al., 2020). Such experiences support wellbeing, whereas misattunements do not (Porges & Furman, 2011). Mentalisation supports wellbeing in multiple ways: when we experience that we feel understood and connected; when we show it to others, other people feel connected to us; and when we have it for ourselves, we can understand our minds and what helps us to move toward wellbeing or away from it. Put simply, the ability to understand the minds of others, to know that others understand us, and that we can outstand ourselves are important sources of wellbeing.

The third major competency is being conscious of being conscious, or aware that we are aware, which introduces new forms of self-awareness. It is the basis for mindfulness (Manuello, Vercelli, Nani, Costa, & Cauda, 2016) and mind awareness (Gilbert, 2019). This competency allows us to have a thought and know we are having a thought, or experience an emotion and know we are having an emotion. We are conscious of having the thought or an emotion in our field of consciousness. Many theorists have pointed out that we could have highly complex forms of reasoning and possibly forms of mentalisation based on algorithms, which artificial intelligence is now exploring, without needing to be conscious of these states. Indeed, we know that consciousness is actually quite a late stage in information processing (Bargh, 2017). There are also debates about the nature of consciousness itself (Harris, 2019). These controversies aside, from the point of view of wellbeing, there is now very good evidence that learning to be mindful of the contents of one's mind and 'being present' are associated with wellbeing (Gu, Strauss, Bond, & Cavanagh, 2015; Ivtzan & Lomas, 2016).

This form of consciousness gives rise to 'knowing intentionality', which in itself is a mystery. For example, lions clearly intend to hunt, kill their prey, and eat but they do not do so knowingly. They cannot observe themselves, question themselves, or decide that hunting is cruel and so they will become vegetarians. It is this knowing intentionality which is so crucial to the way which the human mind works. Psychological wellbeing depends on this competency because it is our knowing awareness that we exist as a self and that we can be in the mental state of happiness or suffering that is central to wellbeing. By being mindful of our actions means that we are more likely to be able to regulate movement in and out of states of wellbeing and distress.

Compassion emerges when caring motives are guided by these three competencies. For example, while we can care for our gardens, cars, or prized possessions, we do not have compassion for them if they are damaged. The concept of compassion is reserved for sentient beings and for the experience of suffering and primarily conscious suffering. Similarly, if we see wellbeing as the opposite of suffering (and this may not be the case in all situations), it only applies to sentient beings that can experience themselves (including their states of suffering versus wellness). Our competencies to mentalise the way we do recruit competencies of our conscious awareness and our abilities for types of reasoning.

In summary, caring becomes compassion when it utilises, on purpose, these competencies of reasoning, empathy/mentalisation, and consciousness of consciousness. We can use our reasoning to work out what will be helpful to ourselves and others and create conditions for wellbeing. Clearly, too, we can use our mentalising skills to work out what will be helpful to ourselves and others that will create the conditions for wellbeing. And we can use these skills with the conscious intention of creating wellbeing. Lacking these competencies would clearly impact our ability to create the conditions for wellbeing.

Figure 4.1 depicts three aspects central to compassion that utilise these competencies. First is *knowing awareness*: that is, we recognise signals of distress or need when we see them and are aware of what it is we are observing. Second, is *empathic awareness*, where we are aware that we can 'feel into' another person's state of mind, or we are aware that we need to find out more about the nature and source of somebody's suffering. Third, we *orientate* ourselves and act in ways with an intention, which in compassion is to address suffering and prevent it. If, on the other hand, the intention is vengeance, then we could use empathy to cause harm rather than relieve it.

Dodge, Daly, Huyton, and Sanders (2012) have proposed that wellbeing arises as:

> The balance point between an individual's resource pool and the challenges faced. . . . Stable wellbeing is when individuals have the psychological, social, and physical resources they need to meet a particular psychological, social, and/or physical challenge. When individuals have more challenges than resources, the see-saw dips, along with their wellbeing. . . . [Conversely] a lack of challenge will lead to stagnation, which will also affect the balance of the see-saw. (p. 230)

Since caring, compassionate connections afford individuals access to psychological, social, and physical resources, they are fundamental to the development of wellbeing.

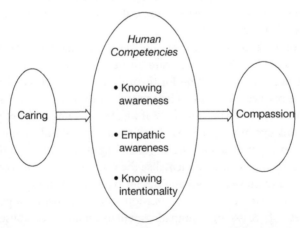

Figure 4.1 Biopsychosocial processes in the links between compassion and wellbeing.

Biological Underpinnings of Compassion and Wellbeing

The algorithms for caring, and its derivative compassion, evolved with a range of physiological systems that influence mental states (Brown & Brown, 2015; Mayseless, 2016), including the hormonal interplay of oxytocin and vasopressin (Carter, Bartal, & Porges, 2017), changes to the frontal cortex and cortical lateralisation (Schore, 2019; Trautwein, Kanske, Böckler, & Singer, 2020), and the myelination of part of the tenth cranial nerve of the parasympathetic system, referred to as the vagus nerve (Petrocchi & Cheli, 2019; Porges, 2007, 2017; Stellar & Keltner, 2017). Interestingly, physiological processes such as oxytocin and the vagus nerve, that evolved as part of caring motivational systems, also underpin different forms of wellbeing (Di Bello et al., 2020; Keltner, Kogan, Piff, & Saturn, 2014). Porges and colleagues (Porges, 2007, 2017; Porges & Furman, 2011) have written extensively on the way the evolution of the myelinated vagus nerve was essential for the development of caring behaviour. It enabled infant and parent to be close to each other and also for the caring behaviours of the parent to regulate the autonomic nervous system of the infant and facilitate experiences of safeness and safety. In this context, infants were liberated from vigilance to threat and able to explore. Hence, the evolution of the vagal nerve enabled positive mental states typically, but not only, stemming from caring and affection.

Not surprisingly, then, today some of our greatest sources of joy, happiness, flourishing, and wellbeing are through caring and compassionate connections. This is an extremely important message because neoliberalism tends to promote the idea that wellbeing and happiness are rooted to individuality, personal effort, and achievement, yet it is clear that individuals without caring connections experience high levels of loneliness and dysfunction (Cacioppo, Capitanio, & Cacioppo, 2014). Indeed, many authors have articulated the link between heart rate variability, positive social relating, and wellbeing (Beauchaine & Thayer, 2015; Di Bello et al., 2020; Keltner et al., 2014, Petrocchi & Cheli, 2019; Porges, 2017; Stellar & Keltner 2017). More recently, social relationships and the quality of our vagal nerve have been shown to play a major role in our abilities to cope both psychologically and physiologically with COVID-19 (Dedoncker, Vanderhasselt, Ottaviani, & Slavich, 2021).

Caring Connections, Biopsychosocial Development, and Wellbeing

The evolution of caring for offspring not only enabled infants to receive help and resources for physical development in the provisioning of food, comfort, and protection but also provided the context for psychosocial development. More than 50 years ago John Bowlby (1969) and Mary Ainsworth (1969) developed what they called *attachment theory* (see Cassidy and Shaver [2016] for a review). This highlighted the fact that (across species) a caring parent provides a number of resources to their young that impact its subsequent psychosocial maturation. These include a 'secure base', which enables the young to rely on the parent to detect threat and offer protection and from which they can begin to explore their environment and return to for support and guidance to learn and practice the skills necessary for adult life. The caring parent also provides a 'safe haven' to comfort the young when distressed or needy, from which the young learn the regulate their own emotions.

In the human context, a secure base and safe haven provide multiple inputs to the child including encouragement and support and also signals of joy, love, and affection. These enable a child to internalise a sense of their own acceptability and lovability in the eyes of others, which builds social confidence (Cassidy & Shaver, 2016; Music, 2017). This is a fundamental platform for later wellbeing because the child has the confidence to build supportive relationships. Sadly, children who do not receive such inputs are more threat sensitive, threat vigilant, and less trusting, each of which can compromise wellbeing (Cassidy & Shaver, 2016; Music, 2017). Stated briefly, then, compassionate care early in life can have a profound effect on our capacities to build wellbeing later in life, while conversely, experiences of early adversity such as child abuse and neglect can increase the risk of mental health problems across the lifespan. Indeed, these impacts can be transmitted beyond the directly affected individual to their offspring (Cowan, Callaghan, Kan, & Richardson, 2016). This intergenerational transmission might be due to behavioural mechanisms (e.g., people with experiences of childhood abuse are at risk of problems in their own parenting, such as higher emotional disengagement) and/or epigenetic pathways. In short, feeling safe and connected in the world impacts greatly on our own physical and mental health and wellbeing and potentially that of subsequent generations (Slavich, 2020).

One way to consider these processes is that early affection, love, and care orientate the child to adopt strategies for *caring and sharing* and building supportive communities around him- or herself. Developing a caring, sharing lifestyle is linked to a greater sense of purpose, wellbeing, and happiness (Mikulincer & Shaver, 2017; Narvaez, 2017; Nelson, Layous, Cole, & Lyubomirsky, 2016; Ryan, 2019). These will marinate the child in the behaviours that stimulate physiological systems that are conducive to positive affect and wellbeing. Individuals who come from less caring and compassionate backgrounds tend to see the world as a more indifferent or competitive place and focus on the need for individual achievement and personal struggle, which increases risk of mental health problems and antisocial behaviour (Cassidy & Shaver, 2016).

The Inter- and Intrapersonal Flows of Compassion and Wellbeing

Most motives and emotions have interpersonal and intrapersonal flow. For instance, I can be angry with you, you can be angry with me, and I can be angry with myself. Compassion also has flow, in that we can be compassionate to others, we can be open and receptive to the compassion from others, and we can be compassionate to ourselves.

Looking briefly at each of these in turn, there is now growing evidence that being compassionate and helpful to others is associated with wellbeing and psychological flourishing (Nelson et al., 2016; Schacter & Margolin, 2019). As is clear from the focus above, there is considerable evidence that having access to caring, supportive relationships and connections has a range of physiological benefits for mental and physical health (Brown & Brown, 2015; Ditzen & Heinrichs, 2014; Slavich, 2020). In addition, feeling socially safe is linked to feeling positively socially connected to others (Kelly, Zuroff, Leybman, & Gilbert, 2012), and social safeness may be an emotion regulation process in its own right (Armstrong, Nitschke, Bilash, & Zuroff, 2020). These, in turn, are linked to the degree to which individuals perceive others as being sensitive to their distress, empathic, and have desires to be helpful. In contrast to these compassion-based connections, we can experience socially disconnecting and uncaring relationships with others such that we experience or anticipate rejection, being criticised or shamed, and feeling isolated and lonely. These processes of social disconnection have long been identified as increasing risks of physical and mental illness and poor wellbeing (Cacioppo & Patrick, 2008).

These processes speak to the availability of caring connections, but there is also the issue of social trust (Luyten et al., 2020) and the openness and responsiveness to receive care and compassion from others (Hermanto, & Zuroff, 2016). Fear of receiving compassion, even if it is available, is associated with mental health problems (Kirby, Day, & Sagar, 2019). People can be frightened to reach out for help because they are ashamed to admit they need it, are ashamed of what they are feeling, or fear becoming obligated.

Last but not least is the finding that how we experience and relate to ourselves plays a fundamental role in wellbeing. We can form compassionate, supportive, and helpful relationships with ourselves and can be sensitive, empathic, and orientated to be helpful to ourselves, with self-compassion found to be associated with wellbeing (Neff, 2011; Zessin et al., 2015).

Compassion as Prevention of Suffering and the Bridge to Wellbeing

In 2013, Gilbert and Choden introduced the concept of prevention into standard definitions of compassion. This produced a significant expansion in the focus and orientation of compassion to address 'needs'. To use a simple illustration, if one does not adequately feed one's baby, then the baby will suffer and potentially die; so, to prevent suffering, a compassionate response must address the need for food. But what about psychological needs? Using the same logic, we can say that if a child's psychological needs, particularly for a secure base and safe haven, are not met, then they will suffer. It is but a small step, then, to see that there are a variety of important psychological needs that, if not met, will generate suffering and, if met, will generate wellbeing. Indeed, in their important integrative chapter on linking compassion and wellbeing, Bohlmeijer and Westerhof (2020) note an important therapeutic observation. While in therapy, we hope to help people work on their mental health problems (e.g., depression and anxiety), but when we think of them in their life beyond therapy we want to think of them as more than just being free of mental health problems; we hope that they will be flourishing. There are many human needs that relate to our psychological wellbeing, and these can include the pursuit of meaning, the ability for creativity and self-expression, and being free from coercion and able to live with autonomy, to name just a few. The fact that intrinsic to compassion is helping ourselves and others to attain these wellbeing needs highlights the close interplay of these two constructs.

CULTIVATING COMPASSION

There are many reasons for cultivating compassion but one of them is the recognition that different motives organise the mind in quite different ways: what we pay attention to, the way we reason, our emotions, and our behavioural impulses will all be different if we are motivated to be, for example, competitive, vengeful, sexual, cooperative, or helpful. Some people with mental health difficulties can be overly rooted in fear-based or competitive motives, such as trying to avoid rejection or feel superior to others.

Compassion-focused therapy is a motivation therapy which aims to switch people's basic orientation from competitive striving and hostile, critical self-evaluation to one of caring and compassion (Gilbert, 2014; Gilbert & Simos, 2022; Sommers-Spijkerman, Trompetter, Schreurs, & Bohlmeijer, 2018). This form of therapy stresses the term 'focused' because it utilises many therapeutic interventions from other approaches but highlights the fact that if we can create a care-compassionate motive and mental state, then the intervention will be more effective. Imagine, for example, helping a person with agoraphobia by engaging in exposure exercises whereby the person enters feared situations such as crowded trains. Now imagine what would happen if you helped that person to understand the value of compassion, create a compassionate inner state to engage with the feared outside, and create an internal voice of kindness and supportiveness with encouragement that acts like a secure base and safe haven. The intervention remains similar, but the preparation and orientation for the intervention are different.

Part of compassion-focused therapy involves helping people understand the nature of our evolved brain, which can be very tricky, and how we can get overly absorbed into motivational systems that can be unhelpful. Insight into this enables clients to begin to recognise the value of switching to and cultivating caring and compassion motives because of their physiological as well as psychological benefits. Hence, psychoeducation plays an important early role in orientating people to compassion training and therapy.

There are then many standard and creative interventions to cultivate and experience the activation of the caring-compassion motivational system which orientates people to try to live to be helpful and not harmful. Compassion-focused therapy and compassionate mind training are multifactorial, encompassing interventions orientated to physiological, psychological, and social processes. Several techniques use the body to support the mind: helping people understand that the states of the brain and the body influence the contents of our minds highlights the importance of attending to them. For example, we now know that diets and breathing techniques can influence the vagus nerve and mental states and wellbeing (Bonaz, Bazin, & Pellissier, 2018; Porges & Dana, 2018). Other practices, such as mindfulness practice, are designed to target our new brain competencies to support mind awareness, mindfulness mentalisation, and rational (helpful) thinking (Gilbert & Choden, 2013). There are also practices for reflecting on the core qualities of compassion and imagining having them, embodying them, and remembering to tune into them and practice thinking and acting from that pattern of self (i.e., the compassionate mind). This is creating a compassionate identity which has considerable overlap with certain Buddhist concepts, particularly Bodhicitta (Gilbert, 2017a). Compassionate letter-writing is one behavioural strategy that can be used to cultivate a more compassionate voice and produce increases in happiness and decreases in depression (Shapira & Mongrain, 2010). Many compassionate practices use visualisations and meditations on a theme of relating. Loving kindness meditations are very common in this regard and entail imagining extending loving kindness and wishes for others to be happy and free of suffering (Neff & Germer, 2018). There is good evidence that practicing these visualisations increases positive emotions (Zeng, Chiu, Wang, Oei, & Leung, 2015) and social connectedness (Hutcherson, Seppala, & Gross, 2008) and triggers beneficial changes in our physiological systems (Hofmann, Grossman, & Hinton, 2011; Matos et al., 2017; Matos, Duarte, Duarte, Gilbert, & Pinto-Gouveia, 2018).

COMPASSION IN SOCIETY

Many commentators have highlighted the fact that COVID-19 witnessed an outpouring of compassion, with people such as frontline healthcare workers risking their health and lives to save others. In fact, these healthcare workers had at least a threefold greater risk of being infected with COVID-19 than the general community (Nguyen et al., 2020). Many others involved themselves in helping people who might need extra support or were living alone. This has raised hope that the tide against neoliberalism and the 'me first' society might be on the turn. Although we can recognise that the world today is considerably more compassionate than it was, for example, during the dominance of the Roman Empire with its slavery, gladiatorial games, and crucifixions, we are also aware that we still have serious inhibitions on compassion at societal and national levels (Gilbert, 2021).

From 'Caring and Sharing' to 'Controlling and Holding'
Evolved Strategies

One of the reasons is because our compassionate mind was 'tuned' in our hunter-gatherer evolutionary period from around 1,000,000 years ago. We are basically designed for small-group living, where caring and sharing are an essential means of survival (Dunbar, 2014; Ryan, 2019). This style of living influenced childcare, which became a community concern and source of social safeness and playfulness (Narvaez, 2017). In addition, humans moved away from the typical primate aggressiveness, as central to the emergence of dominant hierarchies and the regulation of resource access, to an egalitarian care-and-share social structure. Here, status hierarchies were based primarily on how one contributed to the group rather than on what one took out of it. There is increasing evidence that the lives of many (but not all) hunter-gatherers were probably socially less stressful and more cooperative and caring than perhaps we see today. For the majority of people, this is very much reflected today in that we would prefer to have our relationships based on feeling valued, wanted, and desired rather than on people being frightened of us. Indeed, humans compete to be chosen, to be seen as attractive, talented, able and desirable, which also means they will contribute to a relationship rather than take from it.

The advent of agriculture was to change the dynamics of social relating because we went from a context of scarcity and immediate resource use to one of increasing resource availability, storage and wealth accumulation, and group size growth. This context facilitated the re-emergence of aggressive dominant males to control social structure and resource access. All of the major empires have had dominant and often aggressive males (sometimes, but rarely, females) as part of the dominant elite. They operated terror regimes to suppress those below them. Even today there are aggressive male leaders who are killing, locking up, and torturing protesters and opponents. We are inheritors of systems where elites have manipulated both social discourses and persecutory structures that supress the poor. We live in a world of vastly unequal resource access where the elites constantly justify the claim on their millions and billions (Wilkinson & Pickett, 2010). Reich (2018), who was secretary of labour for President Clinton, has documented the extensive and highly callous behaviours in business and politics that have proliferated in the past 40 years, particularly under right-wing regimes. These regimes have seriously moved away from 'working for the common good' to working for pure self-interest only. He outlines in detail the damage this has done to a sense of social trust and the degree to which we perceive politics and business as invested in creating compassionate societies. High-resource environments invite privileged individuals who are relatively ruthless and manipulative and have what are called the 'dark triad' of Machiavellianism, narcissism, and psychopathy (Harrison, Summers, & Mennecke, 2018). These are individuals who are purely self-focused with little interest in the needs of others. They are callous in the sense that they are insensitive to the suffering of others, are not concerned if they cause it, and are not interested in alleviating it. Reich (2018) offers numerous examples from presidents like Richard Nixon, to examples within business and banking and the asset strippers of the 1980s that put many people out of work. Amongst them are individuals who deny problems such as climate change because it interferes with their self-focused narcissistic agendas. Reich (2018) notes that what has been lost is any interest in working for the common good, which is the basis of a compassionate society. In his BBC Reith lectures, previous governor of the Bank of England Mark Carney (2021) made essentially the same point that we have become overly focused on financial values rather than human values to the detriment of all. In addition, there is increasing evidence that, as people become wealthier, they actually become less compassionate not more because they switch to a control and hold (rather than care and share) way of thinking about their relationship to the resources they have (Piff, Kraus, & Keltner, 2018).

Harnessing Compassion to Challenge Harmful Power Structures

One of the key dimensions of a compassionate society, and one that will underpin its wellbeing, is to recall that compassion is partly about the prevention of harm and suffering. Indeed, there is some evidence that hunter-gatherer societies created caring and sharing by suppressing, shunning, and excluding (possibly killing) aggressive, narcissistic individuals. Boehm (1999, 2000) argues that a shift into egalitarian ways of living partly came in the way alliances between the more subordinate individuals could be used to depose bullies. As Boehm (2000) writes,

> Humans can remain egalitarian only if they consciously suppress innate tendencies that otherwise would make for a pronounced social dominance hierarchy. In effect, it is necessary for a large power-coalition (the rank and file of a band) to dominate the group's would-be 'bullies' if egalitarianism is to prevail—otherwise, the group will become hierarchical with marked status differences and strong leadership. On this basis, it can be argued that humans are innately disposed to despotism in Vehrencamp's ethological sense of the word. My point is that humans are not just naturally egalitarian: if we wish to keep social hierarchy at a low level, we must act as intentional groups that vigilantly curtail alpha-type behaviours. This curtailment is accomplished through the cultural agency of social sanctioning . . . , so political egalitarianism is the product of morality. (p. 84)

Increasingly, commentators today are highlighting the fact that if we do not find ways to suppress the narcissism of the dominant elites, then it is difficult to move toward fairer and more caring societies (Reich, 2018; Wilson, 2019). As strange as it may seem, then, a compassionate society progresses not only because of the motivation of individuals but also how it inhibits ruthless narcissism, which is so rampant in Western neoliberal societies, not to mention corruption in many parts of the world. If compassion is seen as somehow weak or simply about kindness, then it completely misses the point that it is one of the most moral and courageous of all of our motivations. It is the motivation that means we cannot stand by while we watch others behave in ways that are destructive and cause suffering to others. As of yet, however, we are wrestling with these problems because, in the face of a right-wing press that constantly stimulates conflict and the rise of populism, those who pursue compassion have their work cut out for them.

Solutions?

Nonetheless, there are solutions (Gilbert, 2021; Wilson, 2019), some examples of which I offer here. First, there are an increasing number of compassion movements including how to build social justice (Atkinson, McKenzie, & Winlow, 2017; Wilson 2019); compassion in farming (www.ciwf.org.uk); creating compassionate-sensitive workplaces (Worline & Dutton, 2017); and cultivating compassionate, sustainable, and moral businesses rather than exploitative ones (Carney, 2021; Friedman, & Gerstein, 2017; Sachs, 2012; Solomon, 2001). For example, Compassion in Politics (www.compassioninpolitics.com) is interacting with members of parliament, highlighting ideas that policies should not be passed which will knowingly cause difficulty to those least able to defend against it. If this had been agreed upon at the time of the global financial crisis, then austerity measures would never have happened because, as the United Nations has pointed out, it was aspects of the elite-run banking and financial services that caused the problem (even though those who suffered the most were the poor while the wealthiest emerged relatively unpunished). As Sachs (2012) highlights, there are problems with the links between political lobbyists, right-wing media, and economic policies, but these can be broken up, and a compassionate economics and politics can become a guiding principle.

Second, although there are problems with leaders within business, there is also an emerging group of leaders who understand the importance of sustainability and that business can support human values, not just finances, and who seek to be a contributor to humanity not harmful to it through business practices (Mellahi, Morrell, & Wood, 2010). A perusal on the Internet will reveal many businesses that are now pursuing what they regard as moral and ethical businesses, building in safeguards against those individuals who can be harmful to business. These businesses not only are mindful of the nature of what they produce and how they produce it but also of those who work for them, and they seek to create supportive working communities (Worline & Dutton, 2017). In addition, stakeholders and shareholders are gradually beginning to think about responsibility and pay attention to the businesses they are involved with, on ethical rather than purely fiscal grounds. Hence the growing interest in green and ethical business (socially responsible) investment (Ransome & Sampford, 2010).

Third is to help build local compassionate communities. For example, Costello (2018) worked with Asian and African countries and developed what he called 'sympathy groups'. These bring people together to inform and then help each other address health problems. One example is facilitating women to come together in certain villages to support childcare that impacts on child complications and postnatal depression difficulties, amongst other problems. Such innovations can be a blueprint for building local compassion communities in general, but they do need facilitators. How these individuals should be trained and funded is a key challenge.

Fourth is recognition that compassion needs to begin in schools by training young people in the nature of a compassionate mind. When I and my children were growing up, there was no insight or education about the most complex and potentially dangerous organ in the universe, which is the human brain. In my involvement with compassion training programmes in schools, there is still resistance because of time pressures and the immense competitiveness that teachers and children are subject to (Coles & Gent, 2020; Gilbert, Matos, Wood, & Maratos, 2020). If we educate children in self-focused competitiveness, which education promotes at the moment, we should not be surprised if that is the type of person who emerges into the working environment, particularly those who come from privileged backgrounds. On the other hand, if we facilitate children to grow in environments of sharing and caring, then those are the values that they are likely to take into their working and social lives (Coles & Gent, 2020).

SUMMARY

This chapter highlighted how compassion evolved out of caring and how both are linked to the organisations of brains, bodies, and minds. It is because compassion is focused on suffering *and* the prevention of suffering, and hence attending to human needs, that it can underpin wellbeing. In addition, when looked at from a prevention of suffering point of view, it offers a lens into multidimensional human activities from politics to businesses to education to personal practices. An understanding of the real nature of compassion offers opportunities for building courageous wisdom as a source of wellbeing in ourselves, our personal relationships, communities, and, ultimately, all nations. The past 20 years have seen many developments in compassion training. Some of these have focused on working with individuals to address stress and mental health problems, but increasingly the psychology of compassion can be used to promote wellbeing in schools, workplaces, social communities, and, ultimately, in nations themselves. Put another way, the social flow of compassion, in how we create caring relations and communities, is one of the most profound sources of wellbeing and happiness.

REFERENCES

Ainsworth, M. D. S. (1969). Object relations, dependency, and attachment: A theoretical review of the infant-mother relationship. *Child Development*, *40*, 969–1025.

Atkinson, R., McKenzie, L., & Winlow, W. (2017). *Building better societies: Promoting social justice in the world falling apart*. Policy Press.

Armstrong III, B. F., Nitschke, J. P., Bilash, U., & Zuroff, D. C. (2020). An affect in its own right: Investigating the relationship of social safeness with positive and negative affect. *Personality and Individual Differences*, 109670. doi:10.1016/j.paid.2019.109670

Bargh, J. (2017). *Before you know it: The unconscious reasons we do what we do*. Simon and Schuster.

Baron-Cohen, S. (2020). *The pattern seekers: A new theory of human invention*. Allen Lane.

Beauchaine, T. P., & Thayer, J. F. (2015). Heart rate variability as a transdiagnostic biomarker of psychopathology. *International Journal of Psychophysiology*, *98*(2), 338–350. doi:10.1016/j.ijpsycho.2015.08.004

Boehm, C. (1999). *Hierarchy in the forest: The evolution of egalitarian behavior*. Cambridge, MA: Harvard University Press.

Boehm, C. (2000). Conflict and the evolution of social control. *Journal of Consciousness Studies*, *7*(1–2), 79–101.

Bohlmeijer, E. T., & Westerhof, G. J. (2020). A new model for sustainable health integrating well-being into psychological treatment. In J. Kirby & P. Gilbert (Eds.), *Making an impact on mental health: The applications of psychological research* (pp. 153–188). Routledge.

Bonaz, B., Bazin, T., & Pellissier, S. (2018). The vagus nerve at the interface of the microbiota-gut-brain axis. *Frontiers in Neuroscience*, *12*, 49. doi:10.3389/fnins.2018.00049

Bowlby, J. (1969). *Attachment and loss, Vol. 1: Attachment*. Basic Books.

Brown, S. L., & Brown, R. M. (2015). Connecting prosocial behavior to improved physical health: Contributions from the neurobiology of parenting. *Neuroscience and Biobehavioral Reviews*, *55*, 1–17. doi:10.1016/j.neubiorev.2015.04.004

Cacioppo, S., Capitanio, J. P., & Cacioppo, J. T. (2014). Toward a neurology of loneliness. *Psychological Bulletin*, *140*(6), 1464–1504. doi:10.1037/a0037618

Cacioppo, J. T., & Patrick, W. (2008). *Loneliness. Human nature and the need for social connection*. W. W. Norton & Company.

Carney, M. (2021). *How we get what we value*. BBC Reith Lectures. https://www.bbc.co.uk/programmes/m000py8t

Carter, S., Bartal, I. B., & Porges, E. (2017). The roots of compassion: an evolutionary and neurobiological perspective. In E. M. Seppälä, E. Simon-Thomas, S. L. Brown, & M. C. Worline (Eds.), *The Oxford handbook of compassion science* (pp. 178–188). Oxford University Press.

Cassidy, J., & Shaver, P. R. (2016). *Handbook of attachment: Theory, research and clinical applications* (3rd ed.). Guilford.

Coles, M. I., & Gent. B. (Eds). (2020). *Education for survival: The pedagogy of compassion*. University College London Institute of Education Press.

Costello, A. (2018). *The social edge: The power of sympathy groups for our health, wealth and sustainable future*. Thornwick.

Cowan, C. S. M., Callaghan, B. L., Kan, J. M., & Richardson, R. (2016). The lasting impact of early-life adversity on individuals and their descendants: Potential mechanisms and hope for intervention. *Genes, Brain and Behavior, 15*(1), 155–168. doi:10.1111/gbb.12263

Dedoncker, J., Vanderhasselt, M. A., Ottaviani, C., & Slavich, G. M. (2021). Mental health during the COVID-19 pandemic and beyond. The importance of the vagus nerve for biopsychosocial resilience. *Neuroscience & Biobehavioral Reviews, 125*, 1–10. doi:10.1016/j.neubiorev.2021.02.010

de Waal, F. B., & Preston, S. D. (2017). Mammalian empathy: Behavioural manifestations and neural basis. *Nature Reviews Neuroscience, 18*(8), 498–509. doi:10.1038/nrn.2017.72

Di Bello, M. D., Carnevali, L., Petrocchi, N., Thayer, J. F., Gilbert, P., & Ottaviani C. (2020). The compassionate vagus: A meta-analysis on the connection between compassion and heart rate variability. *Neuroscience Biobehavioral Review, 116*, 21–30. doi:10.1016/j.neubiorev.2020.06.016

Ditzen, B., & Heinrichs, M. (2014). Psychobiology of social support: The social dimension of stress buffering. *Restorative Neurology and Neuroscience, 32*(1), 149–162. doi:10.3233/RNN-139008

Dodge, R., Daly, A., Huyton, J., & Sanders, L. (2012). The challenge of defining wellbeing. *International Journal of Wellbeing, 2*, 222–235. doi:10.5502/ijw.v2i3.4

Dunbar, R. (2014). *Human evolution: A Pelican introduction*. Penguin.

Friedman, H. H., & Gerstein, M. (2017). Leading with compassion: The key to changing the organizational culture and achieving success. *Psychosociological Issues in Human Resource Management, 5*(1), 160–175.

Geary, D. C. (2000). Evolution and proximate expression of human parental investment. *Psychological Bulletin, 126*, 55–77. doi:10.1037/0033-2909.126.1.55

Gilbert, P. (1989/2016). *Human nature and suffering*. Routledge.

Gilbert, P. (2005). *Compassion: Conceptualisations, research and use in psychotherapy*. Routledge.

Gilbert, P. (2014). The origins and nature of compassion-focused therapy. *British Journal of Clinical Psychology, 53*, 6–41. doi:10.1111/bjc.12043

Gilbert, P. (2017a). Compassion: Definitions and controversies. In P. Gilbert (Ed.), *Compassion: Concepts, research and applications* (pp. 3–15). Routledge/Taylor & Francis Group.

Gilbert, P. (2017b). Compassion as a social mentality: An evolutionary approach. In P. Gilbert (Ed.), *Compassion: Concepts, research and applications* (pp. 31–68). Routledge/Taylor & Francis Group.

Gilbert, P. (2019). Psychotherapy for the 21st century: An integrative, evolutionary, contextual, biopsychosocial approach. *Psychology and Psychotherapy: Theory, Research and Practice, 92*, 164–189. doi:10.1111/papt.12226

Gilbert, P. (2020). Compassion: From its evolution to a psychotherapy. *Frontiers in Psychology, 11*, 3123. doi:10.3389/fpsyg.2020.586161

Gilbert, P. (2021). Creating a compassionate world: Addressing the conflicts between sharing and caring versus controlling and holding evolved strategies. *Frontiers in Psychology, 11*, 3572. doi:10.3389/fpsyg.2020.582090

Gilbert, P. (2022). The evolved functions of caring connections as a basis for compassion. In P. Gilbert & G. Simos (Eds.), *Compassion focused therapy: Clinical practice and applications*. Routledge.

Gilbert, P., & Choden. (2013). *Mindful compassion*. Little Brown.

Gilbert, P., Matos, M., Wood, W., & Maratos, F. (2020). The compassionate mind and the conflicts between competing and caring: Implications for educating young minds. In M. I. Coles & B. Gent (Eds.), *Education for survival: The pedagogy of compassion* (pp. 44–76). Institute of Education Press University College London.

Gilbert, P., & Simos, G. (2022). *Compassion focused therapy: Clinical practice and applications*. Routledge.

Gu, J., Strauss, C., Bond, R., & Cavanagh, K. (2015). How do mindfulness-based cognitive therapy and mindfulness-based stress reduction improve mental health and wellbeing? A systematic review and meta-analysis of mediation studies. *Clinical Psychology Review, 37*, 1–12. doi:10.1016/j.cpr.2015.01.006

Harris, A. (2019). *Consciousness a brief guide of the fundamental mystery of the mind*. HarperCollins.

Harrison, A., Summers, J., & Mennecke, B. (2018). The effects of the dark triad on unethical behavior. *Journal of Business Ethics, 153*, 53–77. doi:10.1007/s10551-016-3368-3

Hermanto, N., & Zuroff, D. C. (2016). The social mentality theory of self-compassion and self-reassurance: The interactive effect of care-seeking and caregiving. *Journal of Social Psychology, 156*(5), 523–535. doi:10.1080/00224545.2015.1135779

Hofer, M. A. (1984). Relationships as regulators: A psychobiologic perspective on bereavement. *Psychosomatic Medicine, 46*, 183–197. doi:10.1097/00006842-1984050000-00001

Hofer, M. A. (1994). Early relationships as regulators of infant physiology and behavior. *Acta Paediatrica, 397*, 9–18. doi:10.1111/j.1651-2227.1994.tb13260.x

Hofmann, S. G., Grossman, P., & Hinton, D. E. (2011). Loving-kindness and compassion meditation: Potential for psychological interventions. *Clinical Psychology Review, 31*, 1126–1132. doi:10.1016/j.cpr.2011.07.003

Hutcherson, C. A., Seppala, M., & Gross, J. J. (2008). Loving-kindness meditation increases social connectedness. *Emotion, 8*, 720–724. doi:10.1037/a0013237

Ivtzan, I., & Lomas, T. (Eds.). (2016). *Mindfulness in positive psychology: The science of meditation and wellbeing*. Routledge.

Kelly, A. C., Zuroff, D. C., Leybman, M. J., & Gilbert, P. (2012). Social safeness, received social support, and maladjustment: Testing a tripartite model of affect regulation. *Cognitive Therapy and Research, 36*, 815–826. doi:10.1007/s10608-011-9432

Keltner, D., Kogan, A., Piff, P. K., & Saturn, S. R. (2014). The sociocultural appraisals, values, and emotions (SAVE) framework of prosociality: Core processes from gene to meme. *Annual Review of Psychology, 65*, 425–460. doi:10.1146/annurev-psych-010213-115054

Kim, S. (2015). The mind in the making: Developmental and neurobiological origins of mentalizing. Personality disorders: *Theory, research, and treatment, 6*(4), 356–365. doi:10.1037/per0000102

Kirby, J. N., Day, J., & Sagar, V. (2019). The 'flow' of compassion: A meta-analysis of the fears of compassion scales and psychological functioning. *Clinical Psychology Review, 70*, 26–39. doi:10.1016/j.cpr.2019.03.001

Lamers, S. M. A., Westerhof, G. J., Glas, C. A. W, &. Bohlmeijer, E. T. (2015). The bidirectional relation between positive mental health and psychopathology in a longitudinal representative panel study. *The Journal of Positive Psychology, 10*, 553–560. doi:10.1080/17439760.2015.1015156

Lunkenheimer, E., Tiberio, S. S., Skoranski, A. M., Buss, K. A., & Cole, P. M. (2018). Parent-child coregulation of parasympathetic processes varies by social context and risk for psychopathology. *Psychophysiology, 55*(2), e12985. doi:10.1111/psyp.12985

Luyten, P., Campbell, C., Allison, E., & Fonagy, P. (2020). The mentalizing approach to psychopathology: State of the art and future directions. *Annual Review of Clinical Psychology, 16,* 297–325. doi:10.1146/annurev-clinpsy-071919-015355

Manuello, J., Vercelli, U., Nani, A., Costa, T., & Cauda, F. (2016). Mindfulness meditation and consciousness: An integrative neuroscientific perspective. *Consciousness and Cognition, 40,* 67–78. doi:10.1016/j.concog.2015.12.005

Mascaro, J. S., Florian, M. P., Ash, M. J., Palmer, P. K., Frazier, T., Condon, P., & Raison, C. (2020). Ways of knowing compassion: How do we come to know, understand, and measure compassion when we see it? *Frontiers in Psychology, 11,* 547241. doi:10.3389/fpsyg.2020.547241

Matos, M., Duarte, C., Duarte, J., Pinto-Gouveia, J., Petrocchi, N., Basran, J., & Gilbert, P. (2017). Psychological and physiological effects of compassionate mind training: A pilot randomised controlled study. *Mindfulness, 8*(6), 1699–1712. doi:10.1007/s12671-017-0745-7

Matos, M., Duarte, J., Duarte, C., Gilbert, P., & Pinto-Gouveia, J. (2018). How one experiences and embodies compassionate mind training influences its effectiveness. *Mindfulness, 9*(4), 1224–1235. doi:10.1007/s12671-017-0864-1

Mayseless, O. (2016). *The caring motivation: An integrated theory.* Oxford University Press.

Mellahi, K., Morrell, K., & Wood, G. (2010). *The ethical business: Challenges and controversies.* Red Globe Press.

Mikulincer, M., & Shaver, P. R. (2017). An attachment perspective on optimism and altruism. In P. Gilbert (Ed.), *Compassion: Concepts, research and applications* (pp. 187–202). Routledge/Taylor & Francis Group.

Music, G. (2017). *Nurturing natures: Attachment and children's emotional, sociocultural and brain development.* (2nd ed.). Routledge.

Narvaez, D. (2017). Evolution, child raising and compassionate morality. In P. Gilbert (Ed.), *Compassion: Concepts, research and applications* (p. 31–68) Routledge/Taylor & Francis Group.

Neff, K. D. (2011). Self-compassion, self-esteem, and well-being. *Social and Personality Psychology Compass, 5*(1), 1–12. doi:10.1111/j.1751-9004.2010.00330.x

Neff, K., & Germer, C. (2018). *The mindful self-compassion workbook: A proven way to accept yourself, build inner strength, and thrive.* Guilford.

Nelson, S. K., Layous, K., Cole, S. W., & Lyubomirsky, S. (2016). Do unto others or treat yourself? The effects of prosocial and self-focused behavior on psychological flourishing. *Emotion, 16*(6), 850–861. doi:10.1037/emo0000178

Nguyen, L., Drew, D., Graham, M., Joshi, A., Guo, C-G., Ma, W., . . . Chan, A. (2020). Risk of COVID-19 among frontline healthcare workers and the general community: A prospective cohort study. *The Lancet: Public Health, 5,* E475–E483. doi:10.1016/S2468-2667(20)30164-X

Petrocchi, N., & Cheli, S. (2019). The social brain and heart rate variability: Implications for psychotherapy. *Psychology and Psychotherapy, 92,* 208–223. doi:10.1111/papt.12224

Piff, P. K., Kraus, M. W., & Keltner, D. (2018). Unpacking the inequality paradox: The psychological roots of inequality and social class. *Advances in Experimental Social Psychology, 57,* 53–124. doi:10.1016/bs.aesp.2017.10.002

Porges, S. W. (2007). The polyvagal perspective. *Biological Psychology, 74*(2), 116–143. Doi:10.1016/j.biopsych.2006.06.009

Porges, S. W. (2017). Vagal pathways: Portals to compassion. In E. M. Seppälä, E. Simon-Thomas, S. L. Brown, M. C. Worline, C. D. Cameron, & J. R. Doty (Eds.), *The Oxford handbook of compassion science* (pp. 189–202). Oxford University Press.

Porges, S. W., & Dana, D. A. (2018). *Clinical applications of the Polyvagal Theory: The emergence of polyvagal-informed therapies.* WW Norton & Company.

Porges, S. W., & Furman, S. A. (2011). The early development of the autonomic nervous system provides a neural platform for social behaviour: A polyvagal perspective. *Infant and Child Development, 20*(1), 106–118. doi:10.1002/icd.688

Ransome, W., & Sampford, C. (2010). *Ethics and socially responsible investment a philosophical approach.* Ashgate Publishing.

Reich, R. B. (2018). *The common good.* Vintage.

Ryan, C. (2019). *Civilized to death: The price of progress.* Avid Reader Press/Simon & Schuster.

Sachs, J. D. (2012). *The price of civilization: Reawakening American virtue and prosperity.* Random House.

Schacter, H. L., & Margolin, G. (2019). When it feels good to give: Depressive symptoms, daily prosocial behavior, and adolescent mood. *Emotion, 19*(5), 923–927. doi:10.1037/emo0000494

Schore, A. N. (2019). *Right brain psychotherapy.* W. W. Norton & Company.

Shapira, L. B., & Mongrain, M. (2010). The benefits of self-compassion and optimism exercises for individuals vulnerable to depression. *Journal of Positive Psychology, 5,* 377–389. doi:10.1080/17439760.2010.516763

Slavich, G. M. (2020). Social safety theory: A biologically based evolutionary perspective on life stress, health, and behavior. *Annual Review of Clinical Psychology, 16,* 265–295. doi:10.1146/annurev-clinpsy-032816-045159

Solomon, R. C. (2001). The moral psychology of business: Care and compassion in the corporation. In J. Dienhart, D. Moberg, & R. Duska (Eds.), *The next phase of business ethics: Integrating psychology and ethics* (vol. 3, pp. 417–438). Emerald Group Publishing.

Sommers-Spijkerman, M. P. J., Trompetter, H. R., Schreurs, K. M. G., & Bohlmeijer, E. T. (2018). Compassion-focused therapy as guided self-help for enhancing public mental health: A randomized controlled trial. *Journal of Consulting and Clinical Psychology, 86*(2), 101–115. doi:10.1037/ccp0000268

Stellar, J. E., & Keltner, D. (2017). Compassion in the autonomic nervous system: The role of the vagus nerve. In P. Gilbert (Ed.), *Compassion: Concepts, research and applications* (pp. 120–134). Routledge/Taylor & Francis Group.

Strauss, C., Taylor, B. L., Gu, J., Kuyken, W., Baer, R., Jones, F., & Cavanagh, K. (2016). What is compassion and how can we measure it? A review of definitions and measures. *Clinical Psychology Review, 47,* 15–27. doi:10.1016/j.cpr.2016.05.004

Suddendorf, T. (2018). Two key features created the human mind: Inside our heads. *Scientific American, 319*(3), 42–47. doi:10.1038/scientificamerican0918-42

Trautwein, F. M., Kanske, P., Böckler, A., & Singer, T. (2020). Differential benefits of mental training types for attention, compassion, and theory of mind. *Cognition, 194*, 104039. doi:10.1016/j.cognition.2019.104039

Wilkinson, R., & Pickett, K. (2010). *The spirit level: Why equality is better for everyone.*

Wilson, D. S. (2019). *This view of life: Completing the Darwinian revolution.* Pantheon Books.

Workman, L., Reader, W., & Barkow, J. H. (Eds.). (2020). *Cambridge handbook of evolutionary perspectives on human behavior.* Cambridge University Press.

Worline, M., & Dutton, J. E. (2017). *Awakening compassion at work: The quiet power that elevates people and organizations.* Berrett-Koehler Publishers.

Zeng, X., Chiu, C. P. K., Wang, R., Oei, T. P. S., & Leung, F. Y. K. (2015). The effect of loving-kindness meditation on positive emotions: A meta-analytic review. *Frontiers in Psychology, 6*, 1693. doi:10.3389/fpsyg.2015.01693

Zessin, U., Dickhäuser, O., & Garbade, S. (2015). The relationship between self-compassion and well-being: A meta-analysis. *Applied Psychology: Health and Well-Being, 7*(3), 340–364. doi:10.1111/aphw.12051

5

Perceived Partner Responsiveness and Wellbeing

HARRY T. REIS AND JENNY D. V. LE ∎

INTRODUCTION

Few questions engage interest more than 'What makes for a happy life?'. Whether in late-night dormitory or pub conversations, self-help books, professionally led therapy, or random musing, people often wonder about the path to happiness. It is fitting, then, that the search for happiness occupies a central role in the writings of religious leaders, philosophers, novelists, and modern-day academics. Among the many classical prescriptions for finding happiness, one can find, for example, the pursuit of a commitment to God (e.g., the Judeo-Christian Bible); perceiving the true nature of reality (Buddhism); living a just, moral life (Plato); and maximising pleasurable activities (Bentham). In more contemporary work, happiness has been theorised to arise, for example, from authenticity to one's true values and interests (Deci & Ryan, 1985), having the right genes (Lykken & Tellegen, 1996) or personality (Anglim, Horwood, Smillie, Marrero, & Wood, 2020), frequently practicing certain cognitive and behavioural strategies (Lyubomirsky, 2008), and residing in one of the Nordic countries (Helliwell et al., 2021).

The rest of this book is devoted to exploring many of these other approaches and scales. In this chapter, we hope to nudge the conversation forward by discussing one factor that has been consistently and robustly associated with happiness: the nature of our close relationships. As we review, extant evidence strongly implicates close relationships as a prime determinant of human wellbeing and happiness. In our view, the cumulative weight of this evidence is sufficiently compelling to insist that researchers move forward to a thornier question: What, more precisely, is it about the existence and nature of close relationships that gives them their power to foster or impair wellbeing? We suggest that research on perceived partner responsiveness, an 'umbrella construct' that integrates many central themes in the literature on close relationships, helps answer this question. After reviewing evidence linking this construct to wellbeing and happiness, we describe the within-person and social-interactive origins of perceived partner responsiveness. The chapter concludes with a brief discussion of several implications of our model that point to potential applications and extensions.

RELATIONSHIPS AND HUMAN WELLBEING

Nearly all theories of human functioning and wellbeing incorporate relationships. In classic psychological theories, relationships figure prominently, such as in early psychoanalytic writing (e.g., by Freud, Adler, Jung, and Horney), object-relations theories (e.g., by Klein, Winnicott, and Sullivan), and, more recently, Bowlby's attachment theory. Similarly, need-based theories always include needs specific to connections with others. For example, Murray (1938) included several needs related to social relations, such as affiliation, rejection, nurturance, and succorance, as did Maslow's (1954) need hierarchy, which generalised such needs under the heading of love and belongingness (although, to be sure, to Maslow, these needs were subordinate to the higher-order needs of self-esteem and self-actualisation).

Contemporary theories also highlight relationships. For example, recent thinking within evolutionary psychology

place social interaction and social relationships squarely within the centre of the action. In particular, social interaction and relationships surrounding mating, kinship, reciprocal alliances, coalitions, and hierarchies are especially critical, because all appear to have strong consequences for successful survival and reproduction. From an evolutionary standpoint, the functions served by social relationships have been central to the design of the human mind. (Buss & Kenrick, 1998, p. 994)

Kenrick, Griskevicius, Neuberg, and Schaller (2010) drew on this principle to revise Maslow's model, putting relational needs at the top of the hierarchy. A different approach, Deci and Ryan's (1985) humanistically based self-determination theory, identifies relatedness as one of three fundamental and intrinsic human needs (the others are autonomy and competence). Baumeister and Leary (1995) summarised these (and many other) theories in describing what they called the *need to belong*:

People seek frequent, affectively positive interactions within the context of long-term, caring relationships.... [This] desire ... may well be one of the most far-reaching and integrative constructs currently available to understand human nature. (p. 522)

It is perhaps no wonder, then, that research on lifespan development consistently finds that success in relationships is a key determinant of wellbeing at all stages of the life cycle (see Hartup & Stevens, 1997, for a review). Likewise, most wellbeing

theories consider positive close relationships as an essential component of happiness (e.g., Diener & Biswas-Diener, 2008; Ryff, 1995; see also Chapter 1, this
volume).

What is the empirical evidence to support these contentions? Although it is beyond the scope of this chapter to comprehensively review this voluminous literature, a few brief examples may help illustrate the strength and breadth with which
existing research documents the impact of relationships on human wellbeing.
For clarity, we subdivide this review into three sections: mental health, subjective
wellbeing, and physical health/mortality.

Mental Health

Researchers have studied the connection between relationships and mental health
in several ways. The most common approach examines ties to marital quality.
Marital problems are robustly associated with a range of mental health disorders
such as depression and anxiety (e.g., Davila, Bradbury, Cohan, & Tochluk, 1997;
Proulx, Helms, & Buehler, 2007; Whisman, 2001), covary with increases in depression symptoms (e.g., Karney, 2001), and predict increases in the risk of having
a major depressive episode within 1 year (Whisman & Bruce, 1999). In a large,
representative sample of Americans, Swindle, Heller, Pescosolido, and Kikuzawa
(2000) found that disruptions of social networks, such as through divorce, death,
or conflict, were the single most common cause of what they called 'nervous
breakdowns'—common language for a major depressive or anxiety episode.
Outside of close relationships, social integration predicts fewer depressive symptoms in adolescents (Ueno, 2005), adults in general (Seeman, 1996; Teo, Choi,
& Valenstein, 2013), and the elderly (Charles & Carstensen, 2010). Even weaker
ties—interactions with acquaintances, co-workers, and strangers—have been
linked to better mental health (Blau & Fingerman, 2010; Sandstrom & Dunn,
2014). Not surprisingly, therefore, troubled relationships have been identified as
the most frequently mentioned reason why people enter psychotherapy (Pinsker,
Nepps, Redfield, & Winston, 1985) and are considered an important resource
for treating emotional disorders (Foran, Whisman, & Beach, 2015; Greenblatt,
Becerra, & Serafetinides, 1982; Weissman, Markowitz, & Klerman, 2007).

One type of mental distress that is closely tied to relational circumstances is
loneliness. Loneliness is not isomorphic with isolation; rather, it occurs when enacted levels of social connection fall short of desired levels (Peplau & Perlman,
1982). As a transitory emotion, loneliness is not considered an emotional disorder; rather, it tends to occur when social networks have been disrupted and
it helps to motivate compensatory actions, such as seeking out social contact
(Hawkley & Cacioppo, 2010). More chronic loneliness, however, is thought to be
a mental health disorder and has been associated with a broad set of emotional
and physical symptoms and even premature death (Holt-Lunstad, Smith, Baker,
Harris, & Stephenson, 2015). Importantly, this more chronic form of loneliness
is strongly correlated with social circumstances, such as low levels of intimacy,

self-disclosure, support (Wheeler, Reis, & Nezlek, 1983) and affection (Arpin & Mohr, 2019), and a cynical, untrusting stance toward others, especially close others (Hawkley, Browne, & Cacioppo, 2005; Tsai & Reis, 2009). The stronger link of loneliness with low-quality social contacts, as opposed to low frequency of social interaction, is particularly evident among elderly persons (Pinquart & Sorenson, 2000).

Subjective Wellbeing

When it comes to subjective wellbeing—people's cognitive and affective evaluation of their life as good (Diener, Lucas, Oishi, & Suh, 2002)—few, if any, factors rival the impact of relationships. In an early study, Glenn and Weaver (1981) concluded that marital happiness was the strongest influence on global happiness. Subsequent studies have shown that relationships are a key predictor of life satisfaction and emotional wellbeing at all stages of the life cycle (e.g., Diener & Biswas-Diener, 2008; Campbell, Converse, & Rodgers, 1976; Diener & Seligman, 2002). For example, among older adults, marital satisfaction and contact with members of one's social network are significant predictors of subjective wellbeing (e.g., Margelisch, Schneewind, Violette, & Perrig-Chiello, 2017; Rafnsson, Shankar, & Steptoe, 2015). A particularly striking result is reported by Sears (1977), who examined late-life retrospections in Terman's 'Gifted Children' sample of men. Even among these highly accomplished individuals, close relationships were endorsed as the number one source of satisfaction in their lives. Consistent with this and much other research, several theorists have defined positive relationships as a necessary component of psychological wellbeing (e.g., Diener & Biswas-Diener, 2008; Ryff, 1995, see also Chapter 1, this volume).

As we elaborate in the next section, it bears noting that research in this area defines 'relationships' in remarkably varied ways, spanning, for example, friendship quality (Demir, Orthel, & Andelin, 2013), frequent social contact (Diener & Seligman, 2002), support availability and receipt (Lakey, 2013), relatedness-need satisfaction in daily life (Reis, Sheldon, Gable, Roscoe, & Ryan, 2000), assistance in mood regulation (Rimé, 2009), social capital (Leung, Kier, Fung, Fung, & Sproule, 2011), and having happy friends (Fowler & Christakis, 2008). Providing a framework that can integrate these diverse conceptualisations is a goal of this chapter.

Physical Health and Mortality

Although strictly speaking subjective wellbeing need not depend on physical health, the link between these constructs is undeniable. For that reason, we include a brief summary of research relating physical health and mortality to relationships. With regard to health, many studies have identified associations between relationship variables and health indicators (both in general and illness-specific). For example, marital strain (defined as dissatisfaction and/or conflict) is associated with the prevalence and severity of cardiovascular disease and poorer endocrine and immunological function (see Robles & Kiecolt-Glaser, 2003, for a review). In one study, marital quality predicted deteriorating health over a 20-year span (Miller, Hollis, Olsen, & Law, 2013), a finding consistent with a meta-analysis conducted by Robles, Slatcher, Trombello, and McGinn (2015). More generally, many studies have documented correlations between specific disease symptoms or disease-related physiological processes and participation in social networks, assessed either quantitatively (i.e., in measures of social integration; see Berkman & Glass, 2000; Seeman, 1996, for reviews) or qualitatively (i.e., measures of social support; see Taylor, 2011, for a review). Some research suggests that these associations are mediated by health behaviours (e.g., Roberson, Shorter, Woods, & Priest, 2018), but other studies point to direct physiological links between inter-personal circumstances and biophysiological processes (see reviews by Uchino, Cacioppo, & Kiecolt-Glaser, 1996; Uchino, Trettevik, de Grey, Cronan, Hogan, & Baucom, 2018). For example, marital conflict down-regulates the immune system (Kiecolt-Glaser et al., 1993).

Studies of premature mortality similarly show strong effects of relationships. For example, in a study that included all first-time cancer patients in the state of California from 2000 to 2009, Martinez et al. (2016) found an elevated risk of death among divorced and never-married cancer patients relative to married patients. King and Reis (2012) found a similar result in a 15-year follow-up of coronary artery bypass surgery patients. Longitudinal studies have also shown increased rates of death among individuals in conflictual or otherwise low-quality marriages (e.g., Bookwala & Gaugler, 2020; Coyne et al., 2001; King & Reis, 2012). It is not just marriage that relates to premature mortality. House, Landis, and Umberson's (1988) classic paper reported a significant increase in the relative risk of early all-cause mortality as a function of low social integration, an effect that has been replicated by other researchers. To put these results into perspective, consider Holt-Lunstad et al.'s (2010) meta-analysis of 148 published studies. They concluded that the relative odds of premature mortality were more substantially reduced by social integration than by not smoking or not being obese. Having supportive relationships conferred similar, albeit somewhat weaker, benefits.

Interim Summary

The selective evidence reviewed above is part of a literature that, in aggregate, supports an incontrovertible conclusion: health and wellbeing are profoundly influenced by the relational circumstances in which people live their lives. Accepting this statement as fact invites a more complex next question: Given the diversity of relational variables that have been studied, how might the various findings be integrated? Which method of conceptualising or describing relational circumstances provides the most useful insights about wellbeing? We turn next to this question.

THE CONSTRUCT OF PERCEIVED
PARTNER RESPONSIVENESS

As the first author of this chapter has argued elsewhere, the progress of relationship science has to some extent been hampered by the absence of 'core organising principles'—that is, a well-defined nomological network that identifies commonalities and connections among the field's many diverse constructs while at the same time noting differences and distinctions (Reis, 2007; 2012; Reis & Mizrahi, 2018).[1] This approach offers several important advantages: it would weave together and integrate seemingly disparate phenomena; it would facilitate generalisation across research topics; it would encourage researchers to consider how their work fits into the field's broader emphasis, contributing to a cumulative science; and, perhaps most importantly, it would ground interventions in a clearly articulated set of principles and empirical findings whose outcomes and potential side-effects can be more precisely anticipated than with the narrower approaches that currently hold sway.

One candidate for a core, organising principle with particular relevance to wellbeing is perceived partner responsiveness. Perceived partner responsiveness is a deliberately broad and inclusive construct encompassing several important themes from the relationship literature. As described more fully later in this chapter, perceived partner responsiveness derives from interactions in which self-disclosures are paired with responsive listening, leading to moments of connection (Reis & Shaver, 1988). When people perceive that their partners have been responsive, they are more willing to be open and emotionally vulnerable, revealing their deepest needs and concerns (Ruan, Reis, Clark, Hirsch, & Bink, 2020). Perceptions of responsiveness have three main attributes: *understanding, validation,* and *caring* (Reis & Shaver, 1988). The first, understanding, refers to the belief that a relationship partner 'gets the facts right' about oneself. Understanding, although valued in and of itself (Gordon & Chen, 2016; Swann, 1990), is useful primarily because it qualifies the partner's response as consistent with self-perceptions—in other words, as empathically accurate. After all, a partner's support and acceptance predicated on a discrepant view of oneself is unlikely to feel relevant or beneficial (see Reis & Clark, 2013, for a review of evidence supporting this proposition). Shared understanding is therefore prerequisite to *validation*, which refers to the belief that partners appreciate and respect one's abilities, traits, and world views. Extensive evidence shows that validation, as distinct from agreeing with the other's position, is a primary contributor to relational intimacy and support (Burleson, 2003; Reis & Shaver, 1988).

The third component of the Reis and Shaver (1988) model, caring, describes the belief that a partner is responsive to one's needs (see also Chapter 4, this volume). It

---

1. Metaphorically speaking, the field might be described as focused more on the trees than the forest, so that our textbooks look more like a lengthy menu-like list of relatively freestanding topics and studies rather than a spider web of interlocking theories and principles.

is the basis of *communal relationships*, which are widely considered to be our most meaningful connections with others (Clark & Aragon, 2013). People routinely list mutual support as integral to their close relationships. In common usage, support refers to assistance, advice, or compassion given during times of stress or need (e.g., Stroebe & Stroebe, 1996), and, when it follows emotional openness, support can help down-regulate stress and anxiety (Slatcher & Selcuk, 2017) and bolster feelings of security (Murray, Bellavia, Rose, & Griffin, 2003). However, support in a time of need is not the only way that partners express caring. A thoughtful gift or a friendly visit may also communicate concern and regard. Even forgiveness and sacrifice can be considered forms of caregiving, in that both involve putting aside personal concerns in order to benefit the partner or relationship. Although usually studied in stressful or difficult circumstances, including illness and injury, caregiving also applies to more positively toned interactions, such as promoting a partner's pursuit of personal goals (Rusbult, Finkel, & Kumashiro, 2009), supporting their exploration of novel pursuits (Feeney & Thrush, 2010), and celebrating their personal accomplishments and good fortune (Gable & Reis, 2010).

Another important theme that contributes to perceived partner responsiveness involves momentary chemistry, or *repeated moments of interactional connection* (Reis, Regan, & Lyubomirsky, 2022). When people respond in an encouraging way to each other's expressions of needs, wishes, or goals, they often experience a palpable sense of connection. Tickle-Degnen and Rosenthal (1987) called this experience *rapport*, comprising affective positivity, mutual attentiveness, and synchrony. A growing literature documents the impact of synchrony, or coordinated affect, movements, and vocalisations, on feelings of connection. For example, interactional synchrony predicts liking in social (Niedenthal, Mermillod, Maringer, & Hess, 2010), romantic (Karremans & Verwijmeren, 2008; Kurtz & Algoe, 2015), and sexual (Birnbaum, Mizrahi, & Reis, 2019) contexts, as well as perceived similarity and compassion (Valdesolo & DeSteno, 2011). Fredrickson (2013) named this construct *positivity resonance* while showing that, as a momentary interpersonal experience, it leads to increased positive emotions, feelings of connectedness over time, and marital satisfaction (Otero et al., 2020). This may be a visceral example of a related, but more cognitive process: *reciprocity of liking*, which is widely accepted as one of the foundational, and best-supported principles of attraction and connection (see Berscheid & Reis, 1998, for a review).

Finally, perceived partner responsiveness is also closely related to a sense of *inclusion and belonging*, both of which are central to social integration. During interaction, the experience of understanding and validation fosters feelings of acceptance and inclusion, meeting basic and presumably innate needs for relatedness and belonging (Baumeister & Leary, 1995; Reis et al., 2000). Aside from their well-known affective impact—inclusion feels good and exclusion feels bad—fulfilment (or not) of belongingness needs has self-regulatory consequences that directly contribute to wellbeing. For example, social exclusion impairs healthy decision-making (Baumeister, DeWall, Ciarocco, & Twenge, 2005) and prosocial behaviour (Twenge, Baumeister, DeWall, Ciarocco, & Bartels, 2007) while increasing aggressiveness (Buckley, Winkel, & Leary, 2004), self-handicapping

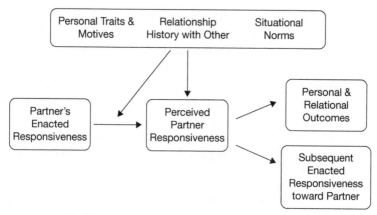

Figure 5.1 A model of the sources of perceived partner responsiveness.

(Twenge, Catanese, & Baumeister, 2002), and substance abuse (Luoma et al., 2007). Exclusion is also a risk factor for psychiatric disorders, such as adolescent depression (Lee et al., 2020). In contrast, social inclusion promotes rational decision-making (Baumeister, Twenge, & Nuss, 2002), empathic concern for others and prosocial behavior (Twenge et al., 2007), adherence to justice norms (van Prooijen, Van den Bos, & Wilke, 2004), and persistence and performance in academic settings (Murphy & Zirkel, 2015).

In sum, perceived partner responsiveness might be thought of as an umbrella construct, encapsulating concepts found throughout the relationships and wellbeing literature. In this role, we construe perceived partner responsiveness as somewhat more of a 'means' than an 'end,' in the sense that this construct describes processes that unfold during interaction and that, when enacted, lead to favourable (or, in their absence, unfavourable) relationship outcomes (as depicted in Figure 5.1). These outcomes are typically broader, more general summary representations of the state of a relationship or social network—for example, that one has social capital or feels a sense of belonging in one's social world.

Of course, although umbrella constructs are useful for highlighting how diverse research programmes may speak to the same underlying process, they are imprecise because they overlook the possibility of subtle yet meaningful conceptual and methodological differences. Therefore, to make a specific case for the contribution of perceived partner responsiveness to wellbeing, we next turn to studies explicitly linking this construct to health and wellbeing.

Perceived Partner Responsiveness and Well-Being

RELATIONSHIP WELLBEING

How does perceived partner responsiveness relate to other operationalisations of relationship quality? In romantic relationships, perceived partner responsiveness has been associated with effective social support (Maisel & Gable, 2009), trust (Rusbult, Kumashiro, & Reis, 2010), commitment (Segal & Fraley, 2016), intimacy (Laurenceau, Barrett, & Rovine, 2005), affectionate touch (Jolink, Chang, & Algoe, 2021), gratitude (Algoe & Zhaoyang, 2016), sexual satisfaction and desire (Birnbaum et al., 2016; Gadassi et al., 2016), forgiveness (Pansera & La Guardia, 2012), security-enhancing interactions (Simpson, Rholes, Oriña, & Grich, 2002), constructive conflict resolution (Overall & McNulty, 2017), and daily experiences of shared reality (Bar-Schacher & Bar-Kalifa, 2021). Another study showed that, in relationship conflict, perceived partner responsiveness prevents power differentials from creating harmful emotional communications (Alonso-Ferres, Righetti, Valor-Segura, & Expósito, 2021). Although studies of nonromantic relationships are rarer, they, too, show broader relational benefits of perceived partner responsiveness; for example, as a predictor of liking among new acquaintances (Sprecher & Treger, 2015), or of communal caregiving between college roommates (Canevello & Crocker, 2010) and friends (Lemay & Clark, 2008). These indicators span a wide conceptual swath, and, for that reason, we suggest that perceived partner responsiveness plays a pivotal role in helping people fulfil their close relationship goals. Moreover, this reasoning also suggests the possibility of targeting perceived partner responsiveness in dyadic and societal interventions, as we discuss in the concluding section of this chapter.

EMOTIONAL WELLBEING

When people perceive that their interaction partners are responsive, they experience positive affect, both in the moment and more generally; in contrast, when they feel that their partners are unresponsive, negative affect typically ensues (Reis & Clark, 2013). In a clinical realm, low levels of perceived partner responsiveness have been linked to symptoms of depression (Whiffen, 2005) and social anxiety (Bar-Kalifa, Hen-Weissberg, & Rafaeli, 2015), although in this work the direction of cause and effect is unclear. Other studies, however, point directly to a causal role for perceived partner responsiveness. For example, in a longitudinal study of Americans, Selcuk, Gunaydin, Ong, and Almeida (2016) found that perceived partner responsiveness from family and friends predicted both hedonic (experiencing pleasure and avoiding pain) and eudaimonic (finding meaning and fulfilment in life; see also Chapter 1, this volume) wellbeing 10 years later.[2] In part, this longitudinal effect was mediated by decreased reactivity to stressors in daily life, consistent with other studies showing that perceived partner responsiveness helps people cope with stressful uncertainty (Dooley, Sweeney, Howell, & Reynolds, 2018), including COVID-related stress (Slatcher, 2021); down-regulate reactions to laboratory stressors (Kane, Wiley, Schetter, & Robles, 2018) and everyday stress (Stanton, Selcuk, Farrell, Slatcher, & Ong, 2019); and, more generally, self-regulate effectively in response to everyday circumstances (Zee, Bolger, & Higgins, 2020). Studies relying on physiological markers—for example, cortisol reactivity (Kane et al., 2018; Slatcher, Selcuk, & Ong, 2015) or sleep quality (Selcuk, Stanton,

---

2. In a single-time study, Tasfiliz et al. (2018) replicated this result in Japan.

Slatcher, & Ong, 2017)—confirm this benefit for stress regulation, ruling out self-report bias as an explanation.

One intriguing mechanism that may account for the emotional benefits of perceived partner responsiveness is suggested by Morelli, Torre, and Eisenberger (2014). In this research, university student participants videorecorded descriptions of a series of important positive and negative events in their lives. Subsequently, while seated in a functional magnetic resonance imaging (fMRI) scanner, they read another student's ostensible reaction to these videorecordings. When the reaction was understanding and validating, neural regions associated with reward and social connection were activated, but when the reaction was nonunderstanding and invalidating, regions associated with negative affect were more active. In another study, perceived responsiveness was associated with naturally circulating oxytocin, a neurohormone thought to regulate pair-bonding (Algoe, Kurtz, & Grewen, 2017). Further support for the idea of a neural basis for the effects of perceived partner responsiveness comes from Wheatley, Kang, Parkinson, and Looser's (2012) proposal that neural synchrony may underpin behavioural synchrony and the experience of 'clicking' with an interaction partner (a conative instantiation of perceived partner responsiveness).

PHYSICAL HEALTH AND MORTALITY

To date, relatively few studies have examined associations between perceived partner responsiveness and health. O'Neill, Mohr, Bodner, and Hammer (2020) found that perceived partner responsiveness predicted lower levels of pain in a sample of military veterans, consistent with Wilson, Martire, and Sliwinski's (2017) finding that osteoarthritis patients had better physical functioning over 18 months when their spouse was responsive to their expressions of pain. Other studies have shown that perceived responsiveness facilitates smoking cessation in the short term (Britton, Haddad, & Derrick, 2019) and over a 9-year span (Derrick, Leonard, & Homish, 2013). In a study of adolescents, higher levels of perceived responsiveness following self-disclosures to various other persons predicted greater health-relevant gene expression and positive affect (Imami et al., 2019).

As for mortality risk, in a large, nationally representative study conducted in the United States, perceived partner responsiveness moderated the association between received partner emotional support and all-cause mortality one decade later (Selcuk & Ong, 2013). For individuals who perceived low partner responsiveness, receiving more emotional support from partners predicted greater mortality risk (presumably because such support came in a conflicted relationship). However, emotional support was unrelated to mortality risk for individuals who perceived high partner responsiveness, presumably because high levels of responsiveness buffers individuals against the potential harm of low support. Both findings held after controlling for demographic factors, physical health, health behaviours, psychological symptoms, and personality traits. A subsequent follow-up study at 20 years found that low partner responsiveness also predicted all-cause mortality, mediated by negative affect reactivity to daily stressors (Stanton et al., 2019). Perceived control has also been identified as a mediator of this association

(Alonso-Ferres, Imami, & Slatcher, 2020), in the sense that responsiveness gives people a sense that they have the means to cope with life's annoyances and adversities.

Child Development

Although this chapter focuses on adults, we briefly review the significant role that responsiveness has played in the parenting literature. Understandably, infants and young children cannot report on their perceptions of parental responsiveness so that research is necessarily based on later retrospections, behavioural observation, and parent's accounts of their enacted behaviour. This very large literature consistently shows that parental responsiveness predicts healthy outcomes for children and throughout later life (see Bugental & Grusec, 2006; van Ijzendoorn, 1995, for reviews).

For example, attachment theorists define responsiveness in terms of caregiver sensitivity to the infant's signals of distress (as well as their signals of other important needs). Sensitive and supportive responses promote infants' confidence that their caregivers will be available and helpful when needed (Ainsworth, Blehar, Waters, & Wall, 1978). This confidence, when elaborated and generalised to other partners, is central to the formation and maintenance of secure internal working models of attachment throughout life—that is, a deeply engrained network of cognitions and emotions indicating that one is worthy of love and capable of establishing and maintaining strong, satisfying adult relationships (Mikulincer & Shaver, 2016; Simpson & Belsky, 2008). In contrast, insensitivity—parental nonresponses or intrusive, noncontingent responses—fosters the development of insecure working models of attachment, which hinder wellbeing in childhood and beyond in various ways; for example, in poorer-quality and more unstable relationships, in a greater prevalence of emotional and behavioural disorders, and in lower subjective wellbeing (see Mikulincer & Shaver, 2016, for a review). For present purposes, we note that *perceptions* of parental responsiveness—that is, retrospections about caregiver responsiveness—figure prominently in mental models of attachment, as featured, for example, in the Adult Attachment Interview (Main, Kaplan, & Cassidy, 1985).

Other developmental frameworks also highlight the importance of responsiveness. Dix (1991), for example, defined parental awareness of and willingness to actively support children's needs, wants, and concerns as a central component of adaptive parenting. Studies in the social-cognitive tradition have shown that warm, responsive parenting is related to a variety of positive socioemotional outcomes in childhood and later life, whereas nonresponsiveness contributes to behavioural and emotional problems (Rothbaum & Weisz, 1994; Thompson, 2015). In accord with our model, developmentalists typically characterise responsive parenting as more than simple warmth, calling attention to behaviours that communicate (in our terminology) understanding, validation, and caring—for example, accurately assessing the child's needs, goals, and abilities; taking the child's perspective into account; and actively encouraging goal-directed strivings and autonomous self-regulation (Deci & Ryan, 1985; Gottman, Katz, & Hooven, 1997).

CLINICAL APPLICATIONS

Clinical interventions illustrate the potential for improving wellbeing by increasing perceived partner responsiveness. For example, many couples therapies emphasise the importance of understanding, validation, and caring. In *emotionally focused couple therapy*, the goal is to recognise and rectify critical failures of expected availability and responsiveness (Johnson, 2004). Similarly, *integrative behavioural couple therapy* stresses the expression of vulnerabilities and acceptance of partners as 'package deals', including strengths and weaknesses, compatibilities and incompatibilities (Christensen, Doss, & Jacobson, 2014). Indeed, *all* couples therapies use responsiveness-related tools, such as the speaker–listener technique in behavioural therapy, a procedure that creates a calm, well-defined structure for communications that are likely to increase understanding and validation (Markman, Stanley, & Blumberg, 1994).

Of course, responsiveness also plays a role in individual therapy, where the therapeutic alliance between client and therapist, a critical component of success, is built on the client's feeling understood, respected, and cared for by the therapist (Hatcher, 2015; Stiles, Honos-Webb, & Surko, 1998). Likewise, in many healthcare settings, the efficacy of the patient–provider relationship depends on patients' feeling listened to, respected, and cared for, qualities nurtured by patient-centred communication (as responsive listening is called in this literature; e.g., Epstein et al., 2005). For example, patients who believe that providers misunderstand their symptoms and needs are less likely to comply with treatment plans than patients who feel understood (Street, Makoul, Arora, & Epstein, 2009).

Interim Summary

Abundant evidence now demonstrates that perceived partner responsiveness promotes healthy outcomes across a broad spectrum of specific behaviours and indicators and hence is an important target in treatments designed to enhance the wellbeing of couples and individuals. Taking this link as a given, the next generation of research questions needs to ask questions about mechanisms (e.g., By what emotional, cognitive, and biological processes does perceived partner responsiveness become entrenched in the individual's makeup?), moderators (e.g., For which individuals and in which contexts are these effects stronger or weaker?), and interventions (How might the conditions that promote perceived partner responsiveness be enhanced in relationships, families, organisations, and cultures?).

WHERE DOES PERCEIVED PARTNER RESPONSIVENESS COME FROM?

Social psychologists, and relationship researchers in particular have long been interested in the interplay of actual interactions and motivated bias in influencing people's perceptions of social behaviour. This interplay seems particularly relevant to judgements about a partner's responsiveness. In general terms, people are more likely to attend to and describe their circumstances accurately when their outcomes depend on a partner's behaviour, as they often do in social interaction (e.g., Berscheid, Graziano, Monson, & Dermer, 1976; Neuberg & Fiske, 1987), as when choosing teammates for an important work project. On the other hand, motivated bias is more likely when behaviours are ambiguous, open to multiple interpretations, and emotionally significant (Chaiken & Maheswaran, 1994; Fiske & Taylor, 1991), as when judging whether an interaction partner is likeable. Both of these perspectives would seem to apply to perceived partner responsiveness. Figure 5.1 depicts a conceptual model of the various sources that contribute to perceived partner responsiveness. We next describe existing research about each of these sources.

Partners' Enacted Responsiveness

To be commonplace, perceptions must be psychologically useful, and, to be useful, they should be grounded in reality. Many studies show that people do judge their partner's responsiveness accurately. For example, Canevello and Crocker (2010) found significant correlations between one roommate's report of enacted responsiveness and the other's perceptions of that behaviour, a result that is consistent with Rusbult et al.'s (2010) studies of romantically involved couples. Laboratory observation studies, in which enacted behaviour is rated by independent observers, have also demonstrated that perceptions of responsiveness reflect a partner's actual behaviour (e.g., Gable, Gonzaga, & Strachman, 2006; Sasaki & Overall, 2021; Simpson, Rholes, & Nelligan, 1992). Studies using a diary format also show correlations between one partner's report of enacted responsiveness and the other's perceptions of that behaviour (e.g., Debrot, Cook, Perrez, & Horn, 2012). Research investigating closely related processes has similarly found evidence for substantial levels of accuracy in perceptions of a partner's caregiving (e.g., Collins & Feeney, 2000), goal-striving (Feeney, 2004), and gratitude (Park, Visserman, Sisson, Le, Stellar, & Impett, 2020).

The benefits of a partner's responsiveness appear to be greater when both partners agree that it has occurred. For example, Reis, Maniaci, and Rogge (2017) found that the emotional boost from compassionate acts and responsiveness were greater when both husbands and wives agreed that these behaviours had taken place. Elsewhere, Pietromonaco, Overall, and Powers (2021) found that one partner's responsiveness, as coded by independent observers, was associated with decreases in the other's depressive symptoms more than a year later, an effect associated with higher marital satisfaction. Although their report does not mention perceived responsiveness, it seems likely that this construct would mediate the observed improvements. In sum, it seems clear that perceived partner responsiveness is, at least in part, an accurate representation of responsive behaviour enacted by a partner.

What kind of behaviours implement responsiveness? These are any behaviours that instil, through interaction, partner feelings of being understood, validated, and cared for. Of course, there are substantial individual and relationship differences regarding which behaviours do so. For example, avoidant individuals tend to see emotional support as intrusive rather than responsive (Simpson et al., 1992). Nevertheless, many behaviours are generally perceived as responsive by most people. Maisel, Gable, and Strachman (2008) provided a list of 19 behaviours that most people see as responsive and that independent coders can quantify by observing laboratory interactions. Similarly, listening research has identified the verbal (e.g., reflections, open questioning, using the speaker's name) and nonverbal (e.g., heading nodding, appropriate facial expressions, forward body lean) behaviours that are likely to engender feeling listened to and hence perceived responsiveness (Itzchakov, Reis, & Weinstein, 2022). Burleson and Samter (1985) took another approach to conceptualising enacted responsiveness, distinguishing levels of supportiveness in personal communications according to their degree of person-centeredness: that is, the extent to which communications recognise and legitimise the other's perspective while helping them understand and cope with relevant feelings. It is important to keep in mind that although most research on enacted responsiveness examines interpersonal communication (i.e., conversation), responsiveness can also be enacted behaviourally; for example, in the purchase of a perfect gift or by babysitting the grandchildren so that their parents can have a much-needed romantic break. In short, to understand whether a particular behaviour is likely to foster perceived partner responsiveness, it is necessary to consider its functional impact on the recipient.

A brief note about the cyclical nature of the model in Figure 5.1 (see right-most lower box). When people experience responsiveness from a partner, they are more likely to enact responsiveness toward that partner in the future. This tendency reflects several processes, including the strong reciprocity norm that regulates social relations, the mutuality inherent in adult communal relationships (Clark & Aragon, 2013), and the reinforcement of intimate commitments that perceived partner responsiveness engenders (Reis & Shaver, 1988). When relationships are viewed temporally, spanning repeated interactions over time, enacted responsiveness is properly construed as a cause and an effect of perceived responsiveness.

Personal Traits and Motives

Here, we refer to the role of individual differences and situationally activated motives in influencing perceptions of a partner's behaviour.[3] In some instances,

---

3. Personality and motives also impel partners to enact (or not enact) responsive behaviour. When these behaviours are perceived, these would be considered examples of accurate perceptions of enacted behaviour, inasmuch as the individual is correctly perceiving the other's behaviour, regardless of its aetiology.

individual differences contribute directly to perceiving responsiveness (in Figure 5.1, the arrow leading directly from this box to perceived partner responsiveness). For example, in general, perceptions of responsiveness tend to be higher among people with high self-esteem (Cortes & Wood, 2018), who are not lonely (Tsai & Reis, 2009), who are securely attached (Beck, Pietromonaco, DeVito, Powers, & Boyle, 2014; Bosisio, Pâquet, Bois, Rosen, & Bergeron, 2020) and trusting (McCarthy, Wood, & Holmes, 2017), and who have more compassionate goals (Canevello & Crocker, 2010; see also Chapter 4, this volume).

Figure 5.1 also includes a certain type of motive, *motivated bias*, as a moderator of perceptions of enacted responsiveness; that is, people's interpretations of their partner's behaviour can be skewed in a direction that helps them accomplish psychologically meaningful goals (e.g., self-esteem maintenance, relationship enhancement or preservation, and so on). Thus, low self-esteem and rejection-sensitive individuals are more likely to interpret their partner's less than fully responsive behaviour as unresponsive (Downey, Freitas, Michaelis, & Khouri, 1998; Gaucher et al., 2012; Murray et al., 2003), and avoidantly attached individuals see their partner's behaviour as less responsive than their partners report (Rodriguez et al., 2019). In these instances, perceiving the partner's behaviour less favourably than objectively warranted serves a self-protective function in the face of potential risk, presumably because dissatisfaction with the relationship can be blamed on the partner rather than oneself. On the other hand, commitment induces partners to view potentially responsive behaviour in a positive light (Rusbult, Olson, Davis, & Hannon, 2001), valuing a partner enhances perceptions that he or she is acting responsively (Lemay, 2014), mindfulness increases the likelihood of acknowledging a partner's expressions of vulnerability (Khalifian & Barry, 2021), and high levels of empathic concern make it easier to recognise genuine responsive caring (Winczewski, Bowen, & Collins, 2016). In these instances, the relatively optimistic interpretations of the partner's behaviour help maintain confidence in the beneficence and security of a relationship.

One form of motivated perception that has received considerable attention is *projection*. When people have behaved responsively toward a partner, or when they anticipate doing so in the future, they are more likely to perceive that partner's behaviour toward themselves as responsive (e.g., Lemay & Clark, 2008; Lemay, Clark, & Feeney, 2007). Presumably, such projection reflects tacit endorsement of reciprocity norms: because communal relationships are based on well-learned expectations of mutual concern (Clark & Aragon, 2013), one's own actions encourage the belief that the partner has, or will shortly, act in kind. This belief helps satisfy trust-relevant motives by enhancing confidence that responsiveness will be provided, should it be needed.[4] Evidence for the impact of projection on

---

4. The fact that perceptions of a partner's responsiveness tend to be more highly correlated with ratings of one's own responsiveness than with the partner's rating of enacted responsiveness might also be due to methodological influences, in that the former correlates two ratings by the same person, whereas the latter correlates ratings from different individuals. Research has not yet sorted out these alternative explanations.

perceived partner responsiveness obtains from diverse studies; for example, a diary study by Debrot et al. (2012) and a laboratory study of parenting by Cross, Overall, Low, and Henderson (2020), who found that parents tended to perceive their co-parents' responsiveness toward their child as similar to their own, over and above actual levels of agreement. Projection effects have also been noted in several related areas of relationship research, such as social support (Brunstein, Dangelmayer, & Schulthiess, 1996) and caring (Kenny & Acitelli, 2001). In these studies, people tend to see correspondence between their own and their partners' provision of support and caring, independent of support and caring that the partner has in actuality provided.

Relationship History with the Other

As noted earlier, perceived partner responsiveness tends to be correlated, often highly so, with other popular relationship processes, such as intimacy, support, and satisfaction. Thus, it is readily apparent that when relationships are high in these qualities, interacting partners are likely to perceive higher levels of responsiveness. For example, friends who are supportive in multiple ways are perceived as more responsive than friends who are supportive in fewer ways (Orehek, Forest, & Wingrove, 2018). Relationship history also matters. As mentioned earlier, attachment experiences in early relationships have substantial influences on adult relationships (see Mikulincer & Shaver, 2016, for a review), but here we call attention to relationship-specific attachments: experiences in a current relationship that affect later experiences in that relationship. For example, avoidant feelings toward a particular partner tended to diminish communal caring in those relationships, whereas relationship-specific anxiety fosters ambivalent feelings about communal care (Bartz & Lydon, 2008). Similarly, the more secure people feel in a particular relationship, relative to other relationships, the more likely they are to see those relationships as fulfilling basic psychological needs such as autonomy, competence, and relatedness (La Guardia, Ryan, Couchman, & Deci, 2000).

It seems likely that prior experiences with a partner will help determine how responsive that partner is seen in a current interaction. We are unaware of research testing this hypothesis, but two contrasting options seem plausible. One might be called *amplification*: if a partner has been responsive in the past, ambiguous behaviours in the present may be interpreted in a positive light. This possibility is consistent with the well-documented idea of *positive illusions*: that the personal attributes of a valued partner are rated more favourably than is objectively warranted (Murray & Holmes, 1997). Of course, the opposite would be true of a previously unresponsive partner whose current attempts to be responsive might be judged more harshly. In this regard, Forest, Kille, Wood, and Holmes (2014) found that partners are less responsive to negative disclosures made by disclosers whom they perceive to express negativity frequently. The other option, which predicts the oppositive effect, is a *contrast effect*: when a partner is usually very responsive, responses that seem to fall short of these lofty expectations might be experienced as relatively disappointing and, as suggested by emotion-in-relationships theorising (Berscheid & Ammazzalorso, 2001), likely to induce a strong, negative emotional reaction.

Finally, relationship history might also help explain how people choose which partner to open up to and, as a consequence, which partners have the opportunity to be responsive (or not). The more responsive that partners have been perceived in the past, the more likely that they will be targeted for disclosures and support-seeking in the future (Clark & Aragon, 2013). Consequently, over time, relationships may develop relatively stable levels of perceived responsiveness.

Situational Norms

By situational norms, we refer to the idea that people normatively expect other persons, including relationship partners, to act responsively (e.g., in an emergency, when a distressing event has occurred, or when a cause for celebration exists). We are unaware of research that explores the influence of norms on perceived responsiveness, but rather draw here on interdependence theory, which examines how people deal with so-called *interdependence dilemmas* (i.e., the choices people make when their own and a partner's preference differ, yet joint action is required). In these situations, norms may help people avoid conflict: whose birthday is it, whose needs are greater, or the Golden Rule (Rusbult et al., 2001). When partners reflect on their partner's responsiveness in these situations, they may focus on the partner's behaviour—that is, whether he or she was responsive or unresponsive—in the context of situationally appropriate norms. For example, if Elaine pays for dinner with Art on a random evening, Art may see her generosity as responsive. But if Elaine buys Art dinner on his birthday, Art may discount her kindness since people commonly treat others to dinner on their birthday (i.e., the behaviour is normative). But making a special dinner might lead to an even stronger attribution of responsiveness if Art has had a bad day and assumes that Elaine is trying to cheer him up (e.g., 'I'm really blown away by your thoughtfulness in trying to help me feel better'). The influence of social norms on judgements of responsiveness seems a direction worthy of future research.

IMPLICATIONS BEYOND PERSONAL RELATIONSHIPS

Although nearly all responsiveness research has studied dyads, our conceptual model may also apply in larger contexts. For example, in schools, students may be more engaged in learning activities when they feel that their teachers and the wider school environment are understanding of and responsive to their needs. Such support is likely to be particularly influential in creating a sense of belonging among students from underrepresented groups, for whom the educational context may be culturally and personally unfamiliar. Teachers, too, benefit from responsiveness conveyed by school administrators, as reflected in lower stress ratings and turnover intentions (Itzchakov et al., 2022).

We also suggest that perceived partner responsiveness would have value in organisational settings, as suggested in two lines of research. First, research indicates that good listening by managers—defined as attentiveness, comprehension, and positive intent in this literature—improves the manager–employee relationship while at the same time improving performance and retention (see review by Kluger & Itzchakov, 2022). Moreover, interventions designed to facilitate high-quality listening in interviews, such as Kluger and Nir's (2010) *feedforward interview*, lead to increases in employee performance. Presumably—and research is needed to examine this conjecture—these gains are mediated by perceived partner responsiveness. A second source of support comes from organisational citizenship research. This construct refers to discretionary behaviours enacted by employees that are not part of any formal reward system, but that nevertheless benefit the organisation (e.g., spending personal time mentoring a junior colleague). Among the documented antecedents of organisational citizenship are constructs familiar to this chapter: leader support, responsive feedback, and personal acceptance of group goals (Organ & Ryan, 1995). We would expect a strong correlation between organisational citizenship and perceived responsiveness, in reference to both the employee's supervisor and the larger organisation.

Perceived responsiveness may also play an influential role in intergroup relations and political life. Feeling misunderstood and disrespected by another social group—that is, believing that others hold a negative stereotype about one's own group—is associated with intergroup tension and enmity (Demoulin, Leyens, & Dovidio, 2009). For example, in a series of five studies, Livingstone, Fernández Rodríguez, and Rothers (2020) found that in-group members who felt misunderstood and disrespected by out-group members were less trusting and more likely to endorse political divisiveness. Relatedly, in the legal realm, Tyler (1990) noted that when people feel listened to and respected, they are more likely to feel justly treated by legal authorities regardless of whatever outcomes occur. Furthermore, conventional wisdom suggests that voters are more likely to endorse political candidates who are, or at least who appear to be, responsive to their needs and priorities—as one voter told a journalist, 'If you want to win my vote, you need to show me that you understand our reality' (The Guardian, 2015). Perhaps a lack of understanding and respect is behind the growth in partisan sectarianism throughout the world today (Finkel et al., 2020).

Finally, it is intriguing to speculate on the implications of our model for responsiveness to (or lack thereof) to the environment. Although we focus on responsiveness among human partners, responsiveness also plays a role in our interaction with our physical environment—the air we breathe, the water we drink, the land on which we live. In these interactions, people rarely consider the planet's response to our actions, which has led directly to the climate crisis that confronts us all today. As a consequence, when catastrophic climate events do occur, we typically do not perceive them as a partner's—that is, the planet's—response to our enacted behaviour. Thus, better understanding of, respect for, and caring toward this interaction partner might set off an interaction sequence, similar to the one depicted in Figure 5.1, that would result in higher wellbeing for our planetary partner and, reciprocally, for ourselves and our children.

SUMMARY

In this chapter, we reviewed the extensive evidence demonstrating the importance of relationships, and particularly perceived partner responsiveness in those relationships, for human wellbeing. The weight of this evidence is compelling: relationships affect our biological, psychological, and social functioning in almost every way that wellbeing traditionally has been assessed: everyday mood, life satisfaction, mental health, physical health, and mortality risk. The term 'relationships' is, of course, expansive and, in the many studies contributing to this conclusion, has been operationalised in myriad ways. This chapter proposes that perceived partner responsiveness can be considered an integrative construct, embodying qualities that bridge the various ways that relationships have been examined and representing the processes likely to make them beneficial or harmful.

In conclusion, we find it striking that a single construct appears to underlie a remarkable range of human connections and their implications for wellbeing—in our families, romantic relationships, and friendships; in our education, work, and healthcare experiences; and in our larger group and political affiliations. Perceiving that others are responsive to the self contributes substantively and substantially to wellbeing across all of these domains. We acknowledge that perceived partner responsiveness is a very broad construct, but it is not an ambiguous one. It has clear and generally recognisable attributes and is engendered when certain interactional circumstances occur, supported by traits and motives that nurture social connections. How might these ideas be used to advance the common good? For researchers, the goal is to better understand and articulate the processes that contribute to perceived partner responsiveness. For practitioners and policymakers, the goal is to implement the results of this research. We hope this chapter provides a framework for facilitating the work of both of these groups.

REFERENCES

Ainsworth, M. D. S., Blehar, M. C., Waters, E., & Wall, S. (1978). *Patterns of attachment: A psychological study of the strange situation.* Erlbaum.
Algoe, S. B., Kurtz, L. E., & Grewen, K. (2017). Oxytocin and social bonds: The role of oxytocin in perceptions of romantic partners' bonding behavior. *Psychological Science, 28*(12), 1763–1772. https://doi.org/10.1177/0956797617716922
Algoe, S. B., & Zhaoyang, R. (2016). Positive psychology in context: Effects of expressing gratitude in ongoing relationships depend on perceptions of enactor responsiveness. *Journal of Positive Psychology, 11*(4), 399–415. https://doi.org/10.1080/17439760.2015.1117131

Alonso-Ferres, M., Imami, L., & Slatcher, R. B. (2020). Untangling the effects of partner responsiveness on health and well-being: The role of perceived control. *Journal of Social and Personal Relationships, 37*(4), 1150–1171. https://doi.org/10.1177/02654 07519884726

Alonso-Ferres, M., Righetti, F., Valor-Segura, I., & Expósito, F. (2021). How power affects emotional communication during relationship conflicts: The role of perceived partner responsiveness. *Social Psychological and Personality Science, 12*(7), 1203–1215. https://doi.org/10.1177/1948550621996496

Anglim, J., Horwood, S., Smillie, L. D., Marrero, R. J., & Wood, J. K. (2020). Predicting psychological and subjective well-being from personality: A meta-analysis. *Psychological Bulletin, 146*(4), 279–323. http://doi.org/10.1037/bul0000226

Arpin, S. N., & Mohr, C. D. (2019). Transient loneliness and the perceived provision and receipt of capitalization support within event-disclosure interactions. *Personality and Social Psychology Bulletin, 45*(2), 240–253. https://doi.org/10.1177/014616721 8783193

Bar-Kalifa, E., Hen-Weissberg, A., & Rafaeli, E. (2015). Perceived partner responsiveness mediates the association between social anxiety and relationship satisfaction in committed couples. *Journal of Social and Clinical Psychology, 34*(7), 587–610. https://doi.org/10.1521/jscp.2015.34.7.587

Bar-Shachar, Y., & Bar-Kalifa, E. (2021). Responsiveness processes and daily experiences of shared reality among romantic couples. *Journal of Social and Personal Relationships.* https://doi.org/10.1177/02654075211017675

Bartz, J. A., & Lydon, J. E. (2008). Relationship-specific attachment, risk regulation, and communal norm adherence in close relationships. *Journal of Experimental Social Psychology, 44*(3), 655–663. https://doi.org/10.1016/j.jesp.2007.04.003

Baumeister, R. F., DeWall, C. N., Ciarocco, N. J., & Twenge, J. M. (2005). Social exclusion impairs self-regulation. *Journal of Personality and Social Psychology, 88*(4), 589–604. https://doi.org/10.1037/0022-3514.88.4.589

Baumeister, R. F., & Leary, M. R. (1995). The need to belong: Desire for interpersonal attachments as a fundamental human motivation. *Psychological Bulletin, 117*(3), 497–529. https://doi.org/10.1037/0033-2909.117.3.497

Baumeister, R. F., Twenge, J. M., & Nuss, C. K. (2002). Effects of social exclusion on cognitive processes: Anticipated aloneness reduces intelligent thought. *Journal of Personality and Social Psychology, 83*(4), 817–827. https://doi.org/10.1037/ 0022-3514.83.4.817

Beck, L. A., Pietromonaco, P. R., DeVito, C. C., Powers, S. I., & Boyle, A. M. (2014). Congruence between spouses' perceptions and observers' ratings of responsiveness: The role of attachment avoidance. *Personality and Social Psychology Bulletin, 40*(2), 164–174. https://doi.org/10.1177/0146167213507779

Berkman, L. F., & Glass, T. (2000). Social integration, social networks, social support, and health. *Social Epidemiology, 1*(6), 137–173.

Berscheid, E., & Ammazzalorso, H. (2001). Emotional experience in close relationships. In G. J. O. Fletcher & M. S. Clark (Eds.), *Blackwell handbook of social psychology* (Vol. 2, pp. 308–330). Blackwell.

Berscheid, E., Graziano, W., Monson, T., & Dermer, M. (1976). Outcome dependency: Attention, attribution, and attraction. *Journal of Personality and Social Psychology, 34*(5), 978–989. https://doi.org/10.1037/0022-3514.34.5.978

Berscheid, E., & Reis, H. T. (1998). Attraction and close relationships. In D. Gilbert, S. Fiske, & G. Lindzey (Eds.), *Handbook of social psychology* (4th ed., pp. 193–281). McGraw-Hill.

Birnbaum, G. E., Mizrahi, M., & Reis, H. T. (2019). Fueled by desire: Sexual activation facilitates the enactment of relationship-initiating behaviors. *Journal of Social and Personal Relationships, 36*(10), 3057–3074. https://doi.org/10.1177/026540751 8811667

Birnbaum, G. E., Reis, H. T., Mizrahi, M., Kanat-Maymon, Y., Sass, O., & Granovski-Milner, C. (2016). Intimately connected: The importance of partner responsiveness for experiencing sexual desire. *Journal of Personality and Social Psychology, 111*(4), 530–546. https://doi.org/10.1037/pspi0000069

Blau, M., & Fingerman, K. L. (2010). *Consequential strangers: The power of people who don't seem to matter . . . but really do.* Norton.

Bookwala, J., & Gaugler, T. (2020). Relationship quality and 5-year mortality risk. *Health Psychology, 39*(8), 633–641. https://doi.org/10.1037/hea0000883

Bosisio, M., Pâquet, M., Bois, K., Rosen, N. O., & Bergeron, S. (2020). Are depressive symptoms and attachment styles associated with observed and perceived partner responsiveness in couples coping with genito-pelvic pain? *Journal of Sex Research, 57*(4), 534–544. https://doi.org/10.1080/00224499.2019.1610691

Britton, M., Haddad, S., & Derrick, J. L. (2019). Perceived partner responsiveness predicts smoking cessation in single-smoker couples. *Addictive Behaviors, 88*, 122–128. https://doi.org/10.1016/j.addbeh.2018.08.026

Brunstein, J. C., Dangelmayer, G., & Schultheiss, O. C. (1996). Personal goals and social support in close relationships: Effects on relationship mood and marital satisfaction. *Journal of Personality and Social Psychology, 71*(5), 1006–1019. https://doi.org/ 10.1037/0022-3514.71.5.1006

Buckley, K. E., Winkel, R. E., & Leary, M. R. (2004). Reactions to acceptance and rejection: Effects of level and sequence of relational evaluation. *Journal of Experimental Social Psychology, 40*(1), 14–28. https://doi.org/10.1016/S0022-1031(03)00064-7

Bugental, D. B., & Grusec, J. E. (2006). Socialization processes. In N. Eisenberg (Ed.), *Handbook of child psychology: Social emotional, and personality development* (6th ed., Vol. 3, pp. 366–428). Wiley.

Burleson, B. R. (2003). The experience and effects of emotional support: What the study of cultural and gender differences can tell us about close relationships, emotion, and interpersonal communication. *Personal Relationships, 10*(1), 1–23. https://doi.org/ 10.1111/1475-6811.00033

Burleson, B. R., & Samter, W. (1985). Consistencies in theoretical and naive evaluations of comforting messages. *Communication Monographs, 52*(2), 103–123. https://doi. org/10.1080/03637758509376099

Buss, D. M., & Kenrick, D. T. (1998). Evolutionary social psychology. In D. Gilbert & S. Fiske (Eds.), *The handbook of social psychology* (4th ed., Vol. 2, pp. 982–1026). McGraw-Hill.

Campbell, A., Converse, P. E., & Rodgers, W. L. (1976). *The quality of American life.* Sage.

Canevello, A., & Crocker, J. (2010). Creating good relationships: Responsiveness, relationship quality, and interpersonal goals. *Journal of Personality and Social Psychology, 99*(1), 78–106. https://doi.org/10.1037/a0018186

Chaiken, S., & Maheswaran, D. (1994). Heuristic processing can bias systematic processing: Effects of source credibility, argument ambiguity, and task importance on attitude judgment. *Journal of Personality and Social Psychology, 66*(3), 460–473. https://doi.org/10.1037/0022-3514.66.3.460

Charles, S. T., & Carstensen, L. L. (2010). Social and emotional aging. *Annual Review of Psychology, 61*, 383–409. https://doi.org/10.1146/annurev.psych.093008.100448

Christensen, A., Doss, B. D., & Jacobson, N. S. (2014). *Integrative behavioral couple therapy.* Norton.

Clark, M. S., & Aragon, O. (2013). Communal (and other) relationships: History, theory development, recent findings, and future directions. In J. A. Simpson & L. Campbell (Eds.), *The Oxford handbook of close relationships* (pp. 255–280). Oxford University Press. https://doi.org/10.1093/oxfordhb/9780195398694.013.0012

Collins, N., & Feeney, B. (2000). A safe haven: An attachment theory perspective on support seeking and caregiving in intimate relationships. *Journal of Personality and Social Psychology, 78*(6), 1053–1073. https://doi.org/10.1037/0022-3514.78.6.1053

Cortes, K., & Wood, J. V. (2018). Is it really "all in their heads"? How self-esteem predicts partner responsiveness. *Journal of Personality, 86*(6), 990–1002. https://doi.org/10.1111/jopy.12370

Coyne, J. C., Rohrbaugh, M. J., Shoham, V., Sonnega, J. S., Nicklas, J. M., & Cranford, J. A. (2001). Prognostic importance of marital quality for survival of congestive heart failure. *American Journal of Cardiology, 88*(5), 526–529. https://doi.org/10.1016/s0002-9149(01)01731-3

Cross, E. J., Overall, N. C., Low, R. S., & Henderson, A. M. (2020). Relationship problems, agreement and bias in perceptions of partners' parental responsiveness, and family functioning. *Journal of Family Psychology, 35*(4), 510–522. https://doi.org/10.1037/fam0000812

Davila, J., Bradbury, T. N., Cohan, C. L., & Tochluk, S. (1997). Marital functioning and depressive symptoms: Evidence for a stress generation model. *Journal of Personality and Social Psychology, 73*(4), 849–861. https://doi.org/10.1037//0022-3514.73.4.849

Debrot, A., Cook, W. L., Perrez, M., & Horn, A. B. (2012). Deeds matter: Daily enacted responsiveness and intimacy in couples' daily lives. *Journal of Family Psychology, 26*(4), 617–627. https://doi.org/10.1037/a0028666

Deci, E. L., & Ryan, R. M. (1985). *Intrinsic motivation and self-determination in human behavior.* Plenum Press.

Demir, M., Orthel, H., & Andelin, A. K. (2013). Friendship and happiness. In S. A. David, I. Boniwell, & A. C. Ayers (Eds.), *The Oxford handbook of happiness* (pp. 860–870). Oxford University Press. https://doi.org/10.1093/oxfordhb/9780199557257.013.0063

Demoulin, S., Leyens, J. P., & Dovidio, J. F. (2009). *Intergroup misunderstandings: Impact of divergent social realities.* Psychology Press.

Derrick, J. L., Leonard, K. E., & Homish, G. G. (2013). Perceived partner responsiveness predicts decreases in smoking during the first nine years of marriage. *Nicotine and Tobacco Research, 15*(9), 1528–1536. https://doi.org/10.1093/ntr/ntt011

Diener, E., & Biswas-Diener, R. (2008). *Rethinking happiness: The science of psychological wealth.* Blackwell.

Diener, E., Lucas, R. E., Oishi, S., & Suh, E. M. (2002). Looking up and looking down: Weighting good and bad information in life satisfaction judgments. *Personality and Social Psychology Bulletin, 28*(4), 437–445. https://doi.org/10.1177/0146167202287002

Diener, E., & Seligman, M. E. (2002). Very happy people. *Psychological Science, 13*(1), 81–84. https://doi.org/10.1111/1467-9280.00415

Dix, T. (1991). The affective organization of parenting: Adaptive and maladaptive processes. *Psychological Bulletin, 110*(1), 3–25. https://doi.org/10.1037/0033-2909.110.1.3

Dooley, M. K., Sweeny, K., Howell, J. L., & Reynolds, C. A. (2018). Perceptions of romantic partners' responsiveness during a period of stressful uncertainty. *Journal of Personality and Social Psychology, 115*(4), 677–687. https://doi.org/10.1037/pspi0000134

Downey, G., & Freitas, A. L., Michaelis, B., & Khouri, H. (1998). The self-fulfilling prophecy in close relationships: Rejection sensitivity and rejection by romantic partners. *Journal of Personality and Social Psychology, 75,* 545–560. https://doi.org/10.1037/0022-3514.75.2.545

Epstein, R. M., Franks, P., Fiscella, K., Shields, C. G., Meldrum, S. C., Kravitz, R. L., & Duberstein, P. R. (2005). Measuring patient-centered communication in patient–physician consultations: Theoretical and practical issues. *Social Science & Medicine, 61*(7), 1516–1528. https://doi.org/10.1016/j.socscimed.2005.02.001

Feeney, B. C. (2004). A secure base: Responsive support of goal strivings and exploration in adult intimate relationships. *Journal of Personality & Social Psychology, 87*(5), 631–648. https://doi.org/10.1037/0022-3514.87.5.631

Feeney, B. C., & Thrush, R. L. (2010). Relationship influences on exploration in adulthood: The characteristics and function of a secure base. *Journal of Personality and Social Psychology, 98*(1), 57–76. https://doi.org/10.1037/a0016961

Finkel, E. J., Bail, C. A., Cikara, M., Ditto, P. H., Iyengar, S., Klar, S., . . . Druckman, J. N. (2020). Political sectarianism in America. *Science, 370*(6516), 533–536. https://doi.org/10.1126/science.abe1715

Fiske, S. T., & Taylor, S. E. (1991). *Social cognition* (2nd ed.). McGraw Hill.

Foran, H. M., Whisman, M. A., & Beach, S. R. (2015). Intimate partner relationship distress in the DSM-5. *Family Process, 54*(1), 48–63. https://doi.org/10.1111/famp.12122

Forest, A. L., Kille, D. R., Wood, J. V., & Holmes, J. G. (2014). Discount and disengage: How chronic negative expressivity undermines partner responsiveness to negative disclosures. *Journal of Personality and Social Psychology, 107*(6), 1013–1032. https://doi.org/10.1037/a0038163

Fowler, J. H., & Christakis, N. A. (2008). Dynamic spread of happiness in a large social network: Longitudinal analysis over 20 years in the Framingham Heart Study. *British Medical Journal, 337,* a2338. https://doi.org/10.1136/bmj.a2338

Fredrickson, B. L. (2013). Positive emotions broaden and build. In M. P. Zanna (Ed.), *Advances in experimental social psychology* (Vol. 47, pp. 1–53). Elsevier Academic Press.

Gable, S., Gonzaga, G., & Strachman, A. (2006). Will you be there for me when things go right? Supportive responses to positive event disclosures. *Journal of Personality and Social Psychology, 91*(5), 904–917. https://doi.org/10.1037/0022-3514.91.5.904

Gable, S. L., & Reis, H. T. (2010). Good news! Capitalizing on positive events in an interpersonal context. In M. P. Zanna (Ed.), *Advances in experimental social psychology* (Vol. 42, pp. 195–257). Elsevier Academic Press.

Gadassi, R., Bar-Nahum, L. E., Newhouse, S., Anderson, R., Heiman, J. R., Rafaeli, E., & Janssen, E. (2016). Perceived partner responsiveness mediates the association between sexual and marital satisfaction: A daily diary study in newlywed couples. *Archives of Sexual Behavior, 45*(1), 109–120. https://doi.org/10.1007/s10 508-014-0448-2

Gaucher, D., Wood, J. V., Stinson, D. A., Forest, A. L., Holmes, J. G., & Logel, C. (2012). Perceived regard explains self-esteem differences in expressivity. *Personality and Social Psychology Bulletin, 38*(9), 1144–1156. https://doi.org/10.1177/014616721 2445790

Glenn, N. D., & Weaver, C. N. (1981). The contribution of marital happiness to global happiness. *Journal of Marriage and the Family, 43*(2), 161–168. https://doi.org/ 10.2307/351426

Gordon, A. M., & Chen, S. (2016). Do you get where I'm coming from?: Perceived understanding buffers against the negative impact of conflict on relationship satisfaction. *Journal of Personality and Social Psychology, 110*, 239–260. https://doi.org/ 10.1037/pspi0000039

Gottman, J. M., Katz, L. F., & Hooven, C. (1997). *Meta-emotion: How families communicate emotionally.* Erlbaum. https://doi.org/10.4324/9780203763568

Greenblatt, M., Becerra, R. M., & Serafetinides, E. A. (1982). Social networks and mental health: An overview. *The American Journal of Psychiatry, 139*(8), 977–984. https://doi.org/10.1176/ajp.139.8.977

Hartup, W. W., & Stevens, N. (1997). Friendships and adaptation in the life course. *Psychological Bulletin, 121*(3), 355–370. https://doi.org/10.1037/0033-2909.121.3.355

Hatcher, R. L. (2015). Interpersonal competencies: Responsiveness, technique, and training in psychotherapy. *American Psychologist, 70*(8), 747–757. https://doi.org/ 10.1037/a0039803

Hawkley, L. C., Browne, M. W., & Cacioppo, J. T. (2005). How can I connect with thee? Let me count the ways. *Psychological Science, 16*(10), 798–804. https://doi.org/ 10.1111/j.1467-9280.2005.01617.x

Hawkley, L. C., & Cacioppo, J. T. (2010). Loneliness matters: A theoretical and empirical review of consequences and mechanisms. *Annals of Behavioral Medicine, 40*(2), 218–227. https://doi.org/10.1007/s12160-010-9210-8

Helliwell, J. F., Layard, R., Sachs, J. D., De Neve, J-E., Aknin, L. B., & Wang, S. (2021). *World happiness report 2021.* https://worldhappiness.report/ed/2021/

Holt-Lunstad, J., Smith, T. B., Baker, M., Harris, T., & Stephenson, D. (2015). Loneliness and social isolation as risk factors for mortality: A meta-analytic review. *Perspectives on Psychological Science, 10*(2), 227–237. https://doi.org/10.1177/174569161 4568352

Holt-Lunstad, J., Smith, T. B., & Layton, J. B. (2010). Social relationships and mortality risk: A meta-analytic review. *PLoS Medicine, 7*(7), e1000316. https://doi.org/ 10.1371/journal.pmed.1000316

House, J. S., Landis, K. R., & Umberson, D. (1988). Social relationships and health. *Science, 241*(4865), 540–545. https://doi.org/10.1126/science.3399889

Imami, L., Stanton, S. C., Zilioli, S., Tobin, E. T., Farrell, A. K., Luca, F., & Slatcher, R. B. (2019). Self-disclosure and perceived responsiveness among youth with asthma: Links to affect and anti-inflammatory gene expression. *Personality and*

Social Psychology Bulletin, 45(8), 1155–1169. https://doi.org/10.1177/014616721 8808497

Itzchakov, G., Reis, H. T., & Weinstein, N. (2022). How to foster perceived partner responsiveness: Listening is key. *Social and Personality Psychology Compass, 16*(1), 1– 16. https://doi.org/10.1111/spc3.12648

Johnson, S. M. (2004). *The practice of emotionally focused couple therapy* (2nd ed.). Taylor & Francis.

Jolink, T. A., Chang, Y. P., & Algoe, S. B. (2021). Perceived partner responsiveness forecasts behavioral intimacy as measured by affectionate touch. *Personality and Social Psychology Bulletin.* https://doi.org/10.1177/0146167221993349

Kane, H. S., Wiley, J. F., Schetter, C. D., & Robles, T. F. (2018). The effects of interpersonal emotional expression, partner responsiveness, and emotional approach coping on stress responses. *Emotion, 19*(8), 1315–1328. https://doi.org/10.1037/emo0000487

Karney, B. R. (2001). Depressive symptoms and marital satisfaction in the early years of marriage: Narrowing the gap between theory and research. In S. R. H. Beach (Ed.), *Marital and family processes in depression: A scientific foundation for clinical practice* (pp. 45–68). American Psychological Association. https://doi.org/10.1037/10350-003

Karremans, J. C., & Verwijmeren, T. (2008). Mimicking attractive opposite-sex others: The role of romantic relationship status. *Personality and Social Psychology Bulletin, 34*(7), 939–950. https://doi.org/10.1177/0146167208316693

Kenny, D. A., & Acitelli, L. K. (2001). Accuracy and bias in the perception of the partner in a close relationship. *Journal of Personality and Social Psychology, 80*(3), 439–448. https://doi.org/10.1037/0022-3514.80.3.439

Kenrick, D. T., Griskevicius, V., Neuberg, S. L., & Schaller, M. (2010). Renovating the pyramid of needs: Contemporary extensions built upon ancient foundations. *Perspectives on Psychological Science, 5*(3), 292–314. https://doi.org/10.1177/17456 91610369469

Khalifian, C. E., & Barry, R. A. (2021). The relation between mindfulness and perceived partner responsiveness during couples' vulnerability discussions. *Journal of Family Psychology, 35*(1), 1–10. https://doi.org/10.1037/fam0000666

Kiecolt-Glaser, J. K., Malarkey, W. B., Chee, M., Newton, T., Cacioppo, J. T., Mao, H. Y., & Glaser, R. (1993). Negative behavior during marital conflict is associated with immunological down-regulation. *Psychosomatic Medicine, 55*(5), 395–409. https://doi.org/10.1097/00006842-199309000-00001

King, K. B., & Reis, H. T. (2012). Marriage and long-term survival after coronary artery bypass grafting. *Health Psychology, 31*(1), 55–62. https://doi.org/10.1037/a0025061

Kluger, A. N., & Itzchakov, G. (2022). The power of listening at work. *Annual Review of Organizational Psychology and Organizational Behavior, 9,* 121–146. https://doi.org/ 10.1146/annurev-orgpsyc-012420-091013

Kluger, A. N., & Nir, D. (2010). The feedforward interview. *Human Resource Management Review, 20*(3), 235–246. https://doi.org/10.1016/j.hrmr.2009.08.002

Kurtz, L. E., & Algoe, S. B. (2015). Putting laughter in context: Shared laughter as behavioral indicator of relationship well-being. *Personal Relationships, 22*(4), 573–590. https://doi.org/10.1111/pere.12095

La Guardia, J. G., Ryan, R. M., Couchman, C. E., & Deci, E. L. (2000). Within-person variation in security of attachment: A self-determination theory perspective on attachment, need fulfillment, and well-being. *Journal of Personality and Social Psychology, 79*(3), 367–384. https://doi.org/10.1037/0022-3514.79.3.367

Lakey, B. (2013). Perceived social support and happiness: The role of personality and relational processes. In S. A. David, I. Boniwell, & A. C. Ayers (Eds.), *The Oxford handbook of happiness* (pp. 847–859). Oxford University Press. https://doi.org/10.1093/oxfordhb/9780199557257.013.0062

Laurenceau, J. P., Barrett, L. F., & Rovine, M. J. (2005). The interpersonal process model of intimacy in marriage: A daily-diary and multilevel modeling approach. *Journal of Family Psychology, 19*(2), 314–323. https://doi.org/10.1037/0893-3200.19.2.314

Lee, H. Y., Jamieson, J. P., Reis, H. T., Beevers, C. G., Josephs, R. A., Mullarkey, M. C., O'Brien, J., & Yeager, D. S. (2020). Getting fewer "likes" than others on social media elicits emotional distress among victimized adolescents. *Child Development, 91*(6), 2141–2159. https://doi.org/10.1111/cdev.13422

Lemay Jr., E. P. (2014). Accuracy and bias in self-perceptions of responsive behavior: Implications for security in romantic relationships. *Journal of Personality and Social Psychology, 107*(4), 638–656. https://doi.org/10.1037/a0037298

Lemay Jr., E. P., & Clark, M. S. (2008). How the head liberates the heart: Projection of communal responsiveness guides relationship promotion. *Journal of Personality and Social Psychology, 94*(4), 647–671. https://doi.org/10.1037/0022-3514.94.4.647

Lemay Jr., E. P., Clark, M. S., & Feeney, B. C. (2007). Projection of responsiveness to needs and the construction of satisfying communal relationships. *Journal of Personality and Social Psychology, 92*(5), 834–853. https://doi.org/10.1037/0022-3514.92.5.834

Leung, A., Kier, C., Fung, T., Fung, L., & Sproule, R. (2011). Searching for happiness: The importance of social capital. *Journal of Happiness Studies, 12*(3), 443–462. https://doi.org/10.1007/s10902-010-9208-8

Livingstone, A. G., Fernández Rodríguez, L., & Rothers, A. (2020). "They just don't understand us": The role of felt understanding in intergroup relations. *Journal of Personality and Social Psychology, 119*(3), 633–656. https://doi.org/10.1037/pspi0000221

Luoma, J. B., Twohig, M. P., Waltz, T., Hayes, S. C., Roget, N., Padilla, M., & Fisher, G. (2007). An investigation of stigma in individuals receiving treatment for substance abuse. *Addictive Behaviors, 32*(7), 1331–1346. https://doi.org/10.1016/j.addbeh.2006.09.008

Lykken, D., & Tellegen, A. (1996). Happiness is a stochastic phenomenon. *Psychological Science, 7*(3), 186–189. https://doi.org/10.1111/j.1467-9280.1996.tb00355.x

Lyubomirsky, S. (2008). *The how of happiness: A scientific approach to getting the life you want*. Penguin.

Main, M., Kaplan, N., & Cassidy, J. (1985). Security in infancy, childhood, and adulthood: A move to the level of representation. *Monographs of the Society for Research in Child Development, 50*(1–2), 66–104. https://doi.org/10.2307/3333827

Maisel, N. C., & Gable, S. L. (2009). The paradox of received social support: The importance of responsiveness. *Psychological Science, 20*(8), 928–932. https://doi.org/10.1111/j.1467-9280.2009.02388.x

Maisel, N. C., Gable, S. L., & Strachman, A. (2008). Responsive behaviors in good times and in bad. *Personal Relationships, 15*(3), 317–338. https://doi.org/10.1111/j.1475-6811.2008.00201.x

Margelisch, K., Schneewind, K. A., Violette, J., & Perrig-Chiello, P. (2017). Marital stability, satisfaction and well-being in old age: Variability and continuity in long-term continuously married older persons. *Aging and Mental Health, 21*(4), 389–398. https://doi.org/10.1080/13607863.2015.1102197

Markman, H. J., Stanley, S., & Blumberg, S. L. (1994). *Fighting for your marriage.* Jossey-Bass.

Martínez, M. E., Anderson, K., Murphy, J. D., Hurley, S., Canchola, A. J., Keegan, T. H., . . . Gomez, S. L. (2016). Differences in marital status and mortality by race/ethnicity and nativity among California cancer patients. *Cancer, 122*(10), 1570–1578. https://doi.org/10.1002/cncr.29886

Maslow, A. H. (1954). *Motivation and personality.* Harper and Row.

McCarthy, M. H., Wood, J. V., & Holmes, J. G. (2017). Dispositional pathways to trust: Self-esteem and agreeableness interact to predict trust and negative emotional disclosure. *Journal of Personality and Social Psychology, 113*(1), 95–116. https://doi.org/10.1037/pspi0000093

Mikulincer, M., & Shaver, P. (2016). *Attachment in adulthood: Structure, dynamics, and change* (2nd ed.). Guilford Press.

Miller, R. B., Hollist, C. S., Olsen, J., & Law, D. (2013). Marital quality and health over 20 years: A growth curve analysis. *Journal of Marriage and Family, 75*(3), 667–680. https://doi.org/10.1111/jomf.12025

Morelli, S. A., Torre, J. B., & Eisenberger, N. I. (2014). The neural bases of feeling understood and not understood. *Social Cognitive and Affective Neuroscience, 9*(12), 1890–1896. https://doi.org/10.1093/scan/nst191

Murphy, M. C., & Zirkel, S. (2015). Race and belonging in school: How anticipated and experienced belonging affect choice, persistence, and performance. *Teacher's College Record, 117*(12), 1–40.

Murray, H. A. (1938). *Explorations in personality.* Oxford University Press.

Murray, S. L., Bellavia, G. M., Rose, P., & Griffin, D. W. (2003). Once hurt, twice hurtful: How perceived regard regulates daily marital interactions. *Journal of Personality and Social Psychology, 84*(1), 126–147. https://doi.org/10.1037/0022-3514.84.1.126

Murray, S. L., & Holmes, J. G. (1997). A leap of faith? Positive illusions in romantic relationships. *Personality and Social Psychology Bulletin, 23*(6), 586–604. https://doi.org/10.1177/0146167297236003

Neuberg, S. L., & Fiske, S. T. (1987). Motivational influences on impression formation: Outcome dependency, accuracy-driven attention, and individuating processes. *Journal of Personality and Social Psychology, 53*(3), 431–444. https://doi.org/10.1037/0022-3514.53.3.431

Niedenthal, P. M., Mermillod, M., Maringer, M., & Hess, U. (2010). The Simulation of Smiles (SIMS) model: Embodied simulation and the meaning of facial expression. *Behavioral and Brain Sciences, 33*(6), 417–433. https://doi.org/10.1017/S0140525X1 0000865

O'Neill, A. S., Mohr, C. D., Bodner, T. E., & Hammer, L. B. (2020). Perceived partner responsiveness, pain, and sleep: A dyadic study of military-connected couples. *Health Psychology, 39*(12), 1089–1099. https://doi.org/10.1037/hea0001035

Orehek, E., Forest, A. L., & Wingrove, S. (2018). People as means to multiple goals: Implications for interpersonal relationships. *Personality and Social Psychology Bulletin, 44*(10), 1487–1501. https://doi.org/10.1177/0146167218769869

Organ, D. W., & Ryan, K. (1995). A meta-analytic review of attitudinal and dispositional predictors of organizational citizenship behavior. *Personnel Psychology, 48*(4), 775–802. https://doi.org/10.1111/j.1744-6570.1995.tb01781.x

Otero, M. C., Wells, J. L., Chen, K.-H., Brown, C. L., Levenson, R. W., & Fredrickson, B. L. (2020). Behavioral indices of positivity resonance associated with long-term marital satisfaction. *Emotion*, *20*(7), 1225–1233. https://doi.org/10.1037/emo0000634

Overall, N. C., & McNulty, J. K. (2017). What type of communication during conflict is beneficial for intimate relationships? *Current Opinion in Psychology*, *13*, 1–5. https://doi.org/10.1016/j.copsyc.2016.03.002

Pansera, C., & La Guardia, J. (2012). The role of sincere amends and perceived partner responsiveness in forgiveness. *Personal Relationships*, *19*(4), 696–711. https://doi.org/10.1111/j.1475-6811.2011.01386.x

Park, Y., Visserman, M. L., Sisson, N. M., Le, B. M., Stellar, J. E., & Impett, E. A. (2020). How can I thank you? Highlighting the benefactor's responsiveness or costs when expressing gratitude. *Journal of Social and Personal Relationships*. https://doi.org/10.1177/0265407520966049

Peplau, L. A., & Perlman, D. (1982). Perspectives on loneliness. In L. A. Peplau & D. Perlman (Eds.), *Loneliness* (pp. 1–18). Wiley.

Pietromonaco, P. R., Overall, N. C., & Powers, S. I. (2021). Depressive symptoms, external stress, and marital adjustment: The buffering effect of partner's responsive behavior. *Social Psychological and Personality Science*. https://doi.org/10.1177/19485506211001687

Pinquart, M., & Sörensen, S. (2000). Influences of socioeconomic status, social network, and competence on subjective well-being in later life: A meta-analysis. *Psychology and aging*, *15*(2), 187–224. https://doi.org/10.1037//0882-7974.15.2.187

Pinsker, H., Nepps, P. Redfield, J., & Winston, A. (1985). Applicants for short-term dynamic psychotherapy. In A. Winston (Ed.), *Clinical and research issues in short-term dynamic psychotherapy* (pp. 104–116). American Psychiatric Association.

Proulx, C. M., Helms, H. M., & Buehler, C. (2007). Marital quality and personal well-being: A meta-analysis. *Journal of Marriage and family*, *69*(3), 576–593. https://doi.org/10.1111/j.1741-3737.2007.00393.x

Rafnsson, S. B., Shankar, A., & Steptoe, A. (2015). Longitudinal influences of social network characteristics on subjective well-being of older adults: Findings from the ELSA study. *Journal of Aging and Health*, *27*(5), 919–934. https://doi.org/10.1177/0898264315572111

Reis, H. T. (2007). Steps toward the ripening of relationship science. *Personal Relationships*, *14*, 1–23. https://doi.org/10.1111/j.1475-6811.2006.00139.x

Reis, H. T. (2012). Perceived partner responsiveness as an organizing theme for the study of relationships and well-being. In L. Campbell & T. J. Loving (Eds.), *Interdisciplinary research on close relationships* (pp. 27–52). APA Books. https://doi.org/10.1037/13486-002

Reis, H. T., & Clark, M. S. (2013). Responsiveness. In J. A. Simpson & L. Campbell (Eds.), *The Oxford handbook of close relationships* (pp. 400–423). Oxford University Press. https://doi.org/10.1093/oxfordhb/9780195398694.013.0018

Reis, H. T., Maniaci, M. R., & Rogge, R. D. (2017). Compassionate acts and everyday emotional well-being among newlyweds. *Emotion*, *17*(4), 751–763. https://doi.org/10.1037/emo0000281

Reis, H. T., & Mizrahi, M. (2018). Whither relationship science? The state of the science and an agenda for moving forward. In A. L. Vangelisti & D. Perlman (Eds.), *The

Cambridge handbook of personal relationships. (pp. 553–564). Cambridge University Press. https://doi.org/10.1017/9781316417867.042

Reis, H. T., Regan, A., & Lyuobomirsky, S. (2022). Interpersonal chemistry: What is it, how does it emerge, and how does it operate? *Perspectives on Psychological Science, 17*(2), 530–558. https://doi.org.10.1177/1745691621994241

Reis, H. T., & Shaver, P. (1988). Intimacy as an interpersonal process. In S. W. Duck (Ed.), *Handbook of personal relationships* (pp. 367–389). John Wiley & Sons.

Reis, H. T., Sheldon, K. M., Gable, S. L., Roscoe, J., & Ryan, R. M. (2000). Daily well-being: The role of autonomy, competence, and relatedness. *Personality and Social Psychology Bulletin, 26*(4), 419–435. https://doi.org/10.1177/0146167200266002

Rimé, B. (2009). Emotion elicits the social sharing of emotion: Theory and empirical review. *Emotion Review, 1*(1), 60–85. https://doi.org/10.1177/1754073908097189

Roberson, P. N. E., Shorter, R. L., Woods, S., & Priest, J. (2018). How health behaviors link romantic relationship dysfunction and physical health across 20 years for middle-aged and older adults. *Social Science and Medicine, 201*, 18–26. https://doi.org/10.1016/j.socscimed.2018.01.037

Robles, T. F., & Kiecolt-Glaser, J. K. (2003). The physiology of marriage: Pathways to health. *Physiology & Behavior, 79*(3), 409–416. https://doi.org/10.1016/s0031-9384(03)00160-4

Robles, T. F., Slatcher, R. B., Trombello, J. M., & McGinn, M. M. (2015). Marital quality and health: A meta-analytic review. *Psychological Bulletin, 140*(1), 140–187. https://doi.org/10.1037/a0031859

Rodriguez, L. M., Fillo, J., Hadden, B. W., Øverup, C. S., Baker, Z. G., & DiBello, A. M. (2019). Do you see what I see? Actor and partner attachment shape biased perceptions of partners. *Personality and Social Psychology Bulletin, 45*(4), 587–602. https://doi.org/10.1177/0146167218791782

Rothbaum, F., & Weisz, J. (1994). Parental converging and child externalizing behavior in non-clinical samples: A meta-analysis. *Psychological Bulletin, 116*(1), 55–74. https://doi.org/10.1037/0033-2909.116.1.55

Ruan, Y., Reis, H. T., Clark, M. S., Hirsch, J. L., & Bink, B. D. (2020). Can I tell you how I feel? Perceived partner responsiveness encourages emotional expression. *Emotion, 20*(3), 329–342. https://doi.org/10.1037/emo0000650

Rusbult, C. E., Finkel, E. J., & Kumashiro, M. (2009). The Michelangelo phenomenon. *Current Directions in Psychological Science, 18*(6), 305–309. https://doi.org/10.1111/j.1467-8721.2009.01657.x

Rusbult, C. E., Kumashiro, M., & Reis, H. T. (2010). The Michelangelo effect and perceived responsiveness. Unpublished manuscript, Vrije Universiteit.

Rusbult, C. E., Olsen, N., Davis, J. L., & Hannon, P. A. (2001). Commitment and relationship maintenance mechanisms. In J. H. Harvey & A. Wenzel (Eds.), *Close romantic relationships: Maintenance and enhancement* (pp. 87–113). Erlbaum.

Ryff, C. D. (1995). Psychological well-being in adult life. *Current Directions in Psychological Science, 4*(4), 99–104. https://doi.org/10.1111/1467-8721.ep10772395

Sandstrom, G. M., & Dunn, E. W. (2014). Social interactions and well-being: The surprising power of weak ties. *Personality and Social Psychology Bulletin, 40*(7), 910–922. https://doi.org/10.1177/0146167214529799

Sasaki, E., & Overall, N. (2021). Partners' withdrawal when actors behave destructively: Implications for perceptions of partners' responsiveness and relationship satisfaction. *Personality and Social Psychology Bulletin, 47*(2), 307–323. https://doi.org/10.1177/0146167220926820

Sears, R. R. (1977). Sources of life satisfactions of the Terman gifted men. *American Psychologist, 32*(2), 119–128. https://doi.org/10.1037/0003-066X.32.2.119

Seeman, T. E. (1996). Social ties and health: The benefits of social integration. *Annals of Epidemiology, 6*(5), 442–451. https://doi.org/10.1016/s1047-2797(96)00095-6

Segal, N., & Fraley, R. C. (2016). Broadening the investment model: An intensive longitudinal study on attachment and perceived partner responsiveness in commitment dynamics. *Journal of Social and Personal Relationships, 33*(5), 581–599. https://doi.org/10.1177/0265407515584493

Selcuk, E., Gunaydin, G., Ong, A. D., & Almeida, D. M. (2016). Does partner responsiveness predict hedonic and eudaimonic well-being? A 10-year longitudinal study. *Journal of Marriage and Family, 78*(2), 311–325. https://doi.org/10.1111/jomf.12272

Selcuk, E., & Ong, A. D. (2013). Perceived partner responsiveness moderates the association between received emotional support and all-cause mortality. *Health Psychology, 32*(2), 231–235. https://doi.org/10.1037/a0028276

Selcuk, E., Stanton, S. C., Slatcher, R. B., & Ong, A. D. (2017). Perceived partner responsiveness predicts better sleep quality through lower anxiety. *Social Psychological and Personality Science, 8*(1), 83–92. https://doi.org/10.1177/1948550616662128

Simpson, J. A., & Belsky, J. (2008). Attachment theory within a modern evolutionary framework. In M. Mikulincer & P. R. Shaver (Eds.), *Handbook of attachment: Theory, research, and clinical applications* (2nd ed., pp. 131–157). Guilford.

Simpson, J. A., Rholes, W. S., & Nelligan, J. S. (1992). Support-seeking and support-giving within couples in an anxiety provoking situation: The role of attachment styles. *Journal of Personality and Social Psychology, 62*(3), 434–446. https://doi.org/10.1037/0022-3514.62.3.434

Simpson, J. A., Rholes, W. S., Oriña, M. M., & Grich, J. (2002). Working models of attachment, support giving, and support seeking in a stressful situation. *Personality and Social Psychology Bulletin, 28*(5), 598–608. https://doi.org/10.1177/0146167202288004

Slatcher, R. (2021). Love in the time of COVID-19: Perceived partner responsiveness buffers people from lower relationship quality associated with COVID-related stressors. Manuscript under review, University of Georgia.

Slatcher, R. B., & Selcuk, E. (2017). A social psychological perspective on the links between close relationships and health. *Current Directions in Psychological Science, 26*(1), 16–21. https://doi.org/10.1177/0963721416667444

Slatcher, R. B., Selcuk, E., & Ong, A. D. (2015). Perceived partner responsiveness predicts diurnal cortisol profiles 10 years later. *Psychological Science, 26*(7), 972–982. https://doi.org/10.1177/0956797615575022

Sprecher, S., & Treger, S. (2015). The benefits of turn-taking reciprocal self-disclosure in get-acquainted interactions. *Personal Relationships, 22*(3), 460–475. https://doi.org/10.1111/pere.12090

Stanton, S. C. E., Selcuk, E., Farrell, A. K., Slatcher, R. B., & Ong, A. D. (2019). Perceived partner responsiveness, daily negative affect reactivity, and all-cause mortality: A 20-year longitudinal study. *Psychosomatic Medicine, 81*(1), 7–15. https://doi.org/10.1097/PSY.0000000000000618

Stiles, W. B., Honos-Webb, L., & Surko, M. (1998). Responsiveness in psychotherapy. *Clinical Psychology: Science and Practice, 5*(4), 439–458. https://doi.org/10.1111/j.1468-2850.1998.tb00166.x

Street Jr., R. L., Makoul, G., Arora, N. K., & Epstein, R. M. (2009). How does communication heal? Pathways linking clinician–patient communication to health outcomes. *Patient Education and Counseling, 74*(3), 295–301. https://doi.org/10.1016/j.pec.2008.11.015

Stroebe, W., & Stroebe, M. S. (1996). The social psychology of social support. In A. Kruglanski & E. T. Higgins (Eds.), *Social psychology: Handbook of basic principles* (pp. 597–621). Guilford.

Swann, W. B., Jr. (1990). To be adored or to be known: The interplay of self-enhancement and self-verification. In R. Sorrentino & E. T. Higgins (Eds.), *Handbook of motivation and cognition* (Vol. 2, pp. 408–448). Guilford.

Swindle Jr, R., Heller, K., Pescosolido, B., & Kikuzawa, S. (2000). Responses to nervous breakdowns in America over a 40-year period: Mental health policy implications. *American Psychologist, 55*(7), 740–749. https://doi.org/10.1037/0003-066X.55.7.740

Taylor, S. E. (2011). Social support: A review. In H. S. Friedman (Ed.), *The Oxford handbook of health psychology* (pp. 189–214). Oxford University Press. https://doi.org/10.1093/oxfordhb/9780195342819.013.0009

Tasfiliz, D., Selcuk, E., Gunaydin, G., Slatcher, R. B., Corriero, E. F., & Ong, A. D. (2018). Patterns of perceived partner responsiveness and well-being in Japan and the United States. *Journal of Family Psychology, 32*(3), 355–365. https://doi.org/10.1037/fam0000378

Teo, A. R., Choi, H. J., & Valenstein, M. (2013). Social relationships and depression: Ten-year follow-up from a nationally representative study. *PLoS ONE, 8*(4), 1–8. https://doi.org/10.1371/journal.pone.0062396

The Guardian. (2015). Only genuine understanding from politicians can save the NHS. http://www.theguardian.com/healthcare-network/views-from-the-nhs-frontline/2015/apr/27/politicians-understanding-save-nhs-election.

Thompson, R. A. (2015). Relationships, regulation, and early development. In M. E. Lamb & R. M. Lerner (Eds.), *Handbook of child psychology and developmental science: Socioemotional processes* (pp. 201–246). John Wiley & Sons. https://doi.org/10.1002/9781118963418.childpsy306

Tickle-Degnen, L., & Rosenthal, R. (1987). Group rapport and nonverbal behavior. In C. Hendrick (Ed.), *Review of personality and social psychology: Vol. 9. Group processes and intergroup relations* (pp. 113–136). Sage.

Tsai, F. F., & Reis, H. T. (2009). Perceptions by and of lonely people in social networks. *Personal Relationships, 16*, 221–238. https://doi.org/10.1111/j.1475-6811.2009.01220.x

Twenge, J. M., Baumeister, R. F., DeWall, C. N., Ciarocco, N. J., & Bartels, J. M. (2007). Social exclusion decreases prosocial behavior. *Journal of Personality and Social Psychology, 92*(1), 56–66. https://doi.org/10.1037/0022-3514.92.1.56

Twenge, J. M., Catanese, K. R., & Baumeister, R. F. (2002). Social exclusion causes self-defeating behavior. *Journal of Personality and Social Psychology, 83*(3), 606–615. https://doi.org/10.1037/0022-3514.83.3.606

Tyler, T. R. (1990). *Why people obey the law.* Yale University Press.

Uchino, B. N., Cacioppo, J. T., & Kiecolt-Glaser, J. K. (1996). The relationship between social support and physiological processes: A review with emphasis on underlying mechanisms and implications for health. *Psychological Bulletin, 119*(3), 488–531. https://doi.org/10.1037/0033-2909.119.3.488

Uchino, B. N., Trettevik, R., Kent de Grey, R. G., Cronan, S., Hogan, J., & Baucom, B. R. W. (2018). Social support, social integration, and inflammatory cytokines: A meta-analysis. *Health Psychology, 37*(5), 462–471. https://doi.org/10.1037/hea0000594

Ueno, K. (2005). The effects of friendship networks on adolescent depressive symptoms. *Social Science Research, 34*(3), 484–510. https://doi.org/10.1016/j.ssresea rch.2004.03.002

Valdesolo, P., & DeSteno, D. (2011). Synchrony and the social tuning of compassion. *Emotion, 11*(2), 262–266. https://doi.org/10.1037/a0021302

van Ijzendoorn, M. H. (1995). Adult attachment representations, parental responsiveness, and infant attachment: A meta-analysis on the predictive validity of the Adult Attachment Interview. *Psychological Bulletin, 117*(3), 387–403. https://doi.org/ 10.1037/0033-2909.117.3.387

Van Prooijen, J. W., Van den Bos, K., & Wilke, H. A. (2004). Group belongingness and procedural justice: Social inclusion and exclusion by peers affects the psychology of voice. *Journal of Personality and Social Psychology, 87*(1), 66–79. https://doi.org/ 10.1037/0022-3514.87.1.66

Weissman, M. M., Markowitz, J. C., & Klerman, G. L. (2007). *Clinician's quick guide to interpersonal psychotherapy.* Oxford University Press.

Wheatley, T., Kang, O., Parkinson, C., & Looser, C. E. (2012). From mind perception to mental connection: Synchrony as a mechanism for social understanding. *Social and Personality Psychology Compass, 6*(8), 589–606. https://doi.org/10.1111/ j.1751-9004.2012.00450.x

Wheeler, L., Reis, H. T., & Nezlek, J. (1983). Loneliness, social interaction and sex roles. *Journal of Personality and Social Psychology, 45*(4), 943–953. https://doi.org/ 10.1037/0022-3514.45.4.943

Whiffen, V. E. (2005). The role of partner characteristics in attachment insecurity and depressive symptoms. *Personal Relationships, 12*(3), 407–423. https://doi.org/ 10.1111/j.1475-6811.2005.00123.x

Whisman, M. A. (2001). The association between depression and marital dissatisfaction. In S. R. H. Beach (Ed.), *Marital and family processes in depression: A scientific foundation for clinical practice* (pp. 3–24). American Psychological Association. https:// doi.org/10.1037/10350-001

Whisman, M. A., & Bruce, M. L. (1999). Marital dissatisfaction and incidence of major depressive episode in a community sample. *Journal of Abnormal Psychology, 108*(4), 674–678. https://doi.org/10.1037//0021-843x.108.4.674

Wilson, S. J., Martire, L. M., & Sliwinski, M. J. (2017). Daily spousal responsiveness predicts longer-term trajectories of patients' physical function. *Psychological Science, 28*(6), 786–797. https://doi.org/10.1177/0956797617697444

Winczewski, L. A., Bowen, J. D., & Collins, N. L. (2016). Is empathic accuracy enough to facilitate responsive behavior in dyadic interaction? Distinguishing ability from motivation. *Psychological Science, 27*(3), 394–404. https://doi.org/10.1177/09567 97615624491

Zee, K. S., Bolger, N., & Higgins, E. T. (2020). Regulatory effectiveness of social support. *Journal of Personality and Social Psychology, 119*(6), 1316–1358. https://doi. org/10.1037/pspi0000235

6

Life Satisfaction, Marital Status, and Partnership Quality

Modelling from Australia

BRUCE CHAPMAN AND NABEEH ZAKARIYYA ∎

INTRODUCTION

For about the past 25 years, the availability of multitudes of unit record data files has led to burgeoning research on many aspects of the life experience. One of the most visited issues relates to the determinants of life satisfaction, on which literally thousands of papers have been written (see also Chapter 3, this volume), even leading to the birth of a new publishing outlet, *The Journal of Happiness Studies*. Part of this upsurge can be explained by the relative ease of the use of ordinary least squares (OLS) regression, in which life satisfaction is treated as the dependent variable, regressed on economic, demographic, health status, and other individual characteristics.

Over time it has become increasingly difficult to find new and interesting life satisfaction issues to explore with this method simply because so much has already been done across a large number of countries. But occasionally an opportunity presents itself, as in the form of the availability of rare information, and this is the motivation for what is presented in this chapter. Specifically, we report on an empirical examination of the associations between relationship status, partner satisfaction, and life satisfaction. Building on the contribution by Chapman and Guven (2016), we analyse data from the Household, Income and Labour Dynamics in Australia (HILDA) survey from 2001 to 2019. HILDA is a large longitudinal dataset that includes a rich set of questions assessing subjective wellbeing, including overall life satisfaction and satisfaction with one's partner. It also includes a significant sample in which both partners in a household are surveyed, providing information which allows us to explore the importance to life satisfaction of both a person's assessment of their partner and their partner's assessment of them, something which has not been previously reported.

RELATIONSHIPS AND LIFE SATISFACTION

There has been considerable research, amounting to hundreds of papers, examining the importance of positive relationships to life satisfaction (for an overview of this research, see Chapter 5, this volume). Empirical tests of the hypothesised role of positive relationships in life satisfaction have taken various forms, many of which focus on the role of the institution of marriage. The simplest form of testing the importance of marriage to life satisfaction follows the approach of Dush and Amato (2005) and Kwon (2021) in which being married is included as a covariant in a single-equation econometric approach to unwrapping the influence of factors also associated with higher levels of life satisfaction. These typically include measures of health, income, age, the presence of children, and education while sometimes also controlling for ethnicity and religiosity (the importance of religion in people's lives). Invariably, on average, marriage is positively associated with higher life satisfaction and often seems to have a fairly large effect.

There are many possible concerns with these typical empirical methods to the issue of the role of marriage. One is related to the question of what economists label 'endogeneity'; that is, there may be a selection bias operating because happier people tend to get married, and this might be the source of the apparent causal association between marriage and life satisfaction. This is a common form of concern with the simple single-equation econometric methods in this area, one that could apply in a general sense to all of this kind of modelling. After all, aren't all of the variables likely to 'explain' life satisfaction related in such a way as to make a single compelling story hard to tell, and isn't it possible that two-way causality is present (such that being more satisfied leads to good health behaviours, higher fertility, greater incomes, and so on)?

It is very likely that the above concerns will remain in this literature, but there have been some attempts to handle the selection process, with two of these being proposed by Grover and Helliwell (2019) and Demir (2008). Through the use of longitudinal data controlling for premarital life satisfaction, the former paper establishes an additional and large effect of being married on life satisfaction, and the latter paper isolates a positive marriage effect after controlling for personality factors.

A different concern with the straightforward tests of the marital status and life satisfaction association focuses on the role of 'partnership/marriage quality', seeking effectively to explore the possibility that the average effect of being married on life satisfaction is complicated or even undermined by there being 'good/happy' and 'poor/unhappy' marriages. This notion is upheld in Demir (2008) and given a strong empirical basis in tests across Germany, the United Kingdom, and the United States by Chapman and Guven (2016), who summarise these findings in stating that, 'People in self-assessed poor marriages are fairly miserable and much less happy than unmarried people, even in the first year of marriage. However, people in self-assessed good marriages are even happier than the literature suggests' (p. 533).

The current chapter builds on these latter studies by moving beyond marital status to also include an aspect of relationships not so far examined: a person's satisfaction with their partner as well as this partner's satisfaction with the person as a partner. Furthermore, we empirically examine satisfaction between partners in a relationship and its association with an individual's overall life satisfaction in comparison with other factors such as socioeconomic status and demographics.

In a notable way, what we are examining empirically are key aspects of the role of perceived partner responsiveness as proposed by Reis and Le (Chapter 5, this volume). What Reis and Le explore in consummate detail is the multidimensional construct of perceived partner responsiveness: that is, the degree to which we see our partners as understanding, respecting, appreciating, and supporting us. What is reported in this chapter could be seen as providing further empirical investigation for their analysis. To elaborate, Reis and Le propose the following sequence (as depicted in Figure 6.1):

1. Partner A demonstrates partner responsiveness to partner B.
2. Partner B perceives this responsiveness.
3. This results in positive outcomes for partner B in terms of relationship satisfaction and their own overall wellbeing.

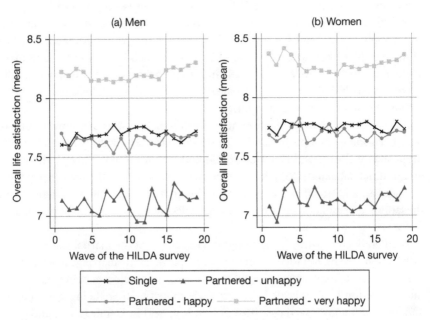

Partnered are gouped according to happiness with relationship.
0–6: Unhappy, 7–8: Happy, 9–10: Very happy

Figure 6.1 Overall life satisfaction for all partnership groups, averaged by HILDA wave.

Our construct of assessing the partner's satisfaction with the respondent can be seen as tapping into this partner's responsiveness to the respondent (especially in terms of the partner's appreciation of the respondent) in accordance with Step 1. Conversely, our construct of assessing the respondent's satisfaction with their partner, as well as the respondent's life satisfaction, would seem to assess the positive outcomes described in Step 3.

The first part of the current exercise is the use of the answers to both questions (i.e., a person's satisfaction with their partner as well as this partner's satisfaction with the person) in the construction of an index reflecting overall partner satisfaction. We take this index to be a reflection of relationship quality, albeit as quite a different representation of this concept to that used and reported in Chapman and Guven (2016). Second, we treat the responses to the questions separately in life satisfaction equations to determine the role of both a respondent's assessment of their partner and the partner's assessment of them. We are able to undertake both approaches separately for men and women and with respect to the use of typical pooled OLS modelling.[1] These disparate exercises allow us to check the robustness of typically used determinants of life satisfaction (such as health, education, income equivalised household income, and age) to the inclusion of unusual and potentially fundamental measures of subjective interest (Ferrer-i-Carbonell & Frijters, 2004).

EMPIRICAL METHODS

In this section, we describe the statistical models we utilised in the analyses that follow. Equation (1) illustrates the usual method, where the dependent variable is the measure of life satisfaction (i.e., happiness), β_m is the coefficient for a marriage dummy. β_j^s are the coefficients for other T control variables (x_j summed to T) in the marriage dummy model.

$$Happiness = \beta_0 + \beta_m X_m + \Sigma_{j=1}^{T} \beta_j X_j \in \tag{1}$$

A more flexible functional form is given by Equation (2) in which γ_i^s are the coefficients for each level of marriage quality, which for our empirical purposes are assumed to number three (as explained below, to correspond to the empirical analysis, 1 = not in a happy relationship, 2 = happy relationship, and 3 = very happy relationship).

$$Happiness = \beta_0 + \gamma_1 X_1 + \gamma_2 X_2 + \gamma_3 X_3 + \Sigma_{j=1}^{T} \beta_j' X_j + \in \tag{2}$$

1. The robustness of all our results has also been verified using fixed-effects estimations. These results are omitted from this chapter and are available from the authors.

In a situation in which the marriage variables are uncorrelated with other control variables, the marriage dummy coefficient from Equation (1) is given by:

$$\beta_m = \bar{\gamma} = \sum_{i=1}^{3} \omega_i \gamma_i,$$

where the weight ω_i is the proportion of the sample for each level of marriage quality. Allowing for some degree of correlation among the regressors, the married dummy can be approximated by:

$$\beta_m \approx \bar{\gamma} = \sum_{i=1}^{3} \omega_i \gamma_i.$$

We are concerned mainly with comparisons of the results of estimations in Equation (1) (with the usual set of right-hand side variables) with the results of various estimations of Equation (2). In a main part of the analysis, we seek to determine the role of marriage quality on happiness, with the clear prediction that $\gamma_1 > \gamma_2 > \gamma_3$. This part of the exercise allows us to illustrate a new range of marriage effects, and this leads to a more disaggregated analysis concerning the effects of different variables on happiness and other differences between people.

Also on method is that the key motivation of this research is to unwrap further the associations between marital status, relationship quality, and life satisfaction. This issue was first explored in Chapman and Guven (2016), in which it was argued that the finding of a significant positive effect of marriage with respect to happiness is unlikely to be the case for couples in unfulfilling marriages, a proposition tested and supported, as previously stated. Specifically, it was found that the happiest people were indeed in happy marriages, but that those in poor-quality relationships were actually less happy than single people.

Our methods extend this work through the use of what we refer to as 'overall partner satisfaction', which uses the responses to questions concerning an individual's view of their happiness with their partner, and their partner's happiness with them. Such an approach has not been done before simply because information on partner's approval of partner has not been available. The current exercise is a richer source of partnership health information since, in the HILDA survey, *both* members of the relationship provide ratings on their satisfaction with their partner on a scale from 0 (*completely dissatisfied*) to 10 (*completely satisfied*).[2]

2. Cassells, Gong, and Keegan (2010) report exercises using the HILDA data on LS and PS. But the methods used are bivariate without econometric application.

While there is a plethora of ways in which basic marital satisfaction might be tested, in a first stage and for simplicity we chose to impose a particular form of partner satisfaction (PS), which is given by:

$$PS = \frac{Satisfaction\ with\ partner + Partner's\ satisfaction\ with\ you}{2}.$$

This form thus implicitly accords equal empirical status to the two partnership satisfaction variables. As well, again for simplicity, we chose to define three categories of partnership quality, labelled 'unhappy', 'medium happy', and 'very happy', according to the following schema:

$$Status = \begin{cases} 0\ if\ single \\ 1\ (unhappy)\ if\ partnered\ and\ PS \in [0,6] \\ 2\ (medium\ happy)\ if\ partnered\ and\ PS \in [7,8] \\ 3\ (very\ happy)\ if\ partnered\ and\ PS \in [9,10] \end{cases}$$

In more accessible parlance, the above means that the three categories are defined in ascending order of satisfaction if the answers measuring PS are, out of 10: 0–6, 7/8, and 9/10, respectively.

While these data impositions are somewhat arbitrary, they have the great advantage of simplicity of both presentation and interpretation. However, it should be noted that we did many and different tests of robustness to variations in the functional form used with respect to partner satisfaction. In the section on 'Results from the Basic OLS Model with Variations', we consider less aggregated forms of the life satisfaction and partner satisfaction associations, illustrating separately the effects on life satisfaction of the separate measures.

DERIVATION OF THE VARIABLES AND DESCRIPTION OF THE RAW DATA

Statistical Characteristics of the Data in Aggregate

In what follows, HILDA data are used to examine several closely related questions. These are annual data, and we have used the 19 waves now available, from 2001 to 2019.

Table 6.1 presents descriptive statistics for the key variables using only the cross-sectional statistics for wave 19 (2019) information (noting that the data from the other waves are quite similar). These data are familiar to researchers focusing on the Australian labour market, with respect to education, income, age, and location. Furthermore, the health status information is consistent with other broad

Table 6.1 DESCRIPTIVE STATISTICS 2019 (MEAN FOR CONTINUOUS VARIABLES, % FOR CATEGORIES)

	Men					Women			
	Single	Unhappy couple	Medium happy couple	Very happy couple	Single	Unhappy couple	Medium happy couple	Very happy couple
Individuals (N)	2,871	500	1,251	3,659	3,572	497	1,257	3,855
Percent of total men/women	34.67	6.04	15.11	44.19	38.91	5.41	13.69	41.99
Continuous variables (mean)								
Overall happiness	7.72	7.15	7.68	8.30	7.74	7.23	7.71	8.36
Happiness with partner	NA	5.07	7.75	9.28	NA	4.26	7.26	9.08
Partner's happiness with you	NA	4.25	7.26	9.19	NA	5.08	7.75	9.34
Household disposable income ($)	62,561	67,728	77,186	75,143	57,936	67,863	77,204	74,793
Age (years)	37.16	48.66	49.22	49.39	45.43	46.21	46.85	47.20
Categorical variables (%)								
Legally married or _de facto_	0.00	70.40	72.98	72.92	0.00	69.62	72.87	72.63
Employed	58.10	75.00	75.30	71.39	52.91	66.60	67.54	62.57
Unemployed	8.57	4.40	2.32	2.27	6.22	2.01	1.91	1.63
Not in labour force	33.33	20.60	22.38	26.35	40.87	31.39	30.55	35.80
Renters	41.43	24.60	23.10	26.96	41.47	24.35	22.91	26.49
Rent to buy scheme	0.00	0.20	0.00	0.08	0.03	0.20	0.00	0.08
Live rent free/life tenure	4.16	1.20	1.04	2.30	3.68	1.01	1.19	2.21
Education:								
Year 11 or below	33.16	17.20	14.71	18.04	33.34	18.71	16.79	22.31
Year 12	23.65	10.80	9.59	11.86	18.03	15.29	11.69	13.05
Certificate/Diploma	28.94	43.60	43.80	41.10	26.76	32.19	31.82	29.83
Graduate or above								
Children:	14.25	28.40	31.89	29.00	21.86	33.80	39.70	34.81

No children	85.79	51.00	56.83	65.76	78.05	50.50	56.80	65.45
One child	9.02	19.80	15.43	12.79	12.51	20.12	15.51	12.94
More than one child	5.19	29.20	27.74	21.45	9.43	29.38	27.68	21.61
Excellent health	13.78	6.04	7.30	12.01	10.21	5.91	5.83	10.78
Very good health	34.21	24.55	33.12	36.33	30.84	27.29	34.66	39.58
Good health	32.97	43.06	41.62	36.42	34.78	41.34	42.17	35.27
Fair health	15.73	19.92	14.76	12.59	18.70	20.16	14.46	11.84
Poor health	3.31	6.44	3.21	2.65	5.47	5.30	2.88	2.53
No others present during interview	80.50	65.79	64.78	61.44	78.11	62.45	59.89	55.92
Major city	65.27	66.40	68.35	64.20	66.61	66.40	68.18	63.96
Inner regional	22.66	22.00	22.22	23.23	22.58	21.93	22.43	23.55
Outer regional	10.60	10.20	8.23	11.00	9.69	10.26	8.19	10.91
Remote Australia	1.46	1.40	1.20	1.56	1.12	1.41	1.19	1.58

Australian data sources, and we are comfortable that the 19 waves of HILDA are an accurate representation of the population as a whole.

With respect to the raw differences between the various marital status and relationship satisfaction variables, the key points are as follows:

1. The majority of couples are married, and the majority of singles have never been in a relationship;
2. Single men are younger than partnered men, and there is no difference in average age between those in different types of relationships;
3. For both men and women, overall measures of life satisfaction appear to be high, with an average figure of around 7.5 out of a range from 0 to 10;
4. For both men and women, the majority of the sample consists of singles (34–39%) and couples in very happy relationships (44%);
5. On average, life satisfaction is lower in couples in unhappy relationships;
6. Couples in medium happy relationships and those who are single have similar overall life satisfaction. In comparison, those who are in very happy relationships have higher life satisfaction than all other groups;
7. Partner's happiness and happiness with partner variables differ between groups. Unsurprisingly, both variables on average record lower scores for unhappy couples;
8. There do not appear to be income differences between all groups; and
9. As would be expected, singles have fewer children than those partnered, and there are no stark differences in the average number of children between couples in happy and unhappy relationships.

Marital Status and Partnership Quality: The Data

Our focus on the role of marriage motivates our interest in presenting the unadjusted data for our derived partner satisfaction categories, with the frequency distributions for Wave 19 presented in Table 6.2. Each cell represents the proportions of the 2019 cross-section in each of the four categories with, for example, about 35–40% of the sample being single, and our life satisfaction categorisation of couples resulting in about 7%, 18%, and 38% of observations in the samples being unhappy, medium happy, and very happy, respectively. There are no

Table 6.2 PERCENTAGE OF MEN AND WOMEN BY RELATIONSHIP STATUS (2019) (%)

	Men	Women	Both
Not in a relationship	34.67	38.91	36.90
In an unhappy relationship	6.27	8.37	7.37
In a medium happy relationship	17.88	17.86	17.87
In a very happy relationship	41.18	34.87	37.86
	100	100	100

important differences in these sample proportions with respect to sex, with the composition for all other waves being fairly similar to this. The unadjusted average data illustrating life satisfaction, with respect to relationship status and relationship satisfaction for all of the 19 waves of HILDA, are presented in Figure 6.1.

The key points are as follows:

1. On average, people in medium happy relationships are about as happy as those who are single;
2. Those in unhappy relationships are unhappier than those who are single; and
3. Those who are in very happy relationships are happier than all other groups.

These data are, of course, raw averages because it is necessary to use econometrics to control for the role of myriad other life satisfaction influences. This is explored in the following section.

RESULTS FROM THE BASIC OLS MODEL WITH VARIATIONS

In our econometric modelling, we chose to follow the methodology supported in Clark, Frijters, and Shields (2008), which is to use a standard OLS regression approach. Table 6.3 presents the marginal effects (and statistical significance) derived from the pooled OLS regressions with life satisfaction as the dependent variable and with all regressions including time fixed effects. The first column of results for men and women shows the baseline model effects, and the second column of results for men and women shows effects including the partner satisfaction categories defined above, with *** denoting significance at the 1% level or lower.

The main findings are as follows. Except for the presence of children, there are no differences in the coefficients for any of the control variables in the baseline models and the partner satisfaction models. For the baseline models, there is a difference in overall happiness between those who have no children and those who do. However, the magnitude of the effects is quite small, with an effect in the order of 0.05 (out of 10) for men and women with one child compared to those with no children. In the baseline model, there is no statistically significant difference between men who have no children and those who have more than one child, whereas the same coefficient for women is highly significant at $p < 0.001$. The importance of children completely disappears for both men and women in the partner satisfaction models, with fairly small coefficients that are not statistically significantly different from zero.

As well, the coefficients on all other control variables are fairly robust to both specifications, and they explain the same relationships that are typically observed

Table 6.3 MARGINAL EFFECTS OF PARTNER SATISFACTION
DETERMINANTS: POOLED OLS

	Baseline	Men Relationship quality	Baseline	Women Relationship quality
[1] Legally married	0		0	
[2] *De facto*	−0.0803***		−0.103***	
[3] Separated	−0.691***		−0.723***	
[4] Divorced	−0.396***		−0.401***	
[5] Widowed	−0.393***		−0.210***	
[6] Never married and not *de facto*	−0.353***		−0.372***	
Single		0		0
Partnered - unhappy		−0.386***		−0.421***
Partnered – medium happy		0.0358		0.0250
Partnered - very happy		0.529***		0.531***
[1] Employed	0	0	0	0
[2] Unemployed	−0.316***	−0.303***	−0.269***	−0.269***
[3] Not in the labour force	0.0255	0.0141	0.121***	0.101***
HH equivalised income (log)	0.0919***	0.0837***	0.109***	0.108***
[1] Own / currently paying off mortgage	0	0	0	0
[2] Rent (or pay board) / Rent-buy scheme	−0.143***	−0.166***	−0.111***	−0.146***
[3] Live here rent free / Life Tenure	−0.108**	−0.127**	−0.0708	−0.0940*
Year 11 or below	0	0	0	0
Year 12	−0.175***	−0.175***	−0.112***	−0.109***
Certificate/Diploma	−0.124***	−0.130***	−0.106***	−0.110***
Graduate or above	−0.280***	−0.270***	−0.195***	−0.190***
Household size (log)	0.0475*	0.103***	−0.00942	0.00907
No children	0	0	0	0
One child	−0.0525**	−0.0198	−0.0526**	−0.00866
More than one child	−0.0308	0.0103	−0.0867***	−0.0211
Excellent health	0	0	0	0
Very good health	−0.467***	−0.450***	−0.467***	−0.445***
Good health	−0.932***	−0.878***	−0.944***	−0.885***
Fair health	−1.526***	−1.454***	−1.576***	−1.500***
Poor health	−2.599***	−2.514***	−2.598***	−2.520***
Age	−0.002***	−0.001***	−0.001***	0.000***
[1] Others present during interview	0	0	0	0
[2] No others present during interview	−0.105***	−0.0804***	−0.0926***	−0.0700***
[9] Don't know - telephone interview	−1.660*	−1.482*	−2.117**	−2.131**
[0] Major Cities of Australia	0	0	0	0
[1] Inner Regional Australia	0.131***	0.116***	0.151***	0.139***
[2] Outer Regional Australia	0.213***	0.188***	0.229***	0.204***
[3] Remote Australia	0.217***	0.198**	0.267***	0.236***

in the literature. In this regard, those who are unemployed are significantly less happy compared to those who are employed (with a magnitude of −0.30 for men and −0.27 for women, both significant at $p < 0.001$). There is no statistically significant difference in overall happiness between employed men and men who are not in the labour force. In contrast, for women, those who are not in the labour force on average are 0.1 points significantly happier than those who are employed. There is a quite large significant difference between homeowners and renters for both men and women. Education contributes negatively to overall happiness. Moreover, the typical statistically significant U-shaped relationship between age and overall happiness is confirmed in our regression.

One particular influence on life satisfaction stands out: self-assessed health. All models confirm a statistically significant and quite large positive relationship between good health and happiness. The magnitude of the effect of self-assessed health is the highest among all variables in the models. Compared to those who report that they are in excellent health, those who report that they are in poor health on average report an overall happiness score that is 2.6 points less. Similarly, those who report fair health report an overall happiness score that is 1.6 points lower, and those in good health report 0.9 points lower. Interestingly, there is a statistically significant difference at $p < 0.001$ even between those who report that they are in very good health and those who report they are in excellent health (with the latter, on average, reporting a happiness score that is 0.5 points higher).

Moving to the first main motivation for our exercise, the role of relationship quality in an assessment of the effect of partnership approval on life satisfaction, the following findings stand out:

1. The baseline models show that, for both men and women, those who are not in a relationship (be they single, separated, divorced, or widowed) are less happy compared to those who are in a relationship. These coefficients are all highly statistically significant with $p < 0.001$;
2. In comparison, the partner satisfaction modelling shows that, compared to those who are single, those who are in an unhappy relationship are significantly unhappier overall, with a magnitude of −0.386 for men and −0.421 for women; and
3. Compared to those who are single, those in a very happy relationship are significantly happier with a magnitude of 0.529 for men and 0.531 for women. This result is highly statistically significant. However, there is no statistically significant difference in overall happiness between those who are single and those who are in a medium happy relationship.

The key finding is that our composite measure of partnership satisfaction has large effects on life satisfaction. To illustrate the size of the effect, we note that those in unhappy relationships are about 0.95 points less happy than those in very happy partnerships, which is an effect of about 12% calculated at the mean. To give this further empirical context, this is about the same effect as having poor health

Table 6.4 COMPARISON OF RELATIONSHIP QUALITY MARGINAL EFFECTS BETWEEN US, UK, GERMAN, AND AUSTRALIAN DATA

	US GSS	BHPS	GSOEP	HILDA	
				Men	Women
Not too happily married	−0.476	−0.547	−0.268	−0.386	−0.421
Pretty happily married	−0.041	−0.177	0.037	0.0358	0.025
Happily married	0.437	0.292	0.343	0.529	0.531

NOTE: Compared to those who are not in a relationship. US GSS, BHPS, GSOEP data are from Chapman and Guven (2014) who estimate marriage quality for both men and women together. For the GSS, happiness is on a scale of 1–3 where (1) not too happy, (2) pretty happy, (3) very happy. GSOEP values were recoded (0–6) not too happy, (7, 8) pretty happy, (9, 10) very happy; and BHPS (1–3) not too happy, (4, 5) pretty happy, (6, 7) very happy. Our HILDA variable is coded similarly to that of GSOEP. The first column is estimated for all the waves of the GSS from 1974 to 2004. The second column is estimated only for the wave (2007) of BHPS. The third column is estimated only for the 25th wave (2007) of GSOEP. Our HILDA estimates are from 2001 to2019.

compared to having fair health and about three times larger than the unhappiness associated with being unemployed. Clearly, our measure of marital quality involving partnership approval is very important in understanding life satisfaction.

All these findings are consistent with the results found in Britain, Germany, and the United States using more conventional measures of marriage quality (Chapman & Guven, 2016). A comparison of the findings is provided in Table 6.4.

The Table 6.4 comparisons reveal the following:

1. The effect of marriage quality on life satisfaction is identical in terms of overall signs (unhappy married people everywhere have statistically significantly lower satisfaction than single people);
2. The effect of marriage quality on life satisfaction is about the same for people who are in the medium happily married category (who do not have statistically different levels of life satisfaction than single people); and
3. Very happily married people (both men and women) in Australia have higher levels of life satisfaction than similarly very happily married people in the United States, Britain, and Germany.

These results affirm the general conclusions of earlier work concerning the broad role of partnership quality even when measured quite differently.

RESULTS FOR DISAGGREGATED MEASURES OF PARTNERSHIP SATISFACTION

The findings reported above relate to estimations of happiness using a composite index that averages couples' satisfaction with each other, which is entirely

Table 6.5 THE EFFECTS ON LIFE SATISFACTION OF PARTNER APPROVAL MEASURES

	Men	Women
Equation 1: Happiness with partner		
Compared to those who are single:		
Unhappy with partner	−0.480***	−0.457***
Medium happy with partner	0.037	0.094***
Very happy with partner	0.606***	0.651***
Equation 2: Partner's happiness with you		
Compared to those who are single:		
Partner unhappy with you	−0.117***	−0.192***
Partner medium happy with you	0.180***	0.151***
Partner very happy with you	0.508***	0.488***

NOTE: For technical reasons, the STATA programme was unable to invert the matrix in a single-stage regression due to collinearity. Consequently, these estimates were obtained from separate regression, which necessarily implies some upwards bias in absolute size of the coefficients and thus marginal effects.

apposite in a context comparing this measure of partnership quality with those reported elsewhere. We now move to a more novel exploration of our unusual data, which is to ask the questions: What effect does a person's satisfaction with their partner have on the person's happiness, and what effect does a partner's satisfaction with the person have on the person's happiness? These enquiries are made possible because each adult in a household is interviewed separately for the HILDA panel.

Given the similarities of the coefficients in this modelling innovation, we chose to not report the estimations in full and instead now examine the separate effects of the different forms of the partner approval measures. These are shown in Table 6.5.

The key findings are as follows:

1. For both men and women, a respondent's satisfaction with their partner is strongly positively associated with their life satisfaction, and there are no differences between the sexes;
2. The orders of magnitude are such that being very happy, compared to being unhappy, with their partner, is associated with a difference of about 1 out of 10 in the life satisfaction measure, which is around 15% calculated at the mean. For context, this is about the same effect on life satisfaction as having fair health compared to poor health and about three times larger than the lower happiness of the unemployed compared to the employed;
3. People whose partners are very happy with them, compared to people whose partners are unhappy with them, have higher life satisfaction, of the order of about 0.6–0.7 out of 10 in the measure. This is just less than 10%, calculated at the mean;

4. The association between approval from one's partner and one's own life satisfaction is seemingly larger for women, with 0.68 higher life satisfaction for women whose partners are very happy with them, compared to 0.62 for the equivalent male comparison;

5. The comparative size of the 'satisfaction with partner' and 'partner's satisfaction with you' life satisfaction association is around double with respect to the former;

6. Compared to being single, people who are very happy with their partner have higher life satisfaction, and people who are very unhappy with their partner have lower life satisfaction; and

7. Compared to being single, people whose partner is very happy with them have higher life satisfaction, and people whose partner is very unhappy with them have lower life satisfaction.

These results, unsurprisingly, are strongly consistent with the findings reported with respect to the composite measure of partnership quality, in effect allowing an unwrapping of the roles of partner approval. An important point is that a respondent's happiness with their partner is associated with about twice the life satisfaction difference when compared to their partner's satisfaction with them.

We have had a close look at the size and significance of all the usual right-hand side variable coefficients in typical LS OLS equations and find close to no difference in them with the inclusion of our measures of partner satisfaction. This allows us to assert with some confidence that happiness modelling lacking measures of partner satisfaction are not compromised without the inclusion of these variables.

SUMMARY

We have used unique data available from the Australian HILDA survey (2001–2019) to explore further the apparent role of measures of partner satisfaction on happiness. At our disposal are measures of a respondent's satisfaction with their partner and their partner's satisfaction with them. Through separate analyses of both a composite index of these two partner satisfaction variables and disaggregated measures of the two variables, we have been able to explore the effect on life satisfaction of these different indicators of partner satisfaction.

A composite index of partner satisfaction is importantly and positively associated with life satisfaction, affirming the findings for Britain, Germany, and the United States reported in Chapman and Guven (2016) and of Diemer (2008). It is clear that these variables, the effect of which has never before been examined in these ways, are strongly associated with relatively large overall life satisfaction differences. In fact, partner satisfaction affects life satisfaction more than the apparent consequences of unemployment and quite similarly to being in fair health compared to being in poor health.

The use of the two different aspects of partner satisfaction adds important new detail to the basic issue of the role of marital status in life satisfaction.

Moreover, our findings further affirm the importance of work conducted by those such as Reis and Le (Chapter 5, this volume) who seek to understand the drivers of partner satisfaction, given the pivotal role of partner satisfaction for life satisfaction.

Appendix Table 6.A1 FULL REGRESSION RESULTS FOR SECTION 5 ESTIMATIONS

	Pooled OLS		Fixed effects	
	Men	Women	Men	Women
Single	0	0	0	0
Both very happy	0.650***	0.685***	0.502***	0.502***
Both happy	0.00428	0.0682**	0.229***	0.230***
Partners - Both unhappy	−0.587***	−0.578***	−0.205***	−0.260***
Respondent unhappy- Partner happy	−0.393***	−0.430***	−0.0244	−0.154***
Respondent unhappy- Partner very happy	−0.423***	−0.381***	−0.00937	−0.0999***
Respondent happy-Partner unhappy	−0.0677*	0.0178	0.131***	0.140***
Respondent happy-Partner very happy	0.0966***	0.122***	0.285***	0.267***
Respondent very happy- Partner unhappy	0.434***	0.428***	0.317***	0.333***
Respondent very happy- Partner happy	0.456***	0.496***	0.403***	0.422***
[1] Employed	0	0	0	0
[2] Unemployed	−0.304***	−0.263***	−0.203***	−0.169***
[3] Not in the labour force	0.00619	0.0918***	−0.0377*	0.0463***
HH equivalized income (log)	0.0879***	0.107***	0.0453***	0.0534***
[1] Own / currently paying off mortgage	0	0	0	0
[2] Rent (or pay board) / Rent-buy scheme	−0.167***	−0.147***	−0.133***	−0.107***
[3] Live here rent free / Life Tenure	−0.133***	−0.0936*	−0.0887**	−0.108***
Year 11 or below	0	0	0	0
Year 12	−0.171***	−0.107***	−0.217***	−0.149***
Certificate/Diploma	−0.122***	−0.107***	−0.248***	−0.125***
Graduate or above	0.249***	−0.190***	−0.325***	−0.200***
Household size (log)	0.100***	0.0259	0.0431**	−0.0238
No children	0	0	0	0
One child	−0.00466	0.000859	0.00679	0.0228
More than one child	0.0272	−0.0134	−0.00236	−0.0269
Excellent health	0	0	0	0
Very good health	−0.437***	−0.428***	−0.200***	−0.227***
Good health	−0.848***	−0.848***	−0.442***	−0.486***
Fair health	−1.409***	−1.453***	−0.814***	−0.877***
Poor health	−2.474***	−2.493***	−1.616***	−1.614***

(continued)

Appendix Table 6.A1 CONTINUED

	Pooled OLS		Fixed effects	
	Men	Women	Men	Women
Age	−0.0556***	−0.0451***	−0.0355***	−0.0222***
Age square/100	0.0674***	0.0573***	0.0389***	0.0260***
[1] Others present during interview	0	0	0	0
[2] No others present during interview	−0.0588***	−0.0409***	−0.0448***	−0.0378***
[9] Don't know - telephone interview	−1.654*	−2.150***	−0.688	−2.122
[0] Major Cities of Australia	0	0	0	0
[1] Inner Regional Australia	0.112***	0.133***	0.0289	0.0532*
[2] Outer Regional Australia	0.180***	0.186***	0.117**	0.0502
[3] Remote Australia	0.200***	0.226***	0.0954	−0.0421
Constant	8.463***	8.128***	8.512***	8.210***
Time fixed effects	Yes	Yes	Yes	Yes
Observations	118979	135119	118979	135119
Adjusted R-squared	0.235	0.230	0.070	0.067

Appendix Table 6.A2 SAMPLE DISTRIBUTIONS FOR DISAGGREGATED PARTNERSHIP SATISFACTION VARIABLES

	Respondent's happiness with partner (Score range)	Partner's happiness with respondent (Score range)	N (For 2019)	% (For 2019)
1. Single	NA	NA	6443	36.90
2. Both very happy	9–10	9–10	5134	29.40
3. Both happy	7–8	7–8	1326	7.59
4. Both unhappy	0–6	0–6	540	3.09
5. Respondent very happy, partner unhappy	9–10	0–6	249	1.43
6. Respondent very happy, partner happy	9–10	7–8	1228	7.03
7. Respondent happy, partner very happy	7–8	0–6	1385	7.93
8. Respondent happy, partner unhappy	7–8	9–10	410	2.35
9. Respondent unhappy, partner very happy	0–6	9–10	339	1.94
10. Respondent unhappy, partner happy	0–6	7–8	408	2.34

REFERENCES

Cassells, R., Gong, H., & Keegan, M. (2010). *The pursuit of happiness: Life satisfaction in Australia*. AMP.

Chapman, B., & Guven, C. (2016). Revisiting the relationship between marriage and wellbeing: Does marriage quality matter? *Journal of Happiness Studies*, *17*(2), 533–551.

Clark, A. E., Frijters, P., & Shields, M. A. (2008). Relative income, happiness, and utility: An explanation for the Easterlin paradox and other puzzles. *Journal of Economic Literature*, *46*(1), 95–144.

Demir, M. (2008). Sweetheart, you really make me happy: Romantic relationship quality and personality as predictors of happiness among emerging adults. *Journal of Happiness Studies*, *9*(2), 257–277.

Dush, C. M. K., & Amato, P. R. (2005). Consequences of relationship status and quality for subjective well-being. *Journal of Social and Personal Relationships*, *22*(5), 607–627.

Ferrer-i-Carbonell, A., & Frijters, P. (2004). How important is methodology for the estimates of the determinants of happiness? *Economic Journal*, *114*(497), 641–659.

Grover, S., & Helliwell, J. F. (2019). How's life at home? New evidence on marriage and the set point for happiness. *Journal of Happiness Studies*, *20*(2), 373–390.

Kwon, H. W. (2021). Are gritty people happier than others?: Evidence from the United States and South Korea. *Journal of Happiness Studies*, *22*, 2937–2959.

7

Indigenous Australian Understandings of Holistic Health and Social and Emotional Wellbeing

HELEN MILROY, KATE DERRY, SHRADDHA KASHYAP,
MONIQUE PLATELL, JOANNA ALEXI, EE PIN CHANG,
AND PAT DUDGEON ∎

INTRODUCTION

Psychological science as a discipline and profession has been complicit in the colonising process, directly through the imposition of Western knowledge systems and indirectly through the devaluing and exclusion of Indigenous knowledges and practices (American Psychological Association, 2021; Australian Psychological Society, 2016; Dudgeon, Rickwood, Garvey, & Gridley, 2014). The evidence hierarchy of the paradigm of science privileges Western conceptualisations of mental health and health in the global community. Yet holistic conceptualisations of wellbeing, based on Indigenous knowledge systems, are shared among Indigenous peoples from different parts of the world (McClintock et al., 2021). An integrated science of wellbeing therefore requires epistemic pluralism: the valuing of Indigenous psychologies and understandings of wellbeing alongside non-Indigenous understandings of wellbeing. This chapter focuses on describing the paradigm of wellbeing as understood by Aboriginal and Torres Strait Islander peoples.

Aboriginal peoples are the Indigenous peoples of mainland Australia and are custodians of the oldest living culture in the world, a culture that has for many centuries prioritised balance and harmony through holistic understandings of wellbeing. The science of wellbeing for Aboriginal and Torres Strait Islander peoples is understood through the model of Social and Emotional WellBeing (SEWB) (Gee, Dudgeon, Schultz, Hart, & Kelly, 2014). While transgenerational experiences of trauma and loss are ubiquitous among Aboriginal and Torres Strait Islander peoples, stories of survival and resilience reflect the continued resistance against colonisation, emergence of Indigenous psychologies, and the significance of SEWB (Dudgeon, Bray, D'costa, & Walker, 2017).

This chapter presents this model of SEWB, which describes the interaction between psychological, physical, societal, cultural, environmental, and spiritual dimensions of wellbeing, alongside the *Dance of Life framework* (Milroy, 2006), which provides avenues for understanding health and wellbeing challenges that are SEWB- and trauma-informed, and it provides pathways toward individual and collective healing. To achieve epistemic pluralism, the discipline of psychology must work to decolonise psychological research and practice by supporting the self-determination and empowerment of Indigenous peoples and the inclusion of Indigenous knowledges and practices (Dudgeon, Rickwood, et al., 2014). SEWB and the Dance of Life enable a more integrated science of wellbeing by demonstrating a holistic and ecological understanding of the human condition and our relationship with the earth and the dynamic world around us.

DECOLONISING PSYCHOLOGY

In Australia, mainstream mental health services and professionals have only recently acknowledged the profound impact of invasion, massacres, attempted genocide, and colonisation on the wellbeing of Aboriginal and Torres Strait Islander peoples and communities (Dudgeon, Rickwood, et al., 2014). A series of Commonwealth and State Acts between 1883 and 1967 saw an extensive period of absolute state control and terror over the lives of Aboriginal and Torres Strait Islander peoples. The direct effects of these legislations include displacement, dispossession of land, forced removal of children and assimilation policies, suppression of language and culture, mistreatment, and pervasive racism and discrimination at the individual, institutional, and system levels (Australian Institute of Health and Welfare, 2018; Dudgeon, Bray, & Walker, 2020). The indirect psychological experiences caused by this colonial legacy also include pervasive grief, trauma, and loss and the silencing and denial of these experiences by the dominant colonial society (Dudgeon & Walker, 2015; Wanganeen, 2014). Consequently, Aboriginal and Torres Strait Islander peoples experience substantially higher rates of psychological distress, hospitalisation for mental and behavioural disorders, self-harm, and suicide (Australian Bureau of Statistics, 2019; Australian Institute of Health and Welfare, 2015, 2020). The social and political factors that have negatively impacted wellbeing, as well as the cultural and community factors that have protected wellbeing, are necessary components of any Indigenous psychology and holistic understandings of wellbeing.

Decolonising psychology refers to recognising Aboriginal and Torres Strait Islander cultural views, conceptual frameworks, and practices based in holistic understandings of health and wellbeing and incorporating them into mainstream mental health services, professional practice and training, and research (Dudgeon & Walker, 2015). As highlighted by Dudgeon and Pickett (2000), 'Australian psychology needs to recognise Australian Indigenous history and cultural difference, and more, to celebrate cultural differences. The understanding of Indigenous history must include awareness about contemporary Indigenous life and the diversity of Indigenous people' (p. 86). Through decolonisation, psychology will be placed to support the empowerment and self-determination of Aboriginal and Torres Strait Islander peoples (Dudgeon, Rickwood, et al., 2014).

Aboriginal and Torres Strait Islander mental health professionals have worked to establish a voice that represents the mental health issues of Aboriginal and Torres Strait Islander peoples in Australia, and Indigenous peoples globally (National Aboriginal and Torres Strait Islander Leadership in Mental Health, 2015). The 200 Years of Unfinished Business report published in 1988 by Aboriginal mental health professional, Pat Swan, is recognised as a pivotal point for change. This text informed the National Aboriginal Health Strategy (NAHS) in 1989, and in the 1991 Royal Commission into Aboriginal Deaths in Custody (RCIADIC) (Dudgeon, Rickwood, et al., 2014). One of the RCIADIC key recommendations was a need for a national consultancy on Aboriginal and Torres Strait Islander peoples' mental health and wellbeing. This culminated in the landmark Ways Forward report (Gee et al., 2014; Swan & Raphael, 1995). This was the first national report to generate a plan of action for the specific mental health needs of Aboriginal and Torres Strait Islander peoples (Swan & Raphael, 1995; Zubrick, Holland, Kelly, Calma, & Walker., 2014). The report highlighted the devastating impact of colonisation and the subsequent social, economic, and health disadvantage that have contributed to widespread mental health challenges experienced by Aboriginal and Torres Strait Islander peoples and communities (Swan & Raphael, 1995; Zubrick et al., 2014). The report emphasised the need for greater understanding among health professionals about the extent and determinants of mental health challenges among Aboriginal and Torres Strait Islander peoples. Furthermore, the report highlighted the need for mental health services to address the underlying grief and psychological distress caused by colonisation and to adopt a holistic view of wellbeing (Swan & Raphael, 1995; Zubrick et al., 2014). The report determined that the 'delineation of mental health problems and disorders must encompass a recognition of the historical and socio-political context of Aboriginal mental health including the impact of colonisation; trauma; loss and grief; separation of families and children; the taking away of land; and the loss of culture and identity; plus the impact of social inequity, stigma, racism and ongoing losses' (Swan & Raphael, 1995, p. 7).

These and many other significant inquiries and reports at the end of the 20th century have enabled a reclaiming of Aboriginal and Torres Strait Islander understandings of wellbeing and national efforts for policy reform (Gee et al., 2014). As a result, the discourse of Aboriginal and Torres Strait Islander mental health has begun to evolve from psychology's traditional disease and deficit models to prioritise wellbeing, holistic health, and cultural responsiveness (Dudgeon, Rickwood, et al., 2014).

A parallel movement of *Indigenous psychology* has also emerged to challenge monocultural narratives about Indigenous peoples across the world that are presented through Western psychology paradigms (Dudgeon, 2017; Dudgeon, Bray, et al., 2017). Indigenous psychology is founded on sovereign Indigenous knowledges, where the historical and contemporary realities of colonisation and the subsequent transgenerational trauma derived from those lived experiences become the relevant contextual lens through which Indigenous peoples' behaviours and responses are interpreted (Dudgeon, Bray, et al., 2017; Dudgeon, Darlaston-Jones, Bray, 2018). Indigenous psychology has been recognised on a global scale with the establishment of the Task Force for Indigenous Psychology in the Society for Humanistic Psychology, Division 32, American Psychological Association. This taskforce describes Indigenous psychology as:

1. A reaction against the colonisation/hegemony of Western psychology
2. The need for non-Western cultures to solve their local problems
3. The need for non-Western culture to recognise itself in the constructs and practices of psychology
4. The need to use Indigenous philosophies and concepts to generate theories of global discourse (American Psychological Association, 2010)

Implicit in these factors is the obligation to 'respect, recognise and uphold Indigenous peoples' individual and collective rights to develop, maintain, and use their own health systems, institutional structures, distinctive customs, spirituality, traditions, procedures and practices in pursuit of their right to health and mental health and wellbeing' (Dudgeon, 2017, p. 252). These obligations have been formalised by the United Nations Declaration on the Rights of Indigenous peoples (2007) and in the Apology to Indigenous peoples given by the Australian Psychological Society (2016) and the American Psychological Association (2021).

Thus, changes in perception toward Aboriginal and Torres Strait Islander concepts of health and wellbeing are underpinned by the principles of empowerment and self-determination (Dudgeon, Rickwood, et al., 2014). Empowerment is described as a means of effecting change through people, organisations, and communities gaining control of their lives (Wallerstein & Bernstein, 1988). The theory of empowerment is critical for Aboriginal and Torres Strait Islander self-determination and individual, family, and community social transformation (Dudgeon, Walker, et al., 2014; Walker, 2005). Self-determination is an ongoing process of choice that ensures Aboriginal and Torres Strait Islander peoples are able to meet their social, cultural, and economic needs, and is a human right (Australian Human Rights Commission, 2013; United Nations, 2007).

Specifically for health and mental health services, this means that mechanisms must be in place to ensure that Aboriginal and Torres Strait Islander peoples are fully involved in any activity or interventions developed for Aboriginal and Torres

Strait Islander peoples and communities (Dudgeon, Rickwood, et al., 2014). This has been epitomised by the phrase adopted by this movement, 'nothing about us without us'. Through empowerment and self-determination, Aboriginal and Torres Strait Islander peoples should be able to lead engagement at all levels of the health system, whether that be interactions between a practitioner and client, developing services and programs, or formulating and implementing policy (Dudgeon, Rickwood, et al., 2014). Self-determination is recognised as best practice toward strengthening wellbeing and decentring the dominance of Western conceptions of racialised deficit (Dudgeon et al., 2018; Dudgeon, Milroy, et al., 2016). However, self-determination can only be wholly achieved when existing government policies reliably encourage and support Aboriginal and Torres Strait Islander governed and culturally based solutions (Horning & Baumbrough, 2020).

SOCIAL AND EMOTIONAL WELLBEING (SEWB)

Indigenous Australian holistic understandings of health and wellbeing are intertwined with Aboriginal and Torres Strait Islander self-hood. The Aboriginal and Torres Strait Islander sense of self is grounded within a collectivist perspective that views self as inseparable from all aspects of life, including community, society, spirituality, culture, and Country (Parker & Milroy, 2014). Each individual's connection to kinship systems and community life has always been central to the functioning of both traditional and contemporary Aboriginal and Torres Strait Islander communities (Dudgeon, Wright, Paradies, Garvey, & Walker, 2014). Kinship systems place each individual securely in relationship to every other individual in their social network and determine the appropriate behaviours of individuals (Dudgeon, Wright, et al., 2014). Community is where participating in kinship networks occurs and where personal connections, obligations, and sociocultural norms are maintained (Dudgeon, Mallard, Oxenham, & Fielder, 2002). In addition, connection to spirituality is the encompassing system that grounds Aboriginal and Torres Strait Islander peoples' cultural worldviews. For Aboriginal and Torres Strait Islander peoples, spirituality is closely linked to their connection to their Country (Gee et al., 2014). Aboriginal and Torres Strait Islander peoples experience the land as a richly symbolic landscape in which land is not owned; rather, individuals belong to the land (Dudgeon, Wright, et al., 2014). To maintain these connections to community, spirituality, culture, and Country, and subsequently to maintain a strong sense of self and cultural identity, it is essential to support Aboriginal and Torres Strait Islander peoples to participate in cultural knowledges and practices that allow them to exercise their cultural rights and responsibilities (Gee et al., 2014). Identifying and engaging with cultural ways of being, knowing, and doing are essential to developing individual, family, and community wellbeing and empowerment (Dudgeon, Gibson, & Bray, 2020; Dudgeon, Walker, et al., 2014).

As can be seen, Aboriginal and Torres Strait Islander whole-of-life views of health extend beyond the physical and emotional wellbeing of an individual and include the social and cultural wellbeing of the whole community, society, and environment (Dudgeon et al., 2018; Gee et al., 2014). This holistic definition of health was first used in the 1989 National Aboriginal Health Strategy (NAHS), and central to this definition of health is SEWB. The concept of SEWB is a positive state of mental health and wellbeing associated with a strong and sustaining cultural identity and community life that provides a source of strength against adversity and other challenges of life (Holland, Dudgeon, & Milroy, 2013). SEWB provides a revolutionary framework which addresses the political and social challenges outlined above, using mechanisms needed to facilitate healing and empowerment by providing a holistic and strengths-based construct which recognises the resilience, abilities, knowledge, and capacities of individuals and communities (Dudgeon, Gibson, et al., 2020). SEWB challenges narrow Western biomedical paradigms and entrenched deficit discourses by providing an alternative language to viewing health and healing and to facilitate empowerment and self-determination for Aboriginal and Torres Strait Islander peoples (Dudgeon, Bray, et al., 2020; Dudgeon, Gibson, et al., 2020; Fogarty, Lovell, Langenberg, & Heron, 2018).

One of the NAHS's key recommendations was for a health framework to be developed by Aboriginal and Torres Strait Islander peoples that recognised the importance of culture and history and which defined health and ill-health from an Aboriginal and Torres Strait Islander perspective (Gee et al., 2014; National Aboriginal Health Strategy Working Party, 1989). Such recommendations culminated in the development of the Ways Forward Report (1995) and the first National Strategic Framework for Aboriginal and Torres Strait Islander People's Mental Health and Social and Emotional Wellbeing 2004–2009 (hereafter referred to as the 2004 MH&SEWB Framework) (Social Health Reference Group, 2004).

The 2004 MH&SEWB Framework was a key guiding document for defining Aboriginal and Torres Strait Islander–specific understandings of SEWB and highlighting the complex, multidimensional nature of this concept of health encompassing connections to land, culture, spirituality, ancestry, family, and community (Social Health Reference Group, 2004). The 2004 MH&SEWB Framework set out the following nine guiding principles, which shape the SEWB concept and describe core Aboriginal and Torres Strait Islander cultural values (Social Health Reference Group, 2004; Swan & Raphael, 1997):

1. Health as holistic
2. The right to self-determination
3. The need for cultural understanding
4. The impact of history in trauma and loss
5. Recognition of human rights
6. The impact of racism and stigma
7. Recognition of the centrality of kinship
8. Recognition of cultural diversity
9. Recognition of Aboriginal strengths

This framework was revolutionary in that it recognised culture as being critically important to building strength, resilience, happiness, identity, and confidence, and it articulated strategies that support self-determination and empowerment (Anderson, 2004; Social Health Reference Group, 2004). It further recognised the impact of trauma, colonisation, and human rights issues on the SEWB of Aboriginal and Torres Strait Islander peoples (Anderson, 2004). The framework highlights that, to facilitate strengthened SEWB for Aboriginal and Torres Strait Islander peoples and communities faced with colonial problems, multidimensional solutions that prioritise empowerment and self-determination are needed for healing. These solutions should build on existing individual, family, and community strengths and capacity and may include Aboriginal and Torres Strait Islander knowledges, psychology, and cultural practices (Social Health Reference Group, 2004). The nine principles have been renewed in the latest 2017–2023 National Strategic Framework for Aboriginal and Torres Strait Islander People's Mental Health and Social and Emotional Wellbeing (Department of Prime Minister and Cabinet, 2017).

The emerging discourse of SEWB and Indigenous wellbeing taking place in Australia and worldwide is part of the global Aboriginal and Torres Strait Islander psychology movement (Dudgeon, Bray, et al., 2017). This movement is promoting the emergence of decolonising psychology, Indigenous self-determination, and transformative Indigenous paradigms that rethink the concept of health and wellbeing (Dudgeon, Bray, et al., 2017).

SEWB and Mental Health

Currently there remains a lack of widespread consensus about the distinctions between SEWB and mental health and how these concepts should coexist or intersect (Atkinson & Kerr, 2003; Hunter, 2004). The 2017 MH&SEWB Framework describes SEWB and mental health as having an interactive relationship, where the two may influence each other (Department of Prime Minister and Cabinet, 2017). SEWB is a complex multidimensional concept of health that extends beyond conventional Western understandings of mental health. While mental health is an important component of SEWB, it should only be viewed as one aspect of health as experienced by Aboriginal and Torres Strait Islander peoples (Gee et al., 2014). Determinants of SEWB include a wide range of issues including collective grief, abuse, substance misuse, physical health problems, child removals, incarceration, systemic racism, and social disadvantage (Barnes & Josefowitz, 2019; Department of Prime Minister and Cabinet, 2017; Menzies, 2019a,b). Reported mental health problems may include anxiety, depression, posttraumatic stress, self-harm, and psychosis (Social Health Reference Group, 2004). Many factors that have a detrimental impact on SEWB, such as abuse, racism, and social disadvantage, are also well-established risk factors for mental health disorders (Gee et al., 2014). In some instances, the development of mental health problems may be symptomatic of a greater SEWB problem (Parker & Milroy, 2014). By viewing mental health within the broader concept of SEWB, life promotion, wellness, and balance are prioritised rather than illness and symptom reduction (Gee et al., 2014). A holistic and ecological view also highlights that, for many Aboriginal and Torres Strait Islander peoples and communities, mental health issues remain linked to the trauma and injustices created by colonisation (Gee et al., 2014).

Conceptualising the SEWB Model

The SEWB construct first outlined in the 2004 MH&SEWB framework was articulated into a model by Aboriginal psychologists Gee, Dudgeon, Schultz, Hart, and Kelly (2014). As shown in Figure 7.1, this model illustrates SEWB in a way that has utility for mental health practitioners and supports the development and implementation of a range of SEWB population health strategies (Gee et al., 2014).

In this model, there are seven interconnected domains of SEWB: Country, spirituality, culture, family and kinship, mind and emotions, and body (Gee et al., 2014). Strong connections to these domains are sources of wellbeing and Aboriginal and Torres Strait Islander identity, which is grounded in a collective perspective. The term 'connections' refers to various ways that diverse Indigenous peoples' experience and express the domains of SEWB across the lifespan and as culture and sense of self evolves. This model recognises that these connections will vary across temporal, geographical, and cultural settings. For many Aboriginal and Torres Strait Islander peoples these connections have been severely disrupted due to intersecting factors associated with colonialism and determinants of health.

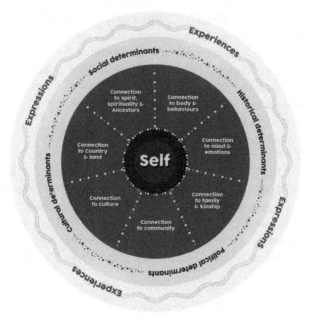

Figure 7.1 Social and emotional wellbeing model.
Adapted from Gee et al. (2014).

These disruptions and subsequent effects on the domains of SEWB may manifest in a number of different ways (Haswell-Elkins et al., 2009). The model emphasises the importance of considering these connections within the broader social, political, historical, and cultural contexts.

Social, Historical, Political, and Cultural Determinants of SEWB

Social determinants of mental health and SEWB for Aboriginal and Torres Strait Islander peoples include socioeconomic status, poverty, unemployment, housing, and educational attainment. Such social determinants do not occur in isolation and have concurrent and cumulative impacts on SEWB. This is important for medical and mental health professionals to consider because this often presents as complex client and family presentations that require a multidisciplinary approach.

Historical determinants refer to the impacts of colonial rule and the extent that historical oppression, racial discrimination, and cultural displacement was and continues to be experienced by individuals, families, and communities. Political determinants of SEWB include unresolved issues related to cultural security, sovereignty, and the rights of self-determination, which contribute to health and wellbeing and would reduce health inequalities for Aboriginal and Torres Strait Islander peoples (Social Health Reference Group, 2004).

Together, historical, social, and political determinants impact cultural determinants and shape the environment and circumstances in which Aboriginal and Torres Strait Islander peoples are born into. *Cultural determinants* originate from a strengths-based perspective, acknowledging the domains of SEWB that build stronger individual and collective identities, resilience, and have a protective influence against the other determinants of health (Lowitja Institute, 2014). These cultural factors, which include an individual's cultural identity, a community's local history of colonisation, and the extent to which a cultural group is able to maintain cultural continuity and retain the right to self-determination, will significantly influence a community's capacity to retain its cultural values, principals, practices, and traditions (Gee et al., 2014).

Cultural continuity has been recognised globally as critical to restoring the SEWB and mental health of Indigenous peoples (Chandler & Lalonde, 1998). To engage practically with these historical and political determinants of SEWB, practitioners must develop knowledge around the history of traditional owner groups in the community they are working in and reflect on the ways in which colonisation has impacted the community (Gee et al., 2014). Therefore, SEWB is an important contribution to overcoming the systematic neglect of culture in health, which has been argued as the foremost barrier to achieving health globally (Napier et al., 2014).

Community Validation of the SEWB Model

The SEWB model discussed above has been validated on a national scale through extensive community consultations. The National Empowerment Project (NEP) led by Professor Dudgeon was an Aboriginal community designed, managed, and led program aimed at understanding SEWB in order to reduce community distress and suicide in Aboriginal communities (Dudgeon, Scrine, Cox, & Walker, 2017). The project's first phase involved community consultations with 11 Aboriginal and Torres Strait Islander communities across Australia to identify the key issues the communities perceived as negatively impacting on the health and wellbeing of individuals, families, and communities as well as solutions to address these challenges (Dudgeon, Bray, et al., 2017). Outcomes of the NEP consultations confirmed the relevance of the seven SEWB domains and the complex interrelationships among social, political, historical, and cultural determinants impacting on SEWB (Dudgeon, Bray, et al., 2017). Participants identified a number of issues which negatively impacted on the wellbeing of individuals, families, and communities and delineated those that were symptomatic or underlying causes and thus comprised key targets for change to enable transformative change (Dudgeon, Bray, et al., 2017).

The findings of the NEP community consultation demonstrated the importance of empowerment and self-determination in promoting healing and health in Aboriginal communities (Dudgeon, Cox, et al., 2014). All communities shared a common belief in the power of a strong cultural identity and connection to culture to improve the lives of individuals, families, and communities. The NEP confirmed that more programs are needed to empower Aboriginal people to heal themselves and have agency over their lives. Consulted communities wanted to take charge to change their lives and those of their families and communities by addressing the specific issues impacting their wellbeing. This had to be done on the communities' terms and through an Aboriginal understanding of healing and wellbeing in order to be effective.

Implementing the SEWB Model in the Health System

The *Dance of Life* (Milroy, 2006; Appendix 2) is an example of a framework which can be used to implement the SEWB model within health and mental health services to provide culturally safe, responsive, and relevant care and thereby avoid further harm to Aboriginal and Torres Strait Islander peoples (see Figure 7.2). The Dance of Life is a multidimensional model, depicted through six images (Figures 7.3–7.8), five of which represent the physical, psychological/emotional, social, spiritual, and cultural dimensions of SEWB. Within each dimension, there are layers to consider, including traditional cultural perspectives, historical understandings, the contemporary context, gaps in knowledge, and a focus on solutions. The sixth image ('The Dance of Life') brings these together to represent the five dimensions in harmony and balance. In this way, the Dance of Life is an example of an implementation of the SEWB model portrayed in a culturally relevant medium that uses narratives within the artwork to describe factors contributing to a person's SEWB (e.g., connection to Country, culture, community, etc.). The Dance of Life has been used as a framework for working with Aboriginal consumers of mental health services, as well as for teaching mainstream mental health

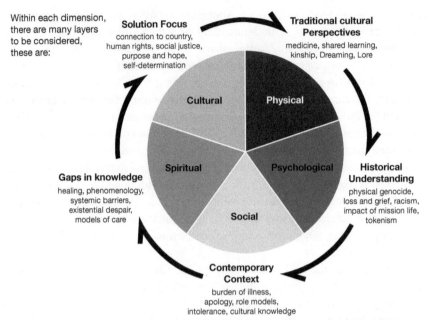

Within each dimension, there are many layers to be considered, these are:

Solution Focus
connection to country, human rights, social justice, purpose and hope, self-determination

Traditional cultural Perspectives
medicine, shared learning, kinship, Dreaming, Lore

Cultural

Physical

Spiritual

Psychological

Historical Understanding
physical genocide, loss and grief, racism, impact of mission life, tokenism

Gaps in knowledge
healing, phenomenology, systemic barriers, existential despair, models of care

Social

Contemporary Context
burden of illness, apology, role models, intolerance, cultural knowledge

[1]The Dance of Life, Milroy, H. (2006). https://www.ranzcp.org/practice-education/aboriginal-torres-strait-islander-mental-health/the-dance-of-life

Figure 7.2 Dance of Life artwork: Understanding layers within dimensions. From Milroy (2006).

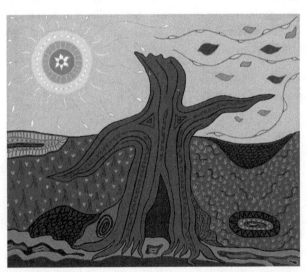

Figure 7.3 Dance of Life artwork: Born from Country: 'We are born from Country and at the end of our days we return to Country'. From Milroy (2006).

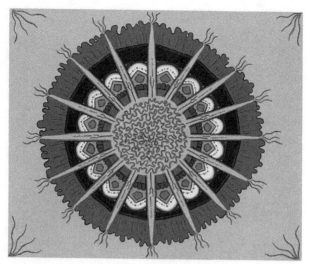

Figure 7.4 Dance of Life artwork: Living Life: 'We experience life through all our senses simultaneously, and the central core of psychological life is alive and constantly growing'. From Milroy (2006).

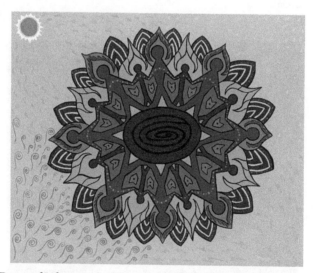

Figure 7.5 Dance of Life artwork: Community Strong Together: 'When a community stands strong together, it blossoms, protects us from adversity, and is a part of our strength and wellbeing going forward . . . the shapes formed in between the figures represent the hearts shared in the community and the notion that to lose one child will destroy more than one heart'.
From Milroy (2006).

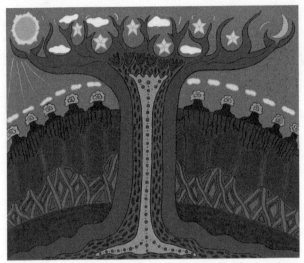

Figure 7.6 Dance of Life artwork: The Tree of Life: 'The tree of life connects the inner dimensions of the earth to the outer dimensions of the universe . . . this timeless dimension with its infinite capacity exists within yet outside of our physical realm, and keeps us connected for eternity'.
From Milroy (2006).

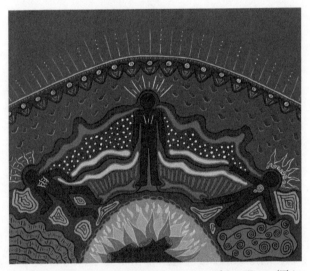

Figure 7.7 Dance of Life artwork: Healing, Ceremony, and Law/Lore: 'This painting takes the form of three figures symbolising healing, ceremony and traditional law/lore. . . . Culture is grounded in the land we belong to as much of the law/lore, ceremony and healing comes from Country'.
From Milroy (2006).

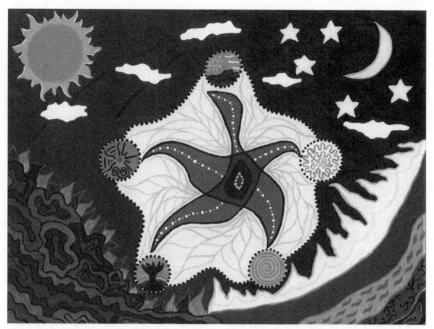

Figure 7.8 Dance of Life artwork: The Dance of Life: 'When we enable a person to restore all the dimensions of their life, then we have achieved a great deal. When all the dimensions are in balance within the universe, we can break free of our shackles and truly dance through life'.
From Milroy (2006).

professionals about culturally responsive and safe ways to work with Aboriginal families and communities.

THE PHYSICAL DIMENSION

Connection to Country is a domain of SEWB and is intertwined with spirituality, family, and culture (Gee et al., 2014). For example, Caring for Country activities such as time on country, gathering food and medicines, ceremony, and protecting sacred sites are important aspects of culture, spirituality, and connectedness to land (Rigby, Rosen, Berry, & Hart, 2011). Indeed, one study suggests that participating in Caring for Country activities was associated with better wellbeing, including less type 2 diabetes and a lower risk of cardiovascular disease (Burgess et al., 2009). Connection to Country is therefore a significant aspect of maintaining wellbeing and can be a source of renewal, while not being able to access familiar surroundings and cultural ways can be a source of significant distress (Milroy, 2006; Marriott & Ferguson-Hill, 2014). In this way, colonisation, cultural genocide, and forced dispossession and displacement of Aboriginal and Torres Strait Islander peoples from traditional lands, kinship systems, and ways of living have contributed to a disproportionate burden of illness. According to the Australian Institute of Health and Welfare (AIHW, 2021), Aboriginal and Torres Strait Islander peoples experience disease burden at 2.3

times the rate for non-Indigenous Australians, where burden of illness refers to the difference between the actual health of a population compared with its ideal health. The five disease groups causing the most burden were mental and substance use disorders, injuries (including suicide), cardiovascular diseases, cancer, and musculoskeletal conditions. It is therefore vital that Aboriginal and Torres Strait Islander knowledges and conceptualisations of health and wellbeing, including the importance of connection to Country, are embedded in all levels of service provision.

The Psychological/Emotional Dimension

Aboriginal and Torres Strait Islander peoples have been exposed to multiple layers of trauma, including intergenerational trauma, ongoing discrimination, and disadvantage, within the context of genocide and colonisation (Menzies, 2019a,b; Milroy et al., 2014; Swan & Raphael, 1997). Despite this, Aboriginal and Torres Strait Islander communities have resisted and survived, and interventions which promote SEWB can build on existing strengths and resilience. It is therefore important for health and mental health service providers to be aware of cultural phenomenology to avoid misdiagnosis, mislabelling, and misunderstanding. For example, within Aboriginal and Torres Strait Islander cultures, it is not unusual to experience voices of ancestors, whereas a Western paradigm of health could view this as psychosis and recommend inappropriate treatment (Parker & Milroy, 2003). Therefore, an understanding of culturally relevant phenomena and an ability to distinguish between symptoms of a disorder, cultural phenomena, or a cultural dimension within a disorder are needed within the health system to provide effective and culturally safe care (Parker & Milroy, 2003).

The Social Dimension

Service providers need to recognise the role of community and kinship systems when working with Aboriginal and Torres Strait Islander communities. For example, health service providers need to understand that some consumers may want their family and extended family members to be involved in decision-making, and that cultural definitions of kinship go beyond the Western definition of immediate family. Working in culturally appropriate and nuanced ways with Aboriginal and Torres Strait Islander communities to promote SEWB requires an understanding of kinship and the connection between community wellbeing and individual wellbeing.

The Spiritual Dimension

Aboriginal peoples are connected to culture, family, and ancestors through spirituality, and while physical bonds between parents and children were broken through the stolen generations, the spiritual connections were not. Spiritual understandings of wellbeing and healing are required for a fuller understanding of healing and recovery. Therefore, understanding this history and dimension is critical to being responsive to the needs and values of Aboriginal and Torres Strait Islander communities and families.

THE CULTURAL DIMENSION

Connection to culture is a determinant of SEWB, and health and mental health systems need to create cultural safety for Aboriginal and Torres Strait Islander consumers throughout the lifespan. Indeed, cultural continuity and higher levels of self-determination among First Nations communities in Canada were associated with a reduced risk of suicide (Chandler & Lalonde, 2008). Making health systems culturally safe requires an understanding of the significance of connection to culture on wellbeing and for health and mental health professionals to take a holistic approach to service provision, not just in a clinical sense, but in a way that is inclusive of culture. Aboriginal and Torres Strait Islander leadership and advocacy, together with the support of non-Indigenous health and mental health professionals, is needed to enable this evolution of the system.

THE DANCE OF LIFE

Health and mental health workers need to be able to tease out the impact of transgenerational disadvantage and discrimination; they need to be able to recognise illness and distress in the midst of cultural, spiritual, and intersectional complexity and ambiguity and attempt to address the many factors impacting on wellbeing. Incorporating historical and cultural perspectives as well as flexibility in approach will enhance a clinician's skills and knowledge and provide a platform for meaningful and respectful cross-cultural exchange.

SUMMARY

This chapter provided an overview of a shifting paradigm of understanding Aboriginal and Torres Strait Islander health and wellbeing and the need to decolonise the science of wellbeing to enable epistemic pluralism and benefit from the wisdom of Indigenous ways of knowing, being, and doing. By the end of the 20th century, continued resistance against colonisation and the monocultural narratives saw a reclaiming and renewing of Aboriginal and Torres Strait Islander peoples' understandings of holistic health and wellbeing and Indigenous psychologies. This movement was underpinned by the principles of empowerment and self-determination, which support the need for Aboriginal and Torres Strait Islander peoples to lead engagement at all levels of the health system. From this movement, the discourse of SEWB emerged to provide an Aboriginal and Torres Strait Islander–specific, holistic, and strengths-based definition of wellbeing and healing. In alignment with the principles of empowerment and self-determination, further work is needed for Aboriginal and Torres Strait Islander knowledges to achieve epistemic equality within, and to complement, Western health and mental health disciplines.

REFERENCES

American Psychological Association. (2010). *Task force on Indigenous psychology.* https://www.indigenouspsych.org

American Psychological Association. (2021). *Apology to People of Color for APA's role in promoting, perpetuating, and failing to challenge racism, racial discrimination, and human hierarchy in the U.S.* https://www.apa.org/about/policy/racism-apology

Anderson, I. (2004). Recent developments in National Aboriginal and Torres Strait islander health strategy. *Australia & New Zealand Health Policy, 1*(3). doi:10.1186/1743-8462-1-3

Atkinson, G., & Kerr, S. (2003). *The Purro Birik social and emotional wellbeing strategy 1999–2002 evaluation report.* Victorian Aboriginal Community Controlled Health Organisations (VACCHO).

Australian Human Rights Commission. (2013). *Right to self determination.* https://humanrights.gov.au/our-work/rights-and-freedoms/right-self-determination

Australian Bureau of Statistics. (2019). *National Aboriginal and Torres Strait Islander health survey.* https://www.abs.gov.au/statistics/people/aboriginal-and-torres-strait-islander-peoples/national-aboriginal-and-torres-strait-islander-health-survey/latest-releasekey-statistics

Australian Institute of Health and Welfare. (2015). *The health and welfare of Australia's Aboriginal and Torres Strait Islander peoples.* https://www.aihw.gov.au/getmedia/584073f7-041e-4818-9419-39f5a060b1aa/18175.pdf.aspx?inline=true

Australian Institute of Health and Welfare. (2018). *Aboriginal and Torres Strait Islander stolen generations and descendants: Numbers, demographic characteristics and selected outcomes.* https://www.aihw.gov.au/getmedia/a6c077c3-e1af-40de-847f-e8a3e3456c44/aihw-ihw-195.pdf.aspx?inline=true

Australian Institute of Health and Welfare. (2020). *Suicide and intentional self-harm.* https://www.aihw.gov.au/reports/australias-health/suicide-and-intentional-self-harm

Australian Institute of Health and Welfare. (2021). *Australian burden of disease study 2018: Key findings for Aboriginal and Torres Strait Islander people.* https://www.aihw.gov.au/getmedia/a0ff4cc7-d02f-4a8d-b737-3052f510688e/aihw-bod-28.pdf.aspx?inline=true

Australian Psychological Society. (2016). *The APS apology to Aboriginal and Torres Strait Islander people.* https://psychology.org.au/community/reconciliation-and-the-aps/aps-apology

Barnes, R., & Josefowitz, N. (2019). Indian residential schools in Canada: Persistent impacts on Aboriginal students' psychological development and functioning. *Canadian Psychology/Psychologie Canadienne, 60*(2), 65.

Burgess, C. P., Johnston, F. H., Berry, H. L., McDonnell, J., Yibarbuk, D., Gunabarra, C., Mileran, A., & Bailie, R. S. (2009). Healthy country, healthy people: The relationship between Indigenous health status and "caring for country". *Medical Journal of Australia, 190*(10), 567–572.

Chandler, M., & Lalonde, C. (1998). Cultural continuity as a hedge against suicide in Canada's First Nations. *Transcultural Psychiatry, 35*(2), 191–219. doi.org/10.1177/136346159803500202

Chandler, M. J., & Lalonde, C. E. (2008). Cultural continuity as a protective factor against suicide in First Nations youth. *Horizons, 10*(1), 68–72.

Department of Prime Minister and Cabinet. (2017). *National strategic framework for Aboriginal and Torres Strait Islander peoples' mental health and social and emotional wellbeing 2017–2023*. https://www.niaa.gov.au/sites/default/files/publications/mhs ewb-framework_0.pdf

Dudgeon, P. (2017). Australian Indigenous psychology. *Australian Psychologist, 52*(4), 251–254. doi:10.1111/ap.12298

Dudgeon, P., Bray, A., D'costa, B., & Walker, R. (2017). Decolonising psychology: Validating social and emotional wellbeing. *Australian Psychologist, 52*(4), 316–325.

Dudgeon, P., Bray, A., & Walker, R. (2020). Self-determination and strengths-based Aboriginal and Torres Strait Islander suicide prevention: An emerging evidence-based approach. In A. Page & W. Stritzke (Eds.), *Alternatives to suicide: Beyond risk and toward a life worth living* (pp. 237–256). Academic Press.

Dudgeon, P., Cox, A., Walker, R., Scrine, C., Kelly, K., Blurton, D., . . . Woods, C. (2014). *Voices of the peoples: The national empowerment project research report*. https://054fc 593-4bdd-4fe8-87ef-100ff1df7134.filesusr.com/ugd/396df4_85c3278f13ce47149 bc394001d69dad6.pdf

Dudgeon, P., Darlaston-Jones, D., Bray, A. (2018). Teaching Indigenous psychology: A conscientisation, de-colonisation and psychological literacy approach to curriculum. In C. Newnes & L. Golding (Eds.), *Teaching critical psychology: International perspectives* (pp. 123–147). Routledge.

Dudgeon, P., Gibson, C., & Bray, A. (2020). Social and emotional well-being: Aboriginal health in Aboriginal hands. In T. Carey & J. Gullifer (Eds.), *Handbook of rural, remote, and very remote mental health* (pp. 1–18). Springer Nature.

Dudgeon, P., Mallard, J., Oxenham, D., & Fielder, J. (2002). Contemporary Aboriginal perceptions of community. In T. Fisher (Ed.), *Psychological sense of community* (pp. 247–267). Plenum Press.

Dudgeon, P., Milroy, J., Calma, T., Luxford, Y., Ring, I., Walker, R., . . . Holland, C. (2016). *Solutions that work - what evidence and our people tell us, Aboriginal and Torres Strait Islander suicide prevention evaluation project report*. https://www.atsispep.sis.uwa. edu.au/__data/assets/pdf_file/0006/2947299/ATSISPEP-Report-Final-Web.pdf

Dudgeon, P., & Pickett, H. (2000). Psychology and reconciliation: Australian perspectives. *Australian Psychologist, 35*(2), 82–87.

Dudgeon, P., Rickwood, D., Garvey, D., & Gridley, H. (2014). A history of Indigenous psychology. In P. Dudgeon, H. Milroy, & R. Walker (Eds.), *Working together: Aboriginal and Torres Strait Islander mental health and wellbeing principles and practice* (pp. 39–54). Commonwealth of Australia.

Dudgeon, P., Scrine, C., Cox, A., & Walker, R. (2017). Facilitating empowerment and self-determination through participatory action research: Findings from the national empowerment project. *International Journal of Qualitative Methods, 16*, 1–11. doi:10.1177/1609406917699515

Dudgeon, P., & Walker, R. (2015). Decolonising Australian psychology: Discourses, strategies, and practice. *Journal of Social and Political Psychology, 3*(1), 276–297.

Dudgeon, P., Walker, R., Scrine, C., Cox, K., D'Anna, D., Dunkley, C., . . . Hams, K. (2014). Enhancing wellbeing, empowerment, healing and leadership. In P. Dudgeon, H. Milroy, & R. Walker (Eds.), *Working together: Aboriginal and Torres Strait Islander mental health and wellbeing principles and practice* (pp. 437–448). Commonwealth of Australia.

Dudgeon, P., Wright, M., Paradies, Y., Garvey, D., & Walker, I. (2014). Aboriginal social, cultural and historical contexts. In P. Dudgeon, H. Milroy, & R. Walker (Eds.), *Working together: Aboriginal and Torres Strait Islander mental health and wellbeing principles and practice* (pp. 3–24). Commonwealth of Australia.

Fogarty, W., Lovell, M., Langenberg, J., & Heron, M. (2018). *Deficit discourse and strengths-based approaches: Changing the narrative of Aboriginal and Torres Strait Islander health and wellbeing.* https://ncis.anu.edu.au/_lib/doc/ddih/Deficit_Disc ourse_and_Strengths-based_Approaches_FINAL_WEB.pdf

Gee, G., Dudgeon, P., Schultz, C., Hart, A., & Kelly, K. (2014). Aboriginal and Torres Strait Islander social and emotional wellbeing. In P. Dudgeon, H. Milroy, & R. Walker (Eds.), *Working together: Aboriginal and Torres Strait Islander mental health and wellbeing principles and practice* (pp. 55–68). Commonwealth of Australia.

Haswell-Elkins, M., Hunter, E., Wargent, R., Hall, B., O'Higgins, C., & West, R. (2009). *Protocols for the delivery of social and emotional wellbeing and mental health services in Indigenous communities: Guidelines for health workers, clinicians, consumers and carers.* https://www.health.qld.gov.au/__data/assets/pdf_file/0029/378731/acknow_ foreward.pdf

Holland, C., Dudgeon, P., & Milroy, H. (2013). *The mental health and social and emotional wellbeing of Aboriginal and Torres Strait Islander peoples, families and communities.* https://www.mentalhealthcommission.gov.au/getmedia/f014d128-ab8a-4a40-b3d2-9a4668a8fd93/Mental-Health-Report-Card-on-Aboriginal-and-Torres-Strait-Islander

Horning, D., & Baumbrough, B. (2020). Contributions to urban Indigenous self-determination: The story of Neeginan and Kaupapa Maori. *Australian Journal of Indigenous Education*, 1–9. doi:doi.org/10.1017/jie.2020.26

Hunter, E. (2004). Commonality, difference and confusion: Changing constructions of Indigenous mental health. *Australian e-Journal for the Advancement of Mental Health, 3*(3), 95–98.

Lowitja Institute. (2014). *Cultural Determinants Roundtable Background Paper.* https://www.lowitja.org.au/content/Document/PDF/Cultural-Determinants-Roundtable-Background-Paper.pdf

Marriott, R., & Ferguson-Hill, S. (2014). Perinatal and infant mental health and wellbeing. In P. Dudgeon, H. Milroy, & R. Walker (Eds.), *Working together: Aboriginal and Torres Strait Islander mental health and wellbeing principles and practice* (pp. 337–354). Commonwealth of Australia.

McClintock, K., King, M., King, A., Connolly, M., Derry, K., & Dudgeon, P. (2021). A collaboration to inform the development of an indigenous wellbeing instrument. *Journal of Indigenous Wellbeing Te Mauri-Pimatisiwin, 6*(3), 31–46.

Menzies, K. (2019a). Understanding the Australian Aboriginal experience of collective, historical and intergenerational trauma. *International Social Work, 62*(6), 1522–1534.

Menzies, K. (2019b). Forcible separation and assimilation as trauma: The historical and socio-political experiences of Australian Aboriginal people. *Social Work & Society, 17*(1).

Milroy, H. (2006). *The dance of life.* https://www.ranzcp.org/practice-education/aborigi nal-torres-strait-islander-mental-health/the-dance-of-life

Milroy, H., Dudgeon, P., & Walker, R. (2014). Community life and development programs–pathways to healing. In P. Dudgeon, H. Milroy, & R. Walker (Eds.),

Working together: Aboriginal and Torres Strait Islander mental health and wellbeing principles and practice (pp. 419–436). Commonwealth of Australia.

Napier, D., Ancarno, C., Butler, B., Calabrese, J., Chater, A., Chatterjee, H., . . . Woolf, K. (2014). Culture and health. *The Lancet, 384*(9954), 1607–1639. doi:10.1016/S0140-6736(14)61603-2

National Aboriginal and Torres Strait Islander Leadership in Mental Health. (2015). *Gayaa Dhuwi (Proud Spirit) Declaration.* https://natsilmh.org.au/sites/default/files/gayaa_dhuwi_declaration_A4.pdf

National Aboriginal Health Strategy Working Party. (1989). *A national Aboriginal health strategy.* Australian Government Department of Aboriginal Affairs.

Parker, R., & Milroy, H. (2003). Schizophrenia and related psychosis in Aboriginal and Torres Strait Islander people. *Aboriginal and Islander Health Worker Journal, 27*(5), 17–19.

Parker, R., & Milroy, H. (2014). Aboriginal and Torres Strait Islander mental health: An overview. In P. Dudgeon, H. Milroy, & R. Walker (Eds.), *Working together: Aboriginal and Torres Strait Islander mental health and wellbeing principles and practice* (pp. 25–38). Commonwealth of Australia.

Rigby, C. W., Rosen, A., Berry, H. L., & Hart, C. R. (2011). If the land's sick, we're sick: The impact of prolonged drought on the social and emotional well-being of Aboriginal communities in rural New South Wales. *Australian Journal of Rural Health, 19*(5), 249–254. https://doi.org/10.1111/j.1440-1584.2011.01223.x

Social Health Reference Group. (2004). *National strategic framework for Aboriginal and Torres Strait Islander peoples' mental health and social and emotional wellbeing 2004–2009.* https://www.niaa.gov.au/sites/default/files/publications/mhsewb-framework_0.pdf

Swan, P., & Raphael, B. (1995). *Ways forward: National consultancy report on Aboriginal and Torres Strait Islander mental health.* http://library.bsl.org.au/jspui/bitstream/123456789/353/1/Ways%20forward_vol.1%20&%202%20_1995.pdf

Swan, P., & Raphael, B. (1997). *Bringing them home: Report of the national inquiry into the separation of Aboriginal and Torres Strait Islander children from their families.* https://humanrights.gov.au/our-work/bringing-them-home-report-1997

United Nations. (2007). *United Nations declaration on the rights of Indigenous peoples.* https://www.un.org/development/desa/indigenouspeoples/declaration-on-the-rights-of-indigenous-peoples.html

Walker, R. (2005). *Transforming strategies in Indigenous education, decolonisation and positive social change.* University of Western Sydney.

Wallerstein, N., & Bernstein, E. (1988). Empowerment education: Freire's ideas adapted to health education. *Health Education & Behaviour, 15*(4), 379–394.

Wanganeen, R. (2014). Seven phases to integrating loss and grief. In P. Dudgeon, H. Milroy, & R. Walker (Eds.), *Working together: Aboriginal and Torres Strait Islander mental health and wellbeing principles and practice* (pp. 475–492). Commonwealth of Australia.

Zubrick, S., Holland, C., Kelly, K., Calma, T., & Walker, R. (2014). The evolving policy context in mental health and wellbeing. In P. Dudgeon, H. Milroy, & R. Walker (Eds.), *Working together: Aboriginal and Torres Strait Islander mental health and wellbeing principles and practice* (pp. 69–89). Commonwealth of Australia.

8

Wellbeing in Higher Education

Evidence- and Policy-Based Strategies to Enhance the Wellbeing of People, Place, and Planet

BRUCE K. CHRISTENSEN AND REBECCA E. KENNEDY ■

INTRODUCTION

As with much discourse on wellbeing, this chapter starts by contemplating its definition, especially in the context of higher education (HE). In 2020, three peak HE organisations[1] from the United States proposed the inter-association definition of wellbeing as 'An optimal and dynamic state that allows people to achieve their full potential; (p. 3). They further specified three, interrelated categories of subjective wellbeing: (1) the perceived assessment of one's own life as being generally happy and satisfying, (2) having one's human rights and needs met, and (3) one's contribution to the community. The definition also recognises the necessity for 'relationships and connectedness, perceived quality of life for all people in the community, and [that] the community meets the needs of all members' (p. 3). We believe that this definition includes many important aspects of wellbeing within the HE context, including the dynamic nature of wellbeing, personal psychological and physical features that promote health and flourishing, essentiality of social justice, importance of subjective quality of life, and need for social harmony and meaning. However, we also seek to take a broader view to include the concentric influences of relationships, communities, culture, society, and the environment, inclusive of their sociopolitical and ecological challenges.

---

1. National Intermural-Recreational Sports Association, Student Affairs Administration in Higher Education, American College Health Association (November 2020). Inter-association definition of wellbeing. Retrieved from www.nirsa.org/hands-in

This perspective has been more roundly adopted in the United Kingdom (e.g., in measuring the nation's wellbeing, the UK Office for National Statistics describes wellbeing as 'how we are doing as individuals, as communities, and as a nation, and how sustainable this is for the future'[2]) and is historically evident in HE policy. For example, in the 1990s, the World Health Organization (WHO) assessed how university environments shape peoples' health and wellbeing, but also sustainable development in the local, regional, and global environments (Dooris, 2001). These efforts suggest that, beyond health, HE wellbeing investment enhances recruitment/retention, institutional productivity, and community sustainability (Dooris & Doherty, 2010a, 2010b). Accordingly, the WHO published the Health Promoting Universities framework (Tsouros, Dowding, Thompson, & Dooris, 1998) outlining a settings-based approach with the following principles: (1) a holistic and socioecological understanding of health; (2) a focus on populations, policy, and environments; (3) equity and social justice; (4) sustainability, community participation, enablement, and empowerment; (5) cooperation, consensus, mediation, and advocacy; and (6) settings as social systems, with sustainable integrative actions and part of an interdependent ecosystem. In response, Dooris et al. (2012) championed the Health Promoting Universities (HPU) movement, which has gained considerable momentum over the past decade and currently consists of 13 national or regional networks.

At the 2015 International Conference on Health Promoting Universities and Colleges, 380 HPU delegates developed, refined, and ratified *The Okanagan Charter: An International Charter for Health Promoting Universities and Colleges*, which sets out a vision to 'transform the health and sustainability of our current and future societies, strength communities and contribute to the wellbeing of people, places, and the planet' (p. 2). The Charter further aspires to the '[infusion] of health into everyday operations, business practices and academic mandates' and the creation of 'compassion, wellbeing, equity and social justice . . . [to] strengthen the ecological, social and economic sustainability of our communities and wider society'.[3] Reflected here is the evolving conception of wellbeing as not merely the absence of illness, but the integration of physical health with mental health, social connectedness and justice, and the sustainability of the planet. This chapter expressly adopts the definition and categories set out by the Okanagan Charter to explore, in turn, the evidence and policy bases for promoting HE wellbeing among its *people*, *places* and, more widely, the *planet*. Before doing so, however, we will document the urgent need for initiatives of this kind by providing an overview of the challenges to wellbeing in the HE setting.

2. For this definition and other details, please see: https://www.ons.gov.uk

3. To access the Okanagan Charter, please see https://www.healthpromotingcampuses.org/okanagan-charter

OVERVIEW AND SCOPE OF THE PROBLEM

Institutes of HE (IHE) are commonly viewed as a nexus of scholarship, creativity, social connection/collaboration, and personal growth; as places of deep meaning and profound impact for those working, learning, and living on campus. Yet, against these celebrated features, IHE have recently been described as environments constituting significant risk for poor wellbeing and mental health (Shaw & Ward, 2014). The largest survey of tertiary students in the United Kingdom (i.e., 37,500 students from 140 universities) found that 20% had a mental health diagnosis, 30% had concerns for which they needed professional help, and approximately 50% had thoughts about self-harm (Pereira et al., 2020). Likewise, a substantial census-matched survey of Australian HE students found that approximately 20% had mental health problems and nearly 70% reported subsyndromal symptoms (Stallman, 2010). The picture is similar in the United States: Kang and colleagues (2021) summarised the prevalence of mental health disorders among undergraduates across 12 separate studies and found highest rates for depression (22%) and eating disorders (19–48%). Results from the Healthy Minds Study, a large longitudinal, online survey (2014–2018) including more than 100 US tertiary institutions and involving more than 50,000 respondents, showed that large segments of students are experiencing moderate to severe depression (31%), an anxiety disorder (26%), and/or nonsuicidal self-injury (36%) (Eisenberg & Lipson, 2016). Importantly, rates of mental health problems are high even when compared to non-students of the same age (Cvetkovski, Revley, & Jorm, 2012; Houghton, Keane, Murphy, Houghton, & Dunne, 2010; Stallman, 2010) and disproportionately impact students who are female, Indigenous, international, younger, from a low-income background, a member of a minority group (e.g., sexually and gender diverse), or from a specific programme (i.e., law, medicine, and doctoral studies). Elevated rates of distress are not limited to undergraduate students. Several studies have demonstrated concerning rates of depression and anxiety among graduate students (Eisenberg, Gollust, Golberstein, & Hefner, 2007; Evans, Bira, Gastelum Weiss, & Vanderford, 2018; Levecque, Anseel, De Beuckelaer, Van der Heyden, & Gisle, 2017) and university faculty and staff[4] (Goodwin et al., 2013; Padilla & Thompson, 2016; Watts & Robertson, 2011).

Poor wellbeing and mental health problems on university campuses have critical implications. They have deleterious effects on students' academic progress (Eisenberg et al., 2007) and their research capacity (Levecque et al., 2017) and are associated with them leaving university (Arria et al., 2013; Devine & Hunter, 2016; Lovitts, 2001), abusing drugs and alcohol (Arria, Barrall, Allen, Bugbee, & Vincent, 2018; Cvetkovski et al., 2012), engaging in self-harm or suicide (Sharp & Theiler, 2018), performing poorly academically (Wyatt & Oswalt, 2013), and

---

4. Please note that, given space restrictions, inclusion of the well-documented risks at IHE for mental health problems among staff and faculty will not be included in the chapter. Interested readers, however, are referred to Morrish (2019).

achieving poor employment outcomes (Jennison, 2004). Higher levels of stress also result in student disengagement, work avoidance, procrastination, and amotivation, each of which erodes student self-efficacy (Evans et al., 2018). Conversely, positive wellbeing has been linked to increased learning (Duckworth & Cara, 2012), innovativeness (Huhtala & Parzefall, 2007), creativity (Ohly & Bledow, 2015), helping behaviours (Grant & Kinman, 2014), socially responsible acts (Crilly, Schneider, & Zollo, 2008), and productivity (Briner & Dewberry, 2007), all of which are catalysts of success in HE environments (Welpe, Wollersheim, Ringelhan, & Osterloh, 2015).

Given scholarship's role as a driver of national intellectual and economic capital, universities and governments are focusing more on the wellbeing of IHE. For society, a well-educated workforce augments the growth and stability of the economy at large and general welfare. Consequently, IHE, apart from their ethical and fiduciary responsibilities to community members, have cast wellbeing as an economic investment and a means of distinguishing themselves in a crowded marketplace. This, coupled with strong campaigns from student groups, unions, and mental health advocacy organisations, has spawned several recent mental health and wellbeing charters from IHE. Examples include the University Mental Health Charter: Principles of Good Practice (2019) from the United Kingdom and the Australian University Mental Health Framework (2020).[5] Both provide evidence-based frameworks for understanding and enhancing the psychological wellbeing of students and staff. Each also emphasises similar foundational perspectives including the importance of whole-of-university approaches, committed, action-oriented leadership, including the student voice and lived experience, fostering diversity and inclusion, co-creation, and providing effective, timely services. The above-noted Okanagan Charter champions just such whole-university strategies for mental health. It also recognises wellbeing as more than individuals' mental health and argues for place-and planet-level interventions. Before addressing the latter, we first review person-level strategies.

PERSON-LEVEL STRATEGIES

To date, the most significant wellbeing investment made by IHE has been through counselling services (Kraft, 2011). It is, therefore, unsurprising that the effectiveness of individual and group based psychological/counselling interventions are among the most studied. The following summary is informed by several narrative/systematic and meta-analytic reviews and organised by treatment approach; it has benefited enormously from the umbrella review performed by Worsley, Pennington, and Corcoran (2020). The reviews collected under this summary

5. For more details regarding the above-noted university mental health frameworks, please see https://universitymentalhealthcharter.org.uk/themes/ and https://www.orygen.org.au/Policy/University-Mental-Health-Framework

have predominantly focused on studies of college students in English-speaking, developed countries who were undergoing interventions aimed at alleviating anxiety, dysphoria, stress/distress, and suicide (both thoughts and behaviour). The quality of these reviews ranges from weak to strong (Worsley et al., 2020), and the studies themselves often have substantial methodological limitations including the lack of appropriate control conditions/groups, random assignment, rigorous sampling frameworks, and evaluation for treatment fidelity. Nevertheless, aggregated results consistently suggest that several interventions have positive effects on the subjective wellbeing of HE students.

Mindfulness

Several reviews have considered the impact of mindfulness-based interventions (MBIs) on the mental health and wellbeing of HE students; four directly studying MBIs (Bamber & Morpeth, 2019; Bamber & Schneider, 2016; Halladay et al., 2019; O'Driscoll, Byrne, McGillicuddy, Lambert, & Sahm, 2017), and seven included in mixed reviews (Breedvelt et al., 2019; Conley, Durlak, & Dickson, 2013; Conley, Durlak, & Kirsch, 2015; Conley, Shapiro, Kirsch, & Durlak, 2017; Huang, Nigatu, Smail-Crevier, Zhang, & Wang, 2018; Litwiller, White, Hamilton-Hinch, & Gilbert, 2018; Regehr, Glancy, & Pitts, 2013). Mindfulness has its origins in the meditative practices of Eastern religions and philosophy and, at its core, describes the process of intentionally focussing attention on the present moment in a non-judgemental manner. MBIs are designed to train people to cultivate mindfulness as a means of coping with psychological distress. Large meta-analyses have shown that MBIs are effective in treating a wide array of psychological problems (Gu, Strauss, Bond, & Cavanagh, 2015). Similarly, reviews of MBIs for HE students have found them to be effective for reducing depression, anxiety, and stress, achieving moderate effect sizes in most meta-analyses.

However, several qualifications are also noted in this literature. First, the positive effects for MBIs were much more likely when compared to passive control conditions (e.g., treatment as usual). Relative to active control conditions, MBIs were sometimes indistinguishable or worse (e.g., relative to art, exercise, music, or peer support—Huang et al., 2018; health education, relaxation or physical activity—Halladay et al., 2019). Second, many studies neglected to examine whether the effects from MBIs were sustained over time, and those that included longitudinal evaluations did so on a timescale of only several months. The results for depressive symptoms were mixed, while those for anxious symptoms were consistent over a 6-month post-intervention period (Halladay, et al., 2019). Third, it is unclear whether the length of intervention and/or the number of sessions makes a difference (e.g., Halladay et al., 2019, vs. Bamber & Morpeth, 2019). Fourth, Conley and colleagues (2013, 2015) found that positive outcomes depended on whether the trial participants were supervised in their mindfulness practice.

Cognitive-Behavioural Interventions

Cognitive-behavioural interventions (CBIs) are built on the foundational observation that the relationship between stressful events and negative emotions/behaviour is mediated by negative (e.g., unrealistic and/or unhelpful) appraisals of these events. Therefore, CBIs focus on modifying unrealistic and/or unhelpful negative thoughts (Beck, 1976). CBIs have proven to be among the most robust forms of psychological treatment for most mental health problems (Hofmann, Asnaani, Vonk, Sawyer, & Fang, 2012). Not surprisingly, CBIs tested in HE contexts have also shown positive results, with most meta-analyses demonstrating moderate to large effects on depression, anxiety, and stress (Conley et al., 2013; Conley et al., 2015; Conley et al., 2017; Cuijpers et al., 2016; Huang et al., 2018; Miller & Chung, 2009; Reavley & Jorm, 2010; Regehr et al., 2013; Winzer, Lindberg, Gulbrandsson, & Sidorchuk, 2018). One review also revealed that CBIs had a moderate effect on academic performance and that positive effects were still present 13–18 months post-intervention (Winzer et al., 2018). Some reviews have found that CBIs provide a superior effect over MBIs in this population and that, although not always as strong as the immediate impact of other interventions (art, exercise, peer support), the longer-term effect for CBIs was greater (Huang et al., 2018). Other variables appear to moderate the positive effect of CBIs. For example, in their review Cuijpers et al. (2016) found that individual CBIs were more effective than those delivered in a group format, and, as with MBIs, Conley et al. (2015) showed that unsupervised CBIs were much less effective. CBIs were also an effective preventative measure for stress reduction (Reavely & Jorm, 2010; Regehr et al., 2013).

Telehealth

Telehealth is the delivery and facilitation of health-related services via tele- and digital communication technologies. Recently, telehealth has gained considerable popularity given its ease of use, wide geographical reach, and utility in the context of COVID-19 restrictions. Commentators have suggested that it may be particularly suitable for HE students given their familiarity with digital technology. In relation to HE, four reviews have investigated the effectiveness of this modality (Conley, Durlak, Shapiro, Kirsch, & Zahniser, 2016; Davies, Morriss, & Glazebrook, 2014; Farrer et al., 2013; Harrer et al., 2018;). Meta-analyses have found moderate, positive effects for telehealth on depression, anxiety, and stress compared with *inactive* controls (Davies et al., 2014); however, relative to *active* controls, telehealth interventions were not effective (Davies et al., 2014). The effects were larger for students already reporting symptoms and interventions targeting skill-training (Conley et al., 2016). A small number of studies reviewed investigated sustained effects and found positive outcomes for periods between 13 and 52 weeks post-intervention (Conley et al., 2016). Farrer and colleagues (2013) conducted a review of randomised control and equivalence trials. Although effective for reducing both anxiety and depression, telehealth was less effective than therapy with human contact.

Psychoeducation

Three reviews included psychoeducational interventions in comparison to other interventions (Conley et al., 2013; Conley et al., 2015; Winzer et al. 2018). The psychoeducation usually included providing information on stress reduction, coping, and relaxation and included perspectives on these processes from CBIs, MBIs, and social skills training. Overall, psychoeducation was rated as less effective than the other methods reviewed above; that is, effect sizes were more often nonsignificant or small in magnitude. Albeit small, the manifest effects were most consistent for common problems, including anxiety, stress, and distress (Conley et al., 2015). One study also found sustained effects at 13–18 months for depression and 7–12 months for anxiety (Winzer et al., 2018).

Relaxation

In a series of meta-analytic studies, Conley and colleagues (2013, 2015) directly tested the impact of relaxation in comparison to other interventions. Relaxation techniques largely comprised the use of guided imagery (i.e., focusing on positive mental images in a relaxed state) and progressive muscle relaxation (i.e., the practice of tightening one muscle group at a time followed by a relaxation phase). Relaxation significantly outperformed all other approaches tested. From this analysis, the rank order of intervention type by effectiveness was relaxation, CBIs, mindfulness, meditation, and psychoeducation (Conley et al., 2015). However, as previously noted, skills-based training was more effective under supervision; when interventions that included supervision were compared, CBIs and MBIs outperformed relaxation (Conley et al., 2013).

Recreation

The activities reviewed under recreational interventions are far-ranging and include yoga, Tai Chi (meditative martial arts), physical activity, and pet interactions. Several reviews included one or more of these interventions for consideration (Breedvelt et al., 2019; Conley et al., 2013; Conley et al., 2015; Huang et al., 2018; Litwiller et al., 2018). In addition, one review concentrated solely on meditation (Shapiro, Brown, & Astin, 2011). In their methodologically strong review and meta-analysis, Huang et al. (2018) found that recreational interventions (physical activity, art, peer support) were effective among students in reducing anxiety and depression. Moreover, recreation interventions produced larger effects for depression and generalised anxiety than did CBIs and MBIs.[6] When comparing across recreation interventions, Breedvelt et al. (2019; yoga, meditation, and MBIs) and Litwiller et al. (2018; MBIs, meditation, Tai Chi, yoga, physical activity, and animal therapy) found no between-condition effects. In contrast, other studies have found that meditation interventions were superior to psychoeducation but less impactful than relaxation, CBIs, or MBIs (Conley et al., 2015).

In addition to its impacts on mental health, participation in campus recreation activities has been associated with increased persistence toward degree completion (Belch, Gebel, & Maas, 2001; Ragheb & McKinney, 1993). A large study commissioned by National Intramural-Recreational Sports Association on the impact of participation in recreation programs on students at 16 selected IHE resulted in interviews with 2,673 students who endorsed the benefits of recreational sports in the following order: (1) improves emotional wellbeing, (2) reduces stress, (3) improves happiness, (4) improves self-confidence, (5) builds character, (6) makes students feel part of the college community, (7) improves interaction with diverse sets of people, (8) is an important part of college social life, (9) teaches team-building skills, (10) is an important part of the learning experience, (11) aids time management, and (12) improves leadership skills. They also found that there was a direct correlation between the level of participation and the degree to which students received these benefits and that benefits were equally strong across gender but stronger for African American, Hispanic, and White students than for Asian students.

Acceptance and Commitment Therapy

Acceptance and commitment therapy (ACT) is a psychological intervention that targets how people relate to their thoughts, emotions, and behaviours rather than their content. These techniques seek to increase psychological flexibility; that is, experiencing the present moment without defence as well as engaging in behaviours in the service of one's chosen values (Hayes, 2004). Howell and Passmore (2018) identified five randomised controlled experiments using ACT as the principal component of interventions for HE students. Their meta-analysis of these studies showed a small but significant positive effect for students receiving these interventions relative to control conditions. These authors note that interventions were generally brief (3–8 weeks), raising questions about the adequacy of dose. In addition, more comprehensive interventions (e.g., online practice of techniques introduced in group sessions) gave rise to larger effects, the operationalisation of ACT varied across studies, and some studies combined ACT with other types of interventions, making it difficult to isolate ACT's specific impact.

---

6. It should be noted that the number of studies reviewed under the recreational domain was low relative to other interventions, and, therefore, these results should be considered with caution.

Suicide Prevention

Harrod and colleagues (2014) focussed their meta-analytic assessment on the prevention of suicide, one of the chief causes of death among persons under 25 (Wasserman & Wasserman, 2010). Across eight studies, which were heterogeneous in design, the effects of classroom instruction, institutional policies, and gatekeeper training programs (i.e., teaching community members to recognise and respond to people at risk of suicide) were analysed. The results suggest that classroom instruction increased short-term knowledge of suicide and suicide prevention. Only one study evaluated institutional policy (i.e., restricting access to laboratory cyanide), which was significantly associated with reduced suicides. Four studies looked at the impact of gatekeeper training and indicated small to medium improvements in knowledge about suicide and self-reported confidence in being able to prevent suicide. Based on her review of mental health gatekeeper training for teenagers and young adults, Lipson (2014) concludes that there are positive (but inconsistent) influences on self-rated knowledge, attitudes, and behavioural intentions, but without comparable effects on action. Moreover, positive training effects appear to diminish over time. This review warns that the implementation of gatekeeper programs for young people is ahead of the research and that most studies are of low methodological quality, fail to measure objective skills, and ignore population outcomes such as health service utilisation.

Wellbeing Courses

Studies investigating the effects of wellbeing courses were most often uncontrolled, longitudinal studies with pre- and post-intervention testing. Consequently, these results should be viewed with caution. Nevertheless, wellbeing courses correlate with gains in mental health knowledge (Becker et al., 2008), social connectedness and hope (Shek, 2012, 2013), psychological quality of life, mood, and emotional control (Hassed, Lisle, Sullivan, & Pier, 2009), mindfulness and self-compassion (Bergen-Cico, Possemato, & Cheon, 2013), and happiness and wellbeing (Lambert, Passmore, & Joshanloo, 2019).

An alternative pedagogical approach is to infuse wellbeing curricula into existing courses. For example, Bughi and colleagues (2006) assessed the wellbeing-related impact of a single lecture on stress management among medical students and found that, 1 month later, self-reported stressed had decreased by 47%. In another study, first-year students who received a manual on coping during their first tutorial and SMS text prompts to cultivate positive emotions demonstrated improved psychological wellbeing (Foster, Allen, Oprescu, & McAllister, 2014).

A strength of the findings in this domain is the ubiquity of positive outcomes across varied interventions and populations. At the same time, however, this literature is small, lacks replication, is poorly controlled, and has done little to isolate the specific mechanisms underlying positive change. The need for further high-quality research in this area is underscored by the value students place on wellbeing courses (Khan & Rieger, 2021; Lee & Graham, 2001). Moreover, the design of these courses can be enhanced through joining with students as co-creators. For instance, students report appreciating the efficiency of addressing wellbeing within a course structure and are favourable about content that combines practicality and application with critical science (Khan & Rieger, 2021).

First-Year Transition Support

Research shows that the transition from secondary to HE contexts is associated with reduced student wellbeing (Fisher & Hood, 1987). Several qualitative studies indicate that social support was the most crucial element facilitating a positive transition to the first year (and success across students' entire program), while its absence predicted negative transitions (Hughes & Smail, 2015; Tett, Cree, & Christie, 2017; Wilcox, Winn, & Fyvie-Gauld, 2005). Students also identified a positive mindset, confidence from relevant adults, orientation to available support, setting expectations, understanding university systems, developing study skills, and a healthy lifestyle (e.g., moderate drinking and regular physical activity) as important. Interestingly, at least in one study (Hughes & Smail, 2015), academic concerns did not emerge as a particular concern among students entering university for the first time.

In concert with these findings, a few studies have investigated interventions to increase social belonging and connectedness.[7] For example, several studies have found positive effects among randomly assigned students to social group interventions (Lamothe et al., 1995; Oppenheimer, 1984). An even briefer intervention (approximately 1 hour) provided students with a third-person narrative from a senior student that framed social adversity as shared and short-lived (Walton & Cohen, 2011). That is, the narrative encouraged students to attribute adversity to common and transient adjustment processes and not to personal deficits or ethnic identity. Participants were also required to write an essay conveying their own experiences that echoed those in the narrative and convert the essay into a speech, which was delivered to a video camera. The intervention improved academic performance via its enhancement of students' sense of belonging and worked to buffer the effects of social adversity on subjective construal (i.e., seeing adversity as an indictment of their belonging). These beneficial effects were still detectable 3 years post-intervention. Moreover, these effects were exaggerated for African American students. Additionally, Dutch researchers developed a pre-academic programme aimed at changing students' perceptions of effective learning, sense of belonging, social interactions with peers and faculty, and academic

7. It should be noted that intervention studies reviewed here do not specifically target at-risk student groups (e.g., those with social anxiety). In this way, they are not selected strategies; however, they are included here because they hold promise in their logical extension for use with at-risk HE populations, especially in the social domain.

performance (van Herpen, Meeuwisse, Adriaan, & Severiens, 2020). The 4-day intervention delivered lectures, assignments, and activities designed to persuade students that social adversity among university students is common and transient, studying at university is a social process, and effective learning is their responsibility. Students enrolled in the programme had better interactions with faculty and peers and achieved better grades.

PLACE-LEVEL STRATEGIES

Place-based approaches generally target larger sections of the campus, are more salutogenic than person-based approaches, and emphasise environmental, economic, social, and cultural determinants of wellbeing. There is much that goes into creating environments that cultivate wellbeing at IHE, including student support services/resources, classroom and curricular approaches, specialised programs, and the campus climate. Rankin and Reason (2008) define campus climate as the attitudes, behaviours, standards, and practices of IHE community members, especially in relation to access, inclusion, and level of respect for individual and group needs, abilities, and potential. In their review, Pascarella and Terenzini (2005) suggest that campus climate is strongly linked to student success and persistence, especially among marginalised students. The built and natural environments of an IHE are also place-level strategies. Here, we review these place-level components and the research and policy evidence that support their effectiveness in promoting wellbeing at IHE.

Health and Counselling Centres

Student support services, such as health and counselling centres, grew out of the necessity to care for the physical health of students (Christmas, 1995; Kraft, 2011). To date, there are nearly 2,000 on-campus medical and mental health services at US colleges alone (American College Health Association, 2016). The American College Health Assessment/National College Health Assessment (ACHA-NCHA) has been used since 2000 to assess the health needs of students, and now more than 1.4 million students from more than 740 IHE across the United States and Canada have taken the survey.[8] Although more than 100 research articles using NCHA data have been published, no studies have reported the effectiveness of student health centres for promoting the health and wellbeing of students. Indirect positive evidence comes from the College Health Surveillance Network, which demonstrated high levels of usage of student health centres by evaluating

8. Results from the ACHA-NCHA surveys can be accessed at https://www.acha.org/NCHA/About_ACHA_NCHA/Participation_History/NCHA/About/Participation_History.aspx?hkey=992b3d9a-9d22-46b8-911c-1f187dd5fb6c

the utilisation patterns of 800,000 students (Turner & Keller, 2015). In addition, qualitative accounts from professional organisations suggest that 'college health plays a critical role in the retention, progression, and graduation of students by providing access to and/or coordination of quality, affordable, convenient health and wellness services and programs delivered by professionals who are attuned to the unique stressors and needs of college students' (Turner & Keller, 2015, p. 1). Moreover, investigations evaluating the outsourcing of health and counselling services (Eddy, Spaudling, & Murphy, 1996; Widseth, Webb, & John, 1997) suggest that privatisation of HE healthcare is disadvantageous.

Classroom and Curricular Approaches

The idea that teaching techniques and curriculum design might positively impact student wellbeing is popular. However, empirical undertakings in this area are scant. One approach that has garnered empirical support, however, is the grading systems by which students are assessed. In general, binary systems (e.g., pass/fail) facilitate greater wellbeing (including higher social cohesion and less stress, burnout, emotional exhaustion, and depersonalisation) as opposed to continuous or multi-interval systems, and without impacting academic performance (Bloodgood, Short, Jackson, & Martindale, 2009; Reed et al., 2011; Rohe et al., 2006).

The few studies exploring the wellbeing benefits of curriculum design have predominantly targeted professional programs (i.e., law and medicine). Typically, these studies implemented several changes at once and, therefore, specific influences are difficult to ascertain. For example, Slavin et al. (2014) reduced student stress, depression, and anxiety after (1) instituting a pass/fail grading system, (2) reducing contact hours, (3) introducing more longitudinal electives, (4) establishing learning communities of staff and students, and, (5) offering a mandatory course on mindfulness and resilience. Similarly, Tang and Ferguson (2014) evaluated sweeping curricular changes in an Australian law school that included online learning, simulated legal transactions, and small-group mentorship. These changes buffered students against the psychological distress observed in the traditional program. Another study documented lower distress and fewer academic concerns after a student-centred, problem-based curriculum replaced the traditional curriculum in a Scottish nursing programme (Jones & Johnston, 2006).

However, not all curricular modifications have been positive. For example, researchers compared traditional and adapted medical curricula that integrated basic sciences with clinical information, increased problem-based and small-group learning, and used a pass/fail grading system (Tucker, Jeon-Slaughter, Sener, Arvidson, & Khalfian, 2015). Unexpectedly, students completing the adapted curriculum scored higher on measures of depression and stress. It should be noted, however, that the sample size for this study was small and interventions were not randomly assigned across students, thereby undermining the validity of these results.

Climate for Ethnic and Racial Diversity

The negative experiences of ethnic and racial minority students at IHE are well-documented. Smith (2009) highlights the concept of racial battle fatigue (i.e., the physical and emotional exhaustion experienced from the cumulative negative effect of racial microaggressions), while others emphasise that social inequality and discrimination at IHE foster poor self-efficacy and coping (Manejwala & Abu-Ras, 2019; Oliver, Datta, & Baldwin, 2019). Patton et al. (2019) comprehensively reviewed research focused on formalised diversity, inclusion, equity, and justice initiatives implemented in IHE over a 50-year period. They identified four main categories of initiatives: (1) student support services (i.e., diversity programs or advocacy offices; racial and cultural awareness workshops), (2) curricular initiatives (i.e., diversity requirements and diversity-related courses), (3) administration and leadership initiatives (i.e., faculty/staff training and the appointment of a chief diversity officer to executive leadership), and (4) institutional policy initiatives (i.e., affirmative action and institution-wide diversity strategies). Overall, the majority of the studies reviewed focused on cross-cultural engagement for White students and do little to critically analyse systems of oppression or transform the campus climate to address injustices. Patton and colleagues criticise the IHE tendency to add support programs for marginalised students and add diversity education and training for majority members rather than work to change the systems both within our IHE and larger society. The researchers do not evaluate the effectiveness of various additive programs or policy initiatives and instead suggest that future research address the dismantling of structural racism, institutional resistance to changing systems of oppression, and promoting change.

Similarly, Iverson (2012), using policy discourse analysis to review 20 IHE diversity action plans, suggests that the most common response to issues of inclusion is to assemble task forces and develop diversity action plans. She notes that, despite burgeoning diversity action plans, university campuses continue to struggle with challenges to achieve institutional diversity. Iverson's analysis reveals that these plans hold the underrepresented group as outsiders, situated against the majority. She notes that diversity action plans should preserve individuality but consider ways to disrupt the insider–outsider distinction that supports exclusion and inequity. In this vein, Miller (2014) provides a general review of the literature on campus climate relating to gender and racial minorities. He argues that IHE can improve by becoming deliberate agents of social change, taking a multidimensional approach focusing on policies and practices but also through the recruitment and support of diverse students, staff, and faculty.

Climate for Sexual and Gender Diversity

Sexually and gender diverse (SGD) students report significant harassment and discrimination in HE (Ferfolja, Asquith, Hanckel, & Brady, 2020; Manning, Pring, & Glider, 2014; Woodford, Kulick, Garvey, Sinco, & Hong, 2018). Numerous studies have also documented higher rates of mental health problems and lower wellbeing among SGD students (Crawford & Ridner, 2018; Greathouse et al., 2018). What is less understood is the aetiology of these differences. In this regard, some research suggests that animosity toward non-heterosexuality (heterosexist harassment) is directly related to SGD students' academic satisfaction and desire to stay at their college (Morris & Lent, 2019).

In the wake of these findings, there is growing support for inclusive policies, awareness programs, and SGD centres/resources that promote acceptance, challenge heterosexism, and provide support for SGD students (Ecker, Rae, & Bassi, 2015; Hafford-Letchfield, Pezzella, Cole, & Manning, 2017; Hatzenbuehler, 2014; Hatzenbuehler & Pachankis, 2016; Pitcher, Camacho, Renn, & Woodford, 2018; Schenk, Sasso, & González-Morales, 2020; Woodford et al., 2016). For example, a study of 58 IHE found that institutional policies and programs protect SGD students from heterosexist discrimination and lead to lower distress and higher self-acceptance (Woodford et al., 2018). Garvey and Dolan (2021) provide a substantial review of SGD student success and conclude that (1) non-discrimination policies are viewed positively by SGD students as evidence of an affirming climate, (2) gender-inclusive housing options reduce SGD student isolation and improve academic outcomes, (3) gender-inclusive restrooms improve SGD safety and perceived inclusiveness, (4) student health plans that cover SGD services (e.g., hormone therapy, gender-affirming surgeries) and employ affirming/non-heterosexist staff increase SGD student support, (5) campuses that collect data on SGD students are better able to meet student needs, and (6) HE records should provide options for students to appropriately identify their chosen name, pronouns, and gender identity.[9]

Climate for Students with Disabilities

Despite widespread legislation prohibiting discrimination based on disability and requiring reasonable accommodations for qualified students, many of these students do not register for or receive appropriate accommodations and supports (Barnard-Brak, Lechtenberger, & Lan, 2010; Herbert, Coduti, & Fleming, 2020; Marshak, Van Wieren, Ferrell, Swiss, & Dugan, 2010; Stein, 2013). Studies generally note the negative experiences of students with disabilities (Cook, Rumrill, & Tankersley, 2009; Vogel, Leyser, Burgstahler, Sligar, & Zecker, 2006) and cite lower wellbeing and increased mental health problems for these students (e.g., Durlak, Rose, & Bursuck, 1994).

Importantly, literature is accumulating on how best to support students with disabilities (Moriña & Biagiotti, 2021). For example, Schreffler et al. (2019) showed

---

9. Garvey and Dolan (2021) also review three inventories for SGD services and make recommendations for IHE on how to initiate and sustain institutional reform to positively transform campus by enacting more socially just policies and practices.

that Universal Design for Learning (i.e., where instructors present the curriculum in multiple ways to engage all learners) was associated with positive academic and psychological outcomes such as enhanced self-regulation and behavioural confidence among students with disabilities. Qualitative research shows that students with disabilities experience faculty as having limited understanding of disability law, disabilities, and how to support disabled students (Herbert et al., 2020). They suggest several remedies (including greater staff empathy/knowledge and course structures to support all student) and underscore the need for research assessing (1) the effectiveness of faculty/staff training models; (2) models to determine how training enhances self-determination, social networks, and academic achievement; (3) the impact of general education courses that address disability topics intended for the general student population; and (4) university-wide efforts to improve disability climate. Unfortunately, the current literature lacks an empirical analysis of the most effective, polices, training, resources, or supports for students with disabilities.

Climate for Substance Abuse and Misuse

Since the early 2000s, research has supported the use of environmental management to reduce substance abuse at IHE. In this vein, the US Higher Education Center for Alcohol and Other Drug Abuse and Violence Prevention proposed five strategies for the environmental management of substance abuse: (1) offer alcohol-free social, extracurricular, and public service options; (2) create a health-promoting normative environment; (3) restrict the marketing and promotion of alcoholic beverages both on and off campus; (4) limit alcohol availability; and (5) increase the enforcement of alcohol and drug laws and policies.[10] Similarly, in 2007, the US National Institute on Alcohol Abuse and Alcoholism published a report advocating that interventions be simultaneously geared to the individual, student body, and campus community and campus–community partnerships that focus on awareness, education, and responsible beverage service. The report also noted that social norms approaches (strategies that use social and traditional marketing interventions) have mixed support but are most effective when combined with other interventions and are utilized on campuses with lower alcohol outlet density and lower levels of drinking.[11]

Universities have also used environmental management to curb smoking. According to the American Non-Smokers' Rights Foundation, as 2021, at least 2,537 US HE campuses were smoke-free and smoking bans on campus are

10. For more details regarding these prevention strategies, please see (https://safesupportivel earning.ed.gov/sites/default/files/hec/product/em101.pdf).

11. For access to this report and more detailed recommendations, please refer to https://www. collegedrinkingprevention.gov/niaaacollegematerials/publications/WhatCollegesNeedtoK now.aspx)

effective. Similarly, a systematic review and meta-analysis of the acceptability and effectiveness of university smoke-free policies found that the majority of students and faculty support such policies and that student smoking prevalence was reduced following implementation of smoking bans (Lupton & Townsend, 2015). Smoke-free policies also affect attitudes about and the initiation of smoking at IHE. For instance, Lechner and colleague (2012) examined smoking behaviour over 4 years following a smoke-free policy and found that smoking decreased and students were less accepting of second-hand smoke exposure. Moreover, the implementation of a tobacco-free policy at three campuses in Alaska resulted in both greater smoking cessation and less smoking initiation (Garcia, Mapaye, Lopez, Roxbury, & Tabatabai-Yazdi, 2020).

Prevention of Sexual Violence

Sexual assault and harassment are significant problems at IHE worldwide (DeGue et al., 2014). The magnitude of these problems led the US Department of Education to take bold action in 2011 by yoking federal funding to IHE's handling of sexual misconduct in order to encourage consistency in the processing of cases. Unfortunately, there are no systematic studies of the impact of this policy on the wellbeing of sexual assault survivors. DeGue et al. (2014) provide a systematic review of 140 evaluations of strategies to reduce sexual violence. Of the 11 that were implemented with HE students, however, none was effective or produced inconclusive results secondary to methodological limitations. A notable exception is the NOMORE Men's Program, which the authors deem as potentially harmful for sexual violence behavioural outcomes since sexually violent behaviours were significantly increased at follow-up among high-risk men.

At least three bystander intervention programs and two self-defence programs for IHE students have been shown to reduce rates of sexual violence. The bystander programs include Green Dot (Coker et al., 2011, 2015), Bringing in the Bystander (Banyard, Moynihan, & Plante, 2007; Cares et al., 2015; Moynihan, Banyard, Arnold, Eckstein, & Stapleton, 2011), and RealConsent (Salazar, Vivolo-Kantor, Hardin, & Berkowitz, 2014). The self-defence programs include Enhanced Access, Acknowledge (Senn et al., 2021), and Sexual Assault Risk Reduction (Gidycz et al., 2015). Among these, RealConsent is the only programme that works to directly reduce rates of perpetration of sexual violence by programme participants. A content analysis of 10 years of sexual violence research at IHE concluded that, 'research on campus sexual violence is dominated by heterosexual cisgender white women as victims and alcohol as a risk factor for sexual violence' (Linder, Grimes, Williams, Lacy, & Parker, 2020, p. 1031). These authors noted that only 10% of articles focused on perpetrators and that IHE research needs to shift away from preventing individual instances of sexual violence (e.g., with bystander intervention or self-defence) and toward addressing the roots causes of sexual violence.

Eisenberg, Lust, Hannan, and Porta (2016) examined data from the College Student Health Survey (CSHS) to establish the relationship between IHE sexual violence resources and mental health outcomes. There were six types of resources assessed: (1) paid staff dedicated to addressing sexual violence, (2) a hotline or 24-hour contact, (3) a safe walk or escort service, (4) activities or events to raise students' awareness of sexual violence issues, (5) support groups or counselling for survivors of sexual violence, and (6) pamphlets or posters around campus. Women with access to more sexual violence resources had better mental health; the review did not, however, evaluate which of these resources had the largest effect.

Built and Natural Environments

A number of community planning principles are applicable to IHE, including physical spaces with good air and water quality; low levels of light and noise pollution; access to safe, affordable housing; and access to healthy, affordable, and convenient food. Additionally, there is evidence to support designing environments with greenspace and provisions for physical activity and transport in the wellbeing of IHE communities. The International WELL Building Institute (IWBI; 2022) outlines a WELL Building Standard based on research to promote the health and subjective wellbeing of people who use a given space.[12] They have developed 10 areas for which they provide associated standards (i.e., air, water, nourishment, light, movement, thermal comfort, sound, materials, mind, community, and innovation). These standards are being used across an array of global settings but also as a guide for the design of buildings on IHE campuses. To date, however, the impact and efficacy of these applications await research.

IHE campuses, once known for poor-quality food outlets (e.g., cafeterias), now routinely offer premier dining facilities and options that include a myriad of healthy foods. Despite these improvements, however, IHE have arguably further to go to improve health. The US Department of Agriculture conducted a multistate research project to promote healthy eating and prevent weight gain across 15 IHE campuses (Horacek et al., 2012b). They found that no IHE received acceptable scores for bikeability, and nearly half scored below an acceptable level for pedestrian facilities, pedestrian/biker and motor vehicle conflict, cross-walk quality, and night-time safety. They also studied the on-campus dining establishments and found that there was limited support for healthy eating habits (Horacek et al., 2012a). Structural elements of the built environment also impact the wellbeing of students. Research shows that students' weight was higher the closer they lived to on-campus dining, but lower the closer they lived to a grocery store. Moreover, students' who lived closer to a gym exercised more often (Kapinos, Yakusheva, & Eisenberg, 2014). Living on campus, the presence of active travel infrastructure, and access to fitness facilities were associated with increased physical activity and

---

12. For more details on the WELL Program, please see: https://v2.wellcertified.com/wellv2/en/overview

health (Ajibade, 2011; Bird et al., 2018; Peachey & Baller, 2015; Shaffer, Bopp, Papalia, Sims, & Bopp, 2017; see also Chapter 9, this volume).

Green space and the ability for active transport have positive physical and mental health outcomes for students across IHE (Baur, 2020; Bird et al., 2018 Hipp, Gulwadi, Alves, & Sequeira, 2016; McFarland, Waliczek, & Zajicek, 2008). Generally, this research is correlational, showing that students who frequently engage with green spaces report higher quality of life, better mood, and lower overall perceived stress (e.g., Holt, Lomard, Best, Smiley-Smith, & Quinn, 2019). In a large-scale UK study, White et al. (2019) found that those who spent at least 120 minutes a week in nature had higher rates of subjective wellbeing. Rakow and Eells (2019) map out 10 steps to developing a 'Nature Rx' programme where students are prescribed more time in nature as a means of promoting mental health. Although they provide examples from IHE, they have yet to publish empirical validation for this approach. Other researchers have focused on what kinds of physical spaces help HE students alleviate stress. Girang, Chu, Endrinal, and Canoy (2020) identified three overarching spatial experiences of stress alleviation for students: (1) being away from stressful places, (2) being present but mentally away from a place, or (3) being engaged within communal spaces. Seitz, Reese, Strack, Frantz, and West (2014) provide similar results; however, they found students prefer green spaces with a human touch such as a bench, fountain, or swing and that co-occupying green spaces with a friend improved wellbeing.

PLANET-LEVEL STRATEGIES

There is growing recognition that wellbeing is possible only within healthy ecosystems (Helne & Hirvilammi, 2015). The UN Educational, Scientific and Cultural Organization (UNESCO) Earth Charter,[13] which has been endorsed by thousands of organisations internationally, states that 'The resilience of the community of life and the wellbeing of humanity depend upon preserving a healthy biosphere with all its ecological systems, a rich variety of plants and animals, fertile soils, pure waters, and clean air'. It recognises the interdependence of all beings and the planet and also calls on educators to provide students with the knowledge, values, and skills needed for a sustainable way of life. As early as the Stockholm Conference of 1972, the United Nations recognised the role of HE in fostering the wellbeing of the planet (Lozano ct al., 2015). Similarly, the 2020 UNESCO Global Education Meeting emphasized IHE's role in redesigning curriculum to support sustainable development.

IHE play an important role in the creation of a well planet, providing much of the research and scholarship on Earth's ecosystems, building students' worldview

---

13. For more details on UNESCO's view of the role of HE in the sustainability of Earth, please see   https://en.unesco.org/news/hesi-highlights-role-higher-education-building-better-world-current-and-future-generations

and personal identity as actors in our planet's future, and underscoring the ethical imperative of sustainable management of the environment (Dagiliute, Liobikiene, & Minelgaite, 2018). A review by Lozano et al. (2015) found that many IHE are engaged in sustainability efforts; however, IHE with an already high commitment to sustainability tended to be the ones that signed such charters and that those lagging in commitment were unlikely to sign. Cheeseman et al. (2019) reviewed 91 peer-reviewed articles on sustainability in HE and highlighted several barriers including apathy from leadership and the need for policies with more 'teeth' such as regional and/or international partnerships resulting in cost savings. Building Research Establishment Environmental Assessment Method (BREEAM), established in the UK in 1990, and Leadership in Energy and Environmental Design (LEED), established in the United States in 1998, are two internationally recognised sets of guidelines (Cole & Valdebenito, 2013). BREEAM and LEED standards, in addition to the WELL standards previously noted, help support the wellbeing of communities and their environments. LEED is one of the most common green certification systems, but little has been published on its use with IHE. In this vein, Kim, Son, and Son (2020) studied 62 Canadian IHE and found that, from an economic standpoint, LEED-certified buildings have a positive impact on school facilities. Yet they note that more research is needed to identify the impact over time on the health and wellbeing of people who live and work in LEED-certified buildings.

According to Kjell (2011), the literature on wellbeing on IHE campuses tends to be quite compartmentalised, with few researchers connecting sustainability to subjective and psychological wellbeing. There are, however, a number of high-profile movements for sustainability on IHE campuses. One example is the American College and University Presidents' Climate Commitment (ACUPCC).[14] In 2006, a group of 12 US institutions signed the agreement to take immediate action to reduce greenhouse gas, move toward carbon neutrality, and integrate sustainability into the curriculum. To date, nearly 700 US IHE have signed on to this effort. This impressive climate commitment is focused solely on climate neutrality and, as yet, devoid of any connection to other campus wellbeing initiatives. The commitment to carbon neutrality signals a recognition of the science around climate change and its eventual impact on people; however, research is needed to connect a well planet to a well people.

Both Kjell (2011) and Helne and Hirvilammi (2015) make compelling arguments that sustainability and wellbeing approaches have the common aim to increase wellbeing. They note that hedonic and eudemonic wellbeing are often decontextualised and investigated individualistically, as if humans are solely interested in individual gain rather than as a 'more holistically complex picture that, for example, also includes human preferences for altruism, cooperation and morality' (Kjell, 2011, p. 258). They note that someone's happiness can lead to another's unhappiness and suggest that wellbeing viewed comprehensively

14. For more information on the ACUPCC, please see https://sustainabledevelopment.un.org/partnership/?p=2375

takes into account this interdependence and how concerns for others portends a wider sense of belonging. Furthermore, they note that decontextualised person-focused conceptualisations of wellbeing suppose that persons could get along without nature and that nature is just a commodity, when it is quite clear that, without nature, persons will perish. Helne and Hirvilammi (2015) note that 'in order to be sustainable, the pursuit of wellbeing and the struggle to meet the needs of mankind should be grounded in a balanced and responsible human–nature relationship' (p. 170). The Okanagan Charter connects planetary well-being with the wellbeing of people, but a literature review conducted by these authors supports the authors' conclusion; that is, much of the wellbeing litera-ture is focused on the psychological wellbeing of persons. One notable excep-tion is a study that outlines how three IHE campuses in California have worked together to study the impact of a one-unit 'foodprint' seminar designed to teach students about food, environment, and society (Malan et al., 2020). These re-searchers found that students who took the class significantly increased their vegetable consumption and decreased their consumption of ruminant meat and sugar-sweetened beverages, positively impacting both their physical health and the environment.

SUMMARY

In his closing prayer at the 2015 International Conference on Health Promoting Universities and Colleges, Okanagan Nation Elder, Grouse Barnes, remarked, 'This land doesn't belong to us. This land belongs to seven generations down the road'. The wellbeing of our planet and its people is arguably the most important challenge of our time. IHE are embracing this challenge, working to support in-dividuals but also focus upstream in recognising the importance of sustainability, social justice, and inclusion and equity as keys to transforming the health of our current and future societies. Table 8.1 provides a summary of the type of research conducted across the person, place, and planet levels, while evidence-based well-being strategies at each level are summarised in Box 8.1.

For decades now, researchers have diligently worked downstream, developing interventions to help individuals improve coping, mental health, and hedonic and eudemonic wellbeing. Much is known about person-level strategies. For example, there is strong evidence to support individual psychological interven-tions, including MBIs, CBIs, ACT, and telehealth. There is also strong evidence to support using psychoeducation, recreation, relaxation, and suicide prevention to enhance subjective wellbeing. There is a growing body of evidence to support programmes for students entering IHE, student programmes to enhance social belonging/connectedness, and wellbeing courses.[15] These tend to be salutogenic,

15. Undoubtedly, this work will be challenged by current shifts in the pedological landscape caused by the COVID-19 pandemic and the rise in remote and online learning. These impacts will be an important area for future research and policy considerations.

Table 8.1 SUMMARY OF THE KINDS OF EVIDENCE SUPPORTING THE POSITIVE IMPACT OF PERSON-, PLACE-, OR PLANET-LEVEL WELLBEING STRATEGIES EMPLOYED IN INSTITUTIONS OF HIGHER EDUCATION (IHE)

Strategy	Meta-analyses	Systematic/ narrative reviews	Randomised-controlled trials	Correlational/ longitudinal studies	Qualitative studies	Policy-practice-based
Person-level strategies						
Support programs for students entering IHE				✓	✓	✓
Student programs to enhance social connectedness				✓		
Mindfulness-based interventions	✓	✓	✓	✓		✓
Cognitive-behavioural interventions	✓	✓	✓	✓		✓
Telehealth	✓	✓	✓	✓		
Psychoeducation	✓	✓	✓	✓		✓
Recreation	✓	✓		✓	✓	✓
Relaxation	✓	✓		✓		
Acceptance and Commitment-based interventions	✓	✓	✓	✓		
Suicide prevention	✓	✓	✓	✓		
Wellbeing courses		✓		✓	✓	✓

Place-level strategies

Health and counselling centres	✓	✓				
Pass/fail grading systems	✓		✓			
Curriculum design (e.g., small group learning)	✓		✓		✓	
Ethnic and racial diversity	✓	✓	✓		✓	
Sexual and gender diversity	✓	✓	✓		✓	
Support students with disabilities	✓	✓	✓		✓	
Reduce substance abuse and misuse	✓	✓	✓		✓	✓
Reduce smoking	✓		✓		✓	✓
Sexual violence prevention	✓	✓	✓		✓	
Built and natural environments	✓	✓	✓			

Planet-level strategies

		✓	✓		✓	

Box 8.1

EVIDENCE-BASED ACTIONS TO CONSIDER AS PART OF A COMPREHENSIVE
PROGRAM TO ENHANCE WELLBEING ON UNIVERSITY CAMPUSES

Person

- Culturally competent health centres to treat physical illness and provide preventative services and education, including offering health plans with covered services for gender minorities
- Recreation centres able to provide facilities for recreation and exercise as well as other strategies such as yoga and tai chi
- Culturally competent counselling centres able to provide psychotherapy including CBI, ACT, and telehealth, as well as, MBI, suicide prevention, and psychoeducation
- Wellbeing courses that include strategies on coping
- First-year transition support
- Interventions to increase social belongingness and connectedness

Place

- Classroom and curricular approaches such as pass/fail grading systems and learning communities
- Policies and practices to support nondiscrimination for minority students
- Centres to advocate for and support students from marginalized communities (including racial, ethic, sexual, and gender minorities as well as students with disabilities)
- Strategies to increase diversity on campus in students, staff, and faculty
- Diversity curriculum, training, and awareness for students, staff, and faculty
- Gender-inclusive housing options and bathrooms
- Options to identify by chosen name, pronouns, and gender identity
- Environmental management strategies to reduce substance abuse (including offering alcohol-free social, extracurricular, and public service options; creating a health-promoting normative environment; restricting the marketing and promotion of alcoholic beverages both on and off campus; limiting alcohol availability; increasing the enforcement of alcohol and drug laws and policies and campus–community partnerships that focus on awareness, education, and responsible beverage service
- Smoke-free campus policies
- Services to support survivors of sexual violence, such as paid staff dedicated to addressing sexual violence, a hotline or 24-hour contact, a safe walk or escort service, activities or events to raise students' awareness of sexual violence issues, support groups or counselling for survivors of

sexual violence, pamphlets or posters around campus, self-defence classes, and bystander intervention programs
- Healthy food climate and access to fitness facilities
- Means for active transport on campus (walkability and bikeability of campus)
- Green spaces, places to be in nature, to be with others yet have the feeling of being away, and natural places with a human touch, such as a bench or fountain
- Peer support initiatives

Planet

- WELL-, LEED-, or BREEAM-designed buildings
- Sustainability initiatives
- Commitments to reduce greenhouse gas and move toward carbon neutrality
- Curriculum on sustainability, including courses that show the interconnectedness of the people and the planet

Calls to Action from the Literature

- Examine the root causes of sexual violence on campus and focus programs to stop perpetrators from engaging in sexual violence
- Examine the systems and policies that 'other' minorities on campus and support the status quo, dismantle these systems of oppression, and create an inclusive environment
- Get upstream, using settings-based whole-university approaches
- Connect the wellbeing of people, places, and the planet, integrating sustainability and planetary wellbeing within the wellbeing of people

---

and many are delivered to groups of students rather than individually. This excellent work notwithstanding, we have underscored the need and opportunities for future research to extend and strengthen the evidence base for these strategies while also examining the systems and social and natural environments that impact the wellbeing of people.

Researchers and administrators have also recognised the importance of place-level strategies, particularly in the areas of substance abuse prevention, health promotion, and student health and counselling services. Increasingly, they are further considering the built and natural environment and its impact on the health and wellbeing of its community members. There is a growing policy commitment to the inclusion of minoritised students such as ethnic and racial minorities as well as sexual and gender minorities. More recently, however, authors are noting the need to shift policy and research away from additive programmes focussed, for example, on supports for the minoritised student or diversity programming for majority students and toward understanding and remedying institutional and structural imbalances of power that lead to oppression, discrimination, and exclusion (see, for example, Llamas, Nguyen, & Tran, 2019). Also key to this conversation is universally designing structures and environments so that minoritised students from a myriad of identities and intersectionalities can flourish. Similarly, the challenges of sexual violence on our campuses have spawned an emerging literature supporting self-defence programmes and bystander interventions designed to reduce the risk of sexual assault. But few interventions have focused directly on the perpetrators of sexual violence and how to change cultures to eliminate root causes of abuse of power and sexual violence. There is a growing body of evidence on support strategies for the success of students with disabilities and need for the application of universal design as an *a priori* approach in support of the mental health and wellbeing of all students with disabilities.

Finally, in alignment with the Okanagan Charter, IHE must take initiative to ensure the sustainability of our societies and our planet, emphasising the interdependence of the subjective wellbeing with the wellbeing of social groups and the physical environments that nurture them. Researchers, practitioners, and decision-makers are called to discover how systems must change to support the wellbeing of people, places, and the planet and to validate and provide evidence for the best ways to engage everyone across IHE, through a wide range of social and environmental changes, to take an explicit stance in favour of health, equity, social justice, and sustainability for all.

ACKNOWLEDGEMENTS

The authors are grateful for the research and editorial support provided by Tammy Fields, Alison Hassall, Aflaha Khan, and Erin Parker.

REFERENCES

Ajibade, P. (2011). Physical activity patterns by campus housing status among African American female college students. *Journal of Black Studies, 42*(4), 548–560.

American College Health Association. (2016). *Framework for a comprehensive health program*. American College Health Association.

Arria, A. M., Barrall, A. L., Allen, H. K., Bugbee, B. A., & Vincent, K. B. (2018). The academic opportunity costs of substance use and untreated mental health concerns among college students. In M. D. Cimini & E. M. Rivero (Eds.), *Promoting behavioral health and reducing risk among college students: A comprehensive approach* (pp. 3–22). Routledge.

Arria, A. M., Caldeira, K. M., Vincent, K. B., Winick, E. R., Baron, R. A., & O'Grady, K. E. (2013). Discontinuous college enrolment: Associations with substance use and mental health. *Psychiatric Services, 64*(2), 165–172.

Bamber, M. D., & Morpeth, E. (2019). Effects of mindfulness meditation on college student anxiety: A meta-analysis. *Mindfulness, 10*, 203–214.

Bamber, M. D., & Schneider, J. K. (2016). Mindfulness-based meditation to decrease stress and anxiety in college students: A narrative synthesis of the research. *Educational Research Review, 18*, 1–32.

Banyard, V. L., Moynihan, M. M., & Plante, E. G. (2007). Sexual violence prevention through bystander education: An experimental evaluation. *Journal of Community Psychology, 35*(4), 463–481.

Barnard-Brak, L., Lechtenberger, D., & Lan, W. Y. (2010). Accommodation strategies of college students with disabilities. *The Qualitative Report, 15*(2), 411–429.

Baur, J. (2020). Campus community gardens and student health: A case study of a campus garden and student well-being. *Journal of American College Health*, 1–8.

Beck, A. T. (1976). *Cognitive therapy and the emotional disorders*. International Universities Press.

Becker, C. M., Johnson, H., Vail-Smith, K., Maahs-Fladung, C., Tavasso, D., Elmore, B., & Blumell, C. (2008). Making health happen on campus: A review of a required general education health course. *Journal of General Education, 57*(2), 67–74.

Belch, H. A., Gebel, M., & Maas, G. M. (2001). Relationship between student recreation complex use, academic performance, and persistence of first-time freshmen. *Journal of Student Affairs Research and Practice, 38*(2), 254–268.

Bergen-Cico, D., Possemato, K., & Cheon, S. (2013). Examining the efficacy of a brief mindfulness-based stress reduction (Brief MBSR) program on psychological health. *Journal of American College Health, 61*(6), 348–360.

Bird, E. L., Ige, J. O., Pilkington, P., Pinto, A., Petrokofsky, C., & Burgess-Allen, J. (2018). Built and natural environment planning principles for promoting health: An umbrella review. *BMC Public Health, 18*, 930.

Bloodgood, R. A., Short, J. G., Jackson, J. M., & Martindale, J. R. (2009). A change to pass/fail grading in the first two years at one medical school results in improved psychological well-being. *Academic Medicine, 84*(5), 655–662.

Breedvelt, J. J. F., Amanvermez, Y., Harrer, M., Karyotaki, E., Gilbody, S., Bockting, C. L. H., . . . Ebert, D. D. (2019). The effects of meditation, yoga, and mindfulness on depression, anxiety, and stress in tertiary education students: A meta-analysis. *Frontiers in Psychiatry, 10*, 1–15.

Briner, R., & Dewberry, C. (2007). Staff wellbeing is key to school success: A research study into the links between staff wellbeing and school performance. https://www.teachertoolkit.co.uk/wp-content/uploads/2014/07/5902birkbeckwbperfsummaryfinal.pdf

Bughi, S. A., Sumcad, J., & Bughu, S. (2006). Effect of brief behavioral intervention program in managing stress in medical students from two Southern California universities. *Medical Education Online, 11*, 1–8.

Cares, A. C., Banyard, V. L., Moynihan, M. M., Williams, L. M., Potter, S. J., & Stapleton, J. G. (2015). Changing attitudes about being a bystander to violence: Translating an in-person sexual violence prevention program to a new campus. *Violence Against Women, 21*(2), 165–187.

Cheeseman, A., Sharon Alexandra Wright, T., Murray, J., & McKenzie, M. (2019). Taking stock of sustainability in higher education: A review of the policy literature. *Environmental Education Research, 25*(12), 1697–1712.

Christmas, W. A. (1995). The evolution of medical services for students at colleges and universities in the United States. *Journal of American College Health*, 43(6), 241–246.

Coker, A. L., Cook-Craig, P. G., Williams, C. M., Fisher, B. S., Clear, E. R., Garcia, L. S., & Hegge, L. M. (2011). Evaluation of green dot: An active bystander intervention to reduce sexual violence on college campuses. *Violence Against Women*, 17(6), 777–796.

Coker, A. L., Fisher, B. S., Bush, H. M., Swan, S. C., Williams, C. M., Clear, E. R., & Degue, S. (2015). Evaluation of the Green Dot Bystander Intervention to reduce interpersonal violence among college students across three campuses. *Violence Against Women*, 21(12), 1507–1527.

Cole, R., & Valdebenito, M. J. (2013). The importation of building environmental certification systems: International usages of BEEAM and LEED. *Building Research & Information*, 41(6), 662–676.

Conley, C. S., Durlak, J. A., & Dickson, D. A. (2013). An evaluative review of outcome research on universal mental health promotion and prevention programs for higher education students. *Journal of America College Health*, 61(5), 286–301.

Conley, C. S., Durlak, J. A., & Kirsch, A. C. (2015). A meta-analysis of universal mental health prevention programs for higher education students. *Prevention Science*, 16, 487–507.

Conley, C. S., Durlak, J. A., Shapiro, J. B., Kirsch, A. C., & Zahniser, E. (2016). A meta-analysis of the impact of universal and indicated preventive technology-delivered interventions for higher education students. *Prevention Science*, 17, 659–678.

Conley, C. S., Shapiro, J. B., Kirsch, A. C., & Durlak, J. A. (2017). A meta-analysis of indicated mental health prevention programs for at-risk higher education students. *Journal of Counselling Psychology*, 64(2), 121–140.

Cook, L., Rumrill, P. D., & Tankersley, M. (2009). Priorities and understanding faculty members regarding college students with disabilities. *International Journal of Teaching and Learning in Higher Education*, 21(1), 84–96.

Crawford, T. N., & Ridner, S. L. (2018). Differences in well-being between sexual minority and heterosexual college students. *Journal of LGBT Youth*, 15(3), 243–255.

Crilly, D., Schneider, S. C., & Zollo, M. (2008). Psychological antecedents to socially responsible behaviour. *European Management Review*, 5, 175–190.

Cuijpers, P., Cristea, I. A., Ebert, D. D., Koor, H. M., Auerbach, R. P., Bruffaerts, R., & Kessler, R. C. (2016). Psychological treatment of depression in college students: A meta-analysis. *Depression and Anxiety*, 33(5), 400–414.

Cvetkovski, S., Reavley, N. J., & Jorm, A. F. (2012). The prevalence and correlates of psychological distress in Australian tertiary students compared to their community peers. *Australian and New Zealand Journal of Psychiatry*, 46, 457–467.

Dagiliute, R., Liobikiene, G., & Minelgaite, A. (2018). Sustainability at universities: Students' perceptions from Green and Non-Green universities. *Journal of Cleaner Production*, 181, 473–482.

Davies, B. E., Morriss, R., & Glazebrook, C. (2014). Computer-delivered and web-based interventions to improve depression, anxiety, and psychological well-being of university students: A systematic review and meta-analysis. *Journal of Medical Internet Research*, 16(5), 1–24.

DeGue, S., Valle, L. A., Holt, M. K., Massetti, G. M., Matjasko, J. L., & Tharp, A. T. (2014). A systematic review of primary prevention strategies for sexual violence perpetration. *Aggression and Violent Behavior*, 19(4), 346–362.

Devine, K., & Hunter, K. H. (2016). PhD student emotional exhaustion: The role of supportive supervision and self-presentation behaviours. *Innovations in Education and
Teaching International, 54*(4) 1–10.

Dooris, M. (2001). The "Health Promoting University": A critical exploration of theory
and practice. *Health Education, 101*(2), 51–60.

Dooris, M., & Doherty, S. (2010a). Healthy universities: Current activity and future
directions—findings and reflections from a national-level qualitative research study.
Global Health Promotion, 17, 6–16.

Dooris, M., & Doherty, S. (2010b). Healthy universities – time for action: A qualitative
research study exploring the potential for a national programme. *Health Promotion
International, 25*(1), 94–106.

Dooris, M., Doherty, S., Cawood, J., & Powell, S. (2012). The healthy universities approach: Adding value to the higher education sector. In A. Scriven & M. Hodgins
(Eds.), *Health promotion settings: Principles and practice* (pp. 153–169). Sage.

Duckworth, K., & Cara, O. (2012). The relationship between adult learning and wellbeing: Evidence from the 1958 National Child Development Study. UK Department
for Business, Innovation & Skills. https://assets.publishing.service.gov.uk/governm
ent/uploads/system/uploads/attachment_data/file/34669/12-1241-relationship-
adult-learning-and-wellbeing-evidence-1958.pdf

Durlak, C. M., Rose, E., & Bursuck, W. D. (1994). Preparing high school students with
learning disabilities for the transition to postsecondary education: Teaching the
skills of self-determination. *Journal of Learning Disabilities, 27*(1), 51–59.

Ecker, J., Rae, J., & Bassi, A. (2015). Showing your pride: A national survey of queer
student centres in Canadian colleges and universities. *Higher Education, 70*(5), 881–
898. https://doi.org/10.1007/s10734-015-9874-x

Eddy, J. P., Spaulding, D. J., & Murphy, S. (1996). Privatization of higher education services: Propositional pros and cons. *Education, 116*(4), 578.

Eisenberg, D., Gollust, S. E., Golberstein, E., & Hefner, J. L. (2007). Prevalence and correlates of depression, anxiety, and suicidality among university students. *Journal of
Orthopsychiatry, 77*(4), 534–542.

Eisenberg, D., & Lipson, S. (2016). *Data from the Healthy Minds Network: The economic
case for student health services.* University of Michigan.

Eisenberg, M., Lust, K., Hannan, P., & Porta, C. (2016). Campus sexual violence resources and emotional health of college women who have experienced sexual assault. *Violence and Victims, 31*(2), 274–284.

Evans, T. M., Bira, L., Gastelum, J. B., Weiss, L. T., & Vanderford, N. L. (2018). Evidence
for a mental health crisis in graduate education. *Nature Biotechnology, 36*, 282–284.

Farrer, L., Gulliver, A., Chan, J., Batterham, P. J., Reynolds, J., Calear, A., Tait, R., Bennett,
K., & Griffiths, K. M. (2013). Technology-based interventions for mental health in tertiary students: A systematic review. *Journal of Medical Internet Research, 15*(5), 1–14.

Ferfolja, T., Asquith, N., Hanckel, B., & Brady, B. (2020). In/ visibility on campus? Gender
and sexuality diversity in tertiary institutions. *Higher Education, 80*(5), 933–947.

Fisher, S., & Hood, B. (1987). The stress of the transition to university: A longitudinal
study of psychological disturbance, absent mindedness and vulnerability to home-
sickness. *British Journal of Psychology, 78*, 425–441.

Foster, J., Allen, W., Oprescu, F., & McAllister, M. (2014). Mytern: An innovative approach to increase students' achievement, sense of wellbeing and levels of resilience.
Journal of the Australian and New Zealand Student Services Association, 43, 31–40.

Garcia G. M., Mapaye, J. C., Lopez, V. D., Roxbury, E., & Tabatabai-Yazdi, N. (2020). Impact of campus tobacco-free policy on tobacco and electronic nicotine delivery systems initiation and cessation among students, faculty, and staff. *Journal of Public Health Issues and Practices*, 4(1), 159–165.

Garvey, J. C., & Dolan, C. V. (2021). Queer and trans college student success. *Higher Education: Handbook of Theory and Research*, 161–215.

Gidycz, C. A., Orchowski, L. M., Probst, D. R., Edwards, K. M., Murphy, M., & Tansill, E. (2015). Concurrent administration of sexual assault prevention and risk reduction programming: Outcomes for women. *Violence Against Women*, 21(6), 780–800.

Girang, B. C., Chu, D. P., Endrinal, M. I., & Canoy, N. (2020). Spatializing psychological well-being: A photovoice approach on the experience of stress alleviation among university students. *Qualitative Research in Psychology*, 1–26.

Goodwin, L., Ben-Zion, I., Fear, N. T., Hotopf, M., Stansfeld, S. A., & Wessely, S. (2013). Are reports of psychological stress higher in occupational studies? A systematic review across occupational and population-based studies. *PLoS ONE*, 8(11), e78693.

Grant, L., & Kinman, G. (2014). Emotional resilience in the helping professional and how it can be enhanced. *Health and Social Care Education*, 3(1), 23–34.

Greathouse, M., BrckaLorenz, A., Hoban, M., Huesman, R., Rankin, S., & Stolzenberg, E. B. (2018). A meta-analysis of queer-spectrum and trans-spectrum student experiences at US research universities. *Evaluating Campus Climate at US Research Universities*, 49–75. https://doi.org/10.1007/978-3-319-94836-2_3

Gu, J., Strauss, C., Bond, R., & Cavanagh, K. (2015). How do mindfulness-based cognitive therapy and mindfulness-based stress reduction improve mental health and well-being? A systematic review and meta-analysis of mediation studies. *Clinical Psychology Review*, 37, 1–12.

Hafford-Letchfield, T., Pezzella, A., Cole, L., & Manning, R. (2017). Transgender students in post-compulsory education: A systematic review. *International Journal of Educational Research*, 86, 1–12.

Halladay, J. E., Dawdy, J. L., McNamara, I. F., Chen, A. J., Vitoroulis, I., McInnes, N., & Munn, C. (2019). Mindfulness for the mental health and well-being of postsecondary students: A systematic review and meta-analysis. *Mindfulness*, 10, 397–414.

Harrer, M., Adam, S. H., Baumeister, H., Cuijpers, P., Karyotaki, E., Auerbach, R. P., . . . Ebert, D. D. (2018). Internet interventions for mental health in university students: A systematic review and meta-analysis. *International Journal of Methods in Psychiatry Research*, 28, 1–18.

Harrod, C. S., Goss, C. W., Stallones, L., & DiGuiseppi, C. (2014). Interventions for primary prevention of suicide in university and other post-secondary educational settings. *Cochrane Database of Systematic Reviews*, 10, 1–88.

Hassed, C., Lisle, S., Sullivan, G., & Pier, C. (2009). Enhancing the health of medical student: Outcomes of an integrated mindfulness and lifestyle program. *Advances in Health Science Education*, 14, 387–398.

Hatzenbuehler, M. L. (2014). Structural stigma and the health of lesbian, gay, and bisexual populations. *Current Directions in Psychological Science*, 23(2), 127–132.

Hatzenbuehler, M. L., & Pachankis, J. E. (2016). Stigma and minority stress as social determinants of health among lesbian, gay, bisexual, and transgender youth: Research evidence and clinical implications. *Pediatric Clinics of North America*, 63(6), 985–997.

Hayes, S. C. (2004). Acceptance and commitment therapy, relational frame theory, and the third wave of behavioural and cognitive therapies. *Behavior Therapy*, *35*(4), 639–665.

Helne, T., & Hirvilammi, T. (2015). Wellbeing and sustainability: A relational approach. *Sustainable Development*, *23*, 167–175.

Herbert, J. T., Coduti, W. A., & Fleming, A. (2020). University policies, resources and staff practices: Impact on college students with disabilities. *Journal of Rehabilitation*, *86*(4), 31–41.

Hipp, J. A., Gulwadi, G. B., Alves, S., & Sequeira, S. (2016). The relationship between perceived greenness and perceived restorativeness of university campuses and student-reported quality of life. *Environment and Behavior*, *48*(10), 1292–1308.

Hofmann, S. G., Asnaani, A., Vonk, I. J. J., Sawyer, A. T., & Fang, A. (2012). The efficacy of cognitive behavioral therapy: A review of meta-analyses. *Cognitive Therapy and Research*, *36*(5), 427–440.

Holt, E. W., Lomard, Q. K., Best, N., Smiley-Smith, S., & Quinn, J. E. (2019). Active and passive use of green space, health, and well-being amongst university students. *International Journal of Environmental Research and Public Health*, *6*(3), 424.

Horacek, T., Erdman, M., Byrd-Bredbenner, C., Carey, G., Colby, S., Greene, G., . . . White, A. (2012a). Assessment of the dining environment on and near the campuses of fifteen post-secondary institutions. *Public Health Nutrition*, 16, 1–11.

Horacek, T. M., White, A. A., Greene, G. W., Reznar, M. M., Quick, V. M., Morrell, J. S., . . . Byrd-Bredbenner, C. (2012b). Sneakers and spokes: An assessment of the walkability and bikeability of U.S. postsecondary institutions. *Journal of Environmental Health*, *74*(7), 8–15.

Houghton, F., Keane, N., Murphy, N., Houghton, S., & Dunne, C. (2010). Tertiary level students and the mental health index (MHI-5) in Ireland. *Irish Journal of Applied Social Studies*, *10*(1), Article 7, 40–48.

Howell, A. J., & Passmore, H. (2018). Acceptance and Commitment Training (ACT) as a positive psychological intervention: A systematic review and initial meta-analysis regarding ACT's role in well-being promotion among students. *Journal of Happiness*, *20*(6), 1995–2010.

Huang, J., Nigatu, Y. T., Smail-Crevier, R., Zhang, X., & Wang, J. (2018). Interventions for common mental health problems among university and college students: A systematic review and meta-analysis of randomized controlled trials. *Journal of Psychiatric Research*, *107*, 1–10.

Hughes, G., & Smail, O. (2015). Which aspects of university life are most and least helpful in the transition to HE? A qualitative snapshot of student perceptions. *Journal of Further and Higher Education*, *39*(4), 466–480.

Huhtala, H., & Parzefall, M. (2007). A review of employee well-being and innovativeness: An opportunity for mutual benefit. *Creativity and Innovation Management*, *16*, 299–306.

International WELL Building Institute. (2022). *WELL Building Standard™ version 2 (WELL v2™)*. https://www.wellcertified.com/

Iverson, S. V. (2012). Constructing outsiders: The discursive framing of access in university diversity policies. *The Review of Higher Education*, *35*(2), 149–177.

Jennison, K. M. (2004). The short-term effects and unintended long-term consequences of binge drinking in college: A 10-year follow-up study. *American Journal of Drug and Alcohol Abuse*, *30*(3), 659–684.

Jones, M. C., & Johnston, D. W. (2006). Is the introduction of a student-centred, problem-based curriculum associated with improvements in student nurse well-being and performance? An observational study of effect. *International Journal of Nursing Studies, 43*, 941–952.

Kang, H. K., Rhodes, C., Rivers, E., Thorton, C. P., & Rodney, T. (2021). Prevalence of mental health disorders among undergraduate university students in the United States. *Journal Psychosocial Nursing, 59*(2), 17–24.

Kapinos, K. A., Yakusheva, O., & Eisenberg, D. (2014). Obesogenic environmental influences on young adults: Evidence from college dormitory assignments. *Economics and Human Biology, 12*, 98–109.

Khan, A. R., & Rieger, E. (2021). *Eliciting student perspectives to inform the design of positive psychology courses: A qualitative study* [Manuscript submitted for publication]. Research School of Psychology, Australian National University.

Kim, J.-M., Son, K., & Son, S. (2020). Green benefits on educational buildings according to the LEED Certification. *International Journal of Strategic Property Management, 24*(2), 83–89.

Kjell, O. N. E. (2011). Sustainable well-being: A potential synergy between sustainability and well-being research. *Review of General Psychology, 14*(3), 255–266.

Kraft, D. P. (2011). One hundred years of college mental health. *Journal of American College Health, 59*(6), 477–481.

Lambert, L., Passmore, H. A., & Joshanloo, M. (2019). A positive psychology intervention program in a culturally-diverse university: Boosting happiness and reducing fear. *Journal of Happiness Studies, 20*, 1141–1162.

Lamothe, D., Currie, F., Alisat, S., Sullivan, T., Pratt, M., Pancer, S. M., & Hunsberger, B. (1995). Impact of social support intervention on the transition to university. *Canadian Journal of Community Mental Health, 14*(2), 167–180.

Lechner, W. V., Meier, E., Miller, M. B., Wiener, J. L., & Fils-Aime, Y. (2012). Changes in smoking prevalence, attitudes, and beliefs over 4 years following a campus-wide anti-tobacco intervention. *Journal of American College Health, 60*(7), 505–511.

Lee, J., & Graham, A. V. (2001). Students' perception of medical school stress and their evaluation of a wellness elective. *Medical Education, 35*(7), 652–659.

Levecque K., Anseel, F., De Beuckelaer, A., Van der Heyden, J., & Gisle, L. (2017). Work organization and mental health problems in PhD students. *Research Policy, 46*, 868–879.

Linder, C., Grimes, N., Williams, B. M., Lacy, M. C., & Parker, B. (2020). What do we know about campus sexual violence? A content analysis of 10 years of research. *The Review of Higher Education, 43*(4), 1017–1040.

Lipson, S. K. (2014). A comprehensive review of mental health gatekeeper-trainings for adolescents and young adults. *International Journal of Adolescent Medicine and Health, 26*(3), 309–320.

Litwiller, F., White, C., Hamilton-Hinch, B., & Gilbert, R. (2018). The impacts of recreation programs on the mental health of postsecondary students in North America: An integrative review. *Leisure Sciences*, 1–25.

Llamas, J. D., Nguyen, K., & Tran, A. G. T. T. (2019). The case for greater faculty diversity: Examining the educational impacts of student-faculty racial/ethnic match. *Race Ethnicity and Education, 24*(3), 375–391.

Lovitts, B. E. (2001). *Leaving the ivory tower: The causes and consequences of departure from doctoral study*. Rowman and Littlefield.

Lozano, R., Ceulemans, K., Alonso-Almeida, M., Huisingh, D., Lozano, F. J., Waas, T., . . . Hugé, J. (2015). A review of commitment and implementation of sustainable of development in higher education results from a worldwide survey. *Journal of Cleaner Production, 108*(A), 1–18.

Lupton, J. R., & Townsend, J. L. (2015). A systematic review and meta-analysis of the acceptability and effectiveness of university smoke-free policies. *Journal of American College Health, 63*(4), 238–247.

Malan, H., Challamel, G. A., Silverstein, D., Hoffs, C., Spang, E., Pace, S. A., . . . Jay, J. (2020). Impact of a scalable, multi-campus "foodprint" seminar on college students' dietary intake and dietary carbon footprint. *Nutrients, 12*(9), 2890.

Manejwala, R., & Abu-Ras, W. (2019). Microaggressions on the university campus and the undergraduate experiences of Muslim South Asian Women. *Journal of Muslim Mental Health, 13*(1), 21–39.

Manning, P., Pring, L., & Glider, P. (2014). Wellness for all: Improving campus climate for LGBTQA students as prevention. *Journal of College and Character, 15*(2), 119–124.

Marshak, L., Van Wieren, T., Ferrell, D. R., Swiss, L., & Dugan, C. (2010). Exploring barriers to college student use of disability services and accommodations. *Journal of Postsecondary Education and Disability, 22*(3), 151–165.

McFarland, A. L., Waliczek, T. M., & Zajicek, J. M. (2008). The relationship between student use of campus green spaces and perceptions of quality of life. *HortTechnology, 18*(2), 232–238.

Miller, E. J., & Chung, H. (2009). A literature review of studies of depression and treatment outcomes among US college students since 1990. *Psychiatric Services, 60*(9), 1257–1260.

Miller, R. A. (2014). An overview of campus climate: Dimensions of diversity in higher education. *Texas Education Review, 2*(2), 184–190.

Moriña, A., & Biagiotti, G. (2021). Academic success factors in university students with disabilities: A systematic review. *European Journal of Special Needs Education*, 1–18.

Morris, T. R., & Lent, R. W. (2019). Heterosexist harassment and social cognitive variables as predictors of sexual minority college students' academic satisfaction and persistence intentions. *Journal of Counseling Psychology, 66*(3), 308–316.

Morrish, L. (2019). *Pressure vessels: The epidemic of poor mental health among higher education staff*. Higher Education Policy Institute.

Moynihan, M. M., Banyard, V. L., Arnold, J. S., Eckstein, R. P., & Stapleton, J. G. (2011). Engaging intercollegiate athletes in preventing and intervening in sexual and intimate partner violence. *Journal of American College Health, 59*(3), 197–204.

National Intramural-Recreational Sports Association. (2004). *The value of recreational sports in higher education: Impact on student enrolment, success, and buying power*. Human Kinetics.

O'Driscoll, M., Byrne, S., McGillicuddy, A., Lambert, S., & Sahm, L. J. (2017). The effects of mindfulness-based interventions for health and social care undergraduate students: A systematic review of the literature. *Psychology, Health, & Medicine, 22*(7), 851–865.

Ohly, S., & Bledow, R. (2015). Well-being and performance in creative work. In M. Veldhoven and R. Peccei (Eds.), *Well-being and performance at work: The role of context* (pp. 75–92). Psychology Press.

Oliver, M. D., Datta, S., & Baldwin, D. R. (2019). Wellness among African-American and Caucasian students attending a predominantly white institution. *Journal of Health Psychology, 24*(12), 1637–1645.

Oppenheimer, B. T. (1984). Short-term small group intervention for college freshmen. *Journal of Counselling Psychology, 31*, 45–53.

Padilla, M. A., & Thompson, J. N. (2016). Burning out faculty at doctoral research universities. *Stress & Health, 32*(5), 551–558.

Pascarella, E. T., & Terenzini, P. T. (2005). *How college affects students. A third decade of research.* Jossey-Bass.

Patton, L. D., Sánchez, B., Mac, J., & Stewart, D. L. (2019). An inconvenient truth about "progress": An analysis of the promises and perils of research on campus diversity initiatives. *Review of Higher Education, 42*(5), 173–198.

Peachey, A. A., & Baller, S. L. (2015). Perceived built environment characteristics of on-campus and off-campus neighborhoods associated with physical activity of college students. *Journal of American College Health, 63*(5), 337–342.

Pereira, S., Early, N., Outar, L., Dimitrova, M., Walker, L., & Dzikiti, C (2020). *University Student Mental Health Survey 2020.* https://assets.website-files.com/602d05d13 b303dec233e5ce3/60305923a557c3641f1a7808_Mental%20Health%20Report%202 019%20(2020).pdf

Pitcher, E., Camacho, T., Renn, K., & Woodford, M. R. (2018). Affirming policies, programs and supportive services: Using an organizational perspective to understand SGD college student success. *Journal of Diversity in Higher Education, 11*(2), 117–132.

Ragheb, M. G., & McKinney, J. (1993). Campus recreation and perceived academic stress. *Journal of College Student Development, 34*(1), 5–10.

Rakow, D. A., & Eells, G. T. (2019). *Nature Rx: Improving college-student mental health.* Cornell University Press.

Rankin, S., & Reason, R. (2008). Transformational tapestry model: A comprehensive approach to transforming campus climate. *Journal of Diversity in Higher Education, 1*(4), 262–274.

Reavley, N., & Jorm, A. F. (2010). Prevention and early intervention to improve mental health in higher education students: A review. *Early Intervention in Psychiatry, 4*, 132–142.

Reed, D. A., Shanafelt, T. D., Satele, D. W., Power, D. V., Eacker, A., Harper, W., . . . Dyrbye, I. M. (2011). Relationship of pass/fail grading and curriculum structure with well-being among preclinical medical students: A multi-institutional study. *Academic Medicine, 86*(11), 1367–1373.

Regehr, C., Glancy, D., & Pitts, A. (2013). Interventions to reduce stress in university students: A review and meta-analysis. *Journal of Affective Disorders, 148*, 1–11.

Rohe, D. E., Barrier, P. A., Clark, M. M., Cook, D. A., Vickers, K. S., & Decker, P. A. (2006). The benefits of pass-fail grading on stress, mood, and group cohesion in medical students. *Mayo Clinic Proceedings, 81*(11), 1443–1448.

Salazar, L. F., Vivolo-Kantor, A., Hardin, J., & Berkowitz, A. (2014). A web-based sexual violence bystander intervention for male college students: Randomized controlled trial. *Journal of Medical Internet Research, 16*(9).

Schenk Martin, R., Sasso, T., & González-Morales, M. G. (2020). SGD students in higher education: An evaluation of website data and accessible, ongoing resources in Ontario universities. *Psychology & Sexuality, 11*(1-2), 75–87.

Schreffler, J., Vasquez III, E., Chini, J., & James, W. (2019). Universal design for learning in postsecondary STEM education for students with disabilities: A systematic literature review. *International Journal of STEM Education*, 6(8).

Seitz, C. M., Reese, R. F., Strack, R. W., Frantz, S., & West, B. (2014). Identifying and improving green spaces on a college campus: A photovoice study. *Ecopsychology*, 6(2), 98–108.

Senn, C. Y., Eliasziw, M., Hobden, K. L., Barata, P. C., Radtke, H. L., Thurston, W. E., & Newby-Clark, I. R. (2021). Testing a model of how a sexual assault resistance education program for women reduces sexual assaults. *Psychology of Women Quarterly*, 45(1), 20–36.

Shaffer, K., Bopp, M., Papalia, Z., Sims, D., & Bopp, C. M. (2017). The relationship of living environment with behavioral and fitness outcomes by sex: An exploratory study in college-aged students. *International Journal of Exercise Science*, 10(3), 330–339.

Shapiro, S. L., Brown, K. W., & Astin, J. A. (2011). Toward the integration of meditation into higher education: A review of research. *Teachers College Record*, 11(3), 493–528.

Sharp, J., & Theiler, S. (2018). A review of psychological distress among university students: Pervasiveness, implications and potential points of intervention. *International Journal for the Advancement of Counselling*, 40(3), 193–212.

Shaw, C., & Ward, L. (2014). Dark thoughts: Why mental illness is on the rise in academia. *The Guardian*. https://www.theguardian.com/higher-education-network/2014/mar/06/mental-health-academics-growing-problem-pressure-university

Shek, D. T. (2012). Development of a positive youth development subject in a university context in Hong Kong. *International Journal of Disability and Human Development*, 11(3), 173–179.

Shek, D. T. (2013). Promotion of holistic development in university students: A credit-bearing course on leadership and intrapersonal development. *Best Practices in Mental Health*, 9(1), 48–61.

Slavin, S. J., Schindler, D. L, & Chibnall, J. T. (2014). Medical student mental health 3.0: Improving student wellness through curricular changes. *Academic Medicine*, 89, 573–577.

Smith, W. (2009). Campus wide climate: Implications for African American students. In L. C. Tillman (Ed.), *The SAGE handbook of African American education* (pp. 297–309). SAGE Publications.

Stallman, H. M. (2010). Psychological distress in university students: A comparison with general population data. *Australian Psychologist*, 45(4), 249–257.

Stein, K. F. (2013). DSS and accommodations in higher education. Perceptions of students with psychological disabilities. *Journal of Postsecondary Education and Disability*, 26(2), 145–161.

Tang, S., & Ferguson, A. (2014). The possibility of wellbeing: Preliminary results from surveys of Australian professional legal education students. *QUT Law Review*, 14(1), 27–51.

Tett, L., Cree, V. E., & Christie, H. (2017). From further to higher education: Transition as an on-going process. *Higher Education*, 73, 389–406.

Tsouros, A., Dowding, G., Thompson, J., & Dooris, M. (1998). *Health promoting universities: Concept, experience and framework for action*. WHO Regional office for Europe. https://www.euro.who.int/__data/assets/pdf_file/0012/101640/E60163.pdf

Tucker, P., Jeon-Slaughter, H., Sener, U., Arvidson, M., & Khalafian, A. (2015). Do medical student stress, health, or quality of life foretell step 1 scores? A comparison of students in traditional and revised preclinical curricula. *Teaching and Learning in Medicine, 27*(1), 63–70.

Turner J. C., & Keller, A. (2015). College health surveillance network: Epidemiology and health care utilization of college students at US 4-year universities. *Journal of American College Health, 63*(8), 530–538.

van Herpen, S. G. A., Meeuwisse, M., Adriaan, W. H., & Severiens, S. E. (2020). A head start in higher education: The effect of transition intervention on interaction, sense of belonging, and academic performance. *Studies in Higher Education, 45*(4), 862–877.

Vogel, S. A., Leyser, Y., Burgstahler, S., Sligar, S. R., & Zecker, S. G. (2006). Faculty knowledge and practices regrading students with disabilities in three contrasting institutions of higher education. *Journal of Postsecondary Education and Disability, 18*(2), 109–123.

Walton, G. M., & Cohen, G. L. (2011). A brief social-belonging intervention improves academic and health outcomes of minority students. *Science, 331*, 1447–1451.

Wasserman, D., & Wasserman, C. (2010). *The Oxford textbook of suicidology and suicide prevention: A global perspective.* Oxford University Press.

Watts, J., & Robertson, N. (2011). Burnout in university teaching staff: A systematic literature review. *Educational Research, 53*(1), 33–50.

Welpe, I., Wollersheim, J., Ringelhan, S., & Osterloh, M. (2015). *Incentives and performance: Governance or research organizations.* Springer International.

White, M. P., Alcock, I., Grellier, J., Wheller, B. W., Hartig, T., Warber, S. L., . . . Fleming, L. E. (2019). Spending at least 120 minutes a week in nature is associated with good health and wellbeing. *Scientific Reports, 9*, 7730.

Widseth, J. C., Webb, R. E., & John, K. B. (1997). The question of outsourcing. *Journal of College Student Psychotherapy, 11*, 3–22.

Wilcox, P., Winn, S., & Fyvie-Gauld, M. (2005). 'It was nothing to do with the university, it was just the people': The role of social support in the first-year experience of higher education. *Studies in Higher Education, 30*(6), 707–722.

Winzer, R., Lindberg, L., Gulbrandsson, K., & Sidorchuk, A. (2018). Effects of mental health interventions for students in higher education are sustainable over time: A systematic review and meta-analysis of randomized controlled trials. *PeerJ, 6*, 1–27.

Woodford, M. R., Joslin, J., Renn, K., Pasque, P. A., Ting, M, Ortega, N., & Burkhardt, J. C. (2016). *Transforming understandings of diversity in higher education: Demography, democracy and discourse.* Stylus.

Woodford, M. R., Kulick, A., Garvey, J. C., Sinco, B. R., & Hong, J. S. (2018). LGBTQ policies and resources on campus and the experiences and psychological well-being of sexual minority college students: Advancing research on structural inclusion. *Psychology of Sexual Orientation and Gender Diversity, 5*(4), 445–456.

Worsley, J., Pennington, A., & Corcoran, R. (2020). *What interventions improve college and university students' mental health and wellbeing? A review of the review-level evidence.* Report for What Works Centre for Wellbeing. https://whatworkswellbeing.org/wp-content/uploads/2020/03/Student-mental-health-full-review.pdf

Wyatt, T., & Oswalt, S. B. (2013). Comparing mental health issues among undergraduate and graduate students. *American Journal of Health Education, 44*(2), 96–207.

AND Physical Health and Wellbeing . . .

9

Integrating Across Diverse Perspectives to Improve Health and Wellbeing

Obesity as an Illustrative Case

PAUL DUGDALE, ELIZABETH RIEGER, AND ROBERT DYBALL ■

INTRODUCTION

Obesity is defined as abnormal or excessive body fat accumulation that presents a risk to health (World Health Organization [WHO], 2020). Only recognised as a disease by the American Medical Association in 2013 (American Medical Association, 2013), it has proven to be complex, challenging, and controversial in its conceptualisation, aetiology, and management. The scale of the obesity pandemic and its detrimental effects on individual and population wellbeing have resulted in obesity becoming a major target for health action over the past 50 years. This has been characterised by intensive efforts on the part of researchers, health professionals, public health campaigns, and higher-weight individuals alike. What is seemingly surprising is that these attempts to reduce obesity levels have generally failed, with the prevalence of obesity and its degree of severity continuing to increase over this period.

But perhaps it should not be surprising that the preventive and therapeutic approaches developed and applied have been insufficient and unsuccessful, given that we lack a scientific and political perspective and practice that integrates effectively across the human biological, psychological, social, and environmental domains. This chapter is a step toward addressing this lack and attempts to generate, or at least imagine, insights from an integrated perspective. Because the drivers and effects of obesity intersect with biophysical and psychosocial domains across scales from the individual through households and neighbourhoods to the national and global, policy and governance responses need to blend a wide range of knowledge domains to reflect this complexity. Although we focus on obesity, our approach is consistent with broader calls for a more thoroughgoing integrative approach to health (e.g., the syndemics model proposed by Tsai, Mendenhall, Trostle, & Kawachi, 2017).

Our chapter starts by sampling some of the key adverse consequences of obesity at the biological, psychological, and societal levels. Since an awareness of such costs can degenerate into a blaming response toward higher-weight people, we then address the pernicious issue of weight stigma and highlight its erroneous suppositions by drawing attention to the complex (and still inadequately understood) drivers of obesity that operate at the environmental level in interaction with individual vulnerability. The discussion then moves on to examine obesity intervention approaches across the various psychological, medical, and societal scales. We conclude by offering an integrated model for understanding obesity that can inform coordinated policy and action.

THE CONSEQUENCES OF OBESITY

Globally, obesity rates have tripled since 1975 (WHO, 2020) and have increased in every country studied over this period (NCD Risk Factor Collaboration, 2017) (see Figure 9.1). Currently, an estimated 38% of adults in the United States

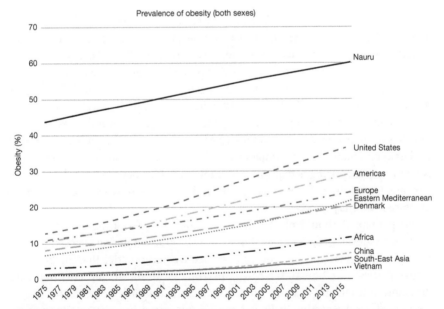

Figure 9.1 The percentage of adults classified in the obese weight range according to the World Health Organization across various countries from 1975 to 2016. Data available at https://ourworldindata.org/obesity

are within the obese weight range (Organisation for Economic Co-operation and Development, 2017).

Such prevalence rates are of significant concern given evidence that obesity (even 'metabolically healthy obesity') substantially increases the risk of developing a wide range of diseases such as type 2 diabetes, cardiovascular diseases, osteoarthritis, and certain cancers (Blüher, 2019; Must et al., 1999; Zhou et al., 2021). More recently, in the convergence between the obesity epidemic and COVID-19 pandemic, obesity was identified in a meta-analysis of 75 studies (Popkin et al., 2020) as a strong risk factor for greater rates of infection, hospitalisation, and mortality from COVID-19. Indeed, one study found that differences in the rates of obesity were the strongest predictor of inter-country variation in COVID-19 death rates (Gardiner, Oben, & Sutcliffe, 2021). The consequences of COVID-19 have in turn been found to result in weight gain among children, adolescents, and adults (Lin, Vittinghoff, Olgin, Pletcher, & Marcus, 2021; Woolford et al., 2021).

In terms of its impact on the global burden of disease, high body weight has been ranked sixth among 67 risk factors, and first (e.g., Australasia) or second (e.g., high-income North America) in many regions (Lim et al., 2012). The increased risk of premature death with high weight was established in a methodologically robust meta-analytic review of 239 studies across four continents (Global BMI Mortality Collaboration, 2016). It was found that mortality risk relative to those in the normal weight range was already higher for people in the overweight range and became greater as body weight increased further.

Obesity confers a risk to health and mortality over and above the negative impacts of poor diet and low levels of physical activity (Valenzuela et al., 2021; Veronese, Li, Manson, Willett, Fontana, & Hu, 2016). For example, a study by Valenzuela et al. (2021) found that people in the obese weight range who were physically active were approximately twice as likely to have elevated cholesterol, five times more likely to have elevated blood pressure, and four times more likely to have type 2 diabetes than inactive people in the normal weight range.

That making changes in diet and physical activity are not sufficient to reduce the greater health risk associated with obesity partly stems from the fact that excess adipose tissue is not benign. Specifically, while adipose tissue was traditionally conceptualised as a passive depository for triglycerides and a store for excess free fatty acids to be released as needed, it is now known to be an active, proinflammatory organ (Lau, Dhillon, Yan, Szmitko, & Verma, 2005). The increased adipose tissue of obesity (especially abdominal obesity) secretes elevated levels of numerous bioactive molecules (e.g., interleukin-6 [IL-6] and tumour necrosis factor-α [TNF-α]) and can impede the secretion of others (e.g., adiponectin), thereby having a negative impact on health through multiple pathways (Van Gaal, Mertens, & De Block, 2006).

Given its adverse health consequences, it is not surprising that obesity imposes a financial burden on affected individuals and society more broadly. For example, in the United States, obesity has been found to double the direct medical costs of adults compared to those in the normal weight range, with these costs comprising more than a twofold increase over the 15-year period investigated (Cawley et al., 2021).

Higher-weight individuals are also vulnerable to various forms of psychological distress. Obesity is associated with poorer quality of life, with people reporting negative impacts of obesity on their occupational, physical, and societal (e.g., adverse reactions from others due to one's weight) functioning (Rieger, Wilfley, Stein, Marino, & Crow, 2005). In addition, a meta-analysis of 17 studies found consistent support for higher body dissatisfaction among people (especially women) in the obese versus normal weight ranges (Weinberger, Kersting, Riedel-Heller, & Luck-Sikorski, 2016). Body dissatisfaction among higher-weight people has, in turn, been found to predict poorer health-related variables such as less readiness for health behaviour change, poorer eating habits, and lower physical fitness (Simões et al., 2021), which likely result in further obesity, thus comprising a negative feedback loop. Obesity is also related to depression, with a meta-analysis of longitudinal studies finding that people classified as overweight were 1.27 times and people classified as obese were 1.55 times more likely to develop depression than their normal-weight counterparts (Luppino et al., 2010).

Unfortunately, acknowledging the diverse and serious consequences of obesity can (and often does) devolve into a blaming response toward higher-weight people in political and popular discourse (Ata & Thompson, 2010). Such responses are harmful and erroneous given (1) the pernicious impacts of weight stigma on targeted individuals and (2) the complex, multidimensional, and multilayered causes of obesity. We consider each of these in turn in the following two sections.

WEIGHT STIGMA

Weight stigma (i.e., prejudicial attitudes and discriminating behaviours) toward higher-weight people is prevalent, pervasive, and, in contrast to other forms of stigma, rising (Andreyeva, Puhl, & Brownell, 2008; Charlesworth & Banaji, 2019; Puhl & Brownell, 2001; Rubino et al., 2020). Among the most disturbing occurrences of weight stigma is in healthcare settings (Gupta, Bombak, Foroughi, & Riediger, 2020), given the purported role of these settings to support health and wellbeing. Experiences of weight stigma from healthcare professionals are prevalent across nations (Puhl, Lessard, Pearl, Himmelstein, & Foster, 2021) and result in higher-weight people being less likely to seek preventive healthcare services (Fontaine, Faith, Allison, & Cheskin, 1998). In this way, weight stigma, together with the biological processes stemming from excess adiposity, contributes to the elevated medical morbidity and mortality experienced by people with obesity. Indeed, it has been estimated through longitudinal research that weight stigma accounts for a substantial proportion of variance (27%) in the negative health outcomes of obesity (Daly, Sutin, & Robinson, 2019), as well as contributing to the occurrence and exacerbation of obesity (Sutin & Terracciano, 2013). Regarding the latter, stigma can contribute to weight gain through multiple, interacting mechanisms (e.g., fear of exercising in public settings, emotional eating, and the physiological impacts of stress on eating and weight regulation) (Brewis, 2014; Lessard, Puhl, Himmelstein, Pearl, & Foster, 2021).

The fact that weight stigma is profoundly damaging to medical and psychosocial health, corrosive of human rights, and (as discussed later) contrary to scientific knowledge in its attribution of blame to higher-weight people underscores its unacceptability. Combating weight stigma is thus a high priority (Rubino et al., 2020). However, not all attempts to mitigate the existence of weight stigma are unproblematic. For instance, to diminish blameworthy attributions, some have argued that claims regarding the negative health consequences of obesity are mistaken (e.g., Campos, Saguy, Ernsberger, Oliver, & Gaesser, 2006). Yet, as Kim and Popkin (2006) argue in their critique of this approach, 'falsely invalidating existing evidence of increasing obesity and its health impact . . . and treating a real health problem as nonexisting is equally irresponsible as blaming the victims' (p. 65).

THE CAUSES OF OBESITY

A more credible and hence convincing approach to undermining weight stigma stems from the sense of shared responsibility that emerges when the complex aetiology of obesity is acknowledged. The drivers of obesity comprise a confluence of environmental, social, biological, and psychological factors. This complexity belies any simplistic 'finger pointing' and instead highlights that effectively supporting the health and wellbeing of higher-weight people necessitates an integrated approach.

Our point of departure is the place of obesity within the global rising tide of chronic diseases. Two historical developments have resulted in a sizable increase in the burden of chronic diseases (Global Burden of Disease Study 2013 Collaborators, 2015). First, demographic transitions led by reduced birth and death rates at all ages have resulted in the ageing of the world's population. Second, this ageing population can be partly attributed to the widespread adoption of technological and medical advances (e.g., the production of penicillin) that have led to a significant reduction in communicable diseases despite their remaining salience (Brachman, 2003). Obesity, one of the most common emergent chronic conditions, does not fit neatly into this narrative since its rise is counter to both of these processes. First, obesity is not commonly a condition of old age, with Class III obesity (defined as a Body Mass Index [BMI] $\geq$40 kg/m^2) falling off sharply after age 65, in part because of its lethality. Second, the obesity pandemic can be understood by technological developments that, while markedly beneficial for health and wellbeing, have nevertheless driven a proliferation of obesogenic environments around the world (Swinburn, Egger, & Raza, 1999). Obesogenic environments highly constrain what is a realistic expectation of outcome regarding body weight, particularly for individuals and communities who are genetically and psychologically vulnerable to their effects (Egger & Swinburn, 2010).

Obesogenic Environments

The rise in obesity rates followed on from a period of immense societal and environmental change that dramatically altered the eating and physical activity patterns of people living in these systems. Individually, the presence or absence of these socioenvironmental factors does not cause a person to become overweight, but they help form a person's preferences and norms and impose significant barriers that work against engagement in health-promoting behaviours. For example, a city that was designed around the car, with little convenient pedestrian access, can make walking or cycling unpleasant or even dangerous. Similarly, having 'just one' beer where the cultural norm is to buy rounds defies convention and invites peer opprobrium.

Marked changes in eating patterns have resulted from food system commodification, the rise in the power and influence of the corporate food retailer, globally extended logistics and supply networks, the power of brand-name and franchise marketing, and lassiez-faire attitudes to market governance (Dyball, Davila, & Wilkes, 2020). Global food supply networks expanded substantially after World War II, distancing food production in time and space from its consumption. Food marketing has created ever new target audiences, including the 'autonomous child decision-maker' (Dixon & Broom, 2007). Commodification of agricultural products (e.g., refined sugars and oils) and globally marketed processed foods that can be transported easily and have long shelf lives have broken many long-standing local food production and consumption patterns and driven dietary patterns toward the frequent consumption of ultra-processed foods that are low cost, energy dense, and highly palatable, thereby fuelling weight gain and obesity (Hall et al., 2019). Consumption of such foods for both children (1 in 5 calories) and adults (1 in 7 calories) has remained high over the past 20-year period (Liu, Lee, Micha, Li, & Mazaffarian, 2021).

This commodification of food has replaced much that was 'home-made' a hundred or so years ago. The latter point is not intended to valorise 'home-made,' as the gendered dimension of traditional roles assigned to this task cannot be ignored. As with housekeeping more generally, food preparation was traditionally seen as a woman's responsibility and demanded long hours in acquisition, preparation, and washing up. Much food marketing, and convenience food in particular, continues to depict women as responsible for 'feeding the family' and targets them accordingly, capitalising on the fact that their engagement in work outside of the home as well their continued greater share of household labour provides fertile ground for marketing ready-made but energy dense substitutes (Dixon & Broom, 2007). Considerations of this type hint at even less obvious elements in the obesity causal sequence, such as trends toward higher costs of home ownership that demand both adults work full-time.

The presence of unseen additives, notably refined sugars, in much food consumed today is particularly true of processed and pre-prepared 'ready meal' options sold as quick, tasty, and convenient supermarket choices and in many fast food options and beverages. These convenience foods are disproportionately aimed at lower socioeconomic groups. Consumption of sugar trends upwards per capita across history, with historical and cultural variations, such as the trade association of the 1700s between Great Britain and US sugar plantations. However, the trend line for obesity increases markedly from the mid-1970s and directly correlates with the introduction of liquid high-fructose corn syrup as an inexpensive enhancer of the taste of many food products. Most significant is its presence in sugar-sweetened soft drinks, the consumption of which is strongly implicated in rising obesity levels across the past 50 years (Johnson, Bell, Zarnowiecki, Rangan, & Golley, 2017; Johnson, Sánchez-Lozada, Andrews, & Lanaspa, 2017).

In addition to their disruption of eating patterns, obesogenic environments are characterised by their impact on average physical activity levels. Reductions in physical activity have been driven by major technology and market trends such as the shift in labour from physical to sedentary work inside and outside the home, from walking/cycling to motorised personal transport with car-dependent urban design and limited bike lane access (Pan et al., 2020), and increasing time spent on screen-based leisure pursuits (Banks, Jorm, Rogers, Clements, & Bauman, 2010; Decelis, Jago, & Fox, 2014). Relative to research on the built environment, associations between obesity and the natural environment (e.g., weather, altitude, air quality, and day length) have received scant attention. However, there is accumulating evidence that both increases and decreases in temperature are associated with decreased physical activity in children (Jia et al., 2020) and that air pollution is associated with the development of obesity in children (de Bont et al., 2021), again possibly due to its negative impact on physical activity. Indeed, there is a growing literature indicating that pollutants and chemical exposure more broadly (e.g., polluted water supplies, transport emissions, agricultural chemicals, and plastics used in food packaging) may act as endocrine-disrupting chemicals to influence the development of obesity in a comparable magnitude to that of unhealthy dietary patterns and sedentary behaviour (Lobstein & Brownell, 2021).

The aforementioned structural features of industrialised societies exert greater effects on those experiencing economic disadvantage, with a negative correlation between socioeconomic status and weight, particularly among women (Newton, Braithwaite, & Akinyemiju, 2017). For example, those with less expendable money are more vulnerable to food insecurity (i.e., restricted or uncertain availability of nutritious food), which is associated with obesity (Adams, Grummer-Strawn, & Chavez, 2003). They also experience greater restrictions in their physical activity options (e.g., the unaffordability of expensive gym memberships and unsafe local environments to exercise, play, or walk/cycle to work in) and poorer infrastructure, including limited access to health-based services and greenspaces (Townshend & Lake, 2017). Research has also demonstrated how the stressors related to socioeconomic hardship can have adverse impacts on the neural pathways regulating an individual's ability to engage in healthy behaviours (Kraft & Kraft, 2021).

Beyond these macro socioenvironmental processes are the micro processes operating at the interpersonal level (i.e., the intersection of the societal and individual scales), with evidence that obesity spreads within social networks.

Specifically, Christakis and Fowler (2007) examined the development of obesity over a 32-year period (1971–2003) among 12,067 participants. The results indicated that an individual's chances of developing obesity increased if those in the individual's social network became obese. For example, a person's chances of becoming obese increased by 171% if they had a mutual friend who became obese. The results suggested that the relevant factor was social connection rather than geographical proximity, raising the intriguing question of what it is about our social ties that could make us vulnerable in this way. Our own research indicates that significant others can engage in a range of behaviours that might either assist (e.g., co-participation in healthy behaviours) or undermine (e.g., weight stigma or modelling unhealthy behaviours) an individual's weight management (Rieger, Lee, Monaghan, Zwickert, & Murray, 2021).

ECOLOGICAL EFFECTS OF OBESOGENIC ENVIRONMENTS

While our focus has thus far been on the impact of socioenvironmental factors that promote obesity, we should also note that there are environmental costs stemming from the production of unhealthy food commodities. Many of these harmful environmental effects stem from the same dominant beliefs about the purpose of food systems that are driving poor health outcomes. Lang and Heasman (2015) call this the 'Productionist' paradigm. At core, this is the notion that food production and distribution is best served by food being treated as an industrialised commodity, like any other consumer good. Characteristic features are to treat agriculture as a process of primary resource extraction, featuring high levels of artificial inputs, typically growing monocultures, and being highly mechanised and energy intensive across all stages in the food supply chain from production, processing, distribution, and retail. In environmental terms, the cost of this has been 40% of the ice-free surface of the planet having been converted to agriculture; 70% of freshwater use being for irrigation; unsustainable linear flows of nutrients, notably nitrogen and phosphorus; estimates of 80% biodiversity loss due to agriculture; and agriculture and emissions from the broader food system accounting for around 25% of anthropocentric greenhouse gas emissions (Campbell et al., 2017).

Biological and Psychological Vulnerability Factors

While overweight and obesity affect the majority of people in developed countries, not all people have been equally vulnerable to the obesogenic environments they inhabit. In this section we highlight, in turn, some of the biological and psychological factors at play in this regard, with an emphasis on factors that interact with the obesogenic environment.

GENETIC FACTORS

The scientific understanding of the biology of obesity has been transformed in the 21st century. Body weight regulation is no longer understood as simply the balance between energy in and energy out, but has moved on to a detailed and still emerging knowledge of the interactions between 12 or more hormones and a set of nested neurological systems spanning neurohormonal control of pituitary hormones, sensory perception, neural reward pathways, and drivers of cortical executive functions, as well as how homeostatic systems might work to defend higher weight (for reviews, see Lowe, Reichelt, & Hall, 2019; Uranga & Keller, 2019; for a lay summary, see Proietto, 2016). As an illustration of the latter, it has been proposed that metabolic adaptation occurs after a period of weight loss in the form of a significant reduction in total energy expenditure as the body works to defend its previous weight, thereby producing resistance to further weight loss and promoting weight regain (Leibel, Rosenbaum, & Hirsch, 1995). The role of metabolic adaptation has been highly contested, with a more recent study showing that it largely disappeared after weight stabilisation and was not predictive of weight regain (Martins, Roekenes, Salamati, Gower, & Hunter, 2020). These findings, however, do not preclude the possible operation of metabolic adaptation during dietary restriction, which would make further weight loss difficult.

Genetic and epigenetic factors underlie some of the heterogenous responses of people to obesogenic environments (Elks et al., 2012). Epigenetic research shows how these environments not only shape changes in eating and physical activity patterns but also alter genetic expression. Epigenetics explores how the genome interacts with the organism and the environment to affect the expression of one's genetic tendency. Epigenetic research has established plausible mechanisms for transgenerational amplification of ancestral obesity through up to three generations, involving DNA methylation mechanisms, adipogenesis (growth of fat storage tissue), glucose and lipid metabolism, and appetite (Youngson & Morris, 2013). Should this intergenerational amplification of obesity prove to be the case (i.e., that exposure during pregnancy to an energy-dense diet causes obesity in the mother, her offspring, and her offspring's offspring), it would add an urgency to effective policies to address obesogenic environments because it may take up to three generations for their impact to wash out of the population's epigenetic structures. As an example of a less obvious candidate in the obesity causal sequence, epigenetic changes in DNA methylation might also be triggered by exposure to environmental chemicals used in food production (e.g., insecticides) (Ruiz-Hernandez et al., 2015), although it is currently unknown whether such changes affect body weight regulation.

The interest in gut microbiota that has risen sharply in the past decade points to the role of not just the human genome (approximately 23,000 genes) in obesity, but also to the genes of our microbiome (approximately 3 million genes) in obesity (Zhao, 2013). While diet can impact on the gut microbiota, these in turn release toxins or beneficial metabolites impacting on health. There is some research that different microbiota can protect against the development of obesity in the context of an energy-dense diet (Maruvada, Leone, Kaplan, & Chang, 2017).

PSYCHOLOGICAL FACTORS

A range of psychological vulnerabilities also act to precipitate weight gain in people who are living in an obesogenic environment. These vulnerabilities include psychological conditions such as depression and binge eating disorder (Fairburn, Cooper, Doll, Norman, & O'Connor, 2000; Luppino et al., 2010), with eating (rendered readily accessible in an obesogenic environment) potentially serving an affect regulation function for people with these conditions (Leehr et al., 2015). Demonstrating the bidirectional nature of such associations, Luppino et al. (2010) found that people with depression were 1.58 times more likely to develop obesity, while people in the obese range were 1.55 times more likely to develop depression, than their normal-weight counterparts. Highlighting the links between weight stigma, depression, and obesity, Adams and Bukowski (2008) found that girls with a BMI in the obese range who experienced weight-based bullying at age 12–13 years reported higher rates of body dissatisfaction at age 14–15 years and had higher depression ratings and BMIs at age 16–17 years.

While obesogenic environments *facilitate* overeating, they conversely work to *undermine* the self-efficacy that is an essential component for sustained engagement in weight management behaviours. In his highly influential 1977 paper, Albert Bandura defined self-efficacy as confidence in one's ability to successfully undertake the behaviours necessary to produce certain outcomes (in our case, the confidence to engage in eating and physical activity patterns conducive to weight management). Bandura (1977) proposed that self-efficacy is fundamental in determining whether or not people will initiate certain behaviours, how much effort they will expend, and how long they will persist with these behaviours in the face of challenges. In the subsequent decades, self-efficacy has been extensively investigated and has been incorporated into the major models used to explain health behaviours (e.g., self-determination theory, protection motivation theory, the theory of planned behaviour, and the transtheoretical model of behaviour change) including weight-related behaviours. For example, in a review of studies addressing 25 predictors of fruit and vegetable consumption among adults, self-efficacy was one of only three factors for which strong evidence was found (Shaikh, Yaroch, Nebleing, Yeh, & Resnicow, 2008). Self-efficacy has also been found to prospectively predict greater engagement in weight control behaviours and greater weight loss among those taking part in a weight loss programme, with effect sizes in the medium range (Linde, Rothman, Baldwin, & Jeffery, 2006). However, sustaining a sense of confidence in one's ability to manage one's weight after leaving a weight loss programme and returning to almost unmitigated exposure to an obesogenic environment is, as we describe in the next section, a major (and for most, a seemingly insurmountable) challenge.

INTERVENTIONS FOR OBESITY

Behavioural Interventions

Behavioural (or lifestyle) interventions support people with obesity to modify their weight control behaviours, with the most effective programmes combining a reduced-calorie diet, increased physical activity, and cognitive-behavioural strategies for altering eating patterns and physical activity. Such programmes typically yield mean weight losses of between 5% and 10% of initial body weight, with associated health benefits and a reduction in risk of many adverse outcomes (Mariam et al., 2021), such as the prevention of 34% of new cases of type 2 diabetes 10 years after treatment (Diabetes Prevention Program Research Group, 2009). They also result in enhanced wellbeing, with a systematic review of 36 studies finding consistent improvements in self-esteem, depression, body image, and health-related quality of life after participation in a behavioural weight loss programme, often of a medium to large effect size (Lasikiewicz, Myrissa, Hoyland, & Lawton, 2014).

Among the crucial challenges for lifestyle programmes is achieving *sustained* weight loss, with weight regain the most common outcome (Butryn, Webb, & Wadden, 2011). As a result, obesity is now widely conceptualised as a chronic condition in which treatment must be long-term, with ongoing patient–clinician contact found to be effective for long-term weight management (e.g., Look AHEAD Research Group, 2014). However, in placing the chronic disease within the individual, this approach minimises or overlooks entirely the chronic pathology that lies within the obesogenic environment, with navigating this environment after treatment ends among the major impediments to long-term weight loss. Those who do manage to maintain at least some of their lost weight over the longer term note, as an enduring and fatiguing challenge, 'the ever presence of hyperpalatable, hypercaloric, inexpensive foods threatening to derail weight loss maintenance on a continuous basis' together with 'unsupportive peers who would discourage, tempt, and pressure [them] to engage in counterproductive activities like overeating and drinking excessively' and 'cultural norms concerning both portions and kinds of food . . . and alcohol consumption' (Spreckley, Seidell, & Halberstadt, 2021, p. 11). In the absence of substantial change at the socioenvironmental level—and we discuss this approach at length below—long-term lifestyle programmes are especially warranted, although the availability of high-intensity lifestyle treatments that can lead to lasting weight loss is woefully inadequate (Heymsfield et al., 2018). This limited access disproportionately impacts on socioeconomically disadvantaged groups, thereby further entrenching health inequities (Coggon & Adams, 2021).

Medical Interventions

For people with clinically severe obesity (defined as a BMI ≥40 or a BMI ≥35 for those with at least one medical complication), treatment from specialist obesity services comprised of multidisciplinary teams (including physicians, surgeons, nurses, dieticians, exercise physiologists, and psychologists) is recommended (Atlantis et al., 2018). Once again, access to these specialist services is highly restricted: in Australia it has been estimated that, even if these services were multiplied 10-fold, it would still take 25 years to treat those with clinically severe obesity.

In specialist obesity services, lifestyle programmes attending to the diet, physical activity, and psychological wellbeing of the patient are supplemented by more intensive interventions appropriate to the specific patient, such as very-low-energy diets (Delbridge & Proietto, 2006), weight loss pharmacotherapies, and bariatric (weight loss) surgery. Bariatric surgery, particularly partial removal of the stomach and its refashioning with a line of surgical staples from a bag to a tube or 'sleeve' (the so-called sleeve gastrectomy), has become one of the most common surgical procedures performed in the developed world. There are problems with both too ready access to it for some and too little access to it for others: many patients have it without proper assessment, preparation, or support, leading to poor results and adverse incidents, whereas others face financial, geographical, or timeliness barriers to access. However, with sound patient selection, patients have negligible mortality, acceptable rates of side effects, and significant and sustained weight loss, at least up to 5 years postoperatively (Hoyuela, 2017; Salminen et al., 2018).

Societal and Environmental Interventions

The pivotal role of the obesogenic environment in driving obesity highlights the dire need for public policy approaches to improve this environment and hence the health of the population. Such improvements are critical in supporting the challenging work undertaken by individuals in managing their weight and broader health. Since the opportunities for intervention at this level are diverse (e.g., health promotion campaigns, food product and menu nutritional labelling, restrictions on advertising of less healthy foods and beverages, and challenging weight bias), only a sample of these will be discussed in this section as a means of proposing some principles for integrated approaches.

The first principle of an integrated approach is to seek approaches whereby targeting one level of the system driving obesity can positively impact on other levels. For example, there has been global action on the taxation of sugar-sweetened beverages to make them less desirable, with approximately 50 countries to date having applied such a tax. The considerable revenue derived from this practice (estimated to be $18 billion across the United States in one taxation model; Powell, Andreyeva, & Isgor, 2020) could be redistributed to build the significantly underresourced healthcare services and programmes for supporting individuals to engage in healthy behaviours and weight management. Therefore, this societal-level intervention not only supports individuals in making healthier choices by altering the obesogenic environment, but also can make individually oriented obesity interventions more accessible for all.

A second principle of an integrated approach is the need to consider individual-level processes in designing public health initiatives to optimise their outcomes (Cory et al., 2021). For instance, one study found that a workplace ban on the sale of sugar-sweetened beverages was minimally effective on its own in reducing consumption among those experiencing strong cravings for these drinks but was highly effective in combination with a brief individual-level intervention designed to increase people's intrinsic motivation to reduce their sugar intake (Mason et al., 2021). These findings underscore the importance of multilevel interventions: without concurrently attending to individual-level factors, public health initiatives will likely be limited in their reach or, at worse, harmful for some (e.g., exacerbating weight concerns and maladaptive dieting among those with or vulnerable to eating disorders) (Treasure & Ambwani, 2021).

To minimise potential harms, an approach that focuses on health promotion for all (i.e., across the body weight spectrum), rather than obesity per se, is recommended. A crucial challenge in this regard is addressing the aforementioned unsustainable food system energy and material flows and restoring them to balance for improving both human and ecological health. Indeed, altering our food practices may well be the single strongest lever we have to optimise human health and environmental sustainability (Willett et al., 2019). This highlights a third principle of an integrated approach to obesity: namely, expanding the endpoint beyond human health to consider the other dimensions of wellbeing such as the health of the planet. A first step in this regard would be to 'eat food, not too much, mostly plants,' as Michael Pollan (2008) succinctly advises (by 'eat food' he means relatively unprocessed meals that our grandparents would recognise as being food). To this we would add, 'and mostly local' since it is at more local scales that food waste (which accounts for as much as 30% of food produced) and transportation and packaging costs and pollutants might be curtailed (Dyball et al., 2020; Ingram et al., 2016). Emerging research is focusing on the best strategies for supporting people to make food choices that support both human and environmental wellbeing (e.g., Cozzio, Volgger, & Taplin, 2021). Societal-level interventions that facilitate physical activity (e.g., creating increased access to bike lanes; Pan et al., 2020) can also have the dual goal of caring for the planet, given the association between lower levels of adiposity and greater access to natural (both green and blue) spaces (Teixeira et al., 2021), and modes of active travel do not generate the pollutants that motorised options create.

A fourth principle of integrated approaches for obesity is that they be sensitive to place in acknowledging the need to design health interventions in light of cultural practices and norms. As just one illustration, ethnographic work highlights the poor fit—and hence lack of success—of Western obesity programmes in the Pacific islands (e.g., dietary changes that are counter to social obligations) (Hardin, McLennan, & Brewis, 2018).

AN INTEGRATED FRAMEWORK FOR INFORMING OBESITY POLICY

In this final section, we discuss interdisciplinary approaches to inform obesity policy that appropriately recognise and address the broader drivers of obesity operating across and between scales. In short, how are we to address the complex skein of issues that bear on slowing and eventually turning around the obesity epidemic? While tuned to obesity, our suggestions may also be useful for other complex system problems.

The policy challenge of achieving good population health outcomes in obeso-genic environments is complex and multifaceted. It necessarily requires know-ledge and strategic contributions from across a range of management sectors. This produces the problems of how to collect, process, integrate, and implement these varied analyses and proposals.

An understandable response to extremely complex problems, as is charac-teristic of obesity and obesogenic environments, is to break their management into discrete parts, dealing with aspects of the problem one by one in isolation. Polycentric government structures attribute responsibility and decision-making into these silos. However, such a strategy will miss important feedback effects by which changes in one part of the system drive changes in other parts. For example, a department of transport may have programmes designed to reduce commute times while a department of health may be concerned with respiratory health impacts of local particulate pollution levels and the effect of motorised travel in discouraging active travel. Although the two departments may see their policy goals as unrelated to each other, the success of the former feeds back to the detriment of the success of the latter.

Policy-makers need an analytical framework through which they can under-stand the interrelationships between sectors and avoid policy interventions in one area that create problematic outcomes for others. *Collaborative conceptual mod-elling* (CCM) is one such framework leading to simple but powerful 'feedback guided analysis' that helps reveal these often unseen feedback processes (Newell & Proust, 2012). CCM also requires participants to generate a 'shared concep-tual repertoire' through which a common understanding of the various special-ised contributions can be gained (Dyball & Newell, 2015). This entails reducing the level of abstraction from the highly technical usage specific to one field of knowledge to more concrete concepts encountered in everyday situations. These low-order conceptual approaches can then allow the depth of knowledge fostered within areas of expertise that operate at higher levels of abstraction to be shared collectively by using accessible and mutually understood terminology. The CCM process simplifies the complexity to a manageable level while at the same time retaining the power of holistic systems thinking by preserving the feedback rela-tionships operating between the main parts. Steps to this 'simple, but powerful' reduction are set out by Newell and Siri (2016).

In *Understanding Human Ecology*, Dyball and Newell (2015) discuss the value of identifying the smallest number of discrete interacting classes of entities driving change in complex human–environmental systems, including obesogenic environments. These are the things representing the state of the environment, both built and natural, that can be thought of as increasing or decreasing over time. Examples of interest to the obesity epidemic could be the number of buses, number of parks, distance to fast-food outlets, and so on. Another set of catego-ries are indicators of health and wellbeing, both physical and psychosocial. As with environmental indicators, this category contains potentially vast numbers of possible factors worthy of attention, and each could be an area of its own know-ledge expertise, policy approaches, public management, and decision-making.

Examples could be people's motivation to engage in physical activity, the energy density of their food choices, and so on.

Central to understanding the behaviour of human systems are the dominant beliefs and values that influence the goals or outcomes set for the system and which inform judgements about whether the state of the system is more or less as it should be. These overarching paradigms are often taken for granted. However, in the face of persistent and intractable problems, such as those caused by obesogenic environments, they need to be surfaced and subjected to critical scrutiny. For example, it might be assumed that the purpose of food systems is to ensure that the community is provided with a range of food choices that deliver nutritional security to its members. But, by many measures, dominant food systems can be characterised as primarily concerned with the industrial production of retail commodities for the purpose of making a profit (Dyball et al., 2020).

Dominant beliefs about what the goal of a system is, or should be, give rise to formal and informal institutions that influence collective human behaviour to achieve those goals. In formal institutions of governance, including governments and their agencies and other legally constituted bodies, these rules for guiding collective behaviour may take the form of defined policy, taxes, regulations, education, and so on that are often written or codified (Fischer et al., 2012). In the context of obesity, formal institutions might include the healthcare system (e.g., what treatments or management regimes are available and what means of access to care a person might have). However, informal institutional arrangements may have an important role in regulating collective behaviour without necessarily being specifically defined. Informal institutional settings can strongly influence what society or peer groups see as 'normal' and appropriate behaviour for a community. Violating these often unwritten and unlegislated standards is not a formal punishable offense but is internalised and 'self-policed' by individuals as they define their own subjectivity in relation to their social context (Foucault, 1977). Informal institutions might, for example, largely determine whether a person presenting with a higher weight would be admired or stigmatised.

These low-order categories of variables can be regarded as common to any human–ecological system. Causal processes drive changes in the strength of dominant attitudes and beliefs, institutional coherence with those beliefs, and outcomes in terms of levels of human health and wellbeing and of environmental health indicators. Feedback from observations and learning about the state of the system's variables may affect those dominant paradigms, reinforcing or eroding them depending on the relative strength of the change process to aspects of social power and policy resistance. Schematically, these interacting categories of variables are shown in the 'cultural adaptation template' in Figure 9.2.

The cultural adaptation template is a valuable framework for organising discussion between multiple stakeholders from different knowledge backgrounds who are seeking to collaborate on tackling complex problems, such as obesity. Participants, who might be practitioners, academics, policy-makers, and community members, can work together to populate the very abstract categories of variables with the knowledge that they have about the levels of specific variables

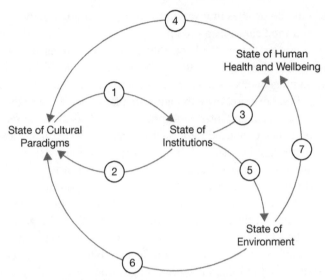

Figure 9.2 A Cultural Adaptation Template. The labels are the main categories of variables that represent the state of the system at any point in time. The arrows represent the causal processes whereby changes in the level or amount of a variable drive changes in the level or amount of the variable to which it is connected. Processes numbered 1, 3, and 5 represent human activities. Processes numbered 2, 4, and 6 represent observation and learning from changes caused by that activity. Process 7 represents the direct influence the state of the environment has on human health and wellbeing. See text for discussion. Adapted from Dyball and Newell (2015).

that fit within those categories. The framework invites attention to be paid to how changes in one set of variables feed back to change others. It also allows consideration to be given to how an intervention to change the level of one variable would also change those others that are connected to that variable. In this way policy 'surprises' (i.e., when undesirable and unintended consequences result from a well-intended intervention) might be avoided. By participating in collectively populating the cultural adaptation template, collaborators are obliged to move between their very detailed abstract disciplinary, practice-based, or experiential knowledge to communicate in simple terms its implication to others. The creation of such a 'shared conceptual repertoire' is a crucial prerequisite to successful collaboration that demands the blending of knowledge from disparate domains. Finally, the framework invites critical discussion around questions of what the behaviour of the system should be, not merely observations on how it is behaving.

Figure 9.3 is an example of the cultural adaptation template populated to represent a system of interest specific to an individual within an obesogenic environment. It serves as a heuristic device to guide a collective management programme.

Working groups and interdepartmental committees (*whole-of-government approaches*) are commonplace in contemporary government. For issues such as obesity and obesogenic environments, these need to be enduring structures, not

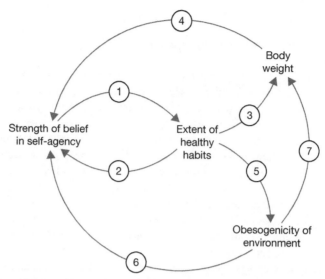

Figure 9.3 An example of the Cultural Adaptation Template applied to obesity showing the structure of the feedback system constraining an individual's body weight. See Table 9.1 for an explanation of the processes represented by the numbered arrows.

Table 9.1 KEY TO THE CULTURAL ADAPTATION TEMPLATE APPLIED TO OBESITY

Link number	Processes represented by each link
L1	The sum of all the processes by which an individual is motivated to align their eating and physical activity habits with whatever their life-world experiences and cultural values normalise as satisfactory body weight.
L2	The process of gauging if the factors regulating an individual's food and physical activity habits cohere with their life world, values, and expectations of what that these behaviours should be. These feedback processes may erode belief in their self-agency if the way they would like their behaviours to be does not align with their actual food habits.
L3	The sum of an individual's food consumption, less energy-expending activities, that directly affects their body weight across time. From a health perspective, the goal of the system should be that body weight is in a state of dynamic equilibrium within what is a healthy weight range for each specific person.
L4	The process of monitoring change in body weight. The extent to which actual body weight aligns with what an individual thinks their weight should be may reinforce or erode their motivation to strive to make further changes. If they are in a healthy weight range this feedback would limit further modification of eating and physical activity habits to maintain that healthy range. However, it is also possible that body weight goals and actual weight fail to align over time, leading to a potential erosion of self-agency and cessation of further attempts at change.

(continued)

Table 9.1 CONTINUED

Link number	Processes represented by each link
L5	The activities an individual takes to modify their relationship with their food systems and the obesogenicity of the food environment within which they live (e.g., where they shop for food and their patronage of fast-food outlets). Their capacity to affect how obesogenic their environment is may include factors outside of their control, for example, whether or not healthy food options are accessible. In terms of energy expenditure, this link also captures the processes whereby an individual can regularly engage in physical activity, given the environmental constraints of their surroundings and personal physical limitations.
L6	The processes of experiencing one's embeddedness in a particular food system environment. This experience may be judged by the individual as being positive, and so tend to reinforce engagement with that food system, or negative, tending to pursue action to change that relationship. An example would be whether buying fresh food directly from a farmer at a farmers' market and preparing from scratch was experienced as a psychosocial reaffirmation of creativity, self-expression, and achievement or of being too onerous, expensive, or time-consuming.
L7	The health benefits or disbenefits that flow from the state of the food system and broader environment in which the individual is embedded. An example would be the time and capacity to access nutritionally balanced fresh food and prepare food in alignment with healthy eating guidelines. If the environment is highly obesogenic, processes captured in this link may well overwhelm any individual efforts made to lower body weight.

ad-hoc and reactive. The systems approach described here helps foster the shared conceptual repertoire necessary to contribute to these collaborative endeavours.

SUMMARY

Obesity poses one of the most concerning and complex public health challenges facing the world today. In this chapter, we have sought to take seriously growing calls for multilevel approaches in conceptualising the aetiology of and interventions for obesity by thinking simultaneously across the biological, psychological, sociocultural, and environmental domains. Our integrated approach makes explicable the fact that, over at least a 30-year period—characterised by intensive efforts on the part of higher-weight individuals, researchers, health professionals, and public health campaigns alike—obesity levels have not declined. It also proposes some ways forward that call for concurrent, connected, compassionate (toward each other), and assertive (toward self-serving commercial interests) action across the individual and societal levels to improve the wellbeing of people and the planet.

REFERENCES

Adams, E. J., Grummer-Strawn, L., & Chavez, G. (2003). Food insecurity is associated with increased risk of obesity in California women. *Journal of Nutrition, 133,* 1070–1074. doi:10.1093/jn/133.4.1070

Adams, R. E., & Bukowski, W. M. (2008). Peer victimization as a predictor of depression and body mass index in obese and non-obese adolescents. *Journal of Child Psychology and Psychiatry, 49,* 858–866. doi:10.1111/j.1469-7610.2008.01886.x

American Medical Association. (2013). *Recognition of obesity as a disease H-440.842.* https://policysearch.ama-assn.org/policyfinder/detail/H-440.842?uri=%2FAMA Doc%2FHOD.xml-0-3858.xml

Ata, R. N., & Thompson, J. K. (2010). Weight bias in the media: A review of recent research. *Obesity Facts, 3,* 41–46. doi:10.1159/000276547

Andreyeva, T., Puhl, R. M., & Brownell, K. D. (2008). Changes in perceived weight discrimination among Americans, 1995–1996 through 2004–2006. *Obesity, 16,* 1129–1134. doi:10.1038/oby.2008.35

Atlantis, E., Kormas, N., Samras, K., Fahey, P., Sumithran, P., Glastras, S., . . . Dixon, J. (2018). Clinical obesity services in public hospitals in Australia: A position statement based on expert consensus. *Clinical Obesity, 8,* 203–210. doi:10.1111/cob.12249

Bandura, A. (1977). Self-efficacy: Toward a unifying theory of behavioural change. *Psychological Review, 84,* 191–215.

Banks, E., Jorm, L., Rogers, K., Clements, M., & Bauman, A. (2010). Screen-time, obesity, ageing and disability: Findings from 91 266 participants in the 45 and Up Study. *Public Health Nutrition, 14,* 34–43. doi:10.1017/S1368980010000674

Blüher, M. (2019). Obesity: Global epidemiology and pathogenesis. *Nature Reviews Endocrinology, 15,* 288–298. doi:10.1038/s41574-019-0176-8

Brachman, P. S. (2003). Infectious diseases—Past, present, and future. *International Journal of Epidemiology, 32,* 684–686. doi:10.1093/ije/dyg282

Brewis, A. A. (2014). Stigma and the perpetuation of obesity. *Social Science & Medicine, 118,* 152–158. doi:10.1016/j.socscimed.2014.08.003

Butryn, M. L., Webb, V., & Wadden, T. A. (2011). Behavioral treatment of obesity. *Psychiatric Clinics of North America, 34,* 841–859. doi:10.1016/j.psc.2011.08.006

Campbell, B. M., Beare, D. J., Bennett, E. M., Hall-Spencer, J. M., Ingram, J. S. I., Jaramillo, F., . . . Shindell, D. (2017). Agriculture production as a major driver of the Earth system exceeding planetary boundaries. *Ecology and Society, 22*(4), Article 8. doi:10.5751/ES-09595-220408

Campos, P., Saguy, A., Ernsberger, P., Oliver, E., & Gaesser, G. (2006). The epidemiology of overweight and obesity: Public health crisis or moral panic. *International Journal of Epidemiology, 35,* 55–60. doi:10.1093/ije/dyi254

Cawley, J., Biener, A., Meyerhoefer, C., Ding, Y., Zvenyach, T., Smolarz, B. G., & Ramasamy, A. (2021). Direct medical costs of obesity in the United States and most populous states. *Journal of Managed Care and Specialty Pharmacy, 27,* 354–366. doi:10.18553/jmcsp.2021.20410

Charlesworth, T. E. S., & Banaji, M. R. (2019). Patterns of implicit and explicit attitudes: I. Long-term change and stability from 2007 to 2016. *Psychological Science, 30,* 174–192. doi:10.1177/095679761881308

Christakis, N. A., & Fowler, J. H. (2007). The spread of obesity in a large social network over 32 years. *New England Journal of Medicine, 357*, 370–379. doi:10.1056/NEJMsa066082

Coggon, J., & Adams, J. (2021). 'Let them choose not to eat cake . . .': Public health ethics, effectiveness, and equity in government obesity strategy. *Future Healthcare Journal, 8*, 1–4. doi:10.7861/fhj.2020-0246

Cory, M., Loiacono, B., Withington, M. C., Herman, A., Jagpal, A., & Buscemi, J. (2021). Behavioral economic approaches to childhood obesity prevention nutrition policies: A social ecological perspective. *Perspectives on Behavior Science, 44*, 317–332. doi:10.1007/s40614-021-00294-y

Cozzio, C., Volgger, M., & Taplin, R. (2021). Point-of-consumption interventions to promote virtuous food choices of tourists with self-benefit or other-benefit appeals: A randomised field experiment. *Journal of Sustainable Tourism*. doi:10.1080/09669582.2021.1932936

Daly, M., Sutin, A. R., & Robinson, E. (2019). Perceived weight discrimination mediates the prospective association between obesity and physiological dysregulation: Evidence from a population-based cohort. *Psychological Science, 30*, 1030–1039. doi:10.1177/0956797619849440

De Bont, J., Díaz, Y., de Castro, M., Cirach, M., Basagaña, X., Nieuwenhuijsen, M., . . . Vrijheid, M. (2021). Ambient air pollution and the development of overweight and obesity in children: A large longitudinal study. *International Journal of Obesity, 45*, 1124–1132. doi:10.1038/s41366-021-00783-9

Decelis, A., Jago, R., & Fox, K. R. (2014). Physical activity, screen time and obesity status in a nationally representative sample of Maltese youth with international comparisons. *BMC Public Health, 14*, 664. doi:10.1186/1471-2458-14-664

Delbridge, E., & Proietto, J. (2006). State of the science: VLED (Very Low Energy Diet) for obesity. *Asia Pacific Journal of Clinical Nutrition, 15*, 49–54.

Diabetes Prevention Program Research Group. (2009). 10-year follow-up of diabetes incidence and weight loss in the Diabetes Prevention Program Outcomes Study. *Lancet, 374*, 1677–1686. doi:10.1016/SO140-6736(09)61457-4

Dixon, J., & Broom, D. (2007). *The seven deadly sins of obesity: How the modern world is making us fat*. UNSW Press.

Dyball, R., Davila Cisneros, F., & Wilkes, B. (2020). A human ecological approach to policy in the context of food and nutrition security. In G. S. Metcalf, K. Kijima, & H. Deguchi (Eds.), *Handbook of systems science* (pp. 1–26). Springer.

Dyball, R., & Newell, B. (2015). *Understanding human ecology: A systems approach to sustainability*. Routledge.

Egger, G., & Swinburn, B. (2010). *Planet obesity: How we're eating ourselves and the planet to death*. Allen & Unwin.

Elks, C. E., den Hoed, M., Zhao, J. H., Sharp, S. J., Wareham, N. J., Loos, R. J. F., & Ong, K. K. (2012). Variability in the heritability of body mass index: A systematic review and meta-regression. *Frontiers in Endocrinology, 3*, 1–16. doi:10.3389/fendo.2012.00029

Fairburn, C., Cooper, Z., Doll, H., Norman, P., & O'Connor, M. (2000). The natural course of bulimia nervosa and binge eating disorder in young women. *Archives of General Psychiatry, 57*, 659–665. doi:10.1001/archpsyc.57.7.659

Fischer, J., Dyball, R., Fazey, I., Gross, C., Dovers, S., Ehrlich, P. R., . . . Borden, R. J. (2012). Human behavior and sustainability. *Frontiers in Ecology and the Environment, 10*(3), 153–160. doi:10.1890/110079

Fontaine, K. R., Faith, M. S., Allison, D. B., & Cheskin, L. J. (1998). Body weight and health care among women in the general population. *Archives of Family Medicine, 7,* 381–384. doi:10.1001/archfami.7.4.381

Foucault, M. (1977). *Discipline and punish: The birth of the prison.* Penguin.

Gardiner, J., Oben, J., & Sutcliffe, A. (2021). Obesity as a driver of international differences in COVID-19 death rates. *Diabetes, Obesity and Metabolism, 23,* 1463–1470. doi:10.1111/dom/14357

Global BMI Mortality Collaboration. (2016). Body mass index and all-cause-mortality: Individual-participant-data meta-analysis of 239 prospective studies in four continents. *Lancet, 388,* 776–786. doi:10.1016/S0140-6736(16)30175-1

Global Burden of Disease Study 2013 Collaborators. (2015). Global, regional, and national incidence, prevalence, and years lived with disability for 301 acute and chronic diseases and injuries in 188 countries, 1990–2013: A systematic analysis for the Global Burden of Disease Study 2013. *Lancet, 386*(9995), 743–800. doi:10.1016/S0140-6736(15)60692-4.

Gupta, N., Bombak, A., Foroughi, I., & Riediger, N. (2020). Discrimination in the health care system among higher-weight adults: Evidence from a Canadian national cross-sectional survey. *Health Promotion and Chronic Disease Prevention in Canada, 40,* 329–335. doi:10.24095/hpcdp.40.11/12.01

Hall, K. D., Ayuketah, A., Brychta, R., Cai, H., Cassimatus, T., Chen, K. Y., . . . Zhou, M. (2019). Ultra-processed diets cause excess calorie intake and weight gain: An in-patient randomized controlled trial of *ad libitum* food intake. *Cell Metabolism, 30,* 67–77. doi:10.1016/j.cmet.2019.05.008

Hardin, J., McLennan, A. K., & Brewis, A. (2018). Body size, body norms and some unintended consequences of obesity intervention in the Pacific Islands. *Annals of Human Biology, 45,* 285–294. doi:10.1080/03014460.2018.1459838

Heymsfield, S., Aronne, L. J., Eneli, I., Kumar, R. B., Michalsky, M., Walker, E., . . . Yanovski, S. (2018). Clinical perspectives on obesity treatment: Challenges, gaps, and promising opportunities. *NAM Perspectives.* Discussion Paper. National Academy of Medicine. doi:10.31478/201809b

Hoyuela, C. (2017). Five-year outcomes of laparoscopic sleeve gastrectomy as a primary procedure for morbid obesity: A prospective study. *World Journal of Gastrointestinal Surgery, 9,* 109–117. doi:10.4240/wjgs.v9.i4.109

Ingram, J., Dyball, R., Howden, M., Vermeulen, S., Garnett, T., Redlingshofer, B., . . . Porter, J. R. (2016). Food security, food systems, and environmental change. *The Solutions Journal, 7*(3), 63–72.

Jia, P., Dai, S., Rohli, K. E., Rohli, R. V., Ma, Y., Yu, C., . . . Zhou, W. (2020). Natural environment and childhood obesity: A systematic review. *Obesity Reviews,* 1–9. doi:10.1111/obr.13097

Johnson, B. J., Bell, L. K., Zarnowiecki, D., Rangan, A. M., & Golley, R. K. (2017). Contribution of discretionary foods and drinks to Australian children's intake of energy, saturated fat, added sugars and salt. *Children, 4,* 104. doi:10.3390/children4120104

Johnson, R. J., Sánchez-Lozada, L. G., Andrews, P., & Lanaspa, M. A. (2017). Perspective: A historical and scientific perspective of sugar and its relation with obesity and diabetes. *Advances in Nutrition, 8,* 412–422. doi:10.3945/an.116.014654

Kim, S., & Popkin, B. M. (2006). Commentary: Understanding the epidemiology of overweight and obesity – a real global public health concern. *International Journal of Epidemiology, 35,* 60–67. doi:10.1093/ije/dyi255

Kraft, P., & Kraft, B. (2021). Explaining socioeconomic disparities in health behaviours: A review of biopsychological pathways involving stress and inflammation. *Neuroscience and Biobehavioral Reviews, 127*, 689–708. doi:10.1016/j.neubiorev.2021.05.019

Lang, T., & Heasman, M. (2015). *Food wars: The global battle for mouths, minds and markets* (2nd ed.). Routledge.

Lasikiewicz, N., Myrissa, K., Hoyland, A., & Lawton, C. (2014). Psychological benefits of weight loss following behavioural and/or dietary weight loss interventions: A systematic research review. *Appetite, 72*, 123–137. doi:10.1016/j.appet.2013.09.017

Lau, D. C. W., Dhillon, B., Yan, H., Szmitko, P. E., & Verma, S. (2005). Adipokines: Molecular links between obesity and atherosclerosis. *American Journal of Physiology – Heart and Circulatory Physiology, 288*, H2031–H2041. doi:10.1152/ajpheart.01058.2004

Lessard, L. M., Puhl, R. M., Himmelstein, M. S., Pearl, R. L., & Foster, G. D. (2021). Eating and exercise-related correlates of weight stigma: A multinational investigation. *Obesity, 29*, 966–970. doi:10.1002/oby.23168

Lobstein, T., & Brownell, K. D. (2021). Endocrine-disrupting chemicals and obesity risk: A review of recommendations for obesity prevention policies. *Obesity Reviews, 22*, e13332. Doi:10.1111/obr.13332

Leehr, E. J., Krohmer, K., Schag, K., Dresler, T., Zipfel, S., & Giel, K. E. (2015). Emotion regulation model in binge eating disorder and obesity – A systematic review. *Neuroscience & Biobehavioral Reviews, 49*, 125–134. doi:10.1016/j.neubiorev.2014.12.008

Leibel, R. L., Rosenbaum, M., & Hirsch, J. (1995). Changes in energy expenditure resulting from altered body weight. *New England Journal of Medicine, 332*, 621–628. doi:10.1056/NEJM199503093321001

Lim, S. S., Vos, T., Flaxman, A. D., Danei, G., Shibuya, K., Adair-Rohani, H., . . . Ezzati, M. (2012). A comparative risk assessment of burden of disease and injury attributable to 67 risk factors and risk factor clusters in 21 regions, 1990–2010: A systematic analysis for the Global Burden of Disease Study 2010. *Lancet, 380*, 2224–2260. doi:10.1016/50140-6736(12)61766-8

Lin, A. L., Vittinghoff, E., Olgin, J. E., Pletcher, M. J., & Marcus, G. M. (2021). Body weight changes during pandemic-related shelter-in-place in a longitudinal cohort study. *JAMA Network Open, 4*, e212536. doi:10.1001/jamanetworkopen.2021.2536

Linde, J., Rothman, A., Baldwin, A., & Jeffery, R. (2006). The impact of self-efficacy on behaviour change and weight change among overweight participants in a weight loss trial. *Health Psychology, 25*, 282–291. doi:10.1037/0278-6133.25.3.282

Liu, J., Lee, Y., Micha, R., Li, Y., & Mozaffarian, D. (2021). Trends in junk food consumption among US children and adults, 2001–2018. *American Journal of Clinical Nutrition, 114*, 1039–1048. doi:10.1093/ajcn/nqab129

Look AHEAD Research Group. (2014). Eight-year weight losses with an intensive lifestyle intervention: The look AHEAD study. *Obesity, 22*, 5–13. doi:10.1002/oby.20662

Lowe, C. J., Reichelt, A. C., & Hall, P. A. (2019). The prefrontal cortex and obesity: A health neuroscience perspective. *Trends in Cognitive Sciences, 23*, 349–361. Doi:10.1016/j.tics.2019.01.005

Luppino, F. S., de Wit, L. M., Bouvy, P. F., Stijnen, T., Cuijpers, P., Penninx, B. W. J. H., & Zitman, F. G. (2010). Overweight, obesity, and depression: A systematic review and meta-analysis of longitudinal studies. *Archives of General Psychiatry, 67*, 220–229. doi:10.1001/archgenpsychiatry.2010.2

Mariam, A., Miller-Atkins, G., Pantalone, K. M., Iyer, N., Misra-Hebert, A. D., Milinovich, A., . . . Rotroff, D. M. (2021). Associations of weight loss with obesity-related comorbidities in a large integrated health system. *Diabetes, Obesity and Metabolism*. 1–10. doi:10.1111/dom.14538

Martins, C., Roekenes, J., Salamati, S., Gower, B. A., & Hunter, G. R. (2020). Metabolic adaptation is an illusion, only present when participants are in negative energy balance. *American Journal of Clinical Nutrition, 112*, 1212–1218. doi:10.1093/ajcn/nqaa220

Maruvada, P., Leone, V., Kaplan, L. M., & Chang, E. B. (2017). The human microbiome and obesity: Moving beyond associations. *Perspective, 22*, 589–599. doi:10.1016/j.chom.2017.10.005

Mason, A. E., Schmidt, L., Ishkanian, L., Jacobs, L. M., Leung, C., Jensen, L., . . . Epel, E. S. (2021). A brief motivational intervention differentially reduces sugar-sweetened beverage (SSB) consumption. *Annals of Behavioral Medicine*. doi:10.1093/abm/kaaa123

Must, A., Spadano, J., Coakley, E. H., Field, A. E., Colditz, G., & Dietz, W. H. (1999). The disease burden associated with overweight and obesity. *JAMA, 282*, 1523–1529. doi:10.1001/jama.282.16.1523

NCD Risk Factor Collaboration. (2017). Worldwide trends in body mass index, underweight, overweight, and obesity from 1975 to 2016: A pooled analysis of 2416 population-based measurement studies in 128.9 million children, adolescents, and adults. *Lancet, 16*, 2627–2642. doi:10.1016/S0140-6736(17)32129-3

Newell, B., & Proust, K. (2012). *Introduction to collaborative conceptual modelling.* Australian National University Open Access Research. https://openresearch-repository.anu.edu.au/handle/1885/9386

Newell, B., & Siri, J. (2016). A role for low-order system dynamics models in urban health policy making. *Environment International, 95*, 93–97. doi:10.1016/j.envint.2016.08.003

Newton, S., Braithwaite, D., & Akinyemiju, T. F. (2017). Socio-economic status over the life course and obesity: Systematic review and meta-analysis. *PLoS One, 12*, e0177151. doi:10.1371/journal.pone.0177151

Organisation for Economic Co-operation and Development. (2017). *Obesity update 2017.* https://www.oecd.org/els/health-systems/Obesity-Update-2017.pdf

Pan, X., Zhao, L., Luo, J., Li, Y., Zhang, L., Wu, T., . . . Jia, P. (2020). Access to bike lanes and childhood obesity: A systematic review and meta-analysis. *Obesity Reviews*, 1–11. doi:10.1111/obr.13042

Pollan, M. (2008). *In defense of food: An eater's manifesto.* Penguin Press.

Popkin, B. M., Du, S., Green, W. D., Beck, M. A., Algaith, T., Herbst, C. H., . . . Shekar, M. (2020). Individuals with obesity and COVID-19: A global perspective on the epidemiology and biological relationships. *Obesity Reviews, 21*, 1–17. doi:10.1111/obr.13128

Powell, L. M., Andreyeva, T., & Isgor, Z. (2020). Distribution of sugar-sweetened beverage sales volume by sugar content in the United States: Implications for tiered taxation and tax revenue. *Journal of Public Health Policy, 41*, 125–138. doi:10.1057/s41271-019-00217-x

Proietto, J. (2016). *Body weight regulation: Essential knowledge to lose weight and keep it off.* Xlibris.

Puhl, R. M., & Brownell, K. D. (2001). Bias, discrimination, and obesity. *Obesity Research*, *9*, 788–805. doi:10.1038/oby.2001.108

Puhl, R. M., Lessard, L. M., Pearl, R. L., Himmelstein, M. S., & Foster, G. D. (2021). International comparisons of weight stigma: Addressing a void in the field. *International Journal of Obesity*, *45*, 1976–1985. Doi:10.1038/s41366-021-00860-z

Rieger, E., Lee, Y. F., Monaghan, C., Zwickert, K., & Murray, K. (2021). *Measuring social processes in weight management: The Weight-Related Interactions Scale (WRIS)*. doi:10.1007/s40519-021-01208-2

Rieger, E., Wilfley, D. E., Stein, R. I., Marino, V., & Crow, S. J. (2005). A comparison of quality of life in obese individuals with and without binge eating disorder. *International Journal of Eating Disorders*, *37*, 234–240. doi:10.1002/eat.20101

Rubino, F., Puhl, R. M., Cummings, D. E., Eckel, R. H., Ryan, D. H., Mechanick, J. I., . . . Rosenbaum, M. (2020). Joint international consensus statement for ending obesity stigma. *Nature Medicine*, *26*, 485–497. doi:10.1038/s41591-020-0803-x

Ruiz-Hernandez, A., Kuo, C. C., Rentero-Garrido, P., Tang, W. T., Redon, J., Ordovas, J. M., . . . Telles-Plaza, M. (2015). Environmental chemicals and DNA methylation in adults: A systematic review of the epidemiologic evidence. *Clinical Epigenetics*, *7*, 55. doi:10.1186/s13148-015-0055-7

Salminen, P., Helmiö, M., Ovaska, J., Juuti, A., Leivonen, M., Peromaa-Haavisto, P., . . . Victorzon, M. (2018). Effect of laparoscopic sleeve gastrectomy vs laparoscopic Roux-en-Y gastric bypass on weight loss at 5 years among patients with morbid obesity: The SLEEVEPASS randomized clinical trial. *JAMA*, *319*, 241–254. doi:10.1001/jama.2017.20313

Shaikh, A., Yaroch, A., Nebeling, L., Yeh, M., & Resnicow, K. (2008). Psychosocial predictors of fruit and vegetable consumption in adults: A review of the literature. *American Journal of Preventive Medicine*, *34*, 535–543. doi:10.1016/j.amepre.2007.12.028

Simões, C. F., Junior, N. N., Locatelli, J. C., de Souza Mendes, V. H., de Oliveira, G. H., Werneck, A. O., . . . Lopes, W. A. (2021). A structural equation modelling associating obesity and body dissatisfaction with health-related biopsychosocial parameters in adolescents. *Current Psychology*. doi:10.1007/s12144-021-01399-y

Spreckley, M., Seidell, J., & Halberstadt, J. (2021). Perspectives into the experience of successful, substantial long-term weight-loss maintenance: A systematic review. *International Journal of Qualitative Studies on Health and Well-being*, *16*, 1–20. doi:10.1080/17482631.2020.1862481

Sutin, A. R., & Terracciano, A. (2013). Perceived weight discrimination and obesity. *PloS ONE*, *8*, e70048–70051. doi:10.1371/journal.pone.0070048

Swinburn, B., Egger, G., & Raza, F. (1999). Dissecting obesogenic environments: The development and application of a framework for identifying and prioritizing environmental interventions for obesity. *Preventive Medicine*, *29*, 563–570. doi:10.1006/pmed.1999.0585.

Teixeira, A., Gabriel, R., Quaresma, L., Alencoão, A., Martinho, J., & Moreira, H. (2021). Obesity and natural spaces in adults and older people: A systematic review. *Journal of Physical Activity and Health*, *18*, 714–727. doi:10.1123/jpah.2020-0589

Townshend, T., & Lake, A. (2017). Obesogenic environments: Current evidence of the built and food environments. *Perspectives in Public Health*, *137*, 38–44. doi:10.1177/1757913916679860

Treasure, J., & Ambwani, S. (2021). Addressing weight stigma and anti-obesity rhetoric in policy change to prevent eating disorders. *The Lancet, 398*, 7–8.

Tsai, A. C., Mendenhall, E., Trostle, J. A., & Kawachi, I. (2017). Co-occurring epidemics, syndemics, and population health. *Lancet, 389*, 978–982. doi:10.1016/S0140-6736(17)30403-8

Uranga, R. M., & Keller, J. N. (2019). The complex interactions between obesity, metabolism and the brain. *Frontiers in Neuroscience, 13*, 513. doi:10.3389/fnins.2019.00513

Valenzuela, P. L., Santos-Lozano, A., Torres Barrán, A., Fernández-Navarro, P., Castillo-García, A., Ruilope, A., . . . Lucia, A. (2021). Joint association of physical activity and body mass index with cardiovascular risk: A nationwide population-based cross-sectional study. *European Journal of Preventive Cardiology*. doi:10.1093/eurpc/zwaa151

Van Gaal, L. F., Mertens, I. L., & De Block, C. E. (2006). Mechanisms linking obesity with cardiovascular disease. *Nature, 44*, 875–880. doi:10.1038/nature5487

Veronese, N., Li, Y., Manson, J., Willett, W. C., Fontana, L., & Hu, F. B. (2016). Combined associations of body weight and lifestyle factors with all cause and cause specific mortality in men and women: Prospective cohort study. *BMC, 355*, i5855. doi:10.1136/bmj.i5855

Weinberger, N. A., Kersting, A., Riedel-Heller, S. G., & Luck-Sikorski, C. (2016). Body dissatisfaction in individuals with obesity compared to normal-weight individuals: A systematic review and meta-analysis. *Obesity Facts, 9*, 424–441. doi:10.1159/000454837

Willett, W., Rockström, J., Loken, B., Springmann, M., Lang, T., Vermeulen, S., . . . Murray, C. J. L. (2019). Food in the Anthropocene: The EAT-*Lancet* Commission on healthy diets from sustainable food systems. *The Lancet, 393*, 447–492. doi:10.1016/S014040-6736(18)31788-4

Woolford, S. J., Sidell, M., Li, X., Else, V., Young, D. R., Resnicow, K., & Koebnick, C. (2021). Changes in body mass index among children and adolescents during the COVID-19 pandemic. *JAMA, 326*, 1434–1436. doi:10.1001/jama.2021.15036

World Health Organization. (2020). *Obesity and overweight*. https://www.who.int/newsroom/fact-sheets/detail/obesity-and-overweight

Youngson, N. A., & Morris, M. J. (2013).What obesity research tells us about epigenetic mechanisms. *Philosophical Transactions of the Royal Society London B Biological Sciences, 368*(1609): 20110337. doi:10.1098/rstb.2011.0337. PMID: 23166398; PMCID: PMC3539363

Zhao, L. (2013). The gut microbiota and obesity: From correlation to causality. *Nature Reviews Microbiology, 11*, 639–647. doi:10.1038/nrmicro3089

Zhou, Z., Macpherson, J., Gray, S. R., Gill, J. M. R., Welsh, P., Celis-Morales, C., . . . Ho, F. K. (2021). Are people with metabolically healthy obesity really healthy? A prospective cohort study of 381,363 UK Biobank participants. *Diabetologia, 64*, 1963–1972. doi:10.1007/s00125-021-05484-6

Wellbeing and Personal Safety

Lessons from Population-Based Strategies to Reduce the Burden of Injury

RUSSELL L. GRUEN, AMIT GUPTA, AND NOBHOJIT ROY ■

INTRODUCTION

During a fundraising campaign for Australia's largest trauma hospital (The Alfred), the people of Melbourne were confronted by a television commercial that opened with a wide-eyed scream and a horrendous crash, followed by smoke, lights and sirens, and emergency teams cutting through twisted metal (see Figures 10.1 and 10.2). It closed with a patient being wheeled into hospital on a trolley, with bloodied bandages, tubes, and monitors, and a nurse leaning over saying reassuringly, 'Don't worry, you're at The Alfred'.

The commercial sent a striking message to all citizens that their personal safety is at risk in activities as mundane as driving from one place to another, but also that help will be there if something terrible happens. It promoted the view that civilised societies protect their citizens from harm and care for them when harmed. Governments do so by providing emergency services, healthcare, and social services. They also regulate products and environments, enforce transport and workplace safety, maintain law and order, and defend against invasion. In Maslow's (1943) famous hierarchy of human needs, safety needs are prerequisite for other forms of fulfilment that ultimately enable people to flourish and realise their potential.

Threats to personal safety are accidental or intentional; can be biological, psychological, social, or environmental in nature; occur in the home, the workplace, in sport and recreation, in public spaces, and in the broader theatres of society; and may be associated with partner and family violence, crime, persecution, terrorism, or war. Fear of being incapacitated is an experience shared by people of all ages and cultures, and, throughout ancient and modern times, people spend

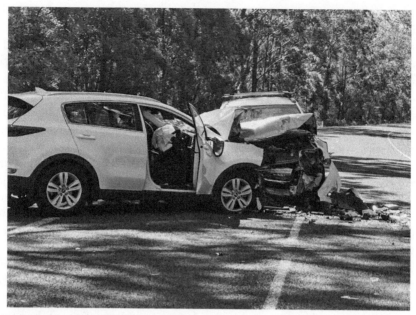

Figure 10.1 Car crash in Victoria, Australia.
Photograph by Jessica Clifford © 2020 ABC. Reproduced by permission of the Australian Broadcasting Corporation—Library Sales.

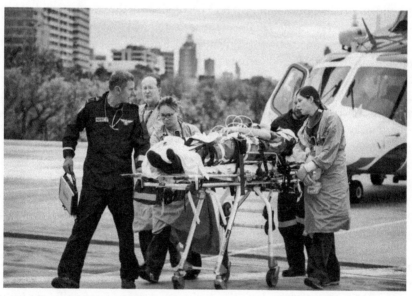

Figure 10.2 Care of the injured by Ambulance Victoria and the Alfred Trauma Service.
Photo by Mark Fitzgerald. Reproduced with permission.

much of their lives trying to recognise, understand, and mitigate its risks. To the degree that subjective wellbeing relates to comfort, health, and happiness at more than a moment in time, and to people's satisfaction with life as a whole, their sense of purpose, and how in control they feel, subjective wellbeing is intimately tied to personal safety (see also Chapter 3, this volume).

Satisfaction with personal safety is included in many scales measuring subjective wellbeing (see, e.g., Australian Unity, 2020). Personal safety differs from other commonly included domains, such as relationships, in that while high satisfaction with relationships is a positive experience (see also Chapter 5 and Chapter 6, this volume), high satisfaction with safety tends to be neutral, and, like pain, its absence is likely to go unnoticed. However, when people feel unsafe it has a large negative impact on individual and community wellbeing. Fear for personal safety impacts wellbeing directly as an unpleasant symptom and also through behavioural responses that aim to avoid or protect in the face of perceived threat (Cummins, 2012).

Much of the research on personal safety and subjective wellbeing has focused on fear of crime, war, or terrorism, especially after the 2001 World Trade Centre attacks. In most communities, such fear is more often based on imagined or anticipatory experience than on actual personal experience. Perceptions of the prevalence of crime or likelihood of a terrorist attack are strongly shaped by media reporting and may be far worse than the actual crime levels or terror risk, causing people to rank their subjective wellbeing lower than it would be if the reporting were more nuanced (Aly, 2012). The policy implications of wellbeing research depend on a rich understanding of how perceptions of the world around us influence people's lives and the validity of the measurement tools employed.

In this chapter, we use trauma systems, which are organised approaches to preventing physical injury and caring for the injured, to consider how cities, states, and nations can advance individual and community wellbeing by promoting individual safety. This selective focus is useful for three reasons. First, most people have direct experience of physical injury and what it is like to be injured. Based in evolutionary biology and survival of the fittest, avoidance of injury is hardwired into our nervous systems, where activation of pain sensors leads to reflex muscle contraction and withdrawal from the stimulus. We pull away even before we have had time to think about it. From infancy we learn to generally avoid sharp, hot, or heavy things that cause pain and injury. Physical injury therefore affords the opportunity to consider how both imagined and actual personal experience might influence subjective wellbeing.

The second reason to take this approach is that trauma systems can influence both individual and community wellbeing in a number of ways. Serious injury, and the ensuing disability, may impact not only on an individual's perceived health and personal safety, but also on the other domains of wellbeing including relationships, achievement in life, standard of living, and future security. Furthermore, while trauma systems primarily serve those who have been injured, their existence reassures the community that help will be provided if and when it is needed in the future. By being there, they promote the wellbeing of all. Research investigating which indicators of the Sustainable Development Goals (SDGs) reliably predict life satisfaction found that road traffic injuries had a significant impact in both developed and developing countries (Kubiszewski, Mulder, Jarvis, & Costanza, 2021; for an overview of the SDGs, see Chapter 21, this volume).

Third, as a public policy intervention designed to improve wellbeing across a jurisdiction by reducing the burden of injury, studying trauma systems provides opportunities for insight about how they work, what it takes to make them work, and what implications there are for other whole-of-population initiatives. Because public media campaigns have often played a significant role in trauma system development, we can learn about the role of media reporting in perceptions of personal safety and subjective wellbeing. And with global interest in injury reduction, we should consider how this knowledge might be transferred and applied in other settings (Bragge & Gruen, 2018).

A SYSTEMS APPROACH TO PREVENTING INJURY AND CARING FOR THE INJURED

Injuries are a major global cause of death and disability. In 2019, an estimated 4.3 million people died following injury, representing 7.6% of all deaths and 11.0% of years of life lost. Furthermore, because they disproportionately affect young people, injuries often result in long-term disability. The three major types—road transport accidents, unintentional injuries, and self-harm and interpersonal violence—each cause approximately one-third of the global burden of injury (GBD 2019 Diseases and Injuries Collaborators, 2020).

Increasing attention to the human and economic consequences led the UN General Assembly to declare two consecutive Decades of Action for Road Safety (2011–2020 and 2021–2030) (United Nations, 2011). The World Health Organization (WHO, 2021) has the ambitious target of halving the absolute number of road traffic deaths and injuries by 2030. Three of the five pillars relate to prevention, including safer roads, safer vehicles, and safer road user behaviour. The other pillars address, first, what happens after someone is injured, referred to as the 'post-crash response' and, second, the overarching governance of all these interrelated activities.

In combination, prevention, post-crash response, and how they are managed are the key components of a trauma system (Figure 10.3). Instead of an isolated specialist hospital, a trauma system is an organised, coordinated effort in a defined geographic area that involves multiple agencies, is integrated with the local public health system, promotes injury prevention, and delivers the full range of care to all injured patients through prehospital, hospital, and rehabilitation services.

High-performing trauma systems have mechanisms to ensure good governance and accountability to their funders, providers, and the communities they serve, and they are underpinned by robust monitoring and incentives for system improvement. Sophisticated trauma registries enable precise definition, collection, reporting, and analysis of data about who is injured and the circumstances

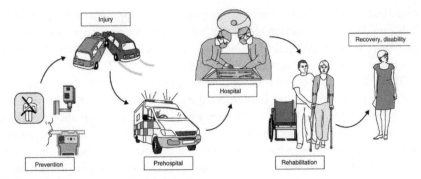

Figure 10.3 Components of a trauma system.
From Gruen et al. (2012). *British Journal of Surgery, 99*(Suppl_1;January 2012), 97–104.
https://doi.org/10.1002/bjs.7754

in which they were injured, what injuries they sustained, how they were treated, and their outcomes (see Australia New Zealand Trauma Registry [ATR], 2022).

Abundant evidence attests to trauma system effectiveness. One of the best systems studied is in Victoria, a southeastern state of Australia that is slightly larger than Great Britain in size (Bragge & Gruen, 2018). In 1969, Victoria had a population of approximately 4 million, and 1,034 people were killed in road traffic crashes, making it a jurisdiction with one of the world's highest per capita rates of road deaths (Figure 10.4). At the time, speed, alcohol, and other risk-taking behaviours were rife, especially among young males, and little attention was paid

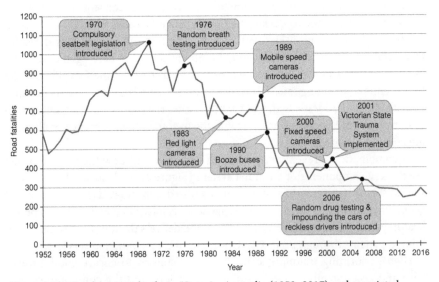

Figure 10.4 Road trauma deaths in Victoria, Australia (1952–2017) and associated legislative interventions.
Figure by author; data from Transport Accident Commission; see Bragge and Gruen (2018).

to safety in vehicle and road design. Carnage ensued for vehicle occupants, pedestrians, and cyclists. The care injured people received was ad hoc, poorly coordinated, and often inadequate to treat the injuries sustained, resulting in much preventable death and disability. In the 50 years since, this situation has been dramatically turned around through safer roads and vehicles, safer road user behaviour (Productivity Commission, 2017), and better trauma care. The per capita death rate has been cut by 85%, and Victorians, living in a state with near double the population that it was in 1969, now take seriously the prospect of eliminating road traffic fatalities altogether.

This achievement is the product of novel and sustained approaches to preventing injury, saving lives, and optimising recovery. Beginning with the world's first compulsory seatbelt legislation in 1970, the Victorian government repeatedly introduced progressive road safety legislation. Standards for road and vehicle design, licensing and regulatory changes, and the introduction and policing of road safety laws all contributed to reducing the road toll.

In 2001, the post-crash response was overhauled, and the Victorian State Trauma System (VSTS) was implemented. It aimed to provide each injured patient with excellent care where and when it was needed, ensuring that the transitions between phases of care were seamless and that existing resources were best integrated to optimise patient outcomes.

Designed to kick in from the moment of injury, a single state-wide emergency number and triage and transfer protocols ensure that each case has the appropriate degree of urgency based on standard criteria. When major trauma criteria are met, on-scene ambulance paramedics liaise directly with a specialised state-wide advisory and retrieval service that coordinates the clinical needs of the patient and the logistics of the retrieval, whether it be by road or by air. Victoria's relatively small geographic size makes most of its population reachable by specialised ambulance helicopters that are able to collect the patient at the roadside and deliver them straight to the helipad of a major trauma centre, bypassing nonspecialist hospitals. Prehospital care is provided at the scene and en route by highly trained ambulance paramedics using robust protocols and advanced technologies. They are trained to perform lifesaving procedures that were previously only provided in hospital settings, such as endotracheal intubation, treatment of collapsed lungs, haemorrhage control and blood transfusions, and advanced life support for cardiac arrest.

The retrieval service not only directs the transfer, but also facilitates preparations at the receiving hospital by providing critical information that enables the emergency department to assemble their team and ready equipment and operating theatres for the patient's arrival. The new state-wide trauma system designated three hospitals (the Alfred Hospital, the Royal Melbourne Hospital, and the Royal Children's Hospital) as major trauma services, to which almost all seriously injured patients are transported. These high-volume services have developed concentrated expertise in caring for the injured, with 24-hour emergency teams and well-rehearsed protocols; experienced specialists in all aspects of resuscitation, surgery, radiology, and critical care; and advanced diagnostic and therapeutic

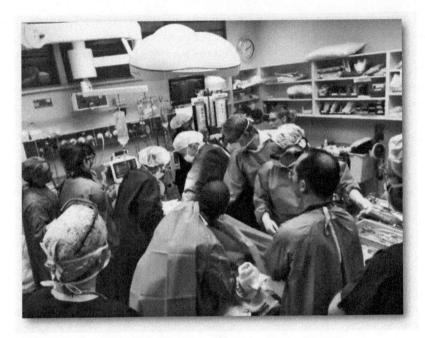

Figure 10.5 Major trauma resuscitations involve many people and concurrent urgent activities.
Photo taken and supplied by Mark Fitzgerald (2018). Reproduced with permission.

modalities (Figure 10.5). This has proven especially important in the team-based resuscitation of severely injured patients in the emergency department, in radiology, or in surgery, where time-critical decisions and skilfully executed interventions are often needed for patient survival.

Following emergency department care, major trauma patients are admitted to hospital. For the most severely injured, this means a period of time in the intensive care unit (ICU), which offers life support, ongoing treatment, continuous monitoring, and intensive nursing. Patients in the ICU may need further surgery and vital organ support, nutrition, bowel and bladder care, and skin care. Visiting family members, who are often coming to terms with the gravity of a loved one's injuries, are also provided with a range of supports.

From the moment that resuscitation is complete, the recovery process begins, aiming to restore the patient as far as possible to their preinjured state. Even while still in ICU each patient is assigned a case manager who begins planning the care that will be needed after hospital. Once weaned off life support, and when intensive care is no longer required, patients are transferred to a hospital ward. Here ongoing medical and nursing care continues, often involving further surgery. Rehabilitation commences on the ward, and sometimes even in the ICU, involving a range of allied health professionals including physiotherapists, occupational therapists, psychologists, social workers, nursing staff, and other specialists.

From soon after arrival at hospital, collaborative multidisciplinary teams foster a shared awareness of each patient's particular medical, physical, mental, emotional, and social needs. When patients no longer need inpatient hospital care they are discharged home or, if necessary, to specialist inpatient rehabilitation or long-term care facilities. Case managers continue to have a significant coordinating role, helping patients and their families navigate the rehabilitation, medical and allied health specialists, and social services involved in supporting their ongoing recovery and disability needs.

In addition to the streamlined system of care, three other components of the new state-wide trauma system are crucial: provider education to support high performance at every stage of care, a new trauma registry, and system governance (Department of Human Services, Victoria, 2009). A next-generation trauma registry was established to collect data—about the circumstances, injuries, care provided, and outcomes for every patient—that could guide all aspects of the system. Until then most trauma centres used 'dead' or 'alive' at the time of hospital discharge as the main outcome measure of trauma care. This is generally inadequate because it says nothing about the premature deaths and the burden of disability among patients who survive to be discharged, nor about the care provided after hospital. These shortfalls were addressed with new ways to collect data, using trained telephone interviewers at regular intervals after injury post-discharge to administer measures of physical capabilities, mental health, pain, return to work and school, use of health and social services, family disruption, and quality of life. The registry is sufficiently resourced to have high coverage, significant precision, and analytic power, and it is an invaluable resource for appreciating the burden of injury, monitoring outcomes, assessing and reporting on performance, diagnosing systemic problems, and guiding innovations and corrective strategies (Figure 10.6).

The trauma registry informs the State Trauma Committee and, ultimately, the Minister for Health, about injury in the state and the performance of its trauma system. In response to that information, the Committee, on which consumers, funders, and provider organisations are represented, recommends protocol changes, service improvements, training activities, and remedial actions, and the registry enables monitoring of impact.

THE IMPACT ON INDIVIDUAL HEALTH AND WELLBEING

In only a few years following its introduction in 2001, the VSTS had significantly reduced the time taken to deliver severely injured and bleeding patients to the necessary level of care. The proportion treated at a major trauma centre increased from less than half to more than 9 out of 10, and many were transferred directly from the crash scene to the trauma centre by helicopter. With timely critical care, lives were saved that would otherwise have been lost. Within a decade of implementation of the new VSTS, the risk that anyone injured would die, all other

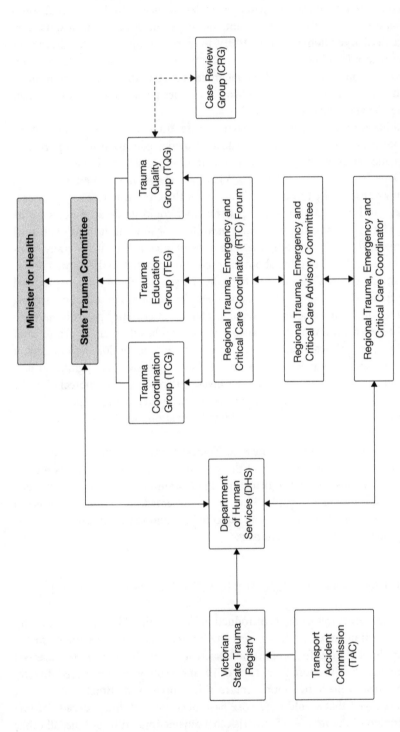

Figure 10.6 Initial governance structure for the Victorian State Trauma System. The State Trauma Committee reports directly to the Minister of Health and receives input about performance from several different sources, including the registry and case reviews. From Victorian Government's 'Trauma towards 2014' report (and 2009).

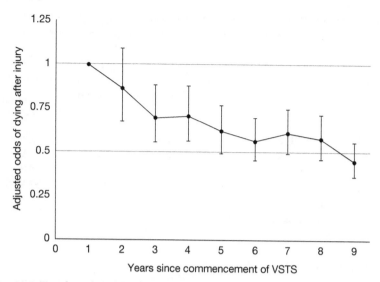

Figure 10.7 Trends in the odds of in-hospital death of major trauma patients adjusted for age, injury severity, head injury, and mechanism in the first 9 years of the VSTS. Reproduced from the Department of Health, Victoria (2011).

things being equal, was halved. Few interventions in medicine have been so effective at reducing mortality (Figure 10.7).

The new trauma registry was also a powerful new tool for understanding survivors' quality of life. As the system matured, it became clear that functional outcomes improved along with survival rates, allaying concerns that the system might be saving lives only for the survivors to remain highly disabled and dependent on long-term supportive care. Instead, the number of severely injured people who were able to return to family, community, and work life increased across the board (Department of Health, Victoria, 2011, 2013). Everyone involved, especially payers, welcomed these findings and the reduced overall societal costs of each case (Gabbe et al., 2014).

On the other hand, the newly available information about the quality of survival also revealed a prolonged and underappreciated burden of injury, especially among patients with brain, spinal cord, or major orthopaedic injuries. One year after 'major trauma', at least one in five patients had not recovered to their preinjury level of function, had not returned to work, were not able to live independently, or were still experiencing significant pain (Table 10.1).

It became clearer that many patients needed ongoing support, some lifelong, after their emergency and hospital care. In light of the data, assessment was made about how well these needs were being met by rehabilitation and support services which, unlike hospitals, had been a range of diffuse and largely uncoordinated community-based public and privately funded providers operating with little oversight, accountability, or quality control. The review found the sector often left patients' needs unmet and their outcomes suboptimal.

Table 10.1 Medium- and longer-term outcomes of survivors of major trauma in Victoria based on data collected on more than 2000 cases from 2006 to 2010

Outcome	Time since injury		
	6 months	12 months	24 months
	%	%	(%)
Incomplete functional recovery	81.9	77.7	72.1
Not yet returned to work	38.4	31.4	27.8
Moderate to severe pain	21.0	20.0	20.0
Moderate to severe disability – physical health (PCS-12)	45.3	40.5	37.4
Moderate to severe disability – mental health (MCS-12)	22.2	23.0	20.4

From Department of Health, Victoria, 2011.

In response, greater use was made of case managers dedicated to coordinating patients' needs and their support services in two specialist streams: 'Recovery', for those for whom full recovery and early return to normal activities were the goals, and 'Independence', for patients in whom full recovery was unlikely and for whom care and support goals were to achieve as much independence as possible.

When the trauma system was first introduced, few stakeholders predicted that after a few years there would be a significant shift in focus from acute life-saving care to the long trail of rehabilitation, recovery, and independence. Gaps were addressed in disability supports that, while apparent to many survivors, were not widely appreciated in government, healthcare services, or the general population. And to the degree that voice was given to caregivers, glimpses were gained of the broader impact of severe trauma on affected families and communities. The proportion of the population continuing to be affected by road trauma, including those who had not fully recovered and their extended families and informal carers, was brought into sharper focus than ever before.

ADVANCING COLLECTIVE WELLBEING THROUGH THE COMMUNITY AS PARTNER

In fact, community engagement has been central to such a major public policy change and health system redesign. In the development of the VSTS over several decades, community engagement led to three critical enablers for lessening the burden of injury. The first was acceptance of injury as a public policy priority, thereby giving permission for successive governments to implement and enforce a range of initiatives even if they came with other types of discomfort or restriction of civil liberties. As a result, Victoria was among the first jurisdictions in the world to enact road safety legislation for compulsory wearing of seatbelts, random blood alcohol and drug testing of drivers, enforcement of speed limit restrictions, and so on, with significant penalties for breaches that included cancellation of driving licences and confiscation of vehicles.

The second enabler was a sustainable no-fault compulsory third-party motor accident insurance scheme that could finance the new trauma system. Introduced in 1985 and administered by a new government agency, the Transport Accident Commission (TAC), the scheme uses a levy on all motor vehicle registrations to finance all emergency, hospital, rehabilitation, and lifelong disability support costs of people sustaining road transport–related injuries, irrespective of whether the victim was the driver, a passenger, or a pedestrian and without regard to whether they were intoxicated, speeding, or had stolen the vehicle. The scheme addressed the problem that trauma care can be expensive and demands immediacy without knowing whether a patient has insurance and can afford it—a situation that had undermined trauma care in many countries because too many patients lacked the means to pay for the care they received. TAC case managers, who oversee and coordinate each patient's specific service needs, improve service efficiency and reduce the financial, emotional, and logistic burden on families. And through prudent financial management and investment in injury prevention, the TAC guarantees continued coverage of current and projected claims well into the future.

The third enabler was recognition of 'preventable deaths' in the 1990s, providing an imperative for change. Although the road toll was portrayed as a tragedy, a sense of inevitability had lingered that bad things would always happen, and there would always be the unlucky ones who found themselves in harm's way. What was unpalatable, however, was the knowledge that deaths were occurring after people had been seriously injured because the emergency care they received was substandard. Neither the public, the medical profession, nor the politicians liked the idea of people dying unnecessarily. Evidence emerged from monthly meetings of trauma care providers throughout the 1990s that one-third of deaths were preventable or potentially preventable if they had received better care, and this rate had changed little over the decade.

Subsequent headlines in Victoria's major newspapers and lobbying by the medical profession galvanised public opinion and demanded a political response. The conservative government of the day ordered a Ministerial Review of Trauma and Emergency Services. The review forensically examined the system and compared it to state-of the-art systems elsewhere, especially making the most of strong professional relationships that Australian doctors had on the US West Coast. In 1999, the reviewers made 120 recommendations that defined a new system of post-crash response in Victoria (Department of Human Services, Victoria, 1999). Even then, change was not assured because the government lost a state election at the very time the new trauma system was on the cusp of being legislated. That an incoming health minister delivered this legislation as almost his first act in office was testament to the credibility of the reforms, the backing of healthcare providers and, importantly, public sentiment demanding an emergency care system second to none in the world.

The successful introduction of new injury-prevention laws that impacted civil liberties, a trauma care financing system funded through introduction of a new tax, and a major restructure of healthcare services for injured patients that could have been at the expense of services for other needy patients all depended on sustained community engagement and favourable public sentiment. For more than half a century strategic publicly funded mass-marketing programmes have been used in Victoria to shape views of public safety.

They began with a celebrated 1970 newspaper campaign, in which the editor-in-chief of Melbourne's *Herald Sun* 'declared war on 1,034' (the number of people killed in road traffic crashes in 1969) by running a front-page story on road trauma every day for 3 months. This set a pattern of mass media engagement that has led to generations of Victorians being exposed to increasingly sophisticated versions of 'it could be you' type messages portraying graphic images and provocative slogans on roadside billboards, at major sporting events, and on television in their living rooms (Figure 10.8).

The TAC's development and placement of road safety advertising material has been a major component of its investment in road safety in Victoria since 1989. Advertisements have targeted specific safety problems (such as drink-driving, speeding, and restraint non-use) and specific target groups (such as younger and novice drivers, older drivers, and rural drivers). They used a range of styles, including provision of specific information about enforcement programmes and advertisements with strong emotive content incorporating graphic crash scenes and the potential consequences of crash involvement. The high-intensity placement of more than 40 television advertisements between 1989 and 2000 won the creators numerous awards and earned global recognition (see, e.g., Transport Accident Commission [TAC], 2010). To all intents and purposes, these

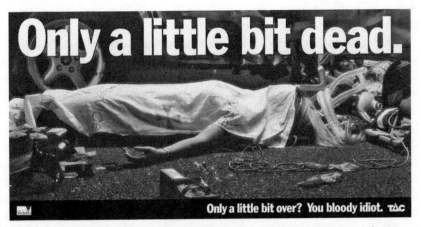

Figure 10.8 Roadside billboard as part of a TAC advertisement campaign combating drink driving. Used with permission from the Transport Accident Commission, Victoria.

commercials have been an integral and inseparable part of a highly effective state-wide programme of legislation, intensive traffic enforcement, and road and vehicle safety improvements that together significantly reduced Victoria's road toll.

The use of shock tactics to motivate individual action was a strategy pioneered two years earlier in the Grim Reaper television advertisements that aired to the Australian public in 1987, to encourage safe behaviours that afford protection from HIV and AIDS. The Grim Reaper was portrayed at a bowling alley with pins represented by average Australians, including mothers and young children. A foreboding voice-over warned that, 'At first, only gays and IV drug users were being killed by AIDS, but now we know every one of us could be devastated by it,' while the Reaper bowled, striking down his victims. The public response was immense, with many complaints that it was too frightening, especially for children, and that it unfairly portrayed gay people. Nonetheless, the campaign was widely recognised as a landmark public health initiative, and it paved the way for a similar strategy in road safety (Magnus, 2006; Double Denim Days, 2020).

The responses to the Grim Reaper advertisement suggested that, in their use of fear as a motivator for change, confronting commercials might negatively influence community perceptions of personal safety. However, there is little evidence available to support this hypothesis. In fact, of the states and territories in Australia, Victoria has among the highest levels of subjective wellbeing, and collective measures of the personal safety component have steadily increased since 2001, when the Australian Unity Wellbeing Index was first implemented (Capic et al., 2016). Attributing this to the development of the state trauma system is impossible, but it is relevant here to consider how 50 years of community-wide messaging may have shaped perceptions. At least there does not appear to be evidence that health outcomes and population-wide perceptions of personal safety are at odds. An evaluation of the TAC approach in 2000 highlighted emotional reactions to the uncomfortable content of the advertisements and also more cognitive responses to the seriousness of the content and how well it was presented. The evaluators made clear to the government sponsors the discomfort they were inflicting on their society, but also their view that the likelihood of an advertisement resulting in a behaviour change depended on its ability to evoke uncomfortable emotions (Harrison & Senserrick, 2000).

While successive governments in Victoria were willing to use shock and fear as a tool to promote public safety, the community was not entirely indifferent to the emotional toll of their campaigns. Once the long-term burden of injury was more fully appreciated, and with greater realisation that physical trauma and psychological trauma can coexist and re-exposure might harm survivors and their families, a subtle but noticeable shift in approaches to community awareness occurred. Alongside the shocking 'it could be you' approaches were campaigns, such as the community support group that led with the slogan 'Touched by the road toll,' which clearly acknowledged that many members of the community had been affected by road trauma, if not through their own experience, then by affecting someone else they knew or had known.

This shift connects with the wider controversy in research on the use of negative emotional messaging in media campaigns. For example, while increasing the intensity of negative imagery depicting vehicle crashes is effective in yielding stronger emotional responses, this does not necessarily translate into stronger intentions to change risky driving behaviours (Borawska, Oleksy, & Maison, 2020). Moreover, the attention-grabbing capacity of such images may be least effective in the very groups they are designed to target, that is, those with a risky driving style. Psychological models developed to predict people's engagement in health-related behaviours (e.g., speeding vs. driving safely) point to a wide range of relevant constructs (e.g., self-efficacy to perform the behaviour and subjective norms regarding the acceptability of the behaviour) in addition to the perception of threat, with research indicating that these constructs may even be more potent predictors than the threat components (e.g., Bui, Mullan, & McCaffery, 2013). Relatedly, research has found that gain-framed messages (e.g., 'respected speed limit = less crashes') result in less speeding than loss-framed messages (e.g., 'exceeded speed limit = more crashes') (Chaurand, Bossart, & Delhomme, 2015). Thus there is greater scope for integration of the extensive psychological literature on models of health behaviours and public media campaigns.

Notwithstanding the ongoing refinement of media messaging, the combination of public health measures, financial enablers, and a political trigger in Victoria led to a rare sustained system-wide transformation, one that has had significant impact on the overall health and wellbeing state-wide. Each of these initiatives was contingent on deliberate sustained community engagement. The development of the VSTS is a valuable case study in public policy and societal change (Bragge & Gruen, 2018).

APPLYING THE LESSONS TO THE GLOBAL BURDEN OF INJURY

It is now widely recognised around the world that the development of civilian trauma systems is the single most significant improvement in the care of injured patients (Pepe, Marttos, Lynn, & Augenstein, 2008). Following the UN Declaration of a Decade of Action, in 2013, the WHO launched its Global Alliance for Care of the Injured (GACI). Informed by the VSTS and others like it, the Global Alliance defined three fundamental tasks for any trauma system: (1) life-saving care at the scene, (2) timely treatment of injuries, and (3) restoration of function and independence (WHO, n.d.) (Figure 10.9).

While the achievements in reduction of injury-related harm in high-income countries were impressive, they exposed some key questions created by a fundamental paradox in road trauma: rapid industrialisation in low-income and middle-income countries has brought with it an epidemic of road traffic injury-related mortality and morbidity, and the greatest burden of injury now exists in countries least prepared to deal with it (e.g., see Tran et al., 2021). Are these achievements relevant and possible in low- and middle-income countries that bear the lion's share

Death rate from road accidents, 2019
The annual number of deaths from road accidents per 100,000 people.
Deaths include those from drivers and passengers, motorcyclists, cyclists and pedestrians.

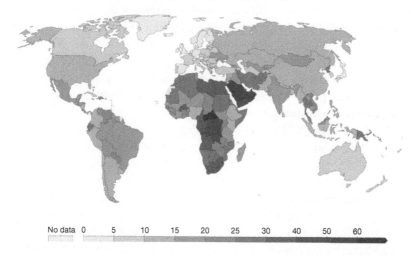

No data   0   5   10   15   20   25   30   40   50   60

OurWorldInData.org/causes-of-death • CC BY
Source: IHME, Global Burden of Disease (2019)
Note: To allow comparisons between countries and over time this metric is age-standardized.

Figure 10.9 Age-standardised death rate from road accidents per 100,000 people, 2019. From Hannah Ritchie and Max Roser (2018). "Causes of death". Published online at OurWorldInData.org. 'https://ourworldindata.org/causes-of-death' [Online Resource] Reproduced under a CC BY 4.0 license.

of the global burden of injury and where helicopter retrieval systems (amongst other resources) are unaffordable? Are there strategies in low-income settings that could be applied without large investments and wholesale health system change? What lessons can we learn, and how can these learnings be applied?

In 2013, the Australian and Indian governments embarked on a collaboration to apply the lessons learned from Victoria in four Indian cities, recognising that, while India had more than 400,000 road trauma deaths per year, trauma care systems were in their infancy (National Trauma Research Institute, 2013). The programme, the Australia–India Trauma Systems Collaboration (AITSC), led to development and implementation of a multi-institutional shared trauma registry and four low-cost but innovative 'best-buy' pre-hospital, hospital, and post-hospital care interventions that could be separately implemented without extensive health system change, that capitalise on new technologies where relevant, and that could be readily evaluated. The interventions were a system of pre-hospital notification to allow the trauma team to assemble prior to patient arrival; a computerised decision support system to reduce errors in complex resuscitation scenarios; institutional quality improvement programmes that asked, for each death, whether care could have been improved; and a simple home-based family-supervised rehabilitation prescription to improve physical recovery of patients with lower-limb injuries (Australia–India Trauma Systems Collaboration [AITSC], 2016).

The programme aimed to rigorously evaluate these four trauma system components as they were introduced in participating sites in India and, at the same time, lay the foundations of a nationally relevant trauma system for the benefit of injured people in India. It used established partnerships and Australian and international injury and trauma systems expertise, combined with an unparalleled living 'laboratory', for understanding the effects of new interventions that high-volume Indian centres provide. It also included putting in place procedures for monitoring system performance; collecting baseline data about injuries, management, and outcomes; consulting about potential feasible interventions; instituting workshops for system-wide capacity building; evaluating interventions, and consulting with key Australian and Indian Government stakeholders (Figure 10.10).

The feasibility and the outcomes of these pilot interventions, as well as data from the trauma registry (Shivasabesan et al. 2019), laid some foundations for a nationally relevant trauma system for the benefit of injured people in India (Mitra et al., 2017; Ministry of Road Transport and Highways, Transport Research Wing, 2018). It has also served to build the capacity of trauma care providers, managers, and government officials for initiating and maintaining better systems of trauma care and improving the quality of existing services (Gruen et al., 2012), and it enhanced knowledge about barriers and facilitators in undertaking system-level change in Indian healthcare settings. Importantly, the partnership created a network of like-minded clinicians, managers, and researchers in Australia and India to further improve care of the injured through future research, policy, and practice partnerships, leading to reductions in preventable deaths and disability after serious injury. The Indian Ministry of Health has prioritised trauma care

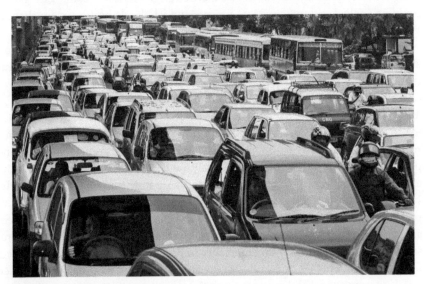

Figure 10.10 Traffic jam in India, 2019.
Photograph by Murali Krishnan © 2017 ABC. Reproduced by permission of the Australian Broadcasting Corporation—Library Sales.

improvement in its 5-year plans and is likely to be receptive to system developments that lead to productivity gains; reduced personal, social, and healthcare costs; and improved community wellbeing.

SUMMARY

In this chapter, we explored the association between injury in ordinary society, its effect on perceived personal safety and other domains of wellbeing, and the relevance of public policy interventions. Even civilian environments present multiple threats to personal safety, among which transport-related injuries are common in urban environments. Many different approaches have advanced safety in the design of roads and vehicles, promoted and enforced safe driver behaviours, and improved emergency care, minimised preventable deaths, and supported eventual recovery. Impact on individual and population-wide health and productivity is evident.

The Victorian case study also makes clear the interdependence of perceptions of injury risk and personal safety and the strategies used to improve safety. Improving safety requires legislative interventions, which in turn require favourable community sentiment, which is principally shaped through public media campaigns. Campaigns that have combined information, threats of penalties, and highly emotive content have been central in attempts to influence safety behaviours and create opportunities for important legislative interventions. But they might also instil community-wide fear that is out of proportion to the risk and exacerbate the psychological and emotional trauma of those who have experienced it before.

Successfully navigating public policy options for enhancing personal safety will increasingly depend on measurement and analysis of a wide range of factors. Much progress has been made in individual-based physical, psychological, and quality of life measures and how they are influenced by a sudden life-changing traumatic event. Efforts are also under way to reduce inequities in personal safety initiatives around the world.

However, there is still much to learn about the community effects of system-wide initiatives and mass marketing strategies, the anxieties and reassurances provided to all citizens by the development of a trauma system 'safety net', cultural nuances and the global applicability of lessons learned in high income countries, and the relative social and economic effects of the various dimensions of subjective wellbeing on which serious injury and its treatment impact. Progress in these areas will advance an integrated science of individual and collective wellbeing.

REFERENCES

Aly, A. (2012). Terror, fear and individual and community well-being. In D. Webb & E. Wills-Herrera (Eds.), *Subjective well-being and security* (pp. 31–43). Springer.

Australia–India Trauma Systems Collaboration (AITSC). (2016). *Australia–India Trauma Systems Collaboration: Reducing the burden of injury in India and Australia.* https://research.monash.edu/en/projects/reducing-the-burden-of-injury-in-india-and-australia-through-deve-2

Australia New Zealand Trauma Registry (ATR). (2022). *The ATR.* https://atr.org.au/

Australian Unity. (2020). *What is the Australian Unity Wellbeing Index?* https://www.australianunity.com.au/wellbeing/What-is-real-wellbeing/What-is-the-Wellbeing-Index

Borawska, A., Oleksy, T., & Maison, D. (2020). Do negative emotions in social advertising really work? Confrontation of classic vs. EEG reaction toward advertising that promotes safe driving. *PLoS ONE, 15*, e0233036. doi:10.1371/journal.pone.0233036

Bragge, P., & Gruen, R. (2018). *From roadside to recovery: The story of the Victorian State Trauma System.* Monash University Publishing.

Bui, L., Mullan, B., & McCaffery, K. (2013). Protection motivation theory and physical activity in the general population: A systematic literature review. *Psychology, Health & Medicine, 18*, 522–542. doi:10.1080/13548506.2012.749354

Capic, T., Cummins, R. A., Silins, E., Richardson, B., Fuller-Tyszkiewicz, M., Hartley-Clark, L., & Hutchinson, D. (2016). *Australian Unity Wellbeing Index Survey 33.0. Report 33.0.*

Chaurand, N., Bossart, F., & Delhomme, P. (2015). A naturalistic study of the impact of message framing on highway speeding. *Transportation Research Part F: Traffic Psychology and Behaviour*, 37–44. doi:10.1016/j.trf.2015.09.001

Cummins, R. A. (2012). Safety and subjective well-being: A perspective from the Australian Unity Wellbeing Index. In D. Webb & E. Wills-Herrara (Eds.), *Subjective well-being and security* (pp. 13–29). Springer.

Department of Health, Victoria. (2013). *Victoria State trauma registry 1 July 2011 to 30 June 2012: Summary report.*

Department of Health, Victoria (Victorian State Trauma Outcome Registry and Monitory Group). (2011). *Victorian State trauma registry 1 July 2009 to 30 June 2010 – summary report.*

Department of Human Services, Victoria. (1999). *Review of trauma and emergency services Victoria 1999: Final report of the Ministerial Taskforce on trauma and emergency services and the Department Working Party on emergency and trauma services.* https://www.health.vic.gov.au/sites/default/files/migrated/files/collections/research-and-reports/t/t2rev---pdf.pdf

Department of Human Services, Victoria. (2009). *Trauma towards 2014: Review and future directions of the Victorian State Trauma System.* https://www.health.vic.gov.au/sites/default/files/migrated/files/collections/policies-and-guidelines/t/trauma_towards_2014---pdf.pdf

Double Denim Days. (2020). *'Grim Reaper' ad campaign (1987).* https://www.youtube.com/watch?v=mSmaWEK_rD4

Gabbe, B. J., Lyons, R. A., Fitzgerald, M. C., Judson, R., Richardson, J., & Cameron P. A. (2014). Reduced population burden of road transport-related major trauma after introduction of an inclusive trauma system. *Annals of Surgery, 261*(3):565–572. doi:10.1097/SLA.0000000000000522

GBD 2019 Diseases and Injuries Collaborators. (2020). Global burden of 369 diseases and injuries in 204 countries and territories, 1990–2019: A systematic analysis for the Global Burden of Disease Study 2019. *Lancet, 396*, 1135–1222.

Gruen, R. L., Gabbe, B. J., Stelfox, H. T., & Cameron, P. A. (2012). Indicators of the quality of trauma care and the performance of trauma systems. *British Journal of Surgery, 99*(Suppl 1), 97–104. doi:10.1002/bjs.7754

Harrison, W. A., & Senserrick. T. M. (2000). *Investigation of audience perceptions of Transport Accident Commission road safety advertising.* Monash University Accident Research Centre Report No. 185.

Kubiszewski, I., Mulder, K., Jarvis, D., & Costanza, R. (2021). better measurement of sustainable development and wellbeing: A small number of SDG indicators reliably predict life satisfaction. *Sustainable Development,* 1–10. doi:10.1002/sd.2234

Magnus, N. (2006). *The AIDS Grim Reaper campaign (A).* The Australian and New Zealand School of Government (ANZCOG) Case Program (2006-90.1).

Maslow, A. H. (1943). A theory of human motivation. *Psychological Review, 50,* 370–396.

Ministry of Road Transport and Highways, Transport Research Wing (2018). *Road accidents in India – 2017.* Government of India.

Mitra, B., Mathew, J., Gupta, A., Cameron, P., O'Reilly, G., Soni, K. D., . . . Fitzgerald, M. (2017). Protocol for a prospective observational study to improve prehospital notification of injured patients presenting to trauma centres in India. *BMJ Open, 7*(7), [e014073]. https://doi.org/10.1136/bmjopen-2016-014073

National Trauma Research Institute. (2013). Australia–India Trauma Systems Collaboration –trauma quality improvement. https://ntri.org.au/trauma-systems/australia-india-trauma-systems-collaboration-trauma-quality-improvement/

Our World in Data. (2020). *Death rate from road accidents, 2019.* https://ourworldindata.org/grapher/death-rates-road-incidents

Pepe, A. M., Marttos, A., Lynn, M., & Augenstein, J. (2008). Trauma systems and trauma triage algorithms. In J. A. Asensio & D. D. Trunkey (Eds.), *Current therapy of trauma and surgical critical care* (pp. 32–46). Elsevier.

Productivity Commission. (2017). *Shifting the dial. 5 year productivity review supporting paper no. 9 – funding and investment for better roads.* Australian Government.

Shivasabesan, G., O'Reilly, G. M., Mathew, J., Fitzgerald, M. D., Gupta, A., Roy, N., Joshipura, M., . . . Australia-India Trauma Systems Collaboration (AITSIC). (2019). Establishing a multicentre trauma registry in India: An evaluation of data completeness. *World Journal of Surgery, 43*(10), 2426–2437. doi:10.1007/s00268-019-05039-2

Tran, T. T., Sleigh, A., & Banwell, C. (2021). Pathways to care: A case study of traffic injury in Vietnam. *BMC Public Health, 21,* 515. doi:10.1186/s12889-021-10539-9

Transport Accident Commission (TAC). (2010, 17 May). *Prestigious international award for TAC ad* [Media release]. http://www.tac.vic.gov.au/about-the-tac/media-and-events/news-and-events/2010-media-releases/prestigious-international-award-for-tac-ad?SQ_ACTION=clear_design name

United Nations. (2011). *Global plan for the decade of action for road safety 2011–2020.* https://cdn.who.int/media/docs/default-source/documents/un-road-safety-collaboration/global_plan_doa_2011-2020.pdf?sfvrsn=a34009ff_3&download=true

World Health Organization. (2021). *Decade of action for road safety 2021–2030).* https://www.who.int/teams/social-determinants-of-health/safety-and-mobility/decade-of-action-for-road-safety-2021-2030

World Health Organization. (n.d.). *WHO global alliance for care of the injured (GACI).* https://www.who.int/initiatives/global-alliance-for-care-of-the-injured

11

An Integrative Perspective on Positive Ageing in Later Life

KANE SOLLY AND NANCY A. PACHANA ■

INTRODUCTION

Life expectancy globally has increased due to successive advancements in disease prevention and management, health promotion, infection control, and public health measures. In 2020, more than 727 million people were aged 65 years and older (9% of the global population), up from 600 million (8%) in 2015 (UN Department of Economic and Social Affairs: Population Dynamics, 2019). This population is predicted to double to 1.5 billion by 2050 (United Nations & Department of Economic and Social Affairs, 2019). The fact that the global population is ageing is a success story, one worth celebrating. Rather than framing ageing as a public health crisis, we should take the time to celebrate the growing normality of reaching old age. Doing so does not detract from the growing issues that arise from an ageing and growing population, including greater demands on healthcare and reduced workforce capacities, but begins combatting the ageist attitudes that so often underlie our societal perceptions and discussions about ageing. Our attention now should be toward supporting older adults to live longer while being healthier, with more meaning, purpose, and self-fulfilment. This need is underscored by the fact that an increase in the quality, meaning, and purpose of life for older adults experiencing an extended lifespan has not been guaranteed and, indeed, has been neglected or undermined by ageist assumptions (Sanyal, 2020). Our current idea of ageing is of a biomedical process of decline and loss, a gradual slide into senility and dependence, while instead we should see ageing for what it is, as an ongoing process of creativity, uniqueness, change, and self-discovery (Sanyal, 2020). We should strive to appreciate the complexity and diversity of the ageing process and recognise, as Sanyal (2020) does, that 'the fruit that an old tree yields [is] an abundance that outweighs the crop of the young' (Sanyal, 2020, p. 5).

There is a light shining on the near horizon. We are seeing global change toward ageing and older adults. We have seen communities and governments collect around older adults in response to the COVID-19 pandemic, we have seen governments globally begin to push for greater care for older adults in the community and in aged care, and the United Nations has declared 2020–2030 the Decade of Healthy Ageing. This is a time for governments, organisations, civil societies, international agencies, academics, professionals, and individuals to collaborate on targeted actions to improve the lives—and our global perception of—older adults. Fundamentally, this is about ensuring that issues pertaining to older adults are front and centre and that, at every level of society, we begin to view ageing as 'the process of developing and maintaining the functional ability that enables wellbeing in older age' (Beard et al., 2015, p. 2151) and to maximise self-determination and wellbeing through the life. The UN decade of healthy ageing seeks to do this through four action areas: addressing societal ageism, developing age-friendly communities, embedding person-centred primary care, and ensuring access to quality residential aged care services to those who need it.

We begin this chapter with a brief overview of these four action areas to clarify the goals being sought for older adults. We then explore the concept of positive ageing, its conception, and its practice globally by organisations and discuss and present how it has been applied within the broader concept of wellbeing. In accordance with our primary aim of providing an integrative lens through which to view wellbeing and ageing across the physical, psychosocial, cultural, and environmental dimensions, we will go on to explore emerging research on the influence of positive ageing on physical, social, and psychological wellbeing and the exciting, new nexus between wellbeing and nature. The opportunities and challenges of ageing demand a systems-level approach to creating contexts in which older individuals can flourish. Our overarching aim is to demonstrate that an integrative approach is necessary to realise the goals of positive ageing.

ACTION AREAS FOR THE DECADE OF HEALTHY AGEING

Changing How We Think, Feel, and Act Toward Age and Ageing

The first goal for the Decade of Healthy Ageing is about addressing societal *ageism*. Ageism is a global issue, manifesting in many overt and covert forms, and this decade is about unveiling these and addressing them at the core. Several identified areas of concern are a lack of agreement about how to define, measure, and analyse central ideas and issues around ageing; a systematic exclusion of older adults from population experiments, including population surveys and clinical trials; and a failure of economic analyses to consider the substantial and diverse contributions older adults make to society, both in paid and un-paid services. Including older adults in the formulation, enactment, and analysis of statistical and experimental data will provide better understanding and appreciation of and for older adults.

This process of challenging and combatting pervasive negative stereotypes is beneficial both for older and younger adults due to the process of internalising ageist stereotypes that eventuate in self-stereotyping in later life (B. R. Levy, 2003). Ageist stereotypes are especially problematic given that they originate in early childhood, develop through reinforcement in adulthood, often operate below awareness, and become self-directed in later life. Thus, left unchallenged, negative attitudes toward ageing and later life eventually become internalised, leading older people to self-discriminate (B. Levy & Schlesinger, 2001). As such, working to challenge these stereotypes and the way we think, feel, and act toward older adults is a political act of self-protection against the harmful effects of ageism that we may all one day be the targets of.

Developing Communities in Ways That Foster the Abilities of Older People

Between 2020 and 2030, the UN is looking to build and maintain the intrinsic capacity of older adults through fostering the development of age-friendly ecosystems/environments. These ecosystems modify existing social and physical services to ensure that older adults can thrive by preserving their functional ability and improving the functional ability of those who have reduced capacity. This goal is multifaceted, with planned improvements seen in the reduction of health risks and also in reducing barriers to and encouraging capacity-enhancing behaviours. Cities and towns should be designed with features ranging from straightforward strategies (e.g., adequate amenities), to accessible transport, to services that foster and celebrate intergenerational engagement. This integrative approach to managing health in ageing through combining both social and health initiatives aims to provide more adaptable and long-term solutions to pervasive issues around ageing.

Delivering Person-Centred, Integrated Care and Primary Health Services That Are Responsive to Older People

Current primary healthcare services are largely unresponsive to the specific needs of older people, and the UN hopes to transform these services so that they deliver person-centred, integrated care to older adults. Redeveloping these systems in ways that do not financially burden the consumer yet focus on the rights and needs of the older person is paramount. There are several strategies identified to achieve this goal: most important is the use of comprehensive assessments to identify frail patients, prevent polypharmacy, and strengthen links between long-term care and health services. This goal also highlights the need to build and sustain an appropriately skilled workforce (Beard et al., 2015).

Providing Older People Access to Long-Term Care When They
Need It

The goal of aged care services should be to facilitate the maintenance of functional ability in older adults who are at high risk of, or currently have, significant
loss of capacity. This should be consistent with the basic rights of the older per-
sona, including ensuring dignity, respect, and fundamental freedoms (e.g., from
harm, neglect, and abuse). However, these systems have many potential benefits
beyond enabling care-dependent older people to live lives of dignity. These benefits include reducing inappropriate use of acute health services, helping families
avoid catastrophic care expenditures, and freeing women in particular to pursue
aspirations beyond caregiving, such as education and formal participation in the
workforce (Beard et al., 2015).

WHAT IS POSITIVE AGEING?

From the global shift against ageist attitudes has sprung a new paradigm that challenges the dominant conceptualisation of ageing that purports ageing to be defined by decline, dysfunction, and social disengagement (Pack, Hand, Rudman,
& Huot, 2019). This new discourse, under the various banners of *positive ageing,
successful ageing,* and *active ageing,* disrupts this idea and reconstructs ageing as a
process determined by individual action, lifestyles, and societal factors, filled with
opportunities for continued enjoyment and flourishment in life. It seeks to create
a more holistic, person-centred, and socially integrated approach to maintaining
wellness across the lifespan.

The Positive Psychology Movement

Positive psychology was first alluded to by Maslow (1954) to combat what was seen
as an almost exclusive focus by psychology at the time on psychopathology and
illness, with little said regarding people's potentialities, virtues, and aspirations—
now dubbed the 'illness ideology' (Maddux, 2008). Positive psychology has thus
attempted to move away from this perspective.

    An important consequence of this focus on disorder and dysfunction has been
the approach and understanding of the concepts of mental illness and mental
health. Mental illness has been the focus of medical and psychological research
for many decades, focusing on abnormality, poor adjustment, sickness, and dysfunction, with little regard for strengths, normality, and health. This has assumed
that mental illness and mental health are points along a continuum, such that
mental illness is the absence of mental health. Recent studies from positive psychology have disconfirmed this idea, finding that mental health (as measured by the

Mental Health Continuum) and mental illness are two distinct yet related constructs (Lamers, Westerhof, Bohlmeijer, ten Klooster, & Keyes, 2011): thus having mental illness does not preclude experiencing mental health. Among a large empirical study of adults experiencing mental illness, more than 14% were experiencing moderate mental health, while almost 2% were flourishing (i.e., experiencing high levels of mental health). This raises an important and meaningful problem in psychology: alleviating mental illness or anguish does not necessitate an equal (or any) improvement in mental health. This has thus become the focus of positive psychology broadly: that is, to focus on the improvement of mental health and wellbeing. A recent systematic review and meta-analysis of positive psychology interventions found that they significantly improved a range of mental health and mental illness measures, including wellbeing, strengths, quality of life, depressive symptoms, anxiety, and stress (Carr et al., 2020). We are beginning to concretely see the benefits of focusing on mental health, as reflected by positive concepts such as quality of life and wellbeing across the population.

Positive Ageing

The goal of positive psychology is to increase the amount of flourishing in an individual's own life and beyond. Positive psychology posits that life transitions need to be interpreted positively in order to maximise wellbeing (Hill, 2010). Positive ageing is thus marked by an ability to engage coping behaviours, flexibility in thought and actions, an affirmation of wellbeing through deciding when to stop activities that are no longer possible, and retaining optimism in the face of decline. It seeks to understand the concepts of recovery, adaptation, and resilience rather than focusing on dysfunction and psychopathology (Bar-Tur & Malkinson, 2014). Positive psychologists argue that wellbeing can be improved, and their research focuses on developing and evaluating interventions and positive psychology exercises that can increase happiness and life satisfaction, thereby encouraging individuals to engage in interesting and meaningful activities (Gallagher & Lopez, 2019). Positive psychology is not simply a psychology of the positive (i.e., happiness, joy, and the range of positive experiences), but rather is about tackling adversity from a strengths-based approach, whereby problems are not viewed as immutable facts but as changeable realities.

Several frameworks have been explored and created to implement positive ageing. Successful ageing was first introduced by Rowe and Kahn (1987, 1997), who described successful ageing as the absence of disease, disability, and risk factors; the maintenance of cognitive and physical functioning; and an active engagement in life. Similarly, the World Health Organization (WHO; 2002a) designed a model of active ageing, which encapsulated all the relevant factors that interact to determine positive ageing including behavioural, social, physical, personal, and economic determinants and health and social services. This model was refined by Paúl, Ribeiro, and Teixeira (2012), incorporating significant contextual

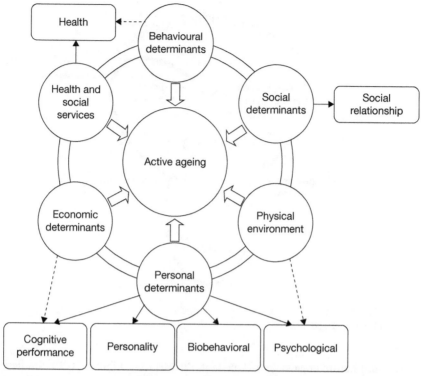

Figure 11.1 Empirically validated WHO active ageing model.
From Paúl, C., Ribeiro, O., & Teixeira, L. (2012). Active ageing: An empirical approach to the WHO model. *Current Gerontology and Geriatrics Research*. https://doi.org/10.1155/2012/382972. Reproduced under a Creative Commons Attribution 3.0 Unported (CC BY 3.0) license.

factors including health, social relationships, cognitive performance, personality, biobehavioural determinants, and psychological determinants (see Figure 11.1). Several other important approaches include productive ageing (Morrow-Howell, Hinterlong, & Sherraden, 2001) and optimal ageing (P. B. Baltes & Baltes, 1990). These models represent how positive ageing is a complex, multifaceted process that incorporates the whole of an individual, not just their physical and mental functioning. As such, positive ageing can be addressed from multiple angles, with each individually varying the value and importance placed on each determinant.

Age-Friendly Ecosystems

The literature around positive ageing interventions is progressively expanding, with a range of interventions and opportunities reported, such as gardening programmes (Scott, Masser, & Pachana, 2015, 2020), physical activity programmes (O'Dwyer, Burton, Pachana, & Brown, 2007), mindfulness activities (Geiger et al.,

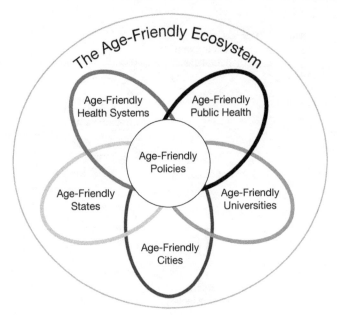

Figure 11.2 The age-friendly ecosystem: A synthesis of age-friendly program. From Fulmer et al. (2020).

2016), and nature engagement (Duedahl, Blichfeldt, & Liburd, 2020). Similarly, positive ageing has been put into practice globally, embodied in several initiatives, one such being the highly successful Age-Friendly Ecosystems (World Health Organization, 2002a). As shown in Figure 11.2, this initiative sought to encourage age-friendly policies and initiatives globally to improve a range of systems, all for the purpose of improving the wellbeing of older adults.

Several initiatives within this broad framework have been successful. For example, age-friendly health systems initiative currently number 625 clinical sites across all 50 states of the United States and in multiple international locations (Fulmer et al., 2020); in 2020, the age-friendly cities and communities initiative included more than 1,000 cities in more than 40 cities, responsible for 240 million people (Fulmer et al., 2020). In addition, there are now more than 70 university institutions putting into practice the age-friendly universities initiative (available at https://www.dcu.ie/agefriendly/age-friendly-members). An example of the guiding principles for age-friendly initiatives is seen in the 10 principles of age-friendly universities, shown in Table 11.1.

Several academics and organisations are also collaborating to incorporate age-friendly philosophies into their practice and to understand how to improve them. For example, the John A. Hartford Foundation worked with five health systems to identify the key starting elements that systems need to provide older adults with the best care. They found that that successful age-friendly healthcare initiatives and interventions have four essential elements, named 'the 4Ms' (see Table 11.2; Fulmer, Mate, & Berman, 2018).

Table 11.1 Age-friendly university principles

1. To encourage the participation of older adults in all the core activities of the university, including educational and research programs
2. To promote personal and career development in the second half of life and to support those who wish to pursue 'second careers'
3. To recognise the range of educational needs of older adults
4. To promote intergenerational learning to facilitate the reciprocal sharing of expertise between learners of all ages
5. To widen access to online educational opportunities for older adults to ensure a diversity of routes to participation
6. To ensure that the university's research agenda is informed by the needs of an ageing society and to promote public discourse on how higher education can better respond to the varied interests and needs of older adults
7. To increase the understanding of students of the longevity dividend and the increasing complexity and richness that ageing brings to our society
8. To enhance access for older adults to the university's range of health and wellness programs and its arts and cultural activities
9. To engage actively with the university's own retired community
10. To ensure regular dialogue with organisations representing the interests of the ageing population

Some Criticisms of Positive Ageing

Despite the successful incorporation of positive ageing concepts on an international scale, several critical gerontologists have disputed some of the central claims and aims of the positive ageing movement. Such gerontologists (e.g., Katz & Calasanti, 2015; Martinson & Berridge, 2015) have drawn attention to the exclusionary potential of some forms of positive ageing discourses. Specifically, discourses surrounding success/health often utilise measures and criteria to

Table 11.2 The '4Ms' for age-friendly healthcare systems

What matters	Know what matters: health outcome goals and care preferences for current and future care, including end of life
	Act on what matters for current and future care, including end of life
Medications	Implement a standard process for age-friendly medication reconciliation
	De-prescribe and adjust doses to be age friendly
Mobility	Implement an individualized mobility plan
	Create an environment that enables mobility
Mentation	Ensure adequate nutrition, hydration, sleep, and comfort
	Engage and orient to maximise independence and dignity
	Identify, treat, and manage dementia, delirium, and depression

Institute for Healthcare Improvement (2019).

determine and assess the quality of how individuals age, suggesting that there is a successful and an unsuccessful way to age. Instead of challenging the prevailing discourse of ageing as a decline, this view may further entrench an ageist perspective, labelling those for whom the effects of ageing are beyond their control as 'unsuccessful'. Assumptions about the ability of individuals across socioeconomic classes to truly be able to 'choose' healthy lifestyles and the 'success' of individuals with longstanding or congenital disorders, for example, are problematic. This has been argued to create a new social duality for ageing—those who age well and those who do not age well—where 'wellness' is measured by the construction of health (Higgs, Leontowitsch, Stevenson, & Jones, 2009) and youthfulness (Gilleard & Higgs, 2000) and defined by meeting certain standards for successful ageing (Crăciun, 2019). The unrealistic nature of these standards is highlighted by the fact that very few older adults have been found to meet them (Hank, 2011). These critiques provide a necessary corrective in calling for an acknowledgement of the physical and mental declines that can occur with ageing while still focusing on optimising the older person's capacity for positive wellbeing, self-fulfilment, and agency (Pack et al., 2019). Nevertheless, it should also be acknowledged that the degree of positive ageing that could be realistically attained by most older adults currently remains unknown given that a thoroughly integrated approach (as we articulate below) has yet to be implemented.

WELLBEING IN LATER LIFE

Positive ageing is largely influenced by the work of positive psychology, which focuses on researching and highlighting the capacities of individuals to strive for wellbeing, acknowledging that individuals do suffer but that this should not be the focus of a holistic and supportive world view. A key focus of positive psychology is wellbeing. There have been several theoretical approaches to wellbeing, including the hedonic/eudaimonic/evaluative wellbeing model and the PERMA model.

The first model of wellbeing categorises wellbeing on three levels: evaluative, hedonic, and eudaimonic (Nikolaev & Nikolaev, 2018; Ryan & Deci, 2001). *Evaluative wellbeing* is best described in terms of people's perceptions of life satisfaction, more commonly labelled as *quality of life*. This type of wellbeing evaluates the overall satisfaction one feels across a range of domains (e.g., health, wealth, social connection, and physical capacity) and across time. It does not assume or designate weights to certain domains, such that life satisfaction captures individuals' satisfaction with the domains that are important to them. Generally, life satisfaction is reflected by a U-shaped curve across the lifespan, peaking in the early years, with a dip between ages 35 and 50, and then increasing again into later life (Blanchflower & Oswald, 2008). A study of Australians older than 50 found that the most valued domains of quality of life were relationships, family, health activities, community, security, belief, independence, and wellbeing (Robleda & Pachana, 2019). For those aged 50–79, family and relationships were valued most highly, while those older than 80 valued health as most important.

Hedonic wellbeing pertains to the generalised feelings and moods that one experiences on a day-to-day basis. In a study by Stone, Schwartz, Broderick, and Deaton (2010) of more than 340,000 individuals in the United States, it was found that hedonic wellbeing was distinctly different from evaluative wellbeing, exhibiting substantially different patterns across the lifespan. Specifically, positively valenced measures (e.g., enjoyment) followed a U-shaped pattern similar to life satisfaction, while negative hedonic measures (e.g., stress) showed either steady decline with age for anger and stress, or an inverted U-shape for worry.

Finally, *eudaimonic wellbeing* is the evaluation of the meaningfulness and purposefulness of life associated with personal and spiritual development (see also Chapter 1, this volume). It involves such broad concepts as self-actualisation (i.e., one's journey to develop and foster creativity, growth, knowledge, and abilities; Ivtzan, Gardner, Bernard, Sekhon, & Hart, 2013). Older adults have been found to have higher levels of and place more importance on the development of self-actualisation than do younger adults (Ivtzan et al., 2013).

The PERMA model of positive wellbeing, also known as 'Flourish' (Seligman, 2011), is a well-established model that frames wellbeing as a process of adaptation, growth, and flourishing while acknowledging health and ageing as integral components that impact one's wellbeing. Seligman has argued that this model is informed by and integrates much of the work of the evaluative/hedonic/eudaimonic model. The PERMA model is composed of five domains: positive emotion, engagement in work and life, positive relationships, meaning in life and work, and accomplishment. It has not been proposed as a new form of wellbeing, but it claims that these five elements constitute the elements of the latent construct of wellbeing (Seligman, 2018). Thus improvement in wellbeing can be achieved through individuals acting in each/any of the domains, as each is intrinsically rewarding in and of itself. The advancement of these domains is suggested to give rise to human flourishing across the lifespan, with the PERMA model used to guide and evaluate positive ageing interventions in older populations. One such positive intervention was the Community Wellbeing and Resilience Program, run by Bartholomaeus, Van Agteren, Iasiello, Jarden, and Kelly (2019). In this study, participants engaged in an 8-week multicomponent wellbeing and resilience programme that utilised weekly training sessions and a peer support component to undertake a community project with the aim to explore how this impacted their wellbeing and resilience. Participants were coached on the development of 10 wellbeing and resilience skills, in ten 90- to 120-minute sessions, including using growth mindsets, cultivating gratitude, responding with interest to others during their interpersonal interactions, and engaging in values-based goals. To assess the effectiveness of this programme in enhancing wellbeing, participants completed the PERMA Profiler (a self-report questionnaire for assessing each of the PERMA domains) at the end of each session. Across two studies, one for the general population and one specifically for older adults, the results found significant effects on the PERMA measures of wellbeing, resilience, and optimism (for the older adults), as well as improvements on a measure of social isolation (in the broader study). In short, this application of the PERMA model found that engaging individuals, and especially older adults, in positive, socially integrated community projects can produce substantial improvements in wellbeing without having to focus on traditional deficit-based models of psychological wellbeing.

PHYSICAL WELLBEING IN LATER LIFE

In 2001, all 191 WHO Member States officially endorsed the WHO's International Classification of Functioning, Disability and Health (ICF), a classification system that provides a standard language and framework to assist in describing health and health-related states (World Health Organization, 2002b). The framework views health and functioning as a complex and dynamic process involving physical changes in body function and structure, along with the capacity of individuals (i.e., the abilities of a person, given a specific health condition) and their level of functioning within their usual environment. The framework acknowledges that ageing may result in a loss of specific functioning, but that individual preferences and intact capacities, as well as environmental factors such as design and accessibility, interact with this. Disability is thus seen as an interaction between health conditions and contextual factors (see Figure 11.3). In this model, physical wellbeing can be seen from three levels: functioning of bodies/body parts, functioning of the whole person, and functioning of the whole person in a social context.

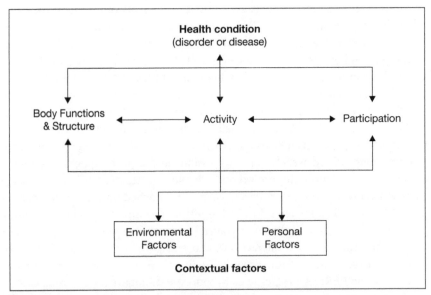

Figure 11.3 Model of disability that is the basis for the ICF.
From World Health Organization. (2002). *Towards a common language for functioning, disability, and health.* WHO. https://cdn.who.int/media/docs/default-source/classificat ion/icf/icfbeginnersguide.pdf. Reproduced under a Creative Commons Attribution-NonCommercial-ShareAlike 3.0 IGO (CC BY-NC-SA 3.0 IGO) license.

Traditionally, physical wellbeing has focused on the former, seeing physical functioning of the body as descriptive of physical wellbeing. This classification allows for the identification of environmental factors that may be facilitating or acting as a barrier to performance.

Starting from this ICF model, we can begin to view ageing in light of the changing capacity of the body and changing performance within the broader environment. As people age, they may experience decreased functioning in certain domains, some of which may result in decreased performance in their regular activities, which will entail a loss of physical wellbeing. Conversely, another individual may experience the same decreased functioning, but it may have no (or minimal) impact on their capacity to perform valued activities, and, as such, physical wellbeing will remain in place. For those with a loss of physical wellbeing, it is useful to look at this through the *Selection, Optimisation, Compensation* (SOC) model.

SOC is a positive ageing model that focuses on the processes that individuals engage in to maximize their gains in response to the changing demands and functionality of ageing (M. M. Baltes & Carstensen, 1996). In this model, *selection* relates to the narrowing of one's life world to fewer domains of functioning, with individuals concentrating on those that are considered most important, though this does not necessitate continuation of the same activities or pastimes (P. B. Baltes & Baltes, 1990). *Optimisation* refers to people's engagement in these specific behaviours and activities that enrich their wellbeing toward self-actualisation. Finally, *compensation* is implemented when there is a loss of functioning that cannot be restored without the provision of some extra resources (physical or mental); this can involve the use of aids or mental strategies. In short, if older adults experience a loss of functioning, they may engage in selection, optimisation, and/or compensation as a way of maintaining positive physical wellbeing.

A large body of literature has examined the role that physical activity plays in keeping healthy in later life. A recent systematic review of studies examining the longitudinal effects of physical activity on healthy ageing found that there is consistent evidence that a range of physical activities is positively associated with healthy ageing across a range of definitions and measurements (Daskalopoulou et al., 2017). A 2013 systematic review of longitudinal cohorts found that physical activity was associated with decreased rates of obesity, weight gain, coronary heart disease, type II diabetes, and dementia (including Alzheimer's disease) (Reiner, Niermann, Jekauc, & Woll, 2013). Another systematic review, though of qualitative studies, found that when older adults engaged in physical activity, they commonly reported regaining feelings of purpose, feeling needed in collective group activity, and creating habitual routines and structures in their day. In overcoming real and perceived barriers to their exercise, and by taking up or sustaining physical activities, older adults can further build self-esteem, all of which contribute to a feeling of greater fulfilment in older age (Morgan, Willmott, Ben-Shlomo, Haase, & Campbell, 2019). Despite the variety of activities available to promote physical wellbeing, there is little consensus around the most effective form of physical activity for older adults (Morgan et al., 2019).

Effective programmes for supporting older adults' physical wellbeing through engagement with social or personal growth activities abound. There are socially minded community programmes, such as gardening (Scott et al., 2015, 2020) and a range of single and multimodal interventions, such as swimming or group-activity programmes (Zubala et al., 2017), and animal-care, animal-assisted activities or pet ownership (see Chowdhury, Nelson, Jennings, Wing, & Reid, 2017; Hughes, Verreynne, Harpur, & Pachana, 2020; Krause-Parello, Gulick, & Basin, 2019). Similarly, the Age Friendly communities initiative described earlier has championed the modification of public services and spaces to accommodate a greater range of physical functioning, with an emphasis on age-friendly structures including simple changes such as wheelchair access. The possibility for engaging older adults in activities that support physical wellbeing are only limited by the imagination. The diverse preferences of older adults, and a focus on their social responsibilities and the value they place on social connection, reflect a need for a whole-system approach that is specifically tailored to meet the social, individual, and environmental needs of older adults rather than focusing on the improvement of their physical wellbeing in isolation. Social policy should be informed by an SOC perspective, creating affordances for older adults to continue or augment their physical performance regardless of their level of physical functioning. This will move our current focus of physical wellbeing away from a medicalised perspective and instead consider physical functioning in relation to the personal and environmental factors that determine physical performance.

SOCIAL WELLBEING AND AGEING

As was evident in our discussion on physical activity, social connection is important to older people, as it is with people of all ages. Our social functioning and our need to feel connected to a larger community does not lessen or change as we age. Humans developed along the evolutionary path consistently engaged with and supported by other humans. Whether through filial or nonfilial connections, and in activities as diverse as social sport, theatre, and the pursuit of knowledge, humans thrive when engaged in social groups. Much research has been done on the development of sociality, from children through to older adults, and social connection is consistently found to be profoundly important. The COVID-19 pandemic heightened and expanded understanding of the value of social connection as people globally were variably under social isolation or lockdown measures. These measures ranged from mandatory masks, social distancing, limited group numbers, and home visits, to whole city lockdowns with forced isolation at home and closure of services, most notably the halting of visitors to aged care facilities. These measures, enacted to try to stop the spread of the virus and preserve the right to life of vulnerable populations, were necessary and effective but also highlighted, on the one hand, the precariousness of our social connections and, on the other hand, our capacity to innovate and develop connections. The COVID-19 social distancing and social isolation measures meant it was more difficult for older adults to engage in social interactions generally. However, a national survey in Australia found older adults (especially those over 75) were less likely to report feeling lonelier within the first 2 months of COVID (Solly & Wells, 2020). Similarly, an American study found that although loneliness increased slightly for older adults, they had a significantly lower average level of loneliness than younger adults (Luchetti et al., 2020). These data are consistent with the general literature that loneliness is more prevalent in most countries in younger people than in those older than age 65 (Barreto, Victor, Hammond, Eccles, Richins, & Qualter, 2021). However, the finding of lower loneliness in older compared to younger people during COVID may also be due to older adults tending to react less to adverse events (Wells, 2017) due to a lifetime of experience in coping with adverse events, with many experiencing World War II, the Cold War, and historical austerity measures. It might also be an example of the adaptability of older adults in utilising the ever-expanding capacities of social media, mobile phones, and video conferencing software to connect with individuals outside of their immediate or local vicinities. Older adults have been one of the main benefactors of this social connection sphere.

That older adults might be more robust against experiences of loneliness is not at all to underestimate the importance of social connection in later life. Indeed, social connection and functioning are especially important in older age as decreases in this are associated with reduced quality of life, including depressive symptoms (Golden et al., 2009); unhealthy behaviours such as smoking, sedentary behaviours, and poor diet (Shankar, McMunn, Banks, & Steptoe, 2011); and reduced physical health such as pain, fatigue, insomnia, and all-cause mortality (Jaremka et al., 2014; Shankar et al., 2011). The importance of social connection and social groups is exemplified by research that has shown that by simply increasing the number of social groups you are a part of or identify with is a protective factor against mortality, enhances wellbeing, and supports better adjustment to retirement (Lam et al., 2018; Steffens, Cruwys, Haslam, Jetten, & Haslam, 2016).

PSYCHOLOGICAL WELLBEING IN LATER LIFE

Psychological wellbeing encompasses the aforementioned components of hedonic, evaluative, and eudaimonic wellbeing. It comes from the complex interplay between multiple facets of one's life—one's physical wellbeing, one's social wellbeing, and also one's internal cognitive processes, appraisals, and evaluations of life events and meaning. People with psychological wellbeing are better able to ride the waves of life, responding constructively to setbacks and savouring successes, to create sustainable and long-term contentment. Much like the previously discussed dimensions of physical and social wellbeing, it is accessible to everyone, regardless of their personal and environmental circumstances. Positive psychology aims to foster and create new adaptive coping behaviours that foster positive mental health.

As people age, they tend to experience a greater number of emotionally stressful events, both positive and negative, with the influx of grandchildren; the loss of siblings, parents, or partners; changing roles through retirement; and health problems, among more seemingly trivial changes such as hair loss, weight gain, or weight loss. These events cause a disruption in the daily psychological equilibrium experienced in the absence of life events, and these can become increasingly difficult to manage when they occur in succession or in tandem. Especially difficult for older adults is a collapse in both physical and social wellbeing (Baker & Procter, 2015; Chapman, 2018; Lavingia, Jones, & Asghar-Ali, 2020). Drastic changes in physical functioning can reduce their perceived ability to engage productively in the world and may create a sense of dependence on and need for social supports. Similarly, as we age and begin losing friends and family, a sense of the finality and closeness of death can be confronting and isolating. Developing positive coping behaviours before and in response to these events is a useful way by which to prepare older adults to cope in the face of changing circumstances.

Laura Carstensen's work on both social relationships and the so-called *positivity effect* contributes to an understanding of the preservation and enhancement of wellbeing in later life. Her *socioemotional selectivity theory* (Carstensen, 1992) posits that one's awareness of a foreshortened future as one ages influences shifts in personal goals and behaviours—and can influence them at any age. For example, younger people tend to pursue goals related to knowledge and older persons tend to prioritise goals linked to meaning. This translates into wider social networks in younger individuals (to best maximise knowledge and information-seeking) and narrowing in later life to those relationships and experiences that are most meaningful. A corollary here is Carstensen's 'positivity effect'—with increasing age, positive memories, stimuli, and relationships become more salient, and negative ones less salient (Carstensen & Mikels, 2005).

In accordance with socioemotional selectivity theory and the positivity effect, research has shown that older adults' social networks, though smaller than those of younger cohorts, provide equal if not greater social support (Lang & Carstensen, 1994). Moreover, older adults actually prune their social networks to maximise positive and meaningful interactions. A focus on the positive has been shown not to be caused by decreasing cognitive capacity in later life; in fact, older adults' relatively greater capacity for cognitive control and emotional regulation actually enhance this ability to focus on the positive (Mather & Carstensen, 2005). Indeed, the waning of negativity found in youth shifting to a positive bias in later life meshes well with positive ageing constructs and potential interventions (Carstensen & DeLiema, 2018).

POSITIVE AGEING IN CULTURAL CONTEXTS

Despite positive psychology's focus on the facilitation and promotion of positive attitudes toward ageing and mental health, several psychologists have questioned the utility of positive psychological perspectives in providing opportunities for cross-cultural applications. Marecek and Christopher (2018) suggest that positive psychology and the discipline of psychology more generally refer to a Western view of mental health, as an individual's functional response to environmental, social, political, and cultural norms, with the role of therapy/interventions to create opportunities for individuals to flourish in their individual contexts and facilitate positive mental health. This view is principally drawn from the ego-centric perspective, as is seen in the previous discussion of the individual's well-being across several domains, and is focused on the individual's capacity for self-determination, differentiation, and growth. Although useful in a Western context, such culturally bound views might resist transcultural application and lack careful consideration of potential transcultural differences—especially in re-lation to the diversity of perspectives, such as sociocentric, cosmocentric, or eco-centric. The discipline of psychology is more culturally bound than is generally acknowledged, reflecting the perspectives of the dominant culture that informs it.

Positive psychology focuses on Western conceptions of positive wellbeing, self-esteem, self-regard, happiness, self-determination, and creation of supportive (and at times larger) social networks. These positive attributes are far from universal, being at times at odds with transcultural understandings of positive mental health and positive attributes. For example, in many Eastern traditions, self-esteem and ego-centred behaviours are seen as traits that should be transcended in order to attain joy, peace, and harmony. Similarly, self-determination and differentiation in social structures is highly valued in Western perspectives of positive psych-ology, while non-Western cultures across Asia and the Americas emphasise the importance of social cohesion and group identities as hallmarks of social func-tioning, wellness, and health. At a minimum, positive psychology must acknow-ledge the culturally bound nature of its beginnings if it is to begin moving toward providing more opportunities for transcultural relevance.

Highlighting the urgency of considering diverse cultural perspectives in the context of positive ageing is that fact that First Nations societies have not shared equally in the longevity benefits of non-Indigenous societies. Steps toward cor-recting this require positive psychology frameworks that avoid further embedding non-Western individuals within Western frames of psychology (Pace & Grenier, 2017). For example, a model of social and emotional wellbeing and mental health was proposed by the Australian Indigenous Psychologists Association to facilitate Indigenous worldviews and culturally relevant perspectives into a holistic psych-ology (Dudgeon & Walker, 2015; Gee, Dudgeon, Schultz, Hart, & Kelly, 2014). Milroy et al. (Chapter 7, this volume) provide a detailed description of this model of social and emotional wellbeing from an Australian Indigenous perspective.

ART, CREATIVITY, AND THE PURSUIT OF BEAUTY

The capacity for human personal expression is a common experience across cul-tural contexts. Globally, art has been used for cultural expression, individual ful-filment, as a method of healing, and as a form of communication. Creative art therapists have been engaging in arts-based community interventions to facilitate mind-body-spirit expression of a range of emotions through the use of expressive practices such as dance, singing, painting, drama, or storytelling (Darewych & Riedel Bowers, 2018). Art is a common form of expression for those experiencing grief, loss, and trauma (Carey, 2006; Thompson & Neimeyer, 2014) and to facilitate developmental changes through adulthood (Darewych, Carlton, & Farrugie, 2015).

In 2000, Gene Cohen released *The Creative Age*, one of the first widely published works championing the creative potential of older adults' lives post-employment (Cohen, 2000). Creativity has been proposed to assist wellbeing in a range of ways, most pertinently through increasing a sense of control and mastery, increasing mind–body coherence, supporting social engagement, and encouraging brain plasticity (Cohen, 2006). It also facilitates the development of problem-solving skills, motivational awareness, and perceptive skills to better manage health and daily experiences (Flood & Phillips, 2007). A 2007 review of creative programmes for older adults found several benefits across art therapy programmes, poetry, journaling, reminiscence, and group activities (Flood & Phillips, 2007).

Artistic expression has been regarded as especially important for older women, who tend to report lower levels of happiness than do their male counterparts (Inglehart, 2002). Negative cultural views of women have contributed to a decreased sense of subjective wellbeing in later life. Yet the capacity for older women to take advantage of changing cultural attitudes to gender as well as tap into their creative endeavours can support meaningful and valued personal pursuits and wellbeing. As such, creating spaces where women are supported to engage in creative tasks and intrinsically motivated activities and identify new activities that facilitate continuation of their self-determined roles is especially important (McHugh, 2016).

WELLBEING THROUGH CONTACT WITH THE NATURAL WORLD

With increasing urbanisation across the globe, we are seeing a rapid receding of green spaces in cities, the loss of nature corridors, and a growing feeling of disconnection from nature. Wellbeing is not only sourced from our intrinsic capacities but also from our environment, including the natural environment. *Biophilia* is the innate human tendency to connect with natural systems and processes, especially with those life and life-like features of non-human environments (Kellert, 2018). This tendency depends on learning, experience, and social support to manifest in daily life and thus requires socially constructed systems that value and encourage nature engagement. Feelings of biophilia have been found to increase across the lifespan (Wickersham, Zaval, Pachana, & Smyer, 2020). This is further supported by findings that physical proximity to nature has been associated with greater longevity (Takano, Nakamura, & Watanabe, 2002) and that, as nature is degraded, health problems and mortality increase (Jardine, Speldewinde, Carver, & Weinstein, 2007; Speldewinde, Cook, Davies, & Weinstein, 2011).

Unfortunately, not all older adults can maintain access to the natural world—this is often the case with residents of aged care facilities. Yet exposure to greenery and nature in these contexts is important and has been found to be supportive of residents' quality of life (Carver, Lorenzon, Veitch, Macleod, & Sugiyama, 2020). These facilities can utilise the 'magic of the mundane', whereby small yet meaningful changes are introduced to increase the exposure of residents to nature. For adults in the community, decreased functionality, especially decreased mobility, is the primary factor that limits whether older adults have connection to nature as they age (Freeman, Waters, Buttery, & van Heezik, 2019). The presence of structures and services informed by age-friendly communities and cities, especially ramps and accessible pathways, are simple measures that can facilitate contact with nature.

Companion pet ownership is a specific instance of biophilia, one involving the human–animal bond, which is important across the lifespan (Pachana, Massavelli, & Robleda-Gomez, 2011). As people age, continuing or beginning pet ownership is a way to express the desire for connection and care of another being. Exposure to animals, whether through ownership or animal-assisted interventions, is beneficial for wellbeing and mental health in older adults (Hughes et al., 2020). The benefits of animal exposure are greatest for live interactions, but simpler interventions including animal calendars and images are also supportive, low-cost measures that are easily implementable in aged care settings.

SUMMARY

The positive ageing movement has important potential impacts on all aspects of later life—from coping with retirement through to maximising creativity and wellbeing. Important theoretical constructs underlie positive psychology and have formed the basis for both effective interventions and policy initiatives. Ageism remains a major barrier to positive ageing, one requiring sustained resistance from those of all generations. While the knowledge silos that exist in research (across psychology, sociology, economics, and so on), policy, and community development have important information, resources, and input to share, what is currently lacking is an integrated and cross-disciplinary taskforce and agenda. Such a multifaceted approach, considering all dimensions of health and wellbeing, will be better placed to develop informed research and policy agendas that reflect the complexity of ageing rather than being focused on any singular feature. Positive ageing cannot be seen as the final movement to conquer the complex beast that is ageing, but merely another stepping-stone along the path of more integrated and informed approaches. As we have discussed, there are many different approaches that have failed to be considered in ageing; with time and humility these approaches may become more predominant and mainstream. More than ever, it is important to recognise that ageing is greater than the sum of its parts, no matter how significant they may seem from our own vantage point. This is particularly important for those from non-majority cultural groups and First Nations people who are disproportionately affected by the dominant discourse and agenda yet have, as of yet, not been given the opportunity to impart their wisdom and perspective and engage with equal grounding.

REFERENCES

Baker, A. E. Z., & Procter, N. G. (2015). 'You just lose the people you know': Relationship loss and mental illness. *Archives of Psychiatric Nursing, 29*(2), 96–101. doi:10.1016/j.apnu.2014.11.007

Baltes, M. M., & Carstensen, L. L. (1996). The process of successful ageing. *Ageing and Society, 16*(4), 397–422. doi:10.1017/S0144686X00003603

Baltes, P. B., & Baltes, M. M. (1990). Psychological perspectives on successful aging: The model of selective optimization with compensation. In M. M. Baltes & P. B. Baltes (Eds.), *Successful aging: Perspectives from the behavioral sciences* (pp. 1–34). Cambridge University Press.

Barreto, M., Victor, C., Hammond, C., Eccles, A., Richins, M. T., & Qualter, P. (2021). Loneliness around the world: Age, gender, and cultural differences in loneliness. *Personality and Individual Differences, 169*, 110066. doi:10.1016/j.paid.2020.110066

Bar-Tur, L., & Malkinson, R. (2014). *The Oxford handbook of clinical geropsychology.* Oxford University Press.

Bartholomaeus, J. D., Van Agteren, J. E. M., Iasiello, M. P., Jarden, A., & Kelly, D. (2019). Positive aging: The impact of a community wellbeing and resilience program. *Clinical Gerontologist, 42*(4), 377–386. doi:10.1080/07317115.2018.1561582

Beard, J. R. D., Officer, A. M. P. H., de Carvalho, I. A. M. D., Sadana, R. S., Pot, A. M. P., Michel, J.-P. M. D., . . . Chatterji, S. M. D. (2015). The world report on ageing and health: A policy framework for healthy ageing. *Lancet, 387*(10033), 2145–2154. doi:10.1016/S0140-6736(15)00516-4

Blanchflower, D. G., & Oswald, A. J. (2008). Is well-being U-shaped over the life cycle? *Social Science & Medicine, 66*(8), 1733–1749. doi:10.1016/j.socscimed.2008.01.030

Carey, L. (2006). *Expressive and creative arts methods for trauma survivors.* Jessica Kingsley Publishers.

Carr, A., Cullen, K., Keeney, C., Canning, C., Mooney, O., Chinseallaigh, E., & O'Dowd, A. (2020). Effectiveness of positive psychology interventions: A systematic review and meta-analysis. *Journal of Positive Psychology*, 1–21. doi:10.1080/17439760.2020.1818807

Carstensen, L. L. (1992). Social and emotional patterns in adulthood: Support for socioemotional selectivity theory. *Psychology and Aging, 7*(3), 331–338. doi:1037//0882-7974.7.3.331

Carstensen, L.L., & DeLiema, M. (2018). The positivity effect: A negativity bias in youth fades with age. *Current Opinion in Behavioral Sciences, 19*, 7–12. doi:10.1016/j.cobeha.2017.07.009

Carstensen, L. L., & Mikels, J. A. (2005). At the intersection of emotion and cognition: Aging and the positivity effect. *Current Directions in Psychological Science, 14*(3), 117–121. doi:10.1111/j.0963-7214.2005.00348.x

Carver, A., Lorenzon, A., Veitch, J., Macleod, A., & Sugiyama, T. (2020). Is greenery associated with mental health among residents of aged care facilities? A systematic search and narrative review. *Aging Mental Health, 24*(1), 1–7. doi:10.1080/13607863.2018.1516193

Chapman, F. (2018). Managing emotional and psychological distress in older people. *Working with Older People, 22*(4), 234–242. doi:10.1108/WWOP-09-2018-0017

Chowdhury, E. K., Nelson, M. R., Jennings, G. L. R., Wing, L. M. H., & Reid, C. M. (2017). Pet ownership and survival in the elderly hypertensive population. *Journal of Hypertension, 35*(4), 769–775. doi:10.1097/HJH.0000000000001214

Cohen, G. D. (2000). *The creative age: Awakening human potential in the second half of life*. William Morrow & Company.

Cohen, G. D. (2006). Research on creativity and aging: The positive impact of the arts on health and illness. *Generations, 30*(1), 7–15.

Crăciun, I. C. (2019). Positive aging theories and views on aging. In I. C. Crăciun (Ed.), *Positive aging and precarity: Theory, policy, and social reality within a comparative German context* (pp. 17–34). Springer International Publishing.

Darewych, O. H., Carlton, N. R., & Farrugie, K. W. (2015). Digital technology use in art therapy with adults with developmental disabilities. *Journal on Developmental Disabilities, 21*(2), 95.

Darewych, O. H., & Riedel Bowers, N. (2018). Positive arts interventions: Creative clinical tools promoting psychological well-being. *International Journal of Art Therapy, 23*(2), 62–69. doi:10.1080/17454832.2017.1378241

Daskalopoulou, C., Stubbs, B., Kralj, C., Koukounari, A., Prince, M., & Prina, A. M. (2017). Physical activity and healthy ageing: A systematic review and meta-analysis of longitudinal cohort studies. *Ageing Research Reviews, 38*, 6–17. doi:10.1016/j.arr.2017.06.003

Dudgeon, P., & Walker, R. (2015). Decolonising Australian psychology: Discourses, strategies, and practice. *Journal of Social and Political Psychology, 3*(1), 276–297.

Duedahl, E., Blichfeldt, B., & Liburd, J. (2020). How engaging with nature can facilitate active healthy ageing. *Tourism Geographies*, 1–21. doi:10.1080/14616688.2020.1819398

Flood, M., & Phillips, K. D. (2007). Creativity in older adults: A plethora of possibilities. *Issues in Mental Health Nursing, 28*(4), 389–411. doi:10.1080/01612840701252956

Freeman, C., Waters, D. L., Buttery, Y., & van Heezik, Y. (2019). The impacts of ageing on connection to nature: The varied responses of older adults. *Health Place, 56*, 24–33. doi:10.1016/j.healthplace.2019.01.010

Fulmer, T., Mate, K. S., & Berman, A. (2018). The age-friendly health system imperative. *Journal of the American Geriatric Society, 66*(1), 22–24. doi:10.1111/jgs.15076

Fulmer, T., Patel, P., Levy, N., Mate, K., Berman, A., Pelton, L., Beard, J., Kalache, A., & Auerbach, J. (2020). Moving toward a global age-friendly ecosystem. *Journal of the American Geriatrics Society, 68*(9), 1936–1940. doi:10.1111/jgs.16675

Gallagher, M. W., & Lopez, S. J. (2019). *Positive psychological assessment: A handbook of models and measures* (2nd ed.). American Psychological Association.

Gee, G., Dudgeon, P., Schultz, C., Hart, A., & Kelly, K. (2014). Aboriginal and Torres Strait Islander social and emotional wellbeing. In P. Dudgeon, H. Milroy, & R. Walker (Eds.), *Working together: Aboriginal and Torres Strait Islander mental health and wellbeing principles and practice* (pp. 55–68). Commonwealth of Australia.

Geiger, P. J., Boggero, I. A., Brake, C. A., Caldera, C. A., Combs, H. L., Peters, J. R., & Baer, R. A. (2016). Mindfulness-based interventions for older adults: A review of the effects on physical and emotional well-being. *Mindfulness, 7*(2), 296–307. doi:10.1007/s12671-015-0444-1

Gilleard, C. J., & Higgs, P. (2000). *Cultures of ageing: Self, citizen, and the body.* Pearson Education.

Golden, J., Conroy, R. M., Bruce, I., Denihan, A., Greene, E., Kirby, M., & Lawlor, B. A. (2009). Loneliness, social support networks, mood and wellbeing in community-dwelling elderly. *International Journal of Geriatric Psychiatry, 24*(7), 694–700. doi:10.1002/gps.2181

Hank, K. (2011). How "successful" do older Europeans age? Findings from SHARE. *Journals of Gerontolology B: Psychologcial Sciences & Social Sciences, 66*(2), 230–236. doi:10.1093/geronb/gbq089

Higgs, P., Leontowitsch, M., Stevenson, F., & Jones, I. R. (2009). Not just old and sick – the 'will to health' in later life. *Ageing and Society, 29*(5), 687–707. doi:10.1017/S0144686X08008271

Hill, R. D. (2010). A positive aging framework for guiding geropsychology interventions. *Behavior Therapy, 42*(1), 66–77. doi:10.1016/j.beth.2010.04.006

Hughes, M. J., Verreynne, M.-L., Harpur, P., & Pachana, N. A. (2020). Companion animals and health in older populations: A systematic review. *Clinical Gerontolology, 43*(4), 365–377. doi:10.1080/07317115.2019.1650863

Inglehart, R. (2002). Gender, aging, and subjective well-being. *International Journal of Comparative Sociology, 43*(3-5), 391–408. doi:10.1177/002071520204300309

Institute for Healthcare Improvement. (2019). *Age-friendly health systems: Guide to using the 4ms in the care of older adults.* http://www.ihi.org/Engage/Initiatives/Age-Friendly-Health-Systems/Documents/IHIAgeFriendlyHealthSystems_GuidetoUsing4MsCare.pdf

Ivtzan, I., Gardner, H. E., Bernard, I., Sekhon, M., & Hart, R. (2013). Wellbeing through self-fulfilment: Examining developmental aspects of self-actualization. *The Humanistic Psychologist, 41*(2), 119–132. doi:10.1080/08873267.2012.712076

Jardine, A., Speldewinde, P., Carver, S., & Weinstein, P. (2007). Dryland salinity and ecosystem distress syndrome: Human health implications. *EcoHealth, 4*(1), 10–17.

Jaremka, L. M., Andridge, R. R., Fagundes, C. P., Alfano, C. M., Povoski, S. P., Lipari, A. M., . . . Kiecolt-Glaser, J. K. (2014). Pain, depression, and fatigue: Loneliness as a longitudinal risk factor. *Health Psychology, 33*(9), 948–957. doi:10.1037/a0034012

Katz, S., & Calasanti, T. (2015). Critical perspectives on successful aging: Does it "appeal more than it illuminates"? *Gerontologist, 55*(1), 26–33. doi:10.1093/geront/gnu027

Kellert, S. (2018). Biophilia. In B. D. Fath (Ed.), *Encyclopedia of ecology* (2nd ed., pp. 247–251). Elsevier.

Krause-Parello, C. A., Gulick, E. E., & Basin, B. (2019). Loneliness, depression, and physical activity in older adults: The therapeutic role of human-animal interactions. *Anthrozoös, 32*(2), 239–254. doi:10.1080/08927936.2019.1569906

Lam, B. C. P., Haslam, C., Haslam, S. A., Steffens, N. K., Cruwys, T., Jetten, J., & Yang, J. (2018). Multiple social groups support adjustment to retirement across cultures. *Social Science & Medicine, 208,* 200–208. doi:10.1016/j.socscimed.2018.05.049

Lamers, S. M. A., Westerhof, G. J., Bohlmeijer, E. T., ten Klooster, P. M., & Keyes, C. L. M. (2011). Evaluating the psychometric properties of the Mental Health Continuum-Short Form (MHC-SF). *Journal of Clinical Psychology, 67*(1), 99–110. doi:10.1002/jclp.20741

Lang, F. R., & Carstensen, L. L. (1994). Close emotional relationships in late life: Further support for proactive aging in the social domain. *Psychology and Aging, 9*(2), 315–324.

Lavingia, R., Jones, K., & Asghar-Ali, A. A. (2020). A systematic review of barriers faced by older adults in seeking and accessing mental health care. *Journal of Psychiatric Practice, 26*(5), 367–382. doi:10.1097/PRA.0000000000000491

Levy, B., & Schlesinger, M. (2001). *Influence of aging self-stereotypes on older individuals' rejecting policy aimed at benefiting the old*. Paper presented at the Annual Scientific Meeting of The Gerontological Society of America.

Levy, B. R. (2003). Mind matters: Cognitive and physical effects of aging self-stereotypes. Journals of Gerontolology B: *Psychologcial Sciences & Social Sciences, 58*(4), P203–211. doi:10.1093/geronb/58.4.P203

Luchetti, M., Lee, J. H., Aschwanden, D., Sesker, A., Strickhouser, J. E., Terracciano, A., & Sutin, A. R. (2020). The trajectory of loneliness in response to COVID-19. *American Psychologist, 75*(7), 897–908. doi:10.1037/amp0000690

Maddux, J. E. (2008). Positive psychology and the illness ideology: Toward a positive clinical psychology. *Applied Psychology, 57*(s1), 54–70. doi:10.1111/j.1464-0597.2008.00354.x

Marecek, J., & Christopher, J. C. (2018). Is positive psychology an indigenous psychology? In N. J. L. Brown, T. Lomas, & F. J. Eiroa-Orosa (Eds.), *The Routledge international handbook of critical positive psychology* (pp. 84–98). Routledge/Taylor & Francis Group.

Martinson, M., & Berridge, C. (2015). Successful aging and its discontents: A systematic review of the social gerontology literature. *Gerontologist, 55*(1), 58–69. doi:10.1093/geront/gnu037

Maslow, A. H. (1954). *Motivation and personality*. Harpers.

Mather, M., & Carstensen, L. L. (2005). Aging and motivated cognition: The positivity effect in attention and memory. *Trends in Cognitive Science, 9*(10), 496–502. doi:10.1016/j.tics.2005.08.005

McHugh, M. C. (2016). Experiencing flow: Creativity and meaningful task engagement for senior women. *Women & Therapy, 39*(3-4), 280–295. doi:10.1080/02703149.2016.1116862

Morgan, G. S., Willmott, M., Ben-Shlomo, Y., Haase, A. M., & Campbell, R. M. (2019). A life fulfilled: Positively influencing physical activity in older adults – A systematic review and meta-ethnography. *BMC Public Health, 19*(1), 362. doi:10.1186/s12889-019-6624-5

Morrow-Howell, N., Hinterlong, J., & Sherraden, M. (2001). *Productive aging*. Johns Hopkins University Press.

Nikolaev, B., & Nikolaev, B. (2018). Does higher education increase hedonic and eudaimonic happiness? *Journal of Happiness Studies, 19*(2), 483–504. doi:10.1007/s10902-016-9833-y

O'Dwyer, S. T., Burton, N. W., Pachana, N. A., & Brown, W. J. (2007). Protocol for Fit Bodies, Fine Minds: A randomized controlled trial on the effect of exercise and cognitive training on cognitive functioning in older adults. *BMC Geriatrics, 4*(7), 23. doi:10.1186/1471-2318-7-23

Pace, J. E., & Grenier, A. (2017). Expanding the circle of knowledge: Reconceptualising successful aging among north American older indigenous peoples. *Journals of*

Gerontology Series B Psychological Sciences and Social Sciences, 72(2), 248–258. doi:10.1093/geronb/gbw128

Pachana, N. A., Massavelli, B. M., & Robleda-Gomez, S. (2011). A developmental psychological perspective on the human-animal bond. In C. Blazina, G. Boyraz, G., & D. Shen-Miller (Eds.), *The psychology of the human-animal bond* (pp. 151–165). Springer.

Pack, R., Hand, C., Rudman, D. L., & Huot, S. (2019). Governing the ageing body: Explicating the negotiation of 'positive' ageing in daily life. *Ageing and Society, 39*(9), 2085–2108. doi:10.1017/S0144686X18000442

Paúl, C., Ribeiro, O., & Teixeira, L. (2012). Active ageing: An empirical approach to the WHO model. *Current Gerontology and Geriatrics Research*, 382972. https://doi.org/10.1155/2012/382972

Reiner, M., Niermann, C., Jekauc, D., & Woll, A. (2013). Long-term health benefits of physical activity: A systematic review of longitudinal studies. *BMC Public Health, 13*(1), 13–813. doi:10.1186/1471-2458-13-813

Robleda, S., & Pachana, N. A. (2019). Quality of life in Australian adults aged 50 years and over: Data using the Schedule for the Evaluation of Individual Quality of Life (SEIQOL-DW). Clinical *Gerontologist, 42*(1), 101–113. doi:10.1080/07317115.2017.1397829

Rowe, J. W., & Kahn, R. L. (1987). Human aging: Usual and successful. *Science, 237*(4811), 143–149. doi:10.1126/science.3299702

Rowe, J. W., & Kahn, R. L. (1997). Successful aging. *Gerontologist, 37*(4), 433–440. doi:10.1093/geront/37.4.433

Ryan, R. M., & Deci, E. L. (2001). On happiness and human potentials: A review of research on hedonic and eudaimonic well-being. *Annual Review of Psychology, 52*(1), 141–166. doi:10.1146/annurev.psych.52.1.141

Sanyal, N. (2020). *Positive ageing: An approach towards transcendence.* Taylor & Francis Group.

Scott, T. L., Masser, B. M., & Pachana, N. A. (2015). Exploring the health and wellbeing benefits of gardening for older adults. *Ageing and Society, 35*(10), 2176–2200. doi:10.1017/S0144686X14000865

Scott, T. L., Masser, B. M., & Pachana, N. A. (2020). Positive aging benefits of home and community gardening activities: Older adults report enhanced self-esteem, productive endeavours, social engagement and exercise. *SAGE Open Med, 8.* doi:10.1177/2050312120901732

Seligman, M. (2018). PERMA and the building blocks of well-being. *Journal of Positive Psychology, 13*(4), 333–335. doi:10.1080/17439760.2018.1437466

Seligman, M. E. P. (2011). *Flourish: A visionary new understanding of happiness and well-being.* Free Press.

Shankar, A., McMunn, A., Banks, J., & Steptoe, A. (2011). Loneliness, social isolation, and behavioral and biological health indicators in older adults. *Health Psychology, 30*(4), 377–385. doi:10.1037/a0022826

Solly, K., & Wells, Y. (2020). How well have senior Australians been coping in the COVID-19 pandemic? *Australasian Journal of Ageing, 39*(4), 386–388. doi:10.1111/ajag.12880

Speldewinde, P. C., Cook, A., Davies, P., & Weinstein, P. (2011). The hidden health burden of environmental degradation: Disease comorbidities and dryland salinity. *EcoHealth, 8*(1), 82–92.

Steffens, N. K., Cruwys, T., Haslam, C., Jetten, J., & Haslam, S. A. (2016). Social group memberships in retirement are associated with reduced risk of premature death: Evidence from a longitudinal cohort study. *BMJ Open*, *6*(2), e010164–e010164. doi:10.1136/bmjopen-2015-010164

Stone, A. A., Schwartz, J. E., Broderick, J. E., & Deaton, A. (2010). A snapshot of the age distribution of psychological well-being in the United States. *Proceedings of the National Academy of Sciences of the United States of America*, *107*(22), 9985–9990. doi:10.1073/pnas.1003744107

Takano, T., Nakamura, K., & Watanabe, M. (2002). Urban residential environments and senior citizens' longevity in megacity areas: The importance of walkable green spaces. *Journal of Epidemiology & Community Health*, *56*(12), 913–918.

Thompson, B. E., & Neimeyer, R. A. (2014). *Grief and the expressive arts: Practices for creating meaning*. Routledge.

UN Department of Economic and Social Affairs: Population Dynamics. (2019). *World population prospect 2019*. https://population.un.org/wpp/Download/Standard/Population/

United Nations, & Department of Economic and Social Affairs. (2019). *World population ageing 2019: Highlights*. https://www.un.org/en/development/desa/population/publications/pdf/ageing/WorldPopulationAgeing2019-Highlights.pdf

Wells, Y. (2017). Life events and older people. In N. Pachana (Ed.), *Encyclopedia of geropsychology* (pp. 1381–1389). Springer.

Wickersham, R. H., Zaval, L., Pachana, N. A., & Smyer, M. A. (2020). The impact of place and legacy framing on climate action: A lifespan approach. *PLoS One*, *15*(2), e0228963. doi:10.1371/journal.pone.0228963

World Health Organization. (2002a). Active ageing: A policy framework. *The Aging Male*, *5*(1), 1–37. doi:10.1080/tam.5.1.1.37

World Health Organization. (2002b). Towards a common language for functioning, disability, and health: ICF. *The International Classification of Functioning, Disability and Health*. https://www.who.int/classifications/icf/icfbeginnersguide.pdf

Zubala, A., MacGillivray, S., Frost, H., Kroll, T., Skelton, D. A., Gavine, A., . . . Morris, J. (2017). Promotion of physical activity interventions for community dwelling older adults: A systematic review of reviews. *PLoS One*, *12*(7), e0180902–e0180902. doi:10.1371/journal.pone.0180902

12

Systems of Care and Experience for Dying Well

MICHAEL CHAPMAN, JENNIFER PHILIP, AND
PAUL KOMESAROFF ■

INTRODUCTION

What does it mean to experience 'wellbeing' as we die? At first sight, this idea appears to be inherently contradictory. However, a moment's reflection reveals several ways in which death and dying may be positively associated with wellbeing. Death and dying are complex experiences and may not be uniformly negative. While they certainly entail loss and frequently suffering, they may also create or reveal meaning. And they may be associated with joyful experiences such as beauty, connection, and love.

In the final pages of Max Porter's *Grief Is the Thing with the Feathers*, Dad narrates as he and the boys say goodbye to their wife and mother by scattering her ashes into the wind on a beach (Porter, 2015, p. 116).

> And the boys were behind me, a tide-wall of laughter and yelling, hugging my legs, tripping and grabbing, leaping, spinning, stumbling, roaring, shrieking and the boys shouted
>
> I LOVE YOU I LOVE YOU I LOVE YOU
>
> and their voice was the life and song of their mother. Unfinished. Beautiful. Everything.

These words express the loving and joyous culmination of a story of grief filled with pain, loss, agonising disconnection, joy, and love, and they capture the complex admixture of these ideas and experiences and the inseparable richness of their combination. Death and dying are suffused with a potential for healing and comfort that is often hidden from view.

The potential coexistence of wellbeing with death and dying also provides some insight into the nature of both. Wellbeing can be understood in part as arising from the impact and responses to the physical, affective, cognitive, social, and spiritual challenges that are familiar and frequent components of human experience. This positions wellbeing as a systemic outcome of interactions involving manifold human systems rather than as a construct wholly arising from individuals. Similarly, the interconnection of social systems, operating in the medium of personal relationships, and communication processes unfolding and interpreted through culture and language contribute to the complexity and depth of the experience of death and dying. Wellbeing is a potential result of these interwoven, ravelled experiences and responses. This notion has critical relevance for understanding the potential for positive experiences relating to death and dying, the breadth of the challenges to these possibilities, and how care can be provided to promote wellbeing, including at the end of life.

Individual subjective concepts of wellbeing and the science and evidence that are applied to evaluate them are largely dependent on a philosophical tradition that assumes individuals to be autonomous, rational agents embedded within communities. While this tradition retains powerful hegemonic force, its limitations have been exposed and alternatives to it proposed in recent critiques. 'Process philosophy' argues against the basic notion that objects or states of affairs can be regarded as static, independent, or 'objective', suggesting instead that they must be regarded as presuppositions of our systems of thought and language. From this perspective, a disjunction between independent persons and the communities or worlds that surround them is artificial because individuals' experiences of self and their worlds are in constant and dynamic flux (Rescher, 1996; Stengers, 2011). In spite of this, research and healthcare practices continue to stress the preponderance of individual experiences over other concerns, limiting the ability to modify the more complex array of variables and their interactions.

Understanding the possibility of wellbeing in death and dying requires a relational notion of experience, inclusive of the relevance of continuous and mutually affecting individual and social systemic processes. It is precisely through this interplay of systemic and interrelated experiences of resources, challenges, and processes that wellbeing is composed in the various systems (people, networks, and communities) linked to death and dying. This chapter explores how a deeper and more relational understanding of wellbeing instils confidence that this state can co-exist with an awareness of our own mortality and be constructively integrated into the more effective provision of care. This argument begins with an exploration of notions of positive aspects of death and dying, exploring different philosophical, literary, cultural, and religious engagements with these ideas. We then explore how these experiences and the experience of wellbeing arise from the interplay of dynamic, living systems, suggesting how wellbeing and death and dying can relate and coexist. Finally, we describe the implications of this understanding for care provision that seeks to support wellbeing within dying.

THE POTENTIAL POSITIVITY OF DEATH AND DYING

Death is not universally associated with the notion of suffering—or perhaps it is better to say that suffering does not make up the totality of how death may be understood. Death and dying are intrinsically normal biological processes that cannot be separated from the lives that they conclude. Our biological lives, regardless of our spiritual or religious beliefs, are bookended by the frail dependencies of our youth and our ageing and culminate in our death, which is a necessary conclusion to our living experience.

Death can be seen as a mechanism for understanding life. The eudaimonia of living a life of meaning and fulfilling one's potential (see also Chapter 1, this volume), sought as an ideal life, was considered by Aristotle to be closely related to dying. The concept related to our total life experience, up to and including our death (Aristotle, 2004). In Aristotle's view, dying could enhance or detract from our eudaimonia depending on how it incorporated the values that we lived by (Dubois, 2014). For him, eudaimonia was also an active telos for the entire process of constructing meaning over the course of our lives, whereby their moral quality could only be ascertained when they had concluded.

Owing to its universal nature, death can also be a source of human connection. Todd May describes death as the 'most important fact about us as human beings' (May, 2009, p. 3). For May, death has the capacity to absorb every other fact about us, and this potency, combined with its inevitability, unpredictability, and tragedy, means that it provides a 'fullness' to life that would not be present without it. Herr Settembrini, in Thomas Mann's *The Magic Mountain*, considers death 'part and parcel of life . . . the inviolable condition of life' but notes that attempts to separate or 'divorce' death from life transforms it in to a feared 'spectre' (Mann, 1927, p. 237). Death is one of the few things that is a universal shared experience. As Lingis (1994) noted, 'We know ourselves in our mortality' (p. 154). Each action we take, and each dwindling moment of time, represents the abatement of the possibilities available to us. While you read this chapter right now, other opportunities are becoming impossibilities. The undeniable certainty of our dying frames and exposes the preciousness of our living actions and experiences as they cumulatively and ceaselessly form the being that we are. Death, and its potent unknowns, can also uncomfortably, but fruitfully, shock us out of expectation of time and the comfortable cloister that habitual patterns of action in our lives can create. We all dwell within vacated spaces. Despite our unique identity, others before us have had our jobs, our experiences, our tasks, and our sense of immortality, and others will again after we are gone. Our lives are built on the lives of others and influence the lives of those to come. Framed within our mortality in this way, our lives bind us to others. Our human kinship is further kindled by the recognition of the shared nature of our mortality within the unique experiences of those around us. Connecting with—touching—others within the shadow of dying is a bonding act of consolation, of solicitude, that can draw us out of the insular shell of our experience. Death as a bedrock of life means that the grief, worry, pain, and loss that I experience was never only mine, but ours.

The relationship between the challenges of death and dying and the possibility of growth and connection can also be seen in many cultural, religious, and spiritual responses to these phenomena. While culture is pervasive, it is not uniform, and multiple cultural facets can influence understandings of dying. For example, Park and Halifax (2021) suggest that those within Western culture reside with a 'taste of grief' due to being conditioned to possess and not let go. For the grief experiences of African Americans and Aboriginal Australians, racism, trauma, and inequity in life and in dying are prominent (Menzies, 2019; Rosenblatt, 2014; see also Chapter 7, this volume). However, the tragic injustice of these experiences does not diminish their potential to be sources of strength. Work with Aboriginal Australians, for instance, suggests that the shared experiences of these adversities and the strengths inherent and developed within cultural practices can lead to the strengthening of communities and further resilience (Usher et al., 2021). The impact of factors such as religiousness and spirituality is similarly complex. Assuming a uniformity of beliefs within faith traditions is reductive and simplistic, given that the interpretation of death, dying, and responses to bereavement can be influenced by many spirituality-associated factors beyond only belonging to a faith (Wortmann & Park, 2008). Nevertheless, religious views often relate to death and dying as events of significant meaning or consolation. Within some Christian views, for instance, death can be seen as the route to a perpetual salvation or as illusory in the sense that the dying person persists through an eternal soul (Park & Halifax, 2021). Suffering and dying are considered universal aspects of living experience in many Buddhist views while also being the root of compassion for ourselves and others and of spiritual transformation (Desjarlais, 2014). Evidence may also suggest that religious belief structures diminish the negative impacts of death on dying. It is important to note that while bereavement studies often suggest a positive relationship between religion-spirituality and adjustment to bereavement, reviews of this literature have stressed the inconsistency of the evidence, and this remains an area requiring further exploration (Park & Halifax, 2021).

The expectation of suffering is commonly associated with death and dying across cultures. The dying process is inevitably associated with innumerable and holistic losses which are of a real and existential nature. Distress and discomfort due to direct experience of changes in our physical being can and often do occur during our dying, along with loss of connection to those or that which is meaningful to us, our cognitive or affective responses to these changes, and how we understand their impact on our sense of identity and wholeness. The challenges and discomforts of death and dying are well understood, even to the point of being anticipated and feared. Whether they always constitute a form of 'suffering', however, requires more thought. Cassell (2004), in his influential work, proposed suffering as a negative state which was a core threat to our intactness, our personhood. Significant physical discomforts (such as the pain of childbirth, for instance) may not therefore constitute suffering as they are not seen as threatening to our integrity or our personhood. In this example, the discomforts of childbirth are also likely to be associated with positive associations, which may influence the experience and meaning of the significant associated discomforts. From this perspective, the potential for wellbeing in death and dying may relate more to how we understand and ascribe meaning to negative experiences usually thought of as 'suffering' (such as pain and loss), rather than our ability to avoid or suppress these experiences.

Suffering and distress during death and dying may also have a more potent relationship to wellbeing than is immediately apparent. To suffer requires a direct and reflective experience of our world. Engagement in, and response to, our experience is necessary for this to occur. This is not comfortable and is rarely sought out and yet, for some, it may still be fruitful. Suffering is the experience of our world where uncertainty and change is predictable and yet often still unexpected. Suffering can express meaning for some if their lifeworld encompasses such a possibility. This might be true, for example, for those with religious interpretations of suffering which embrace its experience as a cleansing punishment. On the other hand, for many, suffering may have no inherent meaning but may still be an avenue for new modalities of understanding and knowledge. For instance, my response to my suffering may enable me to learn about aspects of my identity or the fringes of experience which were previously unavailable to me, or it may connect me to others who respond to my pain or have had similar experiences. A simple and yet hard-won aspect of suffering may be that endurance is thereby rendered possible. Nietzsche (1887) went further, suggesting that suffering, growth, and positive experiences such as joy were inextricably linked to each other—you could not expect or achieve the good without the bad. Suffering may be purposeless. It has been argued by many, including Camus, that suffering and death are irrational with no intrinsic moral meaning. However, even when accepted as intrinsically meaningless, suffering may result in meaningful outcomes. For Camus (1947), knowledge that we will continue to suffer is no reason for 'giving up the struggle' against it (p. 98). As within *The Myth of Sisyphus*, there is an absurd but powerful vitality associated with embracing and bearing up against our frail fates (Camus, 1942/2018). Suffering can also open us to the world and those around us. Cassell (2004) described the 'web of relationships with self and others' necessary for a sense of intactness, coherence, and integrity (the opposite of/antidote to suffering), providing an understanding of the centrality of relationships and interconnections that are necessary for wellbeing (p. 39) (see also Chapter 5, this volume). It can be the 'half-opening that a moan, a cry or a sigh slips through' enabling our openness to the other (Levinas, 2002, p. 158). It can be the naked and raw possibility, the crack where 'the light gets in', transfusing the pain of suffering with hope and potential (Cohen, 1992).

Our relationship with death and dying not only varies across cultures but has changed over time. Dying is increasingly a foretold and expected experience. While human death has always been certain, in current times dying can be predicted with increasing certainty due to the commonality of diagnoses of chronic life-limiting illnesses (Van Der Velden, Francke, Hingstman, & Willems, 2009). Knowledge of the potential contributors to our dying may mean that we can be more prepared for this to occur or, more concerningly, that the distress associated with the knowledge of dying occurs earlier and for longer than it would otherwise.

Preparing for dying in our contemporary age is a topic of increasing discussion in the hope of influencing these responses. In many places, community-level conversations seeking to normalise dying are taking place, and interventions are commonplace to support improvements in care for the dying and the further recognition of the choices and voices of people who are approaching dying. These activities suggest a general recognition that further attention to realising the wellbeing that is latent in dying is needed but, also and most importantly, that improving wellbeing in death and dying is possible.

While the manner of our approaching dying may have changed, the concept that it may entail positive experiences such as growth or healing has deep and ancient roots. The Greek tradition deriving from Hippocrates has been instrumental in the development of modern medicine (Kleisiaris, Sfakianakis, & Papathanasiou, 2014). Hippocrates had a clear awareness that cure was not always possible, and he was of the view that in these situations medicine was 'powerless' (Hurst, Whitmer, Prins, Shepard, & McVey, 2009). In the larger Asklepion tradition, however, there was also the notion that healing may remain possible regardless of the proximity of death (Downie, 2012). Healing here implies the relief of suffering and the importance of the atmosphere and the environment of care in supporting the centrality of the person within this process, as healing is seen as a process that is embodied by a person rather than something that is delivered to or enacted upon a person by an external agent. These ideas can be considered central to the modern practice of palliative care, where it is the person's potential for healing and the supportive presence of those who provide care which are key to best practice (Chapman, Russell, & Philip, 2020; Randall & Downie, 2006).

Similar ideas can be found within non-Western cultures. For example, in Tibetan Buddhism the notion of a 'good death' deeply relates to our personal opportunity to contribute to the experience of our dying rather than external forces. As described in the Tibetan *Book of Living and Dying*, the key aspects of 'whatever we have done in our lives, and what state of mind we are in at that moment' clarify that it is our preparedness for dying and our making sense of our lives that are important for a death that is as good as it can be (Rinpoche, 2002, p. 227). While these traditions suggest some expectation of the potential for positive elements of death and dying, they appear to fall short of the notion of wellbeing in dying, which requires further consideration and exploration.

SYSTEMS OF WELLBEING

Wellbeing has an increasingly important place in how we consider the health, economic status, welfare, and experience of people and populations. As a category that is distinct from, but not fully independent of, disease or illness, it offers specific insights as well as practical directions. To realise such benefits, a rigorous characterisation of its key features is required.

When considered as a field for study and evaluation, subjective wellbeing has been conceptualised in a variety of ways. Two primary historical traditions have conventionally dominated discussion. The hedonic tradition accentuated the relevance of happiness and positive affective states, the minimisation of negative affective states, and satisfaction with existing conditions of life (Dodge, Daly, Huyton, & Sanders, 2012; Kahneman, Diener, & Schwarz, 2003; see also Chapter 3, this volume). By contrast, the eudaimonic tradition has highlighted positive psychological functioning and human growth and development (Waterman, 1993; see also Chapter 1, this volume). Drawing on both these currents of thought, more recent work proposes a nuanced multidimensional understanding of wellbeing which incorporates many of the factors mentioned above (Cummins, 2010; Headley & Wearing, 1992).

These traditional perspectives have been the subject of a radical critique which has suggested the possibility of an alternative theoretical framework that provides novel opportunities for both research and action (Dodge et al., 2012). This theory draws on a systems approach to the understanding of wellbeing. Systems theory conceptualises living systems as reflective, self-interacting processes made up of elements that are interconnected in a manner that can be formally analysed and understood. The system as a whole coheres in a state of dynamic equilibrium that ensures the continuity of its key structural principles. In the course of their development, systems respond to both internal and exogenous influences by displaying innovative relationships while preserving overall stability. Both the responses to such influences or perturbations and the conditions of stability can be interpreted as expressions of a system's purpose. For many systems, their most obvious and superficial purpose is to continue to function as a living system. Systems' reflective responses to perturbations will therefore seek an equipoise where continuation is maintained. A function of a human being, as a living system, is to continue to live. However, considering wellbeing or any number of other purposes, it becomes rapidly clear that this is not the only function of a human system and therefore not the only reflective mediator of its response to perturbations. Systems are therefore reflexively influenced by both multiple conditions and constitute constantly shifting clusters of interactions in a stable, fluctuating unity.

When applied to the concept of wellbeing, systems thinking posits this as a process which perdures as a dynamic equilibrium that balances a variety of forces (Cummins, 2010; Dodge et al., 2012; Headley & Wearing, 1992; see also Chapter 3, this volume). Specifically, wellbeing is seen as a state of dynamic equilibrium within the manifold flux of personal experiences. The latter encompass physical, cognitive, and affective phenomena, which are articulated within a broad context that incorporates social, cultural, and ethical variables. The dynamic processes reflect a person's internal resources as well as their ability to respond to the internal and external challenges to which they are exposed (Cummins, 2010).

These ideas represent the broad scope of the systems interpretation of wellbeing and its far-reaching implications for everyday life. To illustrate the fecundity of this approach, Bertrand Russell's (1930/2006) concept of happiness may be taken as an example. Russell regarded happiness as a state of balance involving many variables. Some of the latter may today appear somewhat anachronistic: for example, the 'plain' (referring to an embodied, physical and 'animal' experience) and the 'fancy' (referring to a more elevated intellectual and spiritual happiness) (p. 71). However, Russell's conclusions were more contemporary. He argued that happiness was not the result of specific, defined contents (such as love or money) but of a dynamic equilibrium among multiple, changing factors. He concluded, for example, that a well-digger or gardener who knew nothing of politics or the wider world could be happy because of the bodily and affective satisfaction derived from life and its tasks. Similarly, an academic, fully absorbed by intellectual pursuits and whose work was valued, may find an intellectually elevated happiness and satisfaction. While Russell's categorisation and examples may seem less convincing with the passage of time, his central point—that happiness or wellbeing represents a state within a dynamic, self-interacting system that manifests itself differently in different factual settings—remains a potent one. To take two more examples: a woman with a job she enjoys and identifies with; who experiences a sense of love, connection, and satisfaction from her relationships with her children, family, and community; and who has access to adequate physical comfort and health may experience a sense of wellbeing from the personally unique combination of these factors, her responses to them, and the resulting balance that is achieved. Although his personal circumstances vary widely, a reclusive man with limited physical comfort or financial resources who passionately identifies with his mission to challenge inequity through political action may also experience a deep sense of wellbeing emerging from the unique play of powerful variables in his life. For resources to act as such they must be sufficient for that personal system, and, while there is likely some theoretical commonality around what denotes minimally 'sufficient' personal systems, the actual outcomes depend on the local specific circumstances in particular cases.

Understanding wellbeing as a reflective result of a myriad of influences opens the potential for it to be maintained despite systemic pressures or disturbances. Our aforementioned political dissident may feel enhanced wellbeing or his experience may become more resilient to future disturbances if he gains resources which affect this systemic experience, such as becoming connected to or accepted by a community of people who share his passionate beliefs. In contrast, our working mother may also continue to experience wellbeing even if some of her systemic resources are lost or threatened (e.g., if her previously good health were to decline as part of an unexpected terminal diagnosis). In such situations, change may occur while the systemic result of wellbeing remains intact. This is because wellbeing is not a singular absolute but a zone of experience self-determined by the system involved. The working mother with the terminal diagnosis may find that the loss of her health is insufficient to destabilise her wellbeing, which is able to endure because of the meaning she derives from the deep love she shares with her family; or she may discover new resources that maintain the wellbeing equilibrium point, such as a new awareness of personal courage or a strength she was previously unaware she possessed. It is also important to note that the achievement of wellbeing does not require that all experiences are concordant with that state. A person approaching dying may have frequent or sustained episodes of physical discomfort, grief, distress, or any number of other challenging experiences which might occur

as part of dying, yet still find themselves in a state of wellbeing if that is the resulting balance of their overall personal system.

A key notion here is, when utilising the systems theoretical lens, that the factors
that influence wellbeing will be determined by the system itself. This approach
has key relevance to the notion of the experience of death and dying and provides an important clue regarding how this might be practically and conceptually
integrated.

SYSTEMIC STRUCTURES FOR PROMOTING WELLBEING IN DYING

A description of wellbeing in the context of death and dying as a systems process requires a characterisation of the structures involved, of the relationships
between them, and of the conditions for stability or equilibrium. Earlier work
has shown that the complex experiences of death and dying and the potential for
wellbeing incorporate a variety of systemic elements (Hodiamont, Jünger, Leidl,
Maier, Schildmann, & Bausewein, 2019). These encompass personal qualities,
such as cognitive and affective capacities and resources; physical experiences and
functions; and spiritual, cultural, or other interpretations. The specific elements
include (among others) embodied experiences of illness and pain; affective experiences such as joy, sadness, and loss; psychological processes such as grief and
mourning; shared social interactions marked by local and wider cultures; and the
processes of understanding that reflect on and draw meaning from all of these.
They do not exist in isolation from each other but cohere in a dynamic, ever-
changing whole, together composing complex unities embedded and subject to
interpretive environments formed by culture and language.

The wellbeing 'systems' are subject to change in response to external forces,
which may result in disruption, evolution, or maintenance of an equilibrium state
(Cummins, 2010). The importance of individual elements for contributing to and
maintaining wellbeing for particular people and communities is highly context-
dependent, varying with the nature and composition of the internal constituents.
Wellbeing in death and dying will not therefore arise from or be attributable to
one factor in one system, or one predictable set of factors in all systems. Different
variables may be influential in different ways in different systems and therefore require specific attention. Cultural contributors to how death and dying are understood, and the language used to describe and interpret the various phenomena,
may contribute in critical and unpredictable ways. The extent to which wellbeing
in death can be achieved, maintained, or supported will vary with the availability
of resources—personal, social, psychological, and financial—that may enable or
limit the dynamic processes and strengthen or undermine the potential for resilient responses to the challenges that inevitably arise.

How, then, can wellbeing in death and dying be fostered, and what should 'care'
include and seek to provide within this context in order to maximise the possibility of wellbeing for a person who is dying and those close to her? Hartogh

(2017) notes that while feeling sad, distressed, or uncomfortable may be unpleasant, efforts to make a person who is approaching death not feel sad, distressed, or uncomfortable may be unrealistic—and may even be unhelpful. This
does not mean that the distress of dying cannot be diminished or that attempts
to reduce distress should not be made, but rather that the removal of distress and
discomfort should not be regarded as a necessary or even expected goal. Distress
and suffering are components of facing the ending of our lives.

Common contributors to suffering in dying, and targets for responses to enhance wellbeing, are often described as falling into several domains, such as the
physical, psychological, social, and spiritual. Physical issues include symptoms
such as pain, nausea, dyspnoea, or fatigue. These are common as death and dying
approaches, particularly with more chronic and advanced illnesses. More complex physical concerns include functional changes and disabilities which are commonly reported as deeply significant for people with advanced illness and those
around them when independence is challenged and reliance upon others for care
increases. The various domains cannot be sharply separated from each other, as
shown by the fact that the functional outcomes of disability are necessarily influenced by other kinds of experience, such as the social and the psychological,
or the critical and less commonly explored community environmental factors to
which they are in turn subject.

Psychological distress associated with death and dying is also commonly described. Biomedical syndromes of distress, such as depression or demoralisa-
tion, are frequently described, and there is evidence these are more common in
the setting of advanced illness. Social distress also commonly occurs and may
be associated with changes in roles, identity, or social status to which the proximity of death can give rise. For example, a dying person's inability to maintain
the identity and status associated with their employment role or their presence
as a parent for their young child can evoke profound distress for all concerned.
Additional social challenges can arise from the need for conversations regarding
end-of-life choices which may have been avoided in the past but which now must
be pursued out of tragic necessity. Changes in personal relationships can also
occur, perhaps prompted by new and possibly unwanted roles, such as the transformation of friends and family into 'carers' owing to a need for intimate physical
care. Spiritual distress likewise is commonly described, often affecting the human
senses of meaning, connection, love, and compassion identified with various different experiences (Edwards, Pang, Shiu, & Chan, 2010; Longaker, 1997).

Approaches to palliative care that are most effective in improving the experiences of people who are close to dying are generally 'holistic' and goal-directed.
Holistic approaches embrace the insight that the separation of suffering, goals,
or preferences into neat domains is no more than an artificial tool to simplify
care delivery. In reality, people (and actual human systems) do not operate in
this way: physical issues cannot be separated from social, psychological, and spiritual meanings, intertwined with the various systems of embodied experience
with which they are linked. Goal-directed strategies ensure that targeting care
toward the achievement of goals identified as relevant to individual patients or

care networks (human systems) will ensure that patients remain the central focus, thereby providing the best chance of achieving outcomes that are both meaningful to them and allow them to preserve some sense of control. A common example of the interplay between holistic and goal-focused aspects of care in practice arises in relation to the familiar work to enable a person approaching dying to be located in their preferred place, such as their home. Similarly, the ability to attend a meaning-making event, such as the wedding of a child or a university graduation ceremony, or to spend a few precious hours with family watching a movie, can be important goals that would have been easy to miss.

The choice of goals often involves a degree of compromise. The decision to spend time doing one thing may require that an alternative has to be foregone. Similarly, the fragility that often accompanies the journey toward dying may mean that particular choices create new risks, as of additional preventable discomfort while outside a healthcare environment, which will need to be explored. A focus on goals that may be difficult or unlikely to be achieved can negatively impact wellbeing. Choices to continue or commence disease-directed therapies of ever-diminishing benefit in the face of progressive deterioration and with potentially distressing side effects are a pertinent example. The goals of such treatments may be improved symptoms, further time, or to maintain hope that there are alternative futures than dying, potentially ephemeral or elusive outcomes with advancing disease. They may, however, risk additional effort, burden, the unnecessary medicalisation of care, space for other priorities, and, for some, harm for patients, families, and healthcare providers. Indeed Cassell (2004) has noted that, in such circumstances, medical treatment itself can be the source of suffering, particularly if its provision is inattentive, unwise, or poorly explained. In this setting, palliative care offers an important response. By deliberately moving the focus from a narrow biomedical disease management approach to a consideration of all aspects of the person in their community, palliative care creates an opening for other areas of development and other modes of wellbeing beyond the reduction in disease or forestalling dying. Supporting people to achieve their goals may therefore simultaneously ameliorate some elements of suffering while potentiating others. In these settings, a judgement must be made about which overall care provision strategy will most effectively improve the systemic wellbeing of the person approaching dying.

These examples show that it is unduly simplistic to assume that wellbeing cannot occur where there is suffering. As we have argued, although suffering relating to death and dying may cause great distress, it can also co-exist with, and in some cases—perhaps ironically—even enhance wellbeing. Distress and suffering may incorporate important systems work undertaken by a dying person and those around them, and so a singular focus on their minimisation or avoidance may not always produce the best outcomes. This is not, of course, to suggest that suffering should not be ameliorated. On the contrary, suffering can cause great and overwhelming pain and eclipse resilience and diminish wellbeing and in these cases is unlikely to contain value. However, the significant experiences of suffering in our lives are mostly not overwhelming and are usually not meaning-depleting.

Michael Kearney (1992) metaphorically suggested that 'the dragon of our suffering' at the end of life may also 'guard a treasure'. Through taking on the battle with suffering, he contends, we may create the necessary space to discover what that treasure is. In a similar vein, Balfour Mount, following the logotherapy of Viktor Frankl, proposed that the quality of our lives in illness is intrinsically associated with a sense of the meaning of both life and suffering (Mount, Boston, & Cohen, 2007). This latter view was supported by evidence from work with people with advanced illness that the potency of a sense of meaning is associated with an experience of integrity, wholeness, and connection. For Nietzsche (1887), suffering is meaningful because it can induce growth and create strength, powerfully influencing those who experience it. Whether this will be the result for personal systems will depend on a host of factors, but the very possibility invites a sense of meaning in suffering and a wellbeing related to suffering that is easily overlooked.

Another important element of care in the support of wellbeing utilising a systemic lens is that it often needs to be extended beyond the individual patient approaching dying. Conceptualising wellbeing as a systemic process encourages us to consider the roles that others in relationship with dying persons may have. A clear and important example of this relates to the grief and bereavement brought about by the death of someone beloved. Living with someone who is dying and experiencing their death inevitably conveys a profound, often lasting impact. Family carers of people who have advanced illnesses where dying is expected, such as advanced cancer, share this experience of illness as grieving observers who know their lives will continue, albeit as forever changed (Murray et al., 2010). In other words, caring for a dying person requires care for those around them, for their whole community. This community, furthermore, may be more extensive than is immediately assumed. A systems approach to wellbeing reinforces the understanding that we are all receivers and providers of care. As Maria Puig de la Bellacasa (2017) observed, 'care is omnipresent, even through the effects of its absence' (p. 1). The experiences of those nominally tasked as care providers (including both clinicians and family caregivers) are entwined with those actually undergoing the process of dying. In turn, carers are often cared for by dying people, as expressed poignantly by Cicely Saunders (1988): 'Sooner or later all who work with dying people know they are receiving more than they are giving as they meet endurance, courage and often humour'.

While most attention, naturally and appropriately, is given to the proximate and direct personal connections between people within networks affected by someone dying, these ideas can be readily extended to a broader context of people. How we think and talk about dying in our society, particularly the intense fear and aversion we habitually associate with it, even in casual conversations, can shape the expectations, anxieties, and choices of those who may later face similar moments. Likewise, how dying is experienced and described by those who have either received care or been affected by its absence may propagate ideas and attitudes throughout the wider society. In this way, a systems understanding of wellbeing in death and dying emphasises a fundamental conclusion: that the community needing and participating in care is everyone.

SUMMARY

Understanding the role of wellbeing in death and dying requires an appreciation of the fecundity and complexity of these experiences and the manner in which they draw on many systems. While suffering is common in dying, this not only does not exclude wellbeing but can often enhance it. Wellbeing, as a continuous systemic process, is a result of many factors which extend well beyond particular individuals, even while the meaning and significance of these factors are highly specific to unique systems and people. Systems can be influenced and adjusted to enhance their potential for realising and supporting wellbeing, and models of palliative care can help facilitate such outcomes. Wellbeing-focused care acts to render suffering less precarious and painful and to realise its latent potential for meaning generation. It recognises that a holistic notion of healing is possible within illness and the proximity of dying. It focuses on goals as a way of making care meaningful to the system. And it acknowledges that care for the dying is care for everyone.

Undoubtedly, further steps are required for such integration to be fully realised. As contributors to a global community touched by death and influencing the distributed experience of death, we have a continuing obligation to learn the lessons (and find the treasures) available to us. Integrating an understanding of wellbeing in death and dying will ultimately require us to become

> a society that acknowledges its own humanity, and neither hides us from it nor it from us; a society of citizens who admit that they are needy and vulnerable, and who discard the grandiose demands for omnipotence and completeness that have been at the heart of so much human misery, both public and private. (Nussbaum, 2004, p. 17)

In short, we are and always will be people, a society caring for and preparing for dying. But recognising this holds a key to our wellbeing.

REFERENCES

Aristotle. (2004). *Nicomachean ethics*. Penguin Books.

Camus, A. (1942/2018). *The myth of Sisyphus*. Vintage International.

Camus, A. (1947). *The plague*. Penguin Modern Classics.

Cassell, E. J. (2004). *The nature of suffering and the goals of medicine* (2nd ed.). https://doi.org/10.1093/acprof:oso/9780195156164.001.0001
10.1093/acprof:oso/9780195156164.003.0003

Chapman, M., Russell, B., & Philip, J. (2020). Systems of care in crisis: The changing nature of palliative care during COVID-19. *Journal of Bioethical Inquiry*. https://doi.org/10.1007/s11673-020-10006-x

Cohen, L. (1992). *Anthem*. Columbia.

Cummins, R. A. (2010). Subjective wellbeing, homeostatically protected mood and depression: A synthesis. *Journal of Happiness Studies, 11*(1), 1–17. https://doi.org/10.1007/s10902-009-9167-0

Desjarlais, R. (2014). Liberation upon hearing: Voice, morality, and death in a Buddhist world. *Ethos, 42*(1), 101–118. https://doi.org/10.1111/etho.12041

Dodge, R., Daly, A., Huyton, J., & Sanders, L. (2012). The challenge of defining wellbeing. *International Journal of Wellbeing, 2*(3), 222–235. https://doi.org/10.5502/ijw.v2i3.4

Downie, R. (2012). Paying attention: Hippocratic and Asklepian approaches. *Advances in Psychiatric Treatment, 18*(5), 363–368. https://doi.org/10.1192/apt.bp.111.009308

Dubois, E. C. (2014). Does happiness die with us? An Aristotelian examination of the fortunes of the deceased. *Journal of Philosophy of Life, 4*(1), 28–37.

Edwards, A., Pang, N., Shiu, V., & Chan, C. (2010). Review: The understanding of spirituality and the potential role of spiritual care in end-of-life and palliative care: A meta-study of qualitative research. *Palliative Medicine, 24*(8), 753–770. https://doi.org/10.1177/0269216310375860

Hartogh, G. D. (2017). Suffering and dying well: On the proper aim of palliative care. *Medicine, Health Care and Philosophy, 20*(3), 413–424. https://doi.org/10.1007/s11019-017-9764-3

Headley, B., & Wearing, A. J. (1992). *Understanding happiness: A theory of subjective well-being.* Longman Cheshire.

Hodiamont, F., Jünger, S., Leidl, R., Maier, B. O., Schildmann, E., & Bausewein, C. (2019). Understanding complexity: The palliative care situation as a complex adaptive system. *BMC Health Services Research, 19*(1), 1–14. https://doi.org/10.1186/s12913-019-3961-0

Hurst, S., Whitmer, M., Prins, M., Shepard, K., & McVey, D. (2009). Medical futility: A paradigm as old as hippocrates. *Dimensions of Critical Care Nursing, 28*(2), 67–71. https://doi.org/10.1097/DCC.0b013e318195d43f

Kahneman, D., Diener, E., & Schwarz, N. (Eds.) (2003). *Well-being: The foundations of hedonic psychology.* Russell Sage Foundation.

Kearney, M. (1992). Palliative medicine: Just another specialty? *Palliative Medicine, 6,* 39–46. https://doi.org/10.1177/02692163200600107

Kleisiaris, C. F., Sfakianakis, C., & Papathanasiou, I. V. (2014). Health care practices in ancient Greece: The Hippocratic ideal. *Journal of Medical Ethics and History of Medicine, 7,* 3–7.

Levinas, E. (2002). Useless suffering. In D. Wood & R. Bernasconi (Eds.), *The provocation of Levinas: Rethinking the other.* Taylor & Francis.

Lingis, A. (1994). *The community of those who have nothing in common.* Indiana University Press.

Longaker, C. (1997). *Facing death and finding hope: A guide to the emotional and spiritual care of the dying.* Random House Publishing Group.

Mann, T. (1927). *The magic mountain.* Actuel Editions.

May, T. (2009). *Death.* Routledge.

Menzies, K. (2019). Understanding the Australian Aboriginal experience of collective, historical and intergenerational trauma. *International Social Work, 62*(6), 1522–1534. https://doi.org/10.1177/0020872819870585

Mount, B. M., Boston, P. H., & Cohen, S. R. (2007). Healing connections: On moving from suffering to a sense of well-being. *Journal of Pain and Symptom Management, 33*(4), 372–388. https://doi.org/10.1016/j.jpainsymman.2006.09.014

Murray, S., Kendall, M., Boyd, K., Grant, L., Highet, G., & Sheikh, A. (2010). Archetypal trajectories of social, psychological, and spiritual wellbeing and distress in family care givers of patients with lung cancer: Secondary analysis of serial qualitative interviews. *BMJ, 340,* c2581. https://doi.org/10.1136/bmj.c2581

Nietzsche, F. (1887). *The gay science.* Amazon Kindle.

Nussbaum, M. C. (2004). *Hiding from humanity: Disgust, shame, and the law.* Princeton University Press.

Park, C. L., & Halifax, R. J. (2021). Religion and spirituality in adjusting to bereavement. In R. A. Neimeyer, D. L. Harris, H. R. Winokuer, & G. F. Thornton (Eds.), *Grief and bereavement in contemporary society* (pp. 355–363). Routledge.

Porter, M. (2015). *Grief is the thing with feathers.* Faber & Faber.

Puig de la Bellacasa, M. (2017). *Matters of care: Speculative ethics in more than human worlds.* University of Minnesota Press.

Randall, F., & Downie, R. S. (2006). *The philosophy of palliative care: Critique and recon-struction.* Oxford University Press.

Rescher, N. (1996). *Process metaphysics: An introduction to process philosophy.* State University of New York Press.

Rinpoche, S. (2002). *The Tibetan book of living and dying.* Rider.

Rosenblatt, P. C. (2014). Grief across cultures: A review and research agenda. In M. S. Stroebe, R. O. Hansson, H. Schut, W. Stroebe (Eds.), *Handbook of bereavement re-search and practice: Advances in theory and intervention* (pp. 207–222). American Psychological Association.

Russell, B. (1930/2006). *The conquest of happiness.* Routledge Classics.

Saunders, C. (1988). Spiritual pain. *Journal of Palliative Care, 4*(3), 29–32. https://doi.org/10.1177/082585978800400306

Stengers, I. (2011). *Thinking with Whitehead.* Harvard University Press.

Usher, K., Jackson, D., Walker, R., Durkin, J., Smallwood, R., Robinson, M., . . . Marriott, R. (2021). Indigenous resilience in Australia: A scoping review using a reflective de-colonizing collective dialogue. *Frontiers in Public Health, 9*(March). https://doi.org/10.3389/fpubh.2021.630601

Van Der Velden, L. F. J., Francke, A. L., Hingstman, L., & Willems, D. L. (2009). Dying from cancer or other chronic diseases in the Netherlands: Ten-year trends derived from death certificate data. *BMC Palliative Care, 8*(1), 4. https://doi.org/10.1186/1472-684X-8-4

Waterman, A. S. (1993). Two conceptions of happiness: Contrasts of personal expres-siveness (eudaimonia) and hedonic enjoyment. *Journal of Personality and Social Psychology, 64*(4), 678–691. https://doi.org/10.1037/0022-3514.64.4.678

Wortmann, J. H., & Park, C. L. (2008). Religion and spirituality in adjustment following bereavement: An integrative review. *Death Studies, 32*(8), 703–736. https://doi.org/10.1080/07481180802289507

AND Societal Wellbeing . . .

13

Wellbeing Frameworks

Emerging Practice, Challenges, and Opportunities

JACKI SCHIRMER, ROBERT TANTON, AND JOHN GOSS ■

INTRODUCTION

The need for an integrated science of wellbeing is nowhere more apparent than in the emerging field of using multi-indicator societal wellbeing frameworks to make positive change in the world. Worldwide, growing numbers of countries, regions, and groups are developing and using these types of wellbeing frameworks to measure the social progress of specific regions or nations and of different groups of people within the regions examined (see Table 13.1). Some frameworks seek to monitor and report change in different aspects of the wellbeing of one or more regions or nations, such as the Organisation for Economic Co-operation and Development (OECD, n.d.) How's Life index or the Canadian Index of Wellbeing (2016). Others aim more specifically to use this information to inform and guide decision-makers as they develop wellbeing budgets and wellbeing-centric policy, such as the New Zealand Living Standards Framework (LSF; NZ Government, 2018) and the Australian Capital Territory (ACT) Wellbeing Framework (ACT Government, 2020). All typically seek to measure multiple aspects of wellbeing using diverse measures that have emerged in very different fields of research, ranging from environmental science to economics, health, and governance studies (Weijers & Morrison, 2018; see also Chapters 14, 17, and 21, this volume).

In this chapter, we examine emerging approaches to integrating the science of wellbeing via the use of societal wellbeing frameworks and highlight priorities for further development. We focus on societal rather than individual wellbeing frameworks. The distinction between these is not always immediately apparent, particularly as many societal frameworks incorporate measurements of aspects of the wellbeing of individuals. However, in general, a societal framework will seek to include a diverse range of measures that examine how well a society provides

Table 13.1 PROMINENT NATIONAL AND INTERNATIONAL WELLBEING FRAMEWORKS IMPLEMENTED SINCE 1990

Year	Wellbeing framework/s	Organisation	Geographic scope	Types of indicators included	Ongoing as of 2021?
1990	Human Development Index	United Nations Development Program	Worldwide	Objective	Yes
1995	Genuine Progress Indicator	Redefining Progress	Used in some countries and US states	Objective	Yes
2001	Vital Signs	Initiated by Canadian Community Foundations	Used by not-for-profit community organisation in multiple countries	Objective and subjective	Yes
2002	Measures of Australia's Progress	Australian Bureau of Statistics	Australia	Objective	No – ceased in 2013
2006	Happy Planet Index	New Economics Foundation NGO	Worldwide	Objective and subjective	Yes
2007-08	National Performance Framework	Scottish Government	Scotland	Objective and subjective	Yes
2008	Gross National Happiness Index	Centre for Bhutan Studies	Bhutan	Objective and subjective	Yes
2009	Canadian Index of Wellbeing	University of Waterloo	Canada	Objective and subjective	Yes
2010	Measuring National Well-being Programme	UK Office for National Statistics	United Kingdom	Objective and subjective	Yes
2011	Better Life Index	Organisation for Economic Cooperation and Development	OECD countries	Objective and subjective	Yes
2012	World Happiness Report	Sustainable Development Solutions Network	Worldwide	Subjective	Yes

2014	Social Progress Index	Social Progress Imperative NGO	Worldwide (with national and regional versions)	Objective	Yes
2015	United Nations Sustainable Development Goals	United Nations	Worldwide	Objective and subjective	Yes
2017	Wellbeing in Germany	German Government	Germany	Objective and subjective	Yes
2018	New Zealand Living Standards Framework	NZ Government	New Zealand	Objective	Yes

References: Canadian Index of Wellbeing, 2016; Die Bundesregierung, 2017; Harrow & Jung, 2016; Helliwell et al. 2020; Hogan et al., 2015; Kubiszewski et al., 2013; NZ Government, 2018; OECD n.d.; Scottish Ministers, 2018; Stanton, 2007; Ura et al., 2012.

for the wellbeing of those who reside in it, as well as some measures of the well-being of those people. Individual wellbeing frameworks focus more specifically on the psychological, social, and other resources available to an individual and how these are used to maintain and build the individual's quality of life. Societal frameworks examine the resources available in a society—from good governance to education and health services, to safe and affordable places to live—their accessibility, and the extent to which these are enabling positive levels of wellbeing for all living in that society. While having some overlap with individual wellbeing frameworks (see also Chapter 1, this volume), societal wellbeing frameworks differ in their scale and the scope of wellbeing resources typically examined.

In this chapter, we briefly trace the evolution of societal wellbeing frameworks in recent decades and how differing processes of development have often led to frameworks that contain similar domains and indicators. The opportunities and challenges of integrating the diverse measures included in these frameworks are then examined.

There are sometimes differing definitions of common terms used to discuss wellbeing frameworks (societal or individual), and this lack of shared meaning is a potential challenge for an integrated science of wellbeing. In this chapter, we use the following terms:

- *Societal wellbeing framework*: An overarching conceptual framework that identifies the aspects of wellbeing to be measured for a given group, region, or country, and (in some cases) how these different aspects can be integrated.
- *Wellbeing domain*: A specific area of wellbeing examined in a framework, usually related to a theorised determinant of wellbeing such as social connections, living standards, safety, or health.
- *Indicator*: A specific aspect of wellbeing that can be measured to identify its state or level. Each domain included in a wellbeing framework typically has multiple indicators.
- *Measure*: The specific data and analytic approach used to populate an indicator.

A BRIEF HISTORY OF SOCIETAL WELLBEING FRAMEWORKS AND THEIR USE

Calls to develop measures of societal progress that go beyond economic growth have a long and storied history. In 1934, Simon Kuznets, one of the architects of the measures of national income subsequently entrenched as measures of social progress, argued that 'the welfare of a nation can scarcely be inferred from a measure of national income' (Jackson, 2010). In 1968, Robert Kennedy famously criticised gross domestic product (GDP) as failing to measure the things that 'make life worthwhile' (Costanza et al., 2014). In 1972, European Commissioner for Agriculture Sicco Mansholt proposed that the European Commission should change its objectives from maximising economic growth to growing 'gross national happiness' (Gómez-Baggethun & Naredo, 2015; Rowan 2020), a statement subsequently made famous through its use by Bhutan's Fourth King, King Jigme Singye Wangchuck (McKay, 2013) As early as 1980, the idea that social progress should be defined based on gross national happiness (GNH) was identified as a guiding principle for Bhutan, although it was the mid-1990s before the concept of GNH was formally embedded in Bhutanese policy and planning (Munro, 2016; see also Chapter 14, this volume).

Despite many calls to go 'beyond GDP', it was the 1990s before the first large-scale attempts to capture broader measures of progress emerged. Frameworks for understanding individual wellbeing emerged somewhat earlier than most societal wellbeing frameworks, with the development of frameworks and measures from Ryff's Psychological Wellbeing Model developed in the 1990s (Ryff & Keyes 1995; see also Chapter 1, this volume), to more recent frameworks such as Seligman's (2018) PERMA framework.

During the 1990s and early 2000s, the first societal wellbeing frameworks emerged that sought to measure multiple dimensions of wellbeing and integrate them in some way, whether through development of a single index combining data from multiple indicators of wellbeing or more qualitatively through decision-makers weighing up the relative importance of data from multiple indicators when identifying actions to improve wellbeing.

Table 13.1 identifies some of the more prominent national and international wellbeing frameworks that have produced data since 1990. It only includes those that have reported data against the specified indicators and provides the year in which data were first produced; in many cases, frameworks were in development for several years prior to this point. While representing a partial list of the many wellbeing frameworks developed, Table 13.1 highlights that, since 2000, and particularly since 2010, the number and type of wellbeing frameworks in use worldwide has grown rapidly. Despite this growth in the development of wellbeing frameworks, the challenges of integrating information from multiple domains and indicators of wellbeing remain significant and are tackled in different ways by different frameworks.

Arguably the first prominent framework to use a wellbeing perspective was the Human Development Index, first produced in 1990. Drawing on Sen's 'capabilities' approach to understanding wellbeing, the Human Development Index measures progress using indicators of life expectancy, education, and household income. These three indicators are combined into a single index measure, with each equally weighted (Stanton, 2007). This approach to integration has been widely discussed and critiqued: some argue that averaging data across three different measures into a single index and using equal weighting of the three oversimplifies the data; these critics instead seek theoretically grounded approaches to weighting. Others argue that the simplicity of using equal weighting, while having limitations, results in a simple and easy to communicate index that can provide a ready alternative to measures of economic growth and be easily used by policymakers (Stanton, 2007).

This type of debate is in no way unique to the Human Development Index: it is typical of the debates that occur when developing any wellbeing framework and of the lack of consensus in this rapidly developing field regarding best-practice approaches. This chapter identifies and discusses common challenges experienced when developing frameworks and when seeking to synthesise and use wellbeing framework data to inform decision-making processes.

THE MEANING OF LIFE: WHAT IS THE PURPOSE OF A WELLBEING FRAMEWORK?

To an extent, all wellbeing frameworks have a shared purpose: they seek to go 'beyond GDP' to present a wider range of measures of societal progress that better reflect the things that matter to human societies. Beyond this general goal, however, the purpose of frameworks often differs significantly—and is often not explicitly stated. Analysis of the frameworks listed in Table 13.1 suggests that societal wellbeing frameworks often have one or more of four purposes: (i) measurement of levels of wellbeing, (ii) achieving outcomes, (iii) supporting decision-making, and/or (iv) communication.

All societal wellbeing frameworks involve measurement of levels of wellbeing: for some this is a means to another end, such as informing policy decisions; for others it is the principal purpose of the framework. Wellbeing frameworks whose purpose is principally measurement and monitoring of change in levels of different aspects of wellbeing do not set specific goals or objectives for wellbeing. They are not designed to inform specific policies or programmes or to measure whether a society is reaching particular objectives. These frameworks typically describe their domains and indicators based on what is being measured rather than on what a society hopes to achieve. For example, the OECD How's Life index, when measuring 'life satisfaction', does not set specific goals for levels of this measure of subjective wellbeing that are being sought, but instead describes what the indicator measures (level of life satisfaction) and produces data on which countries and regions have higher and lower life satisfaction (Durand, 2015).

In contrast, outcome-oriented frameworks are aspirational in nature: they describe their components in terms of what they are trying to achieve and seek to explicitly measure against these outcomes. For example, the third UN Sustainable Development Goal seeks to achieve the aspirational outcome 'good health and wellbeing', with the objective being to 'ensure healthy lives and promote wellbeing for all at all ages' (Howden-Chapman et al., 2017). Specific targets are then set for different aspects of this overall goal. Similarly, the Scottish National Performance Framework is designed around explicit outcomes that 'describe the kind of Scotland we want to see' (Scottish Government, n.d.); these outcomes are reviewed every decade and updated to reflect the changing aspirations of Scotland's population. A potential challenge of outcome-oriented frameworks is the risk of regular change in what is measured: change in desired outcomes may require change in what is measured as part of the framework, and this in turn can risk loss of consistency—and thus comparability—in measurement over time.

Some frameworks incorporate elements of both a focus on measurement and achievement of outcomes in their design. In this type of framework, while each indicator may not be assessed against a specific stated outcome, the framework as a whole is designed to assess whether outcomes considered critical for society are being achieved. The main examples of this are frameworks that explicitly seek to measure both wellbeing outcomes of today and whether there is sufficient wellbeing 'capital' in place to support future wellbeing—notably, the OECD Better Life Index and the New Zealand LSF (Durand, 2015; Hall, 2019). By explicitly measuring both current levels and 'stocks' available for the future, these frameworks are designed to measure the outcome of ensuring sustainable wellbeing for the long term and reduce the risk of prioritising short-term wellbeing outcomes at the expense of the long-term welfare of society as a whole.

While it could be assumed that aspirational, outcome-focused frameworks are specifically designed to support and inform policy and decision-making, this is not necessarily the case. In particular, the UN Sustainable Development Goals are aspirational in nature but are critiqued by some as being 'inspirational rhetoric' that has 'unactionable, unquantifiable targets' instead of comprising indicators that can meaningfully inform and assist decision-makers in achieving these goals (Easterly, 2015). This suggests that not all aspirational, outcomes-focused frameworks are designed specifically to support decision-making.

Thus we argue that a third common objective of wellbeing frameworks is to support decision-making and that this is not necessarily the same as identifying desired outcomes. While all frameworks *can* be used to support decision-making, few have been explicitly designed to be integrated into decision-making processes such as making budget allocation and policy decisions. However, in recent years, more examples are emerging of wellbeing frameworks that have been explicitly designed with decision-making in mind. For instance, New Zealand's LSF was explicitly designed to support the development of wellbeing budget processes: in budget-setting processes, proposed initiatives put forward by ministers and agencies are assessed based on consideration of their likely impacts for the domains included in the LSF (The Treasury, 2019). Interestingly, while designed to support decision-making, the LSF is not outcome-oriented: the LSF does not set a desired outcome for each indicator. Instead, the budget process involves making a case that expenditure will have a positive impact on one or more of the indicators measured as part of the LSF (The Treasury, 2019). This enables the LSF to measure indicators without seeking to measure against set objectives, while objective-setting is incorporated into policy processes that are able to change over time.

The final common purpose of wellbeing frameworks is communication: wellbeing frameworks often have a broader purpose of public education and leadership to inspire action across the public and private sectors (Badham, 2015; Dalziel, Saunders, & Savage, 2019). To achieve this aim, frameworks need to communicate data and information in ways that help engage the broader population in discussions about what is important to quality of life and improve understanding of which people have better and poorer access to a high quality of life. This in turn helps build public understanding and support for the use of wellbeing as a measure of social progress (Durand, 2015). Communication-oriented frameworks seek to ensure that the domains and indicators included can be readily understood not just by experts in the field of wellbeing research, or by policy-makers, but by the broader public. This may mean selecting and presenting measures in ways that ensure that they can be readily understood and interpreted without having a specialist background in the topic of wellbeing.

The varying purposes of different frameworks present both challenges and opportunities for developing an integrated understanding of wellbeing. They provide a diversity of examples of how frameworks can be developed for different purposes. This diversity can present a challenge to developing a shared, integrated understanding of wellbeing yet also ensure that a wider range of perspectives are explored as part of developing an integrated understanding. The type of integration considered appropriate may vary depending on the framework. A framework seeking to communicate to the public may prioritise achieving easy-to-understand, simplified information that enables members of the public to readily compare indicators, even when they draw on data from very different sources and perspectives. This may result in tension between designing frameworks for public communication and designing frameworks that take advantage of the emerging complexity of knowledge about wellbeing across different sciences. Regarding the latter, an integrated understanding of wellbeing may seek to measure a given aspect of wellbeing from differing disciplinary perspectives to better understand how they can be brought together to form an integrated view; however, this increases the complexity of the indicators and may reduce their ease of use by decision-makers or the broader public. For this reason, Costanza et al. (2014) argue that it is critical to invest in 'a sustained, transdisciplinary effort to integrate metrics and build consensus' through both top-down expert-driven processes and 'bottom-up' engagement of civil society to ensure that the resulting approaches are meaningful and useable.

The emergence of multiple outcomes-based frameworks suggests that any approach to wellbeing will need to have mechanisms for engaging with changing values, aspirations, and opportunities that over time lead to evolving views about what it means to achieve 'good' wellbeing—and hence the best indicators of wellbeing. At a minimum, frameworks need to be able to adapt to changing technology and ways of living. For example, the earliest wellbeing frameworks were developed before the advent of the internet or widespread use of mobile phones. In these, having access to telecommunications was not typically considered critical to achieving indicators such as building skills or accessing employment. By 2021, 'digital access' was identified by residents of the Australian Capital Territory in Australia as being critical to their wellbeing and life opportunities and hence was included as a specific indicator in the ACT Wellbeing Framework (ACT Government, 2020). An integrated understanding of wellbeing needs to be flexible enough to understand how the domains and indicators of wellbeing, or the processes by which humans achieve quality of life, change over time, and incorp-orate these into measures used in wellbeing frameworks.

DEVELOPING AND UPDATING WELLBEING FRAMEWORKS: EXPERT VERSUS COMMUNITY-LED PROCESSES

Some wellbeing frameworks have been developed principally by researchers and/or policy-makers with limited input from others; others have been developed as community-led processes in which consultation with key stakeholder groups and the broader community has driven how the framework is conceptualised and de-veloped. Few frameworks have been actively revised since their initial develop-ment: exceptions include ongoing updates to methods and measures used in the Human Development Index (Stanton, 2007) and a review of the Scottish National Outcomes framework 10 years after its initial development to identify changes in desired outcomes across Scottish society (Scottish Ministers, 2018).

The type of process used to develop and review frameworks needs to be con-sidered when seeking to develop an integrated conceptualisation of wellbeing. Should integration be driven by the views of experts (and, if so, by which experts), the general public, specific types of stakeholders, or by a mix of all three? In short, who should have a say on which aspects of wellbeing should be included in a framework and how measures of these different aspects should be integrated and synthesised to form an overall understanding of societal wellbeing? Within this, there are many more specific questions. For example, to what extent should soci-etal frameworks seek to be comparable across regions through use of identical in-dicators versus those specific to the nation or region they examine and the unique values and perspectives residents of that region hold about what it important to their wellbeing? Should indicators be chosen based on the advice of experts, who may have knowledge of the things that influence wellbeing that many citizens of a region may have little conscious awareness of, and/or should they be based on those things citizens are more consciously aware of in terms of their wellbeing?

Many frameworks seek to resolve these questions through ensuring the voices and perspectives of experts, stakeholders, and the public are all provided oppor-tunity to be heard when developing or revising a framework. Examples of wellbe-ing frameworks that have done this include the Bhutan Gross National Happiness Index (see also Chapter 14, this volume), Canadian Index of Wellbeing, German national wellbeing framework, and New Zealand LSF, amongst others (Die Bundesregierung, 2017; Hogan et al., 2015; New Zealand Government, 2018; Ura, Alkire, Zangmo, & Wangdi, 2012). All of these are national frameworks, and this type of multisectoral consultative approach is commonly used to develop these. International wellbeing frameworks, meanwhile, develop domains and indica-tors of wellbeing to be used across multiple countries. The development of these typically relies more on expert advice, or consultation processes between govern-ments. For example, the OECD's Better Life Index and the Social Progress Index were developed primarily using discussions with experts and stakeholders such as national policy-makers and wellbeing researchers (OECD, 2018; Porter & Stern, 2017).

Developing wellbeing frameworks using a collaborative process is argued to build more substantial ownership and 'buy in' to the concept of the framework and to increase the relevance of the framework to the populations it examines. This, in turn, is argued to increase the willingness of decision-makers and the broader public to engage with frameworks and use the data they provide to inform decision-making (Hogan et al., 2015). Hogan et al. (2015) argue that the types of consultative processes commonly used when developing wellbeing frameworks could be better used to integrate the different perspectives on wellbeing that each group can contribute. In particular, they argue that using group design processes for frameworks can 'facilitate joint actions at every level . . . by a variety of stake-holders' (pp. 863–864), particularly if embedded in a systems framework, and they suggest that this provides an opportunity for integrating understandings of different aspects of wellbeing and applying this knowledge to make real world change. However, they also identify significant challenges to achieving this. To succeed, this type of systems-thinking informed collaborative process needs to build a shared understanding of disparate measures of wellbeing drawn from different disciplines, how they relate to each other as part of a system, and how they change over time. This is a challenging undertaking, with many non-experts likely having little to no awareness of many of the factors that may impact their own wellbeing and that of others and many experts having deep but narrow knowledge of different 'slices' of current understandings of wellbeing. The extensive body of work developed in recent decades on transdisciplinary and collaborative learning provides important lessons for those seeking to integrate understandings of wellbeing via this type of process, including multiple methodologies for building shared knowledge (see, e.g., Christinck & Kaufmann, 2017).

A particular challenge is ensuring that the voices of those who have historically been marginalised or ignored are included and prioritised when developing societal wellbeing frameworks. As discussed subsequently, the emergence of societal wellbeing frameworks has been accompanied by concerns that frameworks, if not well designed, risk contributing further to social marginalisation rather than providing a means of highlighting and overcoming disparities in wellbeing opportunities for different groups (Yap & Yu, 2016).

THE EVOLUTION OF DOMAINS AND INDICATORS INCLUDED IN SOCIETAL WELLBEING FRAMEWORKS

As noted earlier, a key attribute of societal wellbeing frameworks is that they examine multiple domains of wellbeing, with several indicators typically measured within each domain. These domains represent different dimensions of or influences on societal wellbeing and typically include areas ranging from the health of the residents of a region, to access to good and fair governance, social connections, standard of living, and the health of the environment, to name a few.

The choice of domains and indicators varies depending on the purpose of the framework (i.e., measurement, outcomes, decision-making, and/or communication), the process used to develop the framework, and, more pragmatically, the availability of data. A key challenge to developing an integrated understanding of wellbeing is the common choice made to limit frameworks to available data: this can result in a bias toward those things already being measured in available datasets, something which typically reflects choices made based on priorities other than the measurement of wellbeing. It can therefore result in a lack of attention to those areas known to be important to wellbeing but for which there is a lack of investment in measurement.

An example is the Index of Wellbeing for Older Australians in Australia. This index was designed using a capabilities framework, an integrative approach to wellbeing that in this case focused on whether older Australians had the capabilities needed across different domains of their life to achieve a positive quality of life. A priority for this index was the production of data for small regions ('small area' data). While a key capability area is health, a lack of small-area health data in Australia meant that the only data able to be reported were those identifying levels of need for assistance with care (Tanton, Miranti, Vidyattama, & Tuli, 2019). Ultimately, the health domain was renamed a 'functional ability' domain to reflect the fact that health data were not available.

Some frameworks exclude domains and indicators for which there is a lack of data; others include them but identify that there is a lack of data. Highlighting data gaps in a framework is preferable to exclusion: identifying gaps encourages investment in filling them, which in turn supports progress toward an integrated conceptualisation of wellbeing.

Figure 13.1 summarises the domains of wellbeing included in 25 wellbeing frameworks. Despite sometimes large differences in the processes used to develop these frameworks, there is often a high degree of similarity between them. Almost all include domains examining standard of living, health, education, and

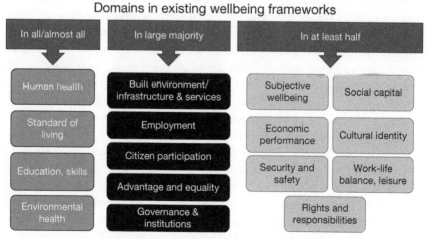

Figure 13.1 Common domains included in wellbeing frameworks in use as of 2021.

environmental health. This likely reflects both that, first, data are more readily available on many of these areas than on other aspects of wellbeing and, second, consensus that these domains are critical determinants of quality of life. Most—but not all—examine access to key infrastructure, services, and/or the quality of the built environment; access to employment; and ability to participate in civic life, as well as quality of governance. This again likely reflects both the availability of data (e.g., measures of employment are typically readily available) and the widely assumed importance of these domains to wellbeing.

Harder to measure domains such as social capital, cultural identity, security and safety, economic performance, work–life balance/leisure, rights and responsibilities, and subjective wellbeing are present in fewer than half of the frameworks. These domains are known to be important to societal wellbeing, but most have not historically been measured as part of national accounts, in national census data, or even in regularly conducted surveys. The importance of some of these areas to wellbeing has only recently been recognised, further contributing to both a common lack of availability of data to include in frameworks and a lack of recognition of these areas in older frameworks. For example, understanding the central importance to wellbeing of being able to safely express and enact cultural identity has emerged more recently than has awareness of the importance of factors such as a person's health and income (e.g., Browne-Yung, Ziersch, Baum, & Gallaher, 2013).

MEASURING INDICATORS

It is common for multiple indicators to be identified as relevant to measuring a domain. For example, an education domain might incorporate indicators of the proportion of adults achieving different levels of formal educational attainment, drop-out rates in high school, performance of current students against standards of literacy and numeracy, and rates of university enrolment. Ideally, the indicators used will represent the domain fully, be well defined, and available in consistent datasets that are consistently and regularly measured over time. In reality, however, as noted above, it is common for limited data to be available to measure indicators. In international wellbeing frameworks, this can mean that the indicators selected for inclusion tend to reflect the countries with the least available data. This limits the indicators that can be used and acts as a barrier to development of an integrated measurement of wellbeing in these frameworks that fully reflects emerging understanding of the diverse things that matter for wellbeing.

A further challenge is that differences across regions can mean an indicator is relevant and suitable for one region while being inappropriate for another. For example, the OECD's Regional Well-Being measures were developed to compare regions within OECD countries. The indicator for the domain 'civic engagement' is 'voter turnout'—the proportion of people who vote (OECD, 2018). This provides a meaningful measure of engagement in regions where voting is voluntary; however, in Australia, where voters are required to vote by law, the rate of close to 100% voter turnout is more likely to reflect a desire to avoid being fined for failing to vote rather than high civic engagement. This suggests a need for differing indicators to be used in different regions, with resulting challenges in comparing findings of different wellbeing frameworks. It may often be unrealistic to have identical indicators across regions within a nation, let alone across multiple nations. This presents a challenge for evolving integrated understandings of wellbeing: rather than reducing wellbeing measurement only to those things that are common across all regions and nations, an integrated approach needs to be able to recognise, celebrate, and engage with these differences in meaningful ways.

Attempts to make wellbeing frameworks comparable can also, if done naïvely, risk further disenfranchising some groups by privileging the indicators that represent the majority at the expense of other groups. Societal wellbeing frameworks should act as mechanisms to shine light on disparities and inequalities in wellbeing. Frameworks that use only data collected by societies that have historically marginalised some groups are unlikely to achieve this goal. This is a critical issue for many groups. For example, Yap and Yu (2016) note that 'parallel to the development of wellbeing frameworks around the world is the emergence of a body of research which questions the utility and relevance of those frameworks in addressing Indigenous aspirations and worldviews about what makes a good life'. As wellbeing science develops, these concerns need to be engaged with and addressed. A growing number of frameworks designed by and for Indigenous peoples highlight the sometimes profound differences in framework domains and indicators that can result from Indigenous-led development processes (Yap & Yu, 2016; see also Chapter 7, this volume). The same is likely to be true for many other groups, and this reinforces the importance to a truly integrated approach to wellbeing of ensuring inclusive processes are used in the development of frameworks.

Beyond the issues of data availability and inclusivity, there remains a lack of consensus around key aspects of wellbeing indicator measurement. These include ongoing debate about the use of objective versus subjective indicators and about whether and how to measure 'sufficiency' (i.e., What is the level of any given indicator needed to provide a 'sufficient' level of wellbeing?). We address each of these issues in turn.

Wellbeing and quality of life can be measured using subjective and objective indicators. Broadly speaking, subjective measures involve people being asked to rate the overall quality of their state of wellbeing or some aspect of it, such as their standard of living, while objective measures involve measuring something that an external observer can measure independently, such as household income, which can be verified by looking at records of payments. Many indicators of wellbeing can be measured using both subjective and objective measures. For example, when measuring household income, it is possible to objectively measure the amount of income earned and identify whether it is sufficient to cover average costs of accommodation, food, and clothing for the household in question. It is also possible to ask members of the household to subjectively rate whether they are very poor, poor, just getting along, reasonably comfortable, very comfortable, or prosperous. Both subjective and objective measures of income have advantages and limitations.

While early wellbeing frameworks predominantly used objective measures, most frameworks developed in recent years have included both subjective and objective measures, following many years of work considering how best to integrate both as part of understanding wellbeing (e.g., Costanza et al. 2007). This likely reflects growing agreement with Diener et al.'s (2009) argument that subjective and objective indicators should be viewed not as 'either/or' options but as being 'best seen as complementary pieces of information that together permit a better understanding of how people are faring in their lives' (p. 45). However, recognising the value of examining both objective and subjective indicators then raises the challenge of how to integrate the different perspectives provided by each. A range of approaches has been proposed to address this: for example, Costanza et al. (2007) provide an integrative definition of quality of life that seeks to identify how objective and subjective wellbeing measures can be used together to understand the 'extent to which objective human needs are fulfilled in relation to personal or group perceptions of subjective well-being' (p. 269). This question has been addressed in a range of ways: some frameworks simply measure a range of indicators, including subjective and objective, and do not attempt to integrate or compare them; others preferentially use objective indicators and only use subjective indicators where there is no alternative; and some generate overall domain-level indicators that are based on integrating both subjective and objective measures (Ura et al., 2012).

There is a similar lack of consensus on whether and how to identify the level of an indicator considered sufficient to support wellbeing. Many frameworks do not set specific thresholds, instead leaving it up to those who are using these measures to determine whether wellbeing is 'good enough' and thus separating the process of measurement from the process of identifying what the objective is for a society or group in terms of a particular indicator. The OECD Better Life Index, for example, does not typically specify how much of each indicator of wellbeing is considered 'enough' for a 'good life', but instead focuses on providing robust measures that enable comparison of different countries and regions (OECD n.d.). This ensures that the objectives set can change over time, while measurement remains standard over time. The Bhutan GNH Index, meanwhile, takes a different approach. Its design includes explicit identification of thresholds considered to represent 'sufficient' wellbeing, followed by gradients of happiness from sufficiency to very high levels. This enables identification of that proportion of the population who are considered to have sufficient happiness, as well as more broadly of those who have differing levels of happiness. The key challenge experienced when defining these thresholds in the GNH index was a lack of evidence regarding what is 'sufficient' for many indicators (Ura et al., 2012). While it is known that simply assuming 'more is better' may often provide a poor or even inaccurate understanding of wellbeing (Reyes-Garcia et al., 2016), there remains a significant lack of evidence-based identification of what constitutes sufficiency and how to identify sufficiency thresholds and gradients. This is the case even for relatively well-studied topics such as an examination of the relationship between income and wellbeing. While it is well-established that the relationship between income and wellbeing is not simple (e.g., Fanning & O'Neill, 2019), there is no consensus about what level of income is needed to support a sufficient level of wellbeing and how to measure this across countries, with debate about the utility of various approaches such as those seeking to measure poverty levels versus living wages (e.g., Rossi & Curtis, 2013) and those seeking to use subjective versus objective assessments of income sufficiency (e.g., Iannello, Sorgente, Lanz, & Antonietti, 2021). Overly simplistic assumptions about the issue of sufficiency, such as the assumption that 'more is better', have significant risk if used in societal wellbeing frameworks, where they risk encouraging investment in increasing levels of things known to influence wellbeing, such as income, beyond the point where this would meaningfully contribute to overall quality of life.

INTEGRATING INDICATORS AND DOMAINS

Beyond the challenges of finding data, determining what measure to use, and identifying thresholds is the overarching question of whether and how to integrate the finding of different indicators and domains to produce index measures of wellbeing. Some wellbeing frameworks present a range of indicators and domains without attempting to integrate them into an overall measure; others have developed and use a range of methods to produce indexes of wellbeing. Some develop indexes for each domain of wellbeing, which are comprised of the indicators within that domain. Other frameworks go further, integrating these domain-level indexes into a single, overall wellbeing index.

The decision to integrate indicators into indexes is a critical one. Some argue that wellbeing frameworks that use a single index measure, such as the Human Development Index, may make it easier to transition to wellbeing over economic measures by providing a similarly easy-to-understand metric (Stanton, 2007). This perspective is likely based in part on the argument that one of the reasons measures of economic growth became almost universally relied on is the relative simplicity of understanding resulting from the synthesis of economic production data into easily understandable metrics of overall economic growth (Costanza, Hart, Talberth, & Posner, 2009). Following this argument, it seems logical that wellbeing metrics should produce similarly simple to interpret measures.

However, while a single index is easier to interpret and analyse, it can hide important information by virtue of combining data about different aspect of wellbeing. For example, a region with an overall high wellbeing index score may have high scores for many dimensions of wellbeing but still have a low score for one domain or indicator of wellbeing. Ideally, indexes should be accompanied by information that allows users of a framework to 'drill down' to understand why an overall index score has grown or declined. Wellbeing frameworks are inherently complex, drawing together data from diverse sources and disciplines: if these diverse data are to be readily accessible, care is needed to ensure that simplicity of interpretation is achieved not only through producing a synthesising index, but also through ensuring the full range of data produced in the framework is readily accessible and easy to interpret. Many examples exist that demonstrate approaches to achieving this: for example, the use of online maps of indexes, domains, and indexes to enable users to easily unpack the content of an index and understand why it is high or low by looking at its constituent elements (Miranti et al., 2021; see also Chapter 21, this volume).

A key challenge in producing an index that is meaningful and able to be 'unpacked' to identify which of its elements is responsible for observed changes is that many wellbeing indicators use different metrics. Combining indicators that are measured using differing metrics (e.g., average dollars of income earned vs. parts per million [ppm] of air pollution) and have different distributions is difficult. One approach is to identify measures that focus on proportions: for example, the percentage of families with low incomes and the percentage ppm in the area. The ACT Wellbeing Framework is an example of this approach (ACT Government, 2020). Another method, used in both the Human Development Index and the Global Youth Development Index (Commonwealth Secretariat, 2021; Stanton, 2007) is to normalise an indicator, so the indicator is

$$Dimension\ Index = \frac{Actual\ Value - Minimum\ Value}{Maximum\ Value - Minimun\ Value}.$$

In this approach, minimum and maximum values are either determined by the designers of the index or calculated from the data. For example, for the Human Development Index, no country in the world in the 20th century had a life expectancy of less than 20 years, so this was set as a minimum; maximum life expectancy is set at 85 as a realistic aspiration for most countries (Stanton, 2007).

However, these methods do not address the question of the relative weighting of different indicators within a domain, or domains within an overall wellbeing index. Many frameworks assume that all indicators are equally important contributors to wellbeing and hence should be weighted equally. This assumption is often a result of a lack of evidence regarding the relative importance of different indicators and wellbeing domains and is also used because equal weighting is conceptually simpler both to apply and to communicate to users of the index while more complex statistical techniques are harder to use and for users to understand. This is, for example, a key reason for the use of equal weighting in the Human Development Index (Stanton, 2007).

However, equal weighting has obvious disadvantages. It is likely that some things are more important to a society's wellbeing than others or that a given amount of change in one indicator has a greater impact on quality of life compared to the same amount of change in another. Use of equal weighting can imply an assumption that one thing is substitutable for another: for example, the synthesis of natural and human-made capital as part of the Genuine Progress Indicator has been criticised because the two are substitutes for each other (Kubiszewski et al., 2013). This then raises the question of how best to determine the relative weight of different indicators in the index. Options include using technical approaches such as principal components analysis to derive an index (Noble et al., 2003). This approach is relatively commonly used by statistical agencies to group indicators of socioeconomic advantage and disadvantage into summary indexes (e.g., Australian Bureau of Statistics, 2018; Fahy, Lee, & Milne, 2017) but, to date, has not typically been used to create indexes that combine indicators in wellbeing frameworks. This approach has the benefit of statistical rigour, but the resulting index is not comparable over time. This significantly reduces its potential for most wellbeing frameworks, which explicitly seek to measure change over time. Ongoing work developing approaches to using statistical techniques that can enable comparison of resulting indexes over time represents an important area for continuing development (McNamara, Tanton, Daly, & Harding, 2009).

Other approaches to weighting different indicators within a domain and different domains within an index include weighting based on views of the community or key stakeholders about the relative importance of different indicators, as was done in the GNH Index, or based on the relative policy importance of differing components (Noble et al., 2003; Ura et al., 2012). The OECD provides an innovative way of combining indicators in their Better Life Index: their interactive website allows users to adjust the weights for each indicator themselves, enabling the user to generate an overall index of wellbeing that reflects their personal views about the relative importance of its different components (OECD, n.d.).

The choices made about whether and how to integrate indicators into domain-level and framework-level indexes will differ depending on the purpose of the framework. There is limited available information on the effectiveness of generating indexes using different approaches and for different purposes: development of evidence-informed practice in this area is an important focus for the further development and refinement of societal wellbeing frameworks.

WELLBEING-DRIVEN POLICY AND ACTION

Whereas early wellbeing frameworks often principally focused on addressing the challenges of measurement and communication, increasing attention is shifting to how best to enable the data reported in societal wellbeing frameworks to be used in decision-making processes. This reflects recognition that while it is critically important to measure and publish wellbeing data that provides a different perspective on progress, 'it is necessary to go beyond simply *making indicators available* to wide audiences' (Exton & Shinwell, 2018, p. 19; emphasis in original), particularly as growing numbers of governments seek to actively use the data produced in wellbeing frameworks to inform their decision-making. Exton and Shinwell (2018) found that amongst those governments that have committed to using wellbeing approaches, wellbeing evidence is used at various stages of the policy cycle in different jurisdictions and often at multiple stages. For example, wellbeing indicators are often used to identify areas where there is greatest need for investment to address low levels of wellbeing, to assess whether a proposed policy or programme is likely to improve wellbeing, and/or to evaluate the effectiveness of policy interventions in 'shifting the dial' for one or more wellbeing indicators.

Exton and Shinwell (2018) identified several common challenges experienced by those seeking to use data from wellbeing frameworks to inform decision-making. In particular, they identified that difficulty occurs when indicators (and a framework more generally) were not developed for policy use. This highlights the importance of clearly identifying the multiple end uses of wellbeing framework data at the framework development stage to ensure that the framework is explicitly designed to produce data that is 'fit for purpose' for these uses.

Another key challenge identified was that of supporting policy-makers to transition from decision-making processes based on criteria other than wellbeing (such as economic growth) to processes that use a wellbeing lens. This is a major shift that requires development of new skills and knowledge amongst the policy-making community, something in an early stage at the time of writing (Dalziel, 2019; Exton & Shinwell, 2018; Reid, 2019). Examples of emerging work include guidance for policy-makers developed by the What Works for Wellbeing Centre in the United Kingdom, which aims to support decision-makers to use wellbeing data in areas as diverse as evaluating the economic outcomes of investments made with a goal of improving wellbeing, to adding life satisfaction measures to surveys, to increasing availability of these data for use in policy evaluation (Wright, Peasgood, & MacLennan, 2017).

It is important to clearly distinguish the purpose and role of a societal wellbeing framework from the more specific monitoring and evaluation frameworks that are necessary for policy development and performance evaluation. It is tempting to seek to replace monitoring and evaluation frameworks with wellbeing frameworks. In our view, it is dangerous to seek to do this: a societal wellbeing framework is not intended to be a specific tool for monitoring and evaluating performance of specific policies, programmes, and actions. We do believe wellbeing frameworks have a role in monitoring and evaluation: the goal of an action may be to achieve growth in an important area of wellbeing, and this overall goal may be measured based partly on identifying whether there is a change in the relevant indicator in a wellbeing framework. However, it is critical to also have a more specific and detailed monitoring and evaluation framework that can interrogate which aspects of a policy, programme, or action were more and less effective, and why—something that sits beyond the role of a framework seeking to measure change in wellbeing consistently over time. The goal is not to have wellbeing frameworks replace existing mechanisms that are effective, but rather to build the linkages needed, for example, through ensuring monitoring and evaluation can be interpreted with reference to an overarching wellbeing framework.

Ultimately, the success or failure of wellbeing frameworks in achieving change rests in large part on whether the new perspectives they provide on progress can be used to inform decision-making and action. This means that continuing to develop a science to guide this type of use of wellbeing framework data is as important as the development of measures of wellbeing.

SUMMARY

The use of societal wellbeing frameworks is growing in popularity worldwide. These frameworks are incorporating a growing number of measures of often highly diverse aspects of wellbeing, from the health of the environment to human health, and from standard of living to a person's ability to safely express their cultural identity, to name a few. The rapid growth in the number and scope of societal wellbeing frameworks is accompanied by multiple challenges and opportunities for advancement of a more integrated understanding of what wellbeing is, how it can be measured, and how this understanding can be used to actively inform decision-making. Existing wellbeing frameworks have a diversity of purposes, ranging from improving availability of measures, to achieving specific wellbeing outcomes, informing decision-making processes, and providing easy-to-understand wellbeing tools and metrics. They are developed using a variety of processes, some focusing more on expert-led development, others more on community-led prioritisation of framework design, and others on a combination of the two. The resulting frameworks have evolved from mostly examining domains of wellbeing for which data are already readily available, such as educational attainment and living standards, to increasingly also measuring things for which data have rarely been previously available, such as time use, social capital, rights and responsibilities, and cultural identity.

Many challenges remain in the development and use of societal wellbeing frameworks. There are often limited data available for many of the indicators known to be important to wellbeing: this results in frameworks that either limit their design to available data or have significant gaps. Lack of data can result in the use of indicators that have less validity than desired or which are relevant in some regions but not in others. Debates persist about the use of subjective versus objective measures of wellbeing, about whether and how to identify 'sufficiency' of levels of wellbeing, and whether and how to integrate indicators into indexes that provide a high-level measure of overall wellbeing.

Many of these challenges appear on the surface to be primarily issues of measurement that are largely in the purview of experts in wellbeing data collection, measurement, and analysis as they develop statistically robust measures of wellbeing. However, they are also questions of value and priority. It is critical to ensure that the processes by which decisions are made about framework development and use are inclusive of those whose wellbeing is being reported on and whose lives are impacted by the decisions made based on information produced in societal wellbeing frameworks.

REFERENCES

ACT Government. (2020). *ACT wellbeing framework*. ACT Government.
Australian Bureau of Statistics. (2018). *Socio-economic indexes for areas (SEIFA) – 2016*. Commonwealth of Australia. https://doi.org/2033.0.55.001

Badham, M. (2015). Democratising cultural indicators: Developing a shared sense of progress. In L. MacDowall, M. Badham, E. Blomkamp, & K. Dunphy (Eds.), *Making culture count: The politics of cultural measurement* (pp. 195–213). Palgrave Macmillan.

Browne-Yung, K., Ziersch, A., Baum, F., & Gallaher, G. (2013). Aboriginal Australians' experience of social capital and its relevance to health and wellbeing in urban settings. *Social Science & Medicine, 97*, 20–28.

Canadian Index of Wellbeing. (2016). *How are Canadians really doing?* Canadian Index of Wellbeing of University of Waterloo.

Christinck, A., & Kaufmann, B. (2017). Facilitating change: Methodologies for collaborative learning with stakeholders. In M. Padmanabhan (Ed.), *Transdisciplinary research and sustainability: Collaboration, innovation and transformation* (pp. 171–190). Routledge.

Commonwealth Secretariat. (2021). *Global Youth Development Index and Report 2020*. Commonwealth Secretariat.

Costanza, R., Fisher, B., Ali, S., Beer, C., Bond, L., Boumans, R., . . . Snapp, R. (2007). Quality of life: An approach integrating opportunities, human needs, and subjective well-being. *Ecological Economics, 61*, 267–276.

Costanza, R., Hart, M., Talberth, J., & Posner, S. (2009). Beyond GDP: The need for new measures of progress. *The Pardee Papers*.

Costanza, R., Kubiszewski, I., Giovannini, E., Lovins, H., McGlade, J., Pickett, K., . . . Wilkinson, R. (2014). Time to leave GDP behind. *Nature, 505*, 283–285.

Dalziel, P. (2019). Wellbeing economics in public policy: A distinctive Australasian contribution? *The Economic and Labour Relations Review, 30*(4), 478–497.

Dalziel, P., Saunders, C., & Savage, C. (2019). *Culture, wellbeing, and the living standards framework: A perspective* (No. 19/02). New Zealand Treasury Discussion Paper.

Die Bundesregierung. (2017). Government report on wellbeing in Germany. https://www.gut-leben-in-deutschland.de/downloads/Government-Report-on-Wellbeing-in-Germany.pdf

Diener, E., Lucas, R., Schimmack, U., & Helliwell, J. (2009). *Well-being for public policy*. Oxford University Press.

Durand, M. (2015). The OECD better life initiative: *How's life?* and the measurement of well-being. *Review of Income and Wealth, 61*(1), 4–17.

Easterly, W. (2015). The SDGs should stand for senseless, dreamy, garbled. *Foreign Policy, 28*.

Exton, C., & Shinwell, M. (2018). *Policy use of well-being metrics: Describing countries' experiences*. OECD Statistics Working Papers 2018/07. OECD Statistics and Data Directorate. https://dx.doi.org/10.1787/d98eb8ed-en

Fahy, K. M., Lee, A., & Milne, B. J. (2017). *New Zealand socio-economic index 2013*. www.stats.govt.nz

Fanning, A. L., & O'Neill, D. W. (2019). The wellbeing–consumption paradox: Happiness, health, income, and carbon emissions in growing versus non-growing economies. *Journal of Cleaner Production, 212*, 810–821.

Gómez-Baggethun, E., & Naredo, J. M. (2015). In search of lost time: The rise and fall of limits to growth in international sustainability policy. *Sustainability Science, 10*(3), 385–395.

Hall, D. (2019). New Zealand's living standards framework: What might Amartya Sen say? *Policy Quarterly*, *15*(1).

Harrow, J., & Jung, T. (2016). Philanthropy and community development: The vital signs of community foundation? *Community Development Journal*, *51*(1), 132–152.

Helliwell, J. F., Huang, H., Wang, S., & Norton, M. (2020). Social environments for world happiness. *World Happiness Report 2020*, 13–45.

Hogan, M. J., Johnston, H., Broome, B., McMoreland, C., Walsh, J. Smale, B., . . . Groarke, A. M. (2015). Consulting with citizens in the design of wellbeing measures and policies: Lessons from a systems science application. *Social Indicators Research 123*, 857–877.

Howden-Chapman, P., Siri, J., Chisholm, E., Chapman, R., Doll, C. N., & Capon, A. (2017). SDG 3: Ensure healthy lives and promote wellbeing for all at all ages. *A guide to SDG interactions: From science to implementation* (pp. 81–126). International Council for Science.

Iannello, P., Sorgente, A., Lanz, M., & Antonietti, A. (2021). Financial well-being and its relationship with subjective and psychological well-being among emerging adults: Testing the moderating effect of individual differences. *Journal of Happiness Studies*, *22*, 1385–1411.

Jackson, T. (2010). Reviewing the research: Report of the Commission on the Measurement of Economic Performance and Social Progress. *Environment*, *53*, 38–40. doi: 10.1080/00139157.2011.539946

Kennedy, R. F. (1968). Remarks of Robert Kennedy at the University of Kansas, March 18, 1968. http://www.glaserprogress.org/program_areas/pdf/Remarks_of_Robert_F_Kennedy.pdf

Kubiszewski, I., Costanza, R., Franco, C., Lawn, P., Talberth, J., Jackson, T., & Aylmer, C. (2013). Beyond GDP: Measuring and achieving global genuine progress. *Ecological Economics*, *93*, 57–68.

McKay, F. (2013). Psychocapital and shangri-las: How happiness became both a means and end to governmentality. *Health, Culture and Society*, *5*(1), 36–50.

McNamara, J., Tanton, R., Daly, A., & Harding, A. (2009). Spatial trends in the risk of social exclusion for Australian children: Patterns from 2001 to 2006. *Child Indicators Research*, *2*, 155–179.

Miranti, R., Tanton, R., Vidyattama, Y., Schimer, J., & Rowe, P. (2021). Examining Evidence of Wellbeing indicators: A Practical Method of Assessment. *Well-being Assessment 4*, 463–494.

Munro, L. T. (2016). Where did Bhutan's gross national happiness come from? The origins of an invented tradition. *Asian Affairs*, *47*(1), 71–92.

Noble, M., Wright, G., Lloyd, M., Dibben, C., Smith, G., Ratcliffe, A., . . . Anttila, C. (2003). *Scottish indices of deprivation 2003*. Social Disadvantage Research Centre.

New Zealand Government. (2018). *Our people, our country, our future. Living Standards Framework: Background and future work*. The Treasury, New Zealand Government. https://treasury.govt.nz/publications/tp/living-standards-frameworkbackground-and-future-work

Porter, M. E., & Stern, S. (2017). *Social progress index 2017*. Social Progress Imperative. https://www2.deloitte.com/content/dam/Deloitte/de/Documents/public-sector/Social-Progress-Index-Findings-Report-SPI-2017.pdf

Organisation for Economic Co-operation and Development (OECD). (2018). *OECD regional well-being: A user's guide. Using data to build better communities*. OECD Publishing.

Organisation for Economic Co-operation and Development (OECD). (n.d.). *Better life index*. http://www.oecdbetterlifeindex.org

Reid, M. (2019). Wellbeing: Adding the local dimension. *Public Sector, 42*(4), 3–5.

Reyes-García, V., Babigumira, R., Pyhälä, A., Wunder, S., Zorondo-Rodríguez, F., & Angelsen, A. (2016). Subjective wellbeing and income: Empirical patterns in the rural developing world. *Journal of Happiness Studies, 17*(2), 773–791.

Rossi, M. M., & Curtis, K. A. (2013). Aiming at half of the target: An argument to replace poverty thresholds with self-sufficiency, or "living wage" standards. *Journal of Poverty, 17*(1), 110–130.

Rowan, K. (2020). The development of well-being policy initiatives. *WellBeing International*. https://wellbeingintl.org/the-development-of-well-being-policy-initiatives/

Ryff, C. D., & Keyes, C. L. M. (1995). The structure of psychological well-being revisited. *Journal of Personality and Social Psychology, 69*(4), 719.

Scottish Government. (n.d.). *National performance framework*. https://nationalperformance.gov.scot/

Scottish Ministers. (2018). *National outcomes for Scotland: Consultation process undertaken to produce draft National Outcomes for Scotland*. Paper presented to Scottish Parliament, March 2018. https://www.parliament.scot/S5_Local_Gov/Inquiries/Updated_National_Outcomes.pdf

Seligman, M. (2018). PERMA and the building blocks of well-being. *The Journal of Positive Psychology, 13*(4), 333–335.

Stanton, E. A. (2007). The human development index: A history. *PERI Working Papers*, 85. Political Economy Research Institute, University of Massachusetts Amherst.

Tanton, R., Miranti, R., Vidyattama, Y., & Tuli, S. (2019). *Index of wellbeing for older Australians (IWOA)*. Commissioned by the Benevolent Society. University of Canberra. https://d3n8a8pro7vhmx.cloudfront.net/benevolent/pages/521/attachments/original/1581053241/Index_of_Wellbeing_for_Older_Australians_%28IWOA%29_FINAL_REPORT.pdf

The Treasury. (2019). *The wellbeing budget*. https://www.treasury.govt.nz/sites/default/files/2019-05/b19-wellbeing-budget.pdf

Ura, K., Alkire, S., Zangmo, T., & Wangdi, K. (2012). *An extensive analysis of GNH index*. The Centre for Bhutan Studies.

Weijers, D., & Morrison, P. S. (2018). Wellbeing and public policy. *Policy Quarterly, 14*(4).

Wright, L., Peasgood, T., & MacLennan, S. (2017). *A guide to wellbeing economic evaluation*. What Works Centre for Wellbeing. https://whatworkswellbeing.org/wp-content/uploads/2020/02/WWCW-Economic-Evaluation-Cost-Effectiveness_Version-1.2-For-website-1.pdf

Yap, M., & Yu, E. (2016). Operationalising the capability approach: Developing culturally relevant indicators of indigenous wellbeing: An Australian example. *Oxford Development Studies, 44*(3), 315–331.

14

Weaving Wellbeing into the Fabric of the Economy

Lessons from Bhutan's Journey Toward Gross National Happiness

JULIA C. KIM, JULIE A. RICHARDSON, AND TSOKI TENZIN ■

INTRODUCTION[1]

Gross national happiness (GNH), as a living experiment in wellbeing economics, has its roots in Bhutan and is now influencing development thinking and practice worldwide. In this chapter, we trace the history of GNH as it emerged from its birthplace in the Himalayan Kingdom of Bhutan and describe how its unique vision has been moving from intention into action. We discuss the GNH Index and how it offers a holistic measurement and policy framework that integrates psychological, physical, societal, and environmental wellbeing. We then explore several unique aspects of GNH, including: (1) prioritising wellbeing—rather than economic growth—as the purpose of the economy, (2) calling attention to addressing both the *outer* conditions (an enabling environment) and *inner* factors (values and mindsets) for a wellbeing economy, and (3) articulating a form of leadership that can be described as 'leadership of the self'. We then describe how GNH is beginning to influence wellbeing initiatives at different levels of scale, including the individual, organisational, national, and global. We argue that, far

1. Aspects of this chapter are included in Julia C. Kim and Amy MacKenzie. Forthcoming. 'Beyond GDP, Beyond Numbers: Bhutan's Journey Towards Gross National Happiness.' In Towards Sustainable Wellbeing: Moving Beyond GDP in Canada and the World, edited by Anders Hayden, Céofride Gaudet, and Jeffrey Wilson. Toronto: University of Toronto Press. This chapter includes updated and new content, including original contributions from new co-authors.

from being a 'luxury' or 'trade-off', the goal of human flourishing is deeply connected to tackling the crisis of sustainability we currently face. Finally, we conclude with reflections on how lessons from Bhutan's experience might help inform and navigate opportunities and challenges going forward, both for Bhutan and for an emerging network of economies of wellbeing worldwide.

FROM ANCIENT ROOTS TO NEW NARRATIVES

GNH emerged in the early 1970s, as the Himalayan Kingdom of Bhutan was beginning to open to greater interaction and exchange with the modern world. It is widely held that the phrase was first expressed by Bhutan's Fourth King, Jigme Singye Wangchuck, when, in response to a reporter's query about his country's gross national product (GDP), he replied that GNH is more important than GNP (Sachs, 2012; Ura, Alkire, & Zangmo, 2012). In so doing, the King succinctly expressed his vision that the country's happiness and wellbeing, rather than simply its economic output, should be the focus of development. In hindsight, it is striking to note that this critical assessment of GNP emanating from the East was being articulated at around the same time as the now historic critique of GNP voiced by Senator Robert Kennedy: 'it measures everything, in short, except that which makes life worthwhile' (Kennedy, 1968, p. 34).

While GNH carries multiple definitions and interpretations, the following has gained wide acceptance: GNH 'measures the quality of a country in a more holistic way [than GNP] and believes that the beneficial development of human society takes place when material and spiritual development occur side by side to complement and reinforce each other' (Ura et al., 2012, p. 111). The underlying roots of GNH can be traced to the Mahayana Buddhist views that historically informed the creation of Bhutan's society and governing structures (Brooks, 2013; Givel M. S., 2015). Although not all Bhutanese are Buddhist, Buddhism's tenets have deeply influenced the country's development philosophy, legal system, and governance for centuries (Brooks, 2013). Happiness as an early guiding principle in Bhutan is visible in the legal code of 1792, which states 'if the Government cannot create happiness (dekid) for its people, there is no purpose for Government to exist' (Ura et al., 2012, p. 111).

Given this context, it is significant that the term 'happiness' in GNH carries a deeper meaning than the fleeting subjective feelings of joy often associated with the word in Western cultures (Ura et al., 2012). In Bhutan, happiness is viewed as being relational and multidimensional, emphasising responsibility, harmony with nature, and concern for the happiness of others (Ura et al., 2012). As Bhutan's first Prime Minister stated in 2008: 'We know that true abiding happiness cannot exist while others suffer, and comes only from serving others, living in harmony with nature, and realising our innate wisdom and the true and brilliant nature of our own minds' (Givel, M., 2015, p. 23). In contrast to a GDP-based paradigm, this concept of happiness suggests a higher purpose for development, one that encompasses the realisation of our individual and collective human potential in balance with the natural world. GNH posits that wellbeing is deeply relational—and therefore supported by connection to oneself, others, and nature. Consequently, the cultivation of inner qualities, such as compassion and wisdom (see also Chapter 4, this volume), are regarded as part of the less tangible but no less significant integration of 'material and spiritual development' that is intrinsic to GNH. In Bhutan, the historical and cultural roots for an economy based on wellbeing run deep. And in modern times, these have been codified in a constitution which proclaims the state's role as striving 'to promote those conditions that will enable the pursuit of Gross National Happiness' (RGOB, 2017, p. 18).

FROM INTENTION TO ACTION

In 2008, Bhutan's Fourth King oversaw a peaceful transition to a constitutional monarchy, with the country's first democratic elections. Until this time, the understanding and application of GNH in Bhutan had been largely intuitive. However, with democratisation and increasing international engagement, there was a need for the GNH vision to be further anchored in specific goals and frameworks for practical application (Choden, 2015). Since then, key aspects for operationalising GNH as a development framework have been articulated and formalised.

GNH: Four Pillars and Nine Domains Create an Enabling Environment for Wellbeing

The core foundations of GNH are based around four pillars: sustainable and equitable socioeconomic development, environmental conservation, preservation and promotion of culture, and good governance. These have subsequently been expanded and measured through the GNH Index, a multidimensional survey tool that is linked with a set of policy and programme screening tools (Ura et al., 2012). The index is informed by periodic national surveys which collect data across nine GNH domains that together create an enabling environment for wellbeing: psychological wellbeing, time use, community vitality, cultural diversity, and resilience, living standards, health, education good governance, and ecological diversity and resilience (see Figure 14.1). The nine domains are measured by 33 clustered indicators that have a total of 124 variables, and all domains are weighted equally because they are viewed as being equally important for achieving happiness (Ura et al., 2012). A threshold level is used to assess sufficiency within the 33 indicators, and, overall, an individual experiencing sufficiency in six or more of the nine domains is considered 'happy'—that is, to have sufficient conditions for happiness. Disaggregating data from the survey allows for comparisons across different groups, such as, by age, gender, educational level, occupation, or geographic district. For example, the most recent GNH survey revealed that, in general, women reported lower happiness levels than men, and farmers lower levels than other occupations. Identifying such gaps should then guide policy-makers

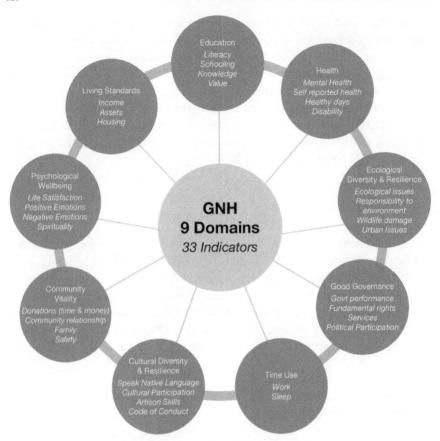

Figure 14.1 Bhutan's Gross National Happiness (GNH) Index.

to direct appropriate funding and interventions toward improving conditions for these groups (CBS, 2016). Taken together, the nine domains represent a holistic measurement and policy framework that integrates psychological, physical, societal, and environmental wellbeing.

Bhutan: Building a Wellbeing Economy at the National Level

To date, Bhutan has conducted three rounds of GNH surveys, including a pilot survey in 2006 and nationwide surveys in 2010 and 2015. Guided by the GNH philosophy, the country has introduced a range of policies to achieve sustainable and equitable development while preserving its cultural traditions. Poverty reduction, universal primary school enrolment, free access to basic health services, distribution of land to landless farmers, expanded public services and infrastructure in rural areas, and increasing women's participation in elected office have been recent priorities. There have been significant improvements in key social indicators including a reduction in poverty and infant mortality rates, rising life

Table 14.1 KEY GROSS NATIONAL HAPPINESS (GNH) INSTITUTIONS IN BHUTAN

Centre for Bhutan and GNH Studies	The GNH Commission	The GNH Centre Bhutan
An autonomous social science research institute established by the government of Bhutan, which conducts and analyzes the national GNH survey, alongside other interdisciplinary research initiatives. https://www.bhutanstudies.org.bt/	The central government body responsible for ensuring all development policies and plans are formulated and implemented in line with the principles of GNH, including through the GNH Policy Screening Tool. https://www.gnhc.gov.bt/en/	A national NGO that aims to translate GNH into practical action at the grassroots level through collaboration with key stakeholders, and through leadership & action-learning programs in Bhutan and internationally. www.gnhcentrebhutan.org

expectancy, and substantial increases in primary school enrolment (World Bank, 2014). Moreover, between 2005 and 2018, Bhutan's Human Development Index increased by 20.5%, positioning the country in the Middle Human Development Category (UNDP Bhutan, 2019).

On the environmental front, Bhutan's Constitution has committed to ensuring that 'a minimum of 60% of the country's land area should be maintained under forest cover for all time' (Royal Government of Bhutan, 2009, p. 1), and Bhutan has attracted attention as the world's first carbon negative country—absorbing more greenhouse gases from the atmosphere than it emits (Climate Council, 2017). To further align government decision-making with GNH values, the GNH Commission (a government planning body) uses a GNH policy-screening tool to provide a systematic appraisal of the potential effects of proposed projects on the nine domains. A policy that fails to receive a sufficiently high score is returned to the proponent agency, outlining why it fell short, along with ways to improve it. The nine GNH domains are also used to guide resource allocation and policy priorities, and, since 2008, targets in the country's Five-Year Plans are based on components of the Index (CBS, 2016). Finally, responding to the need for greater civil society engagement around GNH, the GNH Centre Bhutan (a national nongovernmental organisation [NGO]), has been conducting youth leadership and advocacy programmes, reaching thousands of young people in colleges and schools across Bhutan (Zangmo, 2018). Table 14.1 summarises some of Bhutan's key GNH institutions.

LEADING FROM THE INSIDE OUT

As described above, the GNH approach is unique in several ways. Firstly, it articulates wellbeing (rather than economic growth) as the *purpose* of the economy. GNH is not counter to economic growth, as long as such growth is sustainable and equitable and remains in service to the higher goal of promoting flourishing and wellbeing. Second, GNH places an emphasis on cultivating both the *outer* factors (an enabling environment) and *inner* conditions (values and mindsets) to support a society oriented toward wellbeing. This stands in contrast to more conventional economic development approaches, where values and mindsets are largely considered to be exogeneous, and where emphasis is placed on leveraging external structures, such as policies and market incentives (Nagler, 2020).

A third, and related, aspect of GNH is its reference to cultivating a form of leadership that could be described as 'leadership of the self'. The importance of leading from the inside out is captured in an address by His Majesty the 5th King of Bhutan who urges citizens to live their lives guided by values of kindness, integrity, and justice. As he notes, in order to bring positive change in the world—to eradicate poverty, reduce inequalities, reverse environmental degradation, and improve healthcare—we need to actively seek out 'leadership of the self', rather than leaders to lead the masses (University of Calcutta, 2010, p. 7). In Bhutan, this cultivation of self-leadership has historically been supported by a living tradition of Buddhist ethics, philosophy, meditation, and related spiritual practices. These are seen as vital for cultivating awareness and insight into the interconnectedness of all life and for nourishing compassionate behaviours rooted in appreciation, empathy, and generosity. More recently, such values and skills have been increasingly integrated in a range of secular forms, including the GNH Centre Bhutan's youth leadership programmes, as well as the Ministry of Education's nationwide Educating for GNH initiative (Gyamsho, Sherab, & Maxwell, 2017; Zangmo, 2018).

Beyond Bhutan, it is interesting to note that modern efforts to promote sustainable development have been guided and driven largely by technological, economic, and social interventions and expertise. But, as many are now realising, intellectual understanding and technical interventions, though important, will not be sufficient to inspire the deeply transformative changes required for a paradigm shift toward wellbeing economies (Capra & Luisi, 2014; Green Futures, 2011). Indeed, as some systems thinkers note, one of the critical challenges of the 21st century will be to recognise the interdependence between the socioeconomic systems we ultimately create and the awareness or consciousness of those participating in their creation. In other words, self-leadership matters.

> The success of our actions as change-makers does not depend on *what* we do or *how* we do it, but on the *inner place* from which we operate. . . . We cannot transform the behaviour of systems unless we transform the quality of attention that people apply to their actions within those systems, both individually and collectively. (Scharmer & Kaufer, 2013, pp. 18–19)

Simultaneously, within modern science, we are witnessing a shift in thinking away from reductionist, siloed disciplines and toward more holistic inquiries that recognise the fundamental interdependence of phenomena.

> The new paradigm may be called a holistic world view, seeing the world as an integrated whole rather than a dissociated collection of parts. . . . Deep

ecological awareness recognises the fundamental interdependence of all phenomena and the fact that, as individuals and societies, we are all embedded in (and ultimately dependent on) the cyclical processes of nature. (Capra & Luisi, 2014, p. 12)

This interconnectedness of life is now recognised across many scientific disciplines, including systems thinking and chaos and complexity science. Donella Meadows's seminal paper delineating the range of potential entry points to intervene in complex systems, highlights the nature of such interconnection. In it, she describes nine intervention points (later revised to 12) in order of increasing effectiveness—beginning with outer, material changes (e.g., aiming for greater sustainability by reducing consumption of materials and energy), to relational changes (e.g., improving the flow and feedback of information), to shifting paradigms, and ultimately to shifting inner mindsets and lifestyle aspirations. As she notes, 'because mindsets and paradigms guide behaviours, changing them can have a profound impact. . . . People who manage to intervene in systems at the level of paradigm hit a leverage point that totally transform systems' (Meadows, 1999, p. 18).

Recognising the central role of mindsets in shaping the trajectory of global development interventions and drawing on lessons from GNH, United Nations Development Program (UNDP) Deputy Resident Representative in Bhutan, Jürgen Nagler, has articulated an approach to sustainable development informed by leadership of the self (Box 14.1). As Nagler (2020) notes, to date, development efforts have focused primarily on tackling external and measurable factors, leaving aside an understanding of internal factors and potential underlying root causes of our current health, social, and ecological crises. And while we have

---

Box 14.1

LEADERSHIP OF THE SELF AND SUSTAINABLE DEVELOPMENT

1. Sustainable transformation happens from the inside out.
2. Mindsets matter. They play an important role in human development at the individual, collective and global level.
3. Mindsets can be shifted by increasing awareness, fostering self-reflection and self-responsibility.
4. Solutions need to be co-created which requires a mindset shift of development practitioners themselves.
5. Current development approaches are too materialistic; therefore, they need to move beyond overly focusing on gross domestic product (GDP) and economic development.
6. A new holistic development paradigm should include inner, collective, and planetary wellbeing.

From Nagler, 2020, p. 5.

---

witnessed a flourishing of research into self-empowerment, leadership, and trans-formation in specialised fields including psychology, sociology, philosophy, and neuroscience, these have made minimal direct connection to sustainable devel-opment approaches. This 'blind spot' regarding the role of inner dimensions, such as mindsets, underscores the need for a new holistic approach that takes into account the interaction between internal and external factors in order for development to be transformative and advance sustainable wellbeing for people and planet. There are encouraging signs that global initiatives to address both inner and outer development factors and to cultivate self-leadership are gaining momentum through initiatives such as the UN Sustainable Development Goals Leadership Lab and 'Transforming Systems in the Decade of Action', a collabor-ation between the UNDP and the Presencing Institute (Presencing Institute, 2013; UNDP, 2021).

INTRODUCING WELLBEING ECONOMY PRINCIPLES ACROSS A RANGE OF SECTORS AND SCALES

Bhutan has contributed a wealth of experience through its implementation of GNH as a national-level development strategy, one that expresses a commit-ment to cultivating both the outer and inner conditions for collective wellbeing. As global interest and experience in wellbeing economies deepens, a growing number of governments (including in Costa Rica, New Zealand, Canada, Iceland, Finland, Scotland, and Wales) are prioritising wellbeing at national, regional, and municipal levels (Robert Wood Johnson Foundation, 2018; Wellbeing Economy Alliance, 2021; see also Chapter 13, this volume). Emerging wellbeing economy approaches need not be limited to a national or government mandate and can offer important lessons and applications at different levels of scale. In this section, we explore how emerging initiatives are starting to influence international dis-course and spark innovative applications of wellbeing economy principles at indi-vidual and organisational levels.

Growing Interest in Wellbeing Economies at the International Level

In recent years, Bhutan's efforts have converged with rising global concern re-garding the profound financial, social, and environmental costs of inequitable and unsustainable economic growth. This concern, combined with several high-profile critiques of GDP from respected sources (e.g., Stiglitz, Sen, & Fitoussi, 2010) has brought heightened international interest to Bhutan's experience of GNH. In response, Bhutan has contributed to a range of international initiatives that have brought growing attention to the importance of wellbeing and 'beyond GDP' measures. In 2011, under Bhutan's leadership, the UN General Assembly adopted UN Resolution 65/309 'Happiness: Towards a Holistic Approach to

Development' (United Nations, 2011). The following year, Bhutan convened a High-Level Meeting on Wellbeing and Happiness at the UN Headquarters in New York, bringing together more than 800 delegates and launching a global movement. The vision for a New Development Paradigm was elaborated in a 2013 report, proposing holistic societal happiness as a core development objective in the lead up to the Sustainable Development Goals (NDP Steering Committee and Secretariat, 2013).

Growing global interest in GNH and other 'beyond GDP' approaches has also led to a surge of international conferences and events, in both Bhutan and abroad (CBS, 2016; Robert Wood Johnson Foundation, 2018). In 2013, the GNH Centre Bhutan, together with the Global Leadership Academy (Germany) and the Presencing Institute (United States) launched the 'The Global Wellbeing Lab: Transforming Economy and Society'. Designed as a multistakeholder action-learning platform, the Lab aims to advance new ways of generating and measuring wellbeing at multiple levels of society (Global Wellbeing Lab, 2013). Activating participants from 17 countries, the Lab has inspired new projects and regional initiatives including the Global Wellbeing in Business Lab, the WE-Africa Lab on Building Wellbeing Economies for Africa, and the Wellbeing Economy Alliance (Global Wellbeing Lab, 2016).

GNH at Individual and Organisational Levels

In addition to national or government-led initiatives, the GNH framework can also be applied to cultivating the outer and inner conditions for wellbeing and flourishing at individual and organisational levels. Indeed, this combination of 'top-down' and 'bottom-up' approaches may be a vital strategy for shifting from the current GDP growth paradigm toward an economy centred on wellbeing. In this context, introducing and adapting GNH values, metrics, and approaches across a range of scales can contribute to building a collective *movement* toward wellbeing economies. Reflecting this approach, a GNH and business survey tool was recently launched in Bhutan, with the aim of integrating GNH principles within the country's emerging private sector (CBS, 2017). And in 2016, the GNH Centre Bhutan began a collaboration with a large family-owned, multibusiness corporation based in Thailand to introduce GNH values, practices, and measures into its various companies (Kim J. C., 2017).

The GNH Centre has continued to collaborate with international partners including Schumacher College (United Kingdom) to develop a range of trans-formative action-learning programmes geared toward wellbeing economy innov-ation and leadership at individual and organisational levels. One such initiative, the Right Livelihood and GNH Program, brings together participants from a range of countries and contexts who set out with a personal inquiry or challenge related to cultivating wellbeing in their own life or workplace. After investigating cri-tiques of the current GDP-focused economic paradigm, alternative development approaches including GNH are explored and integrated into a learning journey to Bhutan, to engage experts and key stakeholders and to experience GNH implementation and challenges first-hand. Throughout the programme, both outer and inner dimensions of wellbeing are emphasised, as well as skills and practices to cultivate leadership of the self. Finally, participants are encouraged to deepen and apply their learning in the form of a project or prototype, bringing fresh insight to their original inquiry or challenge. Taken together, this leadership and learning lab allows participants to apply a 'GNH lens' to their own lives and livelihoods, grounding wellbeing economy principles in lived experience and offering a community of practice to test out new ideas and projects.

Over the years, a range of GNH and wellbeing projects have arisen from the Right Livelihood and GNH Program, across a range of sectors and disciplines. By combining inner transformation with outward action, these initiatives are generating insights into how GNH values, principles, and metrics can be adapted and applied at individual and organisational levels (Table 14.2). Beyond the projects themselves, participants have pointed to the value of the peer relationships formed through these experiences. Referring to the resistance they often face in introducing a wellbeing economy approach, many cite these deep, supportive relationships as a key condition for achieving impact in spite of such challenges (Global Wellbeing Lab, 2016). Reflecting the relationship between inner and outer transformation, some participants reported experiences of wellbeing arising from shifts in perception that clarified a sense of purpose and meaning in their own life. This inner alignment in turn equipped them with the motivation, courage, and skills to enact new behaviours and life choices. Follow-up surveys and semi-structured interviews with programme participants revealed a range of positive consequences such as inner shifts relating to values and purpose, as well as experiences of wellbeing that included a range of psychological, physical, societal, and environmental dimensions (Kim & Richardson, forthcoming). Illustrative examples are shown in Tables 14.2 and 14.3.

As this section has highlighted, creating the inner conditions for wellbeing (values and mindsets) can be a powerful agent for shaping wider systems change—beginning with innovative projects and supportive communities of practice—and, ultimately, influencing broader practices, policies, and institutions.

BHUTAN AT A CROSSROADS: NEW CHALLENGES, NEW OPPORTUNITIES

In many ways, GNH is a bold and vitally important work in progress. As acknowledged by the country's first Prime Minister, 'Bhutan is not a country that has attained GNH. . . . Like most developing nations, we are struggling with the challenge of fulfilling the basic needs of our people. What separates us, however, from most others is that we have made happiness—the foundation of human needs—as the goal of societal change' (Royal Government of Bhutan, 2012, p. 108). Moreover, given the interdependence between Bhutan and the global community, it is clear that a movement toward a Wellbeing Economy cannot be pursued in isolation.

Table 14.2 Outer transformation: Creating an enabling
environment for wellbeing through gross national happiness (GNH)
projects and activities

Environment	Converted a land estate to become organic (UK)
	Received a grant for re-wilding land (UK)
	Applied GNH principles to horticultural apprenticeship program (USA)
	Initiated workshops for general public examining links between sense of life purpose and environmental responsibility (UK)
Education	Trained 120 facilitators to use GNH at work (Brazil)
	Retrained as a mindfulness teacher for schools. Started a PhD on holistic education (UK)
	Introduced wellbeing storytelling into educational work (Spain)
	Re-designed engineering curriculum to focus on green technologies & introduced pedagogies encouraging reflection & cooperation rather than competition (Thailand)
	Conducted university-wide GNH survey with undergraduate students (Canada)
	Incorporated principles and practices of GNH into educational curriculum (Spain)
Health	Adapted GNH survey and framework to a hospital (Brazil)
Community vitality	Established community space in city centre offering workshops and events related to wellbeing and sustainability (Hong Kong)
	Established 'Silent Spaces' (quiet, contemplative areas, undisturbed by mobile technology) in 44 gardens across the country (UK)
Business and finance	Hosted Asian Venture Philanthropy event and set up sustainable finance initiative (Hong Kong)
	Worked with businesses to introduce GNH values & principles (Australia)
	Launched social enterprise focusing on youth sports to promote global citizenship, conscious leadership, and sustainable development (Spain)

As one Bhutanese minister expressed, Bhutan 'cannot be a GNH bubble in a GDP world' (Dorji, 2012, p. 8). Here, we explore some of the challenges and opportunities that are becoming apparent as the country modernises.

GNH and Economic Growth: Getting the Balance Right

GNH is not counter to economic growth so long as such growth is viewed 'not as an end in itself but rather as a means to achieve more important ends' (Planning Commission, 1999a, p. 20). Indeed, improving living standards (one of the GNH domains) and reducing poverty and income inequality are important enabling conditions for happiness and wellbeing, as are greater self-reliance, sovereignty,

Table 14.3 INNER TRANSFORMATION AND DIMENSIONS OF WELLBEING EXPERIENCED
BY GROSS NATIONAL HAPPINESS (GNH) PROGRAM PARTICIPANTS

Psychological	'Finding calm inside myself and the courage of stepping out into action.'
	'I am happier at work and have been promoted first to Head of Department and then Head of School.'
	'I experienced boosted confidence and sense of purpose in my work'.
	'Practicing boldness'.
	'My personal journey is to get out of that fear paradigm'.
	'Realising that to change is to become more of who we are'.
	'Finding new purpose in retirement'.
Physical	'The program helped me recover from poor health arising from stress and trauma'.
	'Helped me through my cancer'.
Societal	'I'm involved in many meaningful activities and surrounded with right minded people'.
	'I've found my comrades'.
	'The Right Livelihood tribe is like a community of practice – sharing our paths, growing together and inspiring each other'.
	'The realisation that wellbeing is a social process. Our relationship to self and others is critical to how to positively affect the environment'.
	'I now notice how schools are stressful and sad places – there is a need for new leadership with qualities of empathy'.
	'I began to understand that change doesn't happen at an individual level – it happens in relationship'.
	'We might want to shift our language – what would be sufficient business. What would be enough business for us?'
Environmental	'I felt more deeply connected to nature'.
	'The energy of the forest was extraordinary . . . It made me feel wonderfully alive'.

and security (Planning Commission, 1999b; Hayden, 2015). In 2016, largely due to hydropower expansion, the country experienced an 8% GDP growth rate, making it one of the world's fastest growing economies (Palden, 2019a). This has prompted some to question whether the country may begin to veer toward a more conventional productivist direction (Hayden, 2015). In this context, it is interesting to note that, in 2018, Bhutan's current Prime Minister, Dr. Lotay Tshering and his party campaigned and were elected to office on the promise of 'Narrowing the Gap'; that is, creating a more inclusive society by reducing inequalities and focusing on social investments (Palden T., 2019b). They have subsequently prioritised longer-term social investments in education and health (not necessarily reflected in GDP growth), noting that a more modest growth rate will suffice and that higher rates could widen inequality, causing more disharmony in society (Nima, 2019).

GNH and a Young Democracy

As the country has transitioned to a democratic constitutional monarchy, there is growing awareness that with this comes an important shift in responsibility and the need to exercise new democratic powers wisely. As one expert notes, GNH was quantified to help anchor politicians and bureaucrats to the long-term goals of GNH, in preparation for a time when democratically elected governments could potentially change every 5 years (Palden, S., 2019). And, as another has pointed out, after centuries of isolation, two and a half centuries of constructing a polity, and 100 years of monarchy, the people are mandated to take on new responsibilities and determine where democracy will take Bhutan next (Dorji, 2015). As many are concluding, 'it becomes the responsibility of the citizens who form political parties, elect governments, and function as civil society' to help achieve the vision of GNH (Dorji, 2015, p. 11).

An Expanding Role for Civil Society in Bhutan

To this end, Bhutan's expanding community of civil society organisations (CSOs) stand to play a vital role in ensuring that GNH values and principles are activated at a grassroots level. The concept of a formalised civil society only emerged in Bhutan in the late 1980s. Since 2009, CSOs have been growing and have secured the legal space and mandate to play a greater role in representing the voices and concerns of society (Dorji, 2017). A former GNH Commission Secretary has noted that 'government can't create a GNH society alone. We need active citizen participation' (Colman, 2017, p. 17). While there have been considerable gains in promoting civil society's role within Bhutan, such organisations are still at a fledgling stage, and more support is needed for them to realise their considerable potential (Dorji, 2017).

GNH and the Growing Importance of the Private Sector

Similarly, Bhutan's private sector is growing and has the potential to play a more active role in shaping GNH, and Bhutan's development more broadly. However, this expansion is currently dominated by a few business houses, and there is a need for 'a more balanced spectrum, where artists, intellectuals and diverse professionals can thrive and contribute to the country's growth' (Dorji, 2015, p. 11). The recently launched GNH and Business survey tool (CBS, 2017) encourages businesses to integrate GNH values into their operations. Similarly, in alignment with GNH values and the broader aims of social enterprise, the Loden Foundation seeks to cultivate the ethos of a 'bodhisattva entrepreneur'—evoking the image of a Buddhist hero who has the motivation of serving society and starts a business as a means to that end (Loden Foundation, 2020).

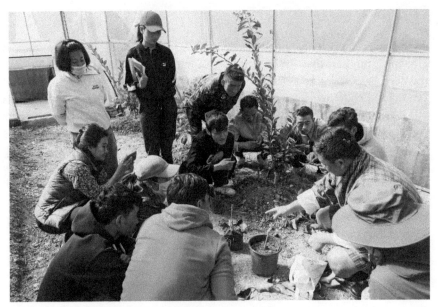

Figure 14.2 Exploring modern gross national happiness (GNH) values: Youth Leadership Program, GNH Centre Bhutan.

Globalisation, Rapid Change, and New Challenges for Bhutan's Youth

Bhutan has a youthful population, with about 56% of the population under age 25 (UNDP Bhutan, 2019) (Figure 14.2). At the same time, this generation faces a rapidly changing landscape driven by increasing exposure to the internet, social media, and globalisation (Phuntsho, 2016). They are now required to 'balance their Bhutanese cultural roots and global citizenship, relate to the past and prepare for the future, make an honest living in a competitive world and uphold lofty ideals and values' (Phuntsho, 2016, p. 16). Most of the challenges they face—unemployment, urbanism, social isolation, loneliness, and the deluge of unverified information—are new problems. At the same time, some are noting a nascent revival of youth interest in Bhutan's traditional practices, spirituality, and culture in response to growing disillusionment with modernity (Phuntsho, 2016).

NAVIGATING THE FUTURE: EMERGING INSIGHTS FOR A GLOBAL NETWORK OF ECONOMIES OF WELLBEING

Drawing from Bhutan's unique heritage and still evolving experience of GNH, it is not feasible or desirable to propose universal lessons to guide other contexts or countries. However, it is possible to reflect on Bhutan's rich experience and draw out key insights that may hopefully inspire courageous experimentation and collaboration toward a global network of economies of wellbeing.

The Importance of Addressing Both the Tangible and Intangible Aspects of Happiness and Wellbeing

One early and enduring contribution of GNH to the Beyond-GDP discourse has been the clear articulation by Bhutan's leaders of the importance of balancing both material and spiritual development or, expressed differently, the tangible and intangible aspects of wellbeing (CBS, 2016). That these are defined and measured through the GNH Index and its nine domains is one factor that distinguishes GNH so clearly from GDP. Although many national surveys routinely collect data on education, health, and living standards, the more intangible domains such as time use, psychological wellbeing, community vitality, and cultural diversity and resilience are equally important in creating an enabling environment for wellbeing (Boniwell, 2009; Layard, Clark, & and Senik, 2012). Beyond promoting an enabling environment, GNH posits that the inner transformation of mindsets and behaviour is as important for human flourishing as the transformation of outer living conditions (NDP Steering Committee and Secretariat, 2013). As noted earlier, Bhutan's rich spiritual heritage draws on diverse traditions of teaching and meditative practices that emphasise the cultivation of wisdom and compassion as means toward genuine happiness (Phuntsho, 2013). Globally, a growing body of interdisciplinary research (neuroscience, positive psychology, sociology, and behavioural economics) highlights the role of wellbeing interventions (including mindfulness, compassion, altruism, volunteering, and other pro-social behaviours) in supporting the physical, psychological, and social aspects of wellbeing and happiness (Goleman & Davidson, 2017; Greenfield & Marks, 2004; Helliwell, Aknin, Shiplett, Huang, & Wang, 2018; Rinpoche, 2007). Thus, addressing both the outer and inner dimensions of wellbeing should be regarded as important and complementary approaches (Diener, 2019).

How Much Is Enough? Notions of Sufficiency, Equity, and Sustainability

The GNH survey applies 'sufficiency thresholds' to calculate whether requisite conditions for happiness have been met. The focus for policy-makers is therefore to enable as many people as possible to meet the threshold fixed for each of the 33 GNH indicators (Penjore, 2017). The underlying principle of sufficiency acknowledges that 'more' does not necessarily translate into enhanced wellbeing. This approach is supported by research showing little, if any, connection between rising per capita income and wellbeing once adequate material living standards have been achieved (Easterlin, McVey, Switek, Sawangfa, & Zweig, 2019). From a sufficiency perspective, one must ask how much is enough and question infinite growth of production and consumption (Deitz & O'Neill, 2013; Princen, 2005). The principle of sufficiency is significant for GNH and for wellbeing economics more broadly because it aims to promote equitable and sustainable socioeconomic development, within the limits of planetary boundaries (Raworth, 2017).

Moving Toward an Eco-centric World View

The nine GNH domains are regarded as being interdependent—a holistic view that does not privilege economic factors above others but places them alongside a range of social and environmental concerns. Moreover, human wellbeing is regarded as intimately interconnected with that of the natural world—an eco-centric rather than an ego-centric view (Scharmer, 2013), where balance among living systems is seen as integral, and the natural world itself has intrinsic value beyond its utility as a natural resource (Figure. 14.3).

In Bhutan, the natural world is still viewed by many as being sacred. For example, in 1994, despite its attractive revenue potential, climbing mountains higher than 6,000 metres was prohibited. Local customs hold such peaks to be the rarefied domain of protective deities and spirits, and, in 2003, mountaineering was banned entirely, leaving Bhutan with some of the highest untouched peaks in the world (Verschuuren, 2016). This sacred view of nature is one shared by many indigenous cultures (see also Chapter 7, this volume) and has likely helped to protect Bhutan's environment well into the present time (Allison, 2017). Similarly, in New Zealand, persistent advocacy and legal cases advanced by Māori people are showing how new policies that respect and protect forests and rivers are codifying such eco-centric cultural narratives. This profound shift in how nature is viewed could have important implications for other countries where dominant narratives and policy currently place people at the 'receiving end' of nature, rather than being part of a vibrant, interdependent whole (Acharya & Ng, 2020).

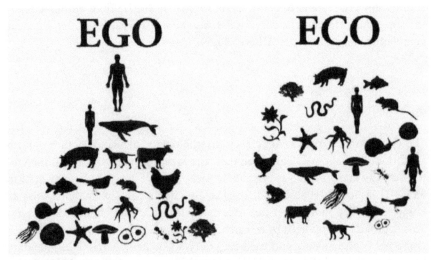

Figure 14.3 From an ego-centric to eco-centric world view.
From Lehmann, S. (2019). Reconnecting with nature: Developing urban spaces in the age of climate change. *Emerald Open Research*, *1*(2). https://doi.org/10.12688/emeraldopen res.12960.1. Reproduced under a Creative Commons Attribution 4.0 International (CC BY 4.0) license.

The Power of a Multisector Approach Crossing Diverse Scales and Contexts

Bhutan's approach to integrating and operationalising GNH (embedding the vision within key legal instruments such as the Constitution, applying new survey and policy-making tools, and engaging influential sectors of society) is instrumental in taking a wellbeing approach beyond vision and into action. It offers a multilevel, multisector approach that provides useful insights for others embarking on a similar course. While starting with a national-level approach may not be feasible or desirable in many countries, this chapter has shown that it is possible to introduce wellbeing metrics and approaches at smaller scales, where innovation and learning can progress in a supportive environment. GNH is not so much a static model that can be standardised and replicated out, but rather points to a profound shift in how the purpose of the economy is viewed, accompanied by a dynamic process that can be applied in response to a specific, evolving context. As this chapter has illustrated, 'starting where you are' and experimenting through an action-research approach can enable GNH to take root in an iterative and locally responsive way. Thus, a *culture of equity and wellbeing* can be grown from the grassroots level, cultivating fertile soil for the seeds of new national-level wellbeing measures and policies to land (Robert Wood Johnson Foundation, 2018). New wellbeing economy communities and networks are already emerging and gaining momentum through initiatives such as the Wellbeing Economy Alliance (Wellbeing Economy Alliance, 2021). As such initiatives grow over time, they can generate practical leverage points and popular support for subsequently mainstreaming new progress measures at a wider, systemic level.

Going Beyond Numbers: The Importance of Transformative Leadership

Experience has shown that, in the absence of deeply internalised values, reporting on measurements can remain an intellectual exercise, open to misinterpretation or manipulation in the service of political agendas (Scharmer C. O., 2013). For this reason, transformative leadership development remains a central component of the GNH Centre's programmes (Global Wellbeing Lab, 2016). As this chapter has demonstrated, it is critical to demystify economics as the abstract purview of academics and politicians and to ground it firmly in the values and lived experiences of everyday life (Figure 14.4). Doing so encourages individuals and communities to apply a 'wellbeing economy lens' to their own contexts, which, in turn, can reveal how a country's narrow pursuit of economic growth has often come at the cost of widening social disparities, loss of work–life balance, diminishing social connection, and worsening psychological wellbeing (Kim & Richardson, forthcoming). This in turn can shift mindsets from a sense of powerlessness to agency and from a position of fear to one of curiosity—not simply asking *what do*

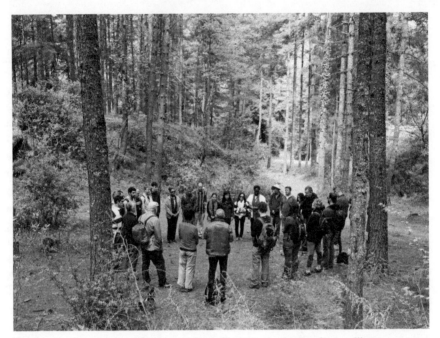

Figure 14.4 The Global Wellbeing Lab: Transformative leadership for a wellbeing economy.

we stand to lose, but what do we *hope to gain* by transitioning toward an economy of greater equity and wellbeing?

In this respect, the notion of 'leadership of the self' has implications for a wellbeing economy beyond the borders of Bhutan. A growing body of research and practice indicates that leading from the inside out requires a new set of skills and capacities that can be cultivated at both individual and collective levels (Nagler, 2020; Shawoo & Thornton, 2019). Bringing together ancient wisdom traditions and findings from modern neuroscience, new initiatives are beginning to strengthen inner leadership capacities including *awareness, connection, insight,* and *purpose* and integrating them within the spheres of education, healthcare, and business (Dahl, 2020). Other innovations in leadership practice include inter-listening (Lipari, 2014), sensing (Scharmer, 2016), reflexive social practice (Cunliffe, 2009; Kaplan & Davidoff, 2014), reciprocity (Scolaro, 2019), and awareness-based systems thinking (Koenig, Seneque, Pomeroy, & Scharmer, 2021). This is a rich and multidisciplinary field where further research and application can make a significant contribution to our collective efforts to cultivate wellbeing at individual, organisational, and systems levels.

SUMMARY

From its early origins in the Himalayas, Bhutan's contribution to our collective understanding of how to create a society based on happiness and wellbeing has steadily advanced. As some note, whether or not Bhutan ultimately manages to blaze a trail toward a desirable post-growth future, it has already integrated environmental considerations and social equity into the development process to a much greater extent than in 'business-as-usual' development strategies. Perhaps most valuable of all, it has elevated the importance, for the rest of the world, of asking critical questions about the ultimate purposes that economic development should serve (Hayden, 2015; Sachs, 2012).

In this chapter, we have shown how GNH should rightly be viewed as a *journey* rather than a final destination. As Bhutan's experience reveals, weaving wellbeing into the fabric of the economy requires bold vision, leadership from the inside out, and an actively engaged range of stakeholders including government, the private sector, and civil society. Moreover, in an increasingly turbulent and interdependent world, it is a journey that cannot be undertaken alone. Bhutan's experience is already revealing important challenges and opportunities for others treading this path, whether at individual, organisational, national, or international levels.

We have highlighted the powerful systems-change leverage points afforded by shifting mindsets and paradigms—describing what is possible when wellbeing is prioritised as the *purpose* of the economy. Furthermore, we have shown how rediscovering the intimate connection between our inner experience and the outer world offers a powerful orientation to shape and amplify emerging economies of wellbeing. The GNH approach expands our traditional economic focus from its narrow, outer manifestation of GDP growth and wealth creation to bring into view the inner dynamics of value creation and social narrative— and how these enable or constrain our individual and collective choices as economic agents. Finally, we have described the importance of 'leading from the inside out', showing how a growing range of experimental GNH initiatives continue to offer alternative economic pathways beyond orthodox GDP-based approaches.

As Bhutan's journey toward GNH illustrates, the goal of human flourishing is profoundly connected to our ability to tackle the urgent crisis of sustainability we now face. Far from being a 'luxury' or 'trade-off' in the face of sustainable development, prioritising wellbeing and reconnecting our inner experience with the external world are *vital* to making the leap from our current economy of consumption toward one of planetary wellbeing. In the words of Andreas Weber, as we contemplate our uncertain future in the age of the Anthropocene,

> The goal of leading a fuller life, is the most important steppingstone toward changing our relationships with the animate earth and among ourselves. If we adopt this perspective, we will begin to see that something is sustainable if it enables more life—for myself, for other human individuals involved, for the ecosystem, on a broader cultural level. It is crucial to rediscover the linkage between our inner experience and the external natural order. (Weber, 2019, p. 35)

REFERENCES

Acharya, K., & Ng, T. (2020). I am the river, the river is me: Prioritizing well-being through water policy. Meeting of the Minds, The Global Water Equity Blog Series. https://meetingoftheminds.org/i-am-the-river-the-river-is-me-prioritizing-well-being-through-water-policy-33035

Allison, E. (2017, Sept 26). Spirits and nature: The intertwining of sacred cosmologies and environmental conservation in Bhutan. *Journal for the Study of Religion, Nature and Culture, 11*(2), 197–226.

Boniwell, I. (2009). *Time for life: Satisfaction with time use and its relationship with subjective wellbeing.* VDM.

Brooks, J. (2013). Avoiding limits to growth: Gross national happiness in Bhutan as a model for sustainable development. *Sustainability, 5*(9), 3640–3664.

Capra, F., & Luisi, P. L. (2014). *The systems view of life: A unifying vision.* Cambridge University Press.

CBS. (2016). *A compass towards a just and harmonious society: 2015 GNH survey report.* The Centre for Bhutan Studies and GNH Research.

CBS. (2017). *Proposed GNH of business.* Centre for Bhutan Studies and GNH Research.

Choden, T. (2015). What would a 21st century Bhutanese identity be? *The Druk Journal, 1*(1). http://drukjournal.bt/what-would-a-21st-century-bhutanese-identity-be/

Climate Council. (2017). Bhutan is the world's only carbon negative country – so how did they do it? https://www.climatecouncil.org.au/bhutan-is-the-world-s-only-carbon-negative-country-so-how-did-they-do-it/

Colman, T. R. (2017). Civil society: Why it matters. *The Druk Journal, 3*(2). http://drukjournal.bt/civil-society-why-it-matters/

Cunliffe, A. L. (2009). Reflexivity, learning and reflexive practice. In S. J. Armstrong, & C. V. Fukami, *The Sage handbook of management, learning, education and development* (pp. 405–418). Sage Publications.

Dahl, C. J.-M. (2020). The plasticity of well-being: A training-based framework for the cultivation of human flourishing. *Proceedings of the National Academy of Sciences, 117*(51), 32197–32206.

Deitz, R., & O'Neill, D. (2013). *Enough is enough: Building a sustainable economy in a world of finite resources.* Berrett-Koehler.

Diener, E. (2019). Well-being interventions to improve societies. In Global Happiness Council, *Global happiness and wellbeing policy report.* Global Council for Happiness and Wellbeing.

Dorji, K. (2012). Why Bhutan? A GNH perspective. *Kuensel.* https://kuenselonline.com/why-bhutan-a-gnh-perspective/

Dorji, K. (2015). What is the "Bhutanese-ness" of the Bhutanese people? *The Druk Journal, 1*(1). http://drukjournal.bt/what-is-the-bhutanese-ness-of-the-bhutanese-people/

Dorji, L. (2017). Emergence of civil society in Bhutan. *The Druk Journal, 3*(2). http://drukjournal.bt/emergence-of-civil-society-in-bhutan/

Easterlin, R. A., McVey, L. A., Switek, M., Sawangfa, O., & Zweig, J. S. (2019). The happiness-income paradox revisited. *Proceedings of the National Academy of Sciences, 107*(52), 22463–22468.

Givel, M. (2015). Mahayana Buddhism and gross national happiness in Bhutan. *International Journal of Wellbeing, 5*(2), 14–27.

Givel, M. S. (2015). Gross national happiness in Bhutan: Political institutions and implementation. *Asian Affairs, 46*(1), 102–117.

Global Wellbeing Lab. (2016). The Global Wellbeing Lab 2.0 - transforming economy and society, summary report. Presencing Institute, GNH Centre Bhutan, GIZ Global Leadership Academy. https://www.we-do-change.org/fileadmin/downloads/Report _The_Global_Wellbeing_Lab_2.pdf?_=1602505636

Goleman, D., & Davidson, R. J. (2017). *Altered traits: Science reveals how meditation changes your mind, brain, and body.* Penguin Random House.

Greenfield, E., & Marks, N. (2004). Formal volunteering as a protective factor for older adults' pscyhological wellbeing. *Journal of Gerontology Series B: Psychological Sciences and Social Sciences, 59*(5), s258–s264.

Green Futures. (2011). Moving mountains: How can faith shape our future? Forum for the Future.

Gyamsho, D. C., Sherab, K., & Maxwell, T. (2017). Teacher learning in changing professional contexts: Bhutanese teacher educators and the Educating for GNH initiative. *Cogent Education.* https://www.cogentoa.com/article/10.1080/2331186X.2017.1384 637.pdf

Hayden, A. (2015). Bhutan: Blazing a trail to a postgrowth future. *Journal of Environment & Development, 24*(2), 161–186.

Helliwell, J., Aknin, L., Shiplett, H., Huang, H., & Wang, S. (2018). Social capital and pro-social behavior as sources of wellbeing. In E. Diener, S. Oishi, & L. Tay (Eds.), *Handbook of wellbeing.* DEF Publishers.

Kaplan, A., & Davidoff, S. (2014). *A delicate activism: A radical approach to change.* Proteus Initiative.

Kennedy, R. F. (1968). Robert F. Kennedy: Remarks at the University of Kansas March 18, 1968. https://www.jfklibrary.org/learn/about-jfk/the-kennedy-family/ robert-f-kennedy/robert-f-kennedy-speeches/remarks-at-the-university-of-kan sas-march-18-1968

Kim, J., & Richardson, J. (forthcoming). *Innovation toward a wellbeing economy: Lessons from the right livelihood and GNH practitioner programs.* GNH Centre Bhutan.

Kim, J. C. (2017). Health, Happiness and Wellbeing: Implications for Public Policy. Happiness: Transforming the Development Landscape. D. K. Ura. Thimphu, Bhutan, Centre for Bhutan Studies and GNH: 169–201. https://eclass.edc.uoc.gr/ modules/document/file.php/DEA110/Happiness_Transforming_the_Developmen t_L%20%282%29.pdf#page=174

Koenig, O., Seneque, M., Pomeroy, E., & Scharmer, O. (2021). Journal of awareness-based systems change: The birth of a journal. *Journal of Awareness-Based Systems Change 1*(1), 1–8. https://doi.org/10.47061/jabsc.v1i1.678

Layard, R., Clark, A., & and Senik, C. (2012). The causes of happiness and misery. In J. F. Helliwell, R. Layard, & J. Sachs (Eds.), *World happiness report* (pp. 58–89).

Lipari, L. (2014). *Listening, thinking, being: Toward an ethics of attunement.* Pennsylvania State University Press.

Loden Foundation. (2020). The Loden report. http://loden.org/wp-content/uploads/ 2020/02/Loden-Anual-Report-2019.pdf

Meadows, D. (1999). *Leverage points: Places to intervene in a system*. Sustainability Institute.

Nagler, J. (2020). *We become what we think: The key role of mindsets in human development*. International Science Council. https://council.science/current/blog/we-become-what-we-think-the-key-role-of-mindsets-in-human-development/

NDP Steering Committee and Secretariat. (2013). *Happiness: Towards a new development paradigm. Report of the Kingdom of Bhutan*. Royal Government of Bhutan.

Nima. (2019). We will not measure country's progress only by GDP: Prime Minister. *Kuensel*. https://www.dailybhutan.com/article/we-will-not-measure-bhutan-s-progress-only-by-gdp-prime-minister-dr-lotay-tshering

Palden, S. (2019). GNH in action. *Kuensel*. http://www.kuenselonline.com/gnh-in-action/

Palden, T. (2019a). Bhutan enters period to shed LDC status. *Kuensel*. http://www.kuenselonline.com/bhutan-enters-preparatory-period-to-shed-lcd-status/

Palden, T. (2019b). Narrowing the poverty gap in the 12th plan. *Kuensel*. https://kuenselonline.com/narrowing-the-poverty-gap-in-the-12th-plan/

Penjore, D. (2017). Sustainable development goals and gross national happiness. *The Druk Journal*, 3(1). http://drukjournal.bt/sustainable-development-goals-and-gross-national-happiness/

Phuntsho, K. (2013). *The history of Bhutan*. Random House India.

Phuntsho, K. (2016). The promise of broken youth: A positive perspective. *The Druk Journal*, 2(2). http://drukjournal.bt/the-promise-of-broken-youth-a-positive-perspective/

Planning Commission. (1999a). *Bhutan 2020 (Part I)*. Bhutan.

Planning Commission. (1999b). *Bhutan 2020 (Part II)*. Bhutan: p. 7.

Presencing Institute. (2013). Global wellbeing and GNH lab. https://vimeo.com/85855298

Princen, T. (2005). *The logic of sufficiency*. MIT Press.

Raworth, K. (2017). *Doughnut economics: Seven ways to think like a 21st-century economist*. Random House.

RGOB. (2017). GNH. The permanent mission of the Kingdom of Bhutan to the United Nations in New York. https://www.mfa.gov.bt/pmbny/?page_id=166

Rinpoche, Y. M. (2007). *The joy of living: Unlocking the secret and science of happiness*. Three Rivers Press.

Robert Wood Johnson Foundation. (2018). Advancing well-being in an inequitable world: Moving from measurement to action. Summary of insights from the Robert Wood Johnson Foundation's Global Conference on Well-being. Robert Wood Johnson Foundation. https://www.rwjf.org/en/library/research/2019/01/advancing-well-being-in-an-inequitable-world.html

Royal Government of Bhutan. (2009). *National forest policy of Bhutan*. Royal Government of Bhutan.

Royal Government of Bhutan. (2012). *Defining a new economic paradigm: Report of the High Level Meeting on Wellbeing and Happiness*. Royal Government of Bhutan.

Sachs, J. (2012). Introduction. In J. Helliwell, R. Layard, & J. Sachs (Eds.), *World happiness report* (pp. 2–9). Columbia Earth Institute.

Scharmer, C. O. (2013). *From ego-system to eco-system economies*. https://www.opendemocracy.net/en/transformation/from-ego-system-to-eco-system-economies/

Scharmer, O. C. (2016). *Theory U leading from the future as it emerges: The social technology of presencing*. Berrett-Koehler.

Scharmer, O., & Kaufer, K. (2013). *Leading from the emerging future: From ego-system to eco-system economies*. Berrett-Koehler.

Scolaro, N. (2019). Paying it forward: Interview with Nipun Mehta. Service Space. http://nipun.servicespace.org/blog.php?src=cf&id=28450

Shawoo, Z., & Thornton, T. F. (2019). The UN local communities and Indigenous peoples' platform: A traditional ecological knowledge-based evaluation. *WIRES Climate Change*.

Stiglitz, J., Sen, A., & Fitoussi, J.-P. (2010). *Mismeasuring our lives: Why GDP doesn't measure up*. The New Press.

UNDP. (2021, Jan 21). *Transforming systems in the decade of action: Global dialogue series*. SparkBlue. https://www.sparkblue.org/transformation-dialogue-1

UNDP Bhutan. (2019). *Bhutan national human development report: Ten years of democracy in Bhutan*. United Nations Development Programme Bhutan & Parliament of the Kingdom of Bhutan.

United Nations. (2011). UN Resolution 65/309: Happiness: Towards a holistic approach to development. https://www.un.org/esa/socdev/ageing/documents/NOTEON HAPPINESSFINALCLEAN.pdf

University of Calcutta. (2010). *Annual convocation address by His Majesty Jigme Khesar Namgyel Wangchuck, King of Bhutan*. University of Calcutta.

Ura, K., Alkire, S., & Zangmo, T. (2012). Case study: Bhutan gross national happiness and the GNH index. In J. Helliwell, J. Sachs, & R. Layard (Eds.), *World happiness report* (pp. 108–159).

Verschuuren, B. (2016). Nye within protected areas of Bhutan. In *Asian Sacred Natural Sites: Philosophy and practice in protected areas and conservation*. Routledge.

Wangdi, T. (2018, July 17). *News and media literacy for CSOs*. Bhutan Centre for Media and Democracy. http://bcmd.bt/news-and-media-literacy-for-csos/

Weber, A. (2019). *Enlivenment: Toward a poetics for The Anthropocene*. MIT Press.

Wellbeing Economy Alliance. (2021). Our vision for a movement to bring about economic system change: Bold, vital, and entirely possible. Wellbeing Economy Alliance.

World Bank. (2014). *Bhutan country snapshot*. World Bank.

Zangmo, R. (2018). *Promoting GNH values among Bhutanese youth*. Kuensel. http://www.kuenselonline.com/promoting-gnh-values-among-young-bhutanese/

15

America's Crisis of Despair

The Case for a Wellbeing-Based Recovery, with Lessons from and for Other Countries

CAROL GRAHAM ■

INTRODUCTION

Despair in the United States is a barrier to reviving labour markets and productivity; jeopardises wellbeing, health, and longevity; and adds to the toxic state of politics. Despair was increasing among Americans well before COVID-19; the virus was an exponential shock. Before COVID, when the United States boasted robust stock markets and record low levels of unemployment, an astounding 20% of prime aged males were out of the labour force. From 2005 to 2019, an average of 70,000 Americans died annually from deaths of despair (suicide, drug overdose, and alcohol and other poisonings). These deaths are concentrated among less than college educated middle-aged Whites, with those who are out of the labour force disproportionately represented (Graham & Pinto, 2019). Low-income minorities are significantly more optimistic than Whites and much less likely to die of these deaths.

This despair reflects the decline of the White working class. It contributes to the country's decreasing geographic mobility (Graham & Pinto, 2021) and has political spillovers. Counties with more people reporting lost hope in the years before 2016 were more likely to vote for Trump, for example, and similar patterns are reflected in the 2020 election outcome. President Biden had most of the support of the most productive and populous counties across the country, while Trump had support in less populous ones with declining economies (Herrin et al., 2018; Pinto, Bencsik, Chuluun, & Graham, 2020). Wellbeing in the United

An earlier and slightly different version of this piece appeared in the Brookings Blueprints for recovery series, a web-based institutional series.

States is more divided across the rich and the poor than in most countries, with the rich in the United States often having higher levels of wellbeing than the rich in other countries, while the US poor have significantly lower levels of wellbeing than do the poor in Latin America, who are materially much more deprived (Graham, 2017).

Unlike many other wealthy (and less wealthy) countries, the United States has yet to embrace societal wellbeing as a central policy priority and to use wellbeing-based metrics to complement and support traditional income-based measures of progress (see also Chapter 17, this volume). Wellbeing metrics allow us to attach relative values to the non-income dimensions of human experience and assess their contributions to quality of life in the moment and to broader cognitive evaluations of life. The use of wellbeing metrics in economic and other analyses has developed in sophistication over the past two decades. It is robust to a range of measurement concerns (discussed below) and has gained traction in mainstream economics as an approach to address an array of questions that cannot be answered by the standard revealed-preference approach in economics (i.e., the approach that underlies neoclassic economics and is based on assessing individual preferences/utility via observable consumption choices within a fixed budget constraint).

The key departure is the use of surveys of self-reports of individual wellbeing, an approach which challenges the assumption that individual decisions are based on maximising utility. Wellbeing metrics allow scholars to test the extent to which individuals value goods such as health, fairness and equity, volunteering, friendships, the arts, and respect and autonomy in the workplace as much or even more than income. This approach is particularly well-suited for addressing the plight of cohorts in despair who are unlikely to respond to financial or other incentives to rejoin the labour market and other aspects of community life. Without taking new approaches, the large cohort of workers that have simply dropped out of the labour force and have lost hope of having a purposeful existence will continue to suffer *and* remain a barrier to a full economic recovery. There are many examples of ways to help the desperate and isolated in the burgeoning field of wellbeing research and policy applications that are relevant to the United States and beyond (Graham & McLennon, 2021).

In this chapter, I propose that the US administration must address the various manifestations of despair, which have been further exacerbated by COVID, as a critical first step to economic and social recovery. This effort would monitor trends and coordinate federal and local efforts, as well as help to incorporate wellbeing-based approaches into them. Policy responses to date have been fragmented, with most focused on drug interdiction rather than on the root cause of despair. Even the public health efforts devoted to the problem do not have a strategy to address these. There are local efforts to boost the wellbeing of vulnerable cohorts, but most are isolated silos. There is no federal-level entity to provide financial or logistical support, nor is there a system that can disseminate relevant information to other communities seeking solutions. While federal agencies—such as the Centers for Disease Control and Prevention (CDC)—track mortality trends, there is no system that tracks the underlying causes of these deaths. Enhancing societal wellbeing would provide the policy frame.

Our research has shown that significant drops in hope among less-educated White males preceded deaths of despair by several decades, and the patterns in reported stress and lack of hope match those in deaths of despair across individuals, race, and place (O'Connor & Graham, 2019). Had the United States been measuring and tracking wellbeing regularly—as do a growing number of other countries (see also Chapter 13, this volume)—it could have helped avert a crisis of premature mortality.

DEATHS OF DESPAIR: WHO AND WHY?

The problem is a crisis of despair and associated premature death among significant parts of the US population. The challenge is how to reduce despair in places and populations where it has been lost. This is not a traditional policy problem. Yet failing to address it will jeopardise labour markets, productivity, and the much needed post–COVID-19 recovery, shorten life spans, exacerbate social and health problems, and continue to poison politics.

Lack of hope is a central issue. The American dream is in tatters, and, ironically, it is worse for Whites (for a review of changing beliefs in the American Dream, see Graham, 2017). The United States has higher levels of wellbeing differences across the rich and the poor than most wealthy countries and Latin America. Americans report more pain than respondents in 30 other wealthy countries (Blanchflower & Oswald, 2019). Whites, and particularly poor rural ones, report more pain than poor minorities, and America's high levels of reported pain are largely driven by middle-aged Whites. As there is no objective reason that Whites should have more pain than minorities who typically have significantly worse working conditions and access to healthcare, this suggests psychological pain as well as physical pain.

The addictive nature of prescribed opioids, meanwhile, has fed into a vicious circle of despair. Those who are out of the labour force, in pain, uneducated, and without a narrative for the future are more likely to request and receive prescription opioids. Whites are much more likely to be prescribed opioids for pain than are minorities, an inequity that has, ironically, been somewhat protective of mental health for minorities. The addiction to opioids and the eventual need to turn to illicit drugs when the prescriptions stop contribute to further despair and addiction.

In addition to the economic and health shocks from COVID-19, the despair among the White working class drives nativist politics, vulnerability to fake news, populist messages, and scepticism about science. Those trends are even evident in response to and compliance with COVID-19 policies, with Whites in general the group that is least likely to wear masks, as we found in our COVID-19 survey (discussed below). Sadly, our society's despair is even a factor in the ideological polarisation that is hampering our response to a deadly pandemic.

There are a number of historical instances in which relative deprivation and insecurity about the future have led to support for extremist politicians (such as Weimar Germany); other recent work documents the links between financial crises (distinct from recessions) and extreme right-wing voting in European countries over the past century (Funke, Shularick, & Trebesch, 2016). The tragic events at the Capitol on January 6—with additional instigation from others such as the then president and a few legislators—are reminiscent. The United States will not emerge from this crisis of despair as a healthy and productive society unless it begins to address its root causes.

Prior to COVID-19, an average 70,000 Americans died annually due to deaths of despair (i.e., suicides, overdoses, and alcohol-related illnesses). The rate of increase is also remarkable: while just under 20,000 people died of overdose in 2020, almost 75,000 did so in 2017. Overdoses kill more Americans than suicides, motor vehicle accidents, firearms, and homicides combined; overdose is now a key contributor to the drop in America's life expectancy.

Since COVID-19, death rates due to overdose have risen significantly due to increased social isolation and joblessness (discussed in detail below). This crisis cannot be solved by simply reducing the supply of drugs. People in despair will inevitably find substitute drugs. Most recently, increasing numbers of individuals with substance use disorders have switched to illegal and more deadly opioid strands such as fentanyl, which is responsible for an increase in overdose deaths nationwide since 2017 (for data on fentanyl deaths, see the CDC annual reports available at https://www.cdc.gov/nchs/fastats/deaths.htm; on the mechanics of addiction, see Satel, 2019).

There are long-term reasons for this. As blue-collar jobs began to decline from the late 1970s on, those displaced workers—and their communities—lost their purpose and identity and lacked a narrative for going forward. For decades, Whites had privileged access to these jobs and the stable communities that came with them. As globalisation led companies to relocate elsewhere, many communities experienced high levels of joblessness, affecting marriages, unions, and civic organisations (Opportunity America, the American Enterprise Institute for Public Policy Research, and the Brookings Institution, 2018; Sawhill, 2018).

Primarily White manufacturing and mining communities—in the suburbs and rural areas and often in the middle of the country—have the highest rates of despair and deaths. In contrast, more diverse urban communities have higher levels of optimism, better health indicators, and significantly lower rates of these deaths. We have developed a vulnerability indicator (available at https://www.brookings.edu/interactives/wellbeing-interactive/) that tracks and visualises these trends in wellbeing and the linkages to deaths of despair and excess deaths due to COVID-19, highlighting the places in the country that are most vulnerable.

White men who are out of the labour force, meanwhile, have the worst health markers in the country, including high levels of opioid addiction and reported pain, and the lowest levels of hope compared to any labour market cohort. They are also much less likely to move to look for jobs. They tend to live in counties where a high percentage of respondents still live in their parents' homes or census tracts (census tracts are an indicator in the US census data that is based on where individual homes are located). These counties tend to be in the same ones that have experienced significant economic decline. The national average percentage of people who live in their parents' census tract, per county, is 26.1, while the maximum level is 61.7—a large divergence across counties and regions. The average percent of people living in their parents' homes as adults is 11.8, while the maximum is 42.9, again reflecting large differences across counties as well as the lack of mobility of those who are out of the labour force, who tend to live in the high-percentage counties (Graham & Pinto, 2021).

The lasting belief in the rewards of individual effort has also eroded in this group, while lack of trust in public safety nets remains. Scepticism of higher education and science leaves them less-equipped to navigate a future in which the nature of work—and particularly low-skilled jobs—is changing. High levels of addiction and despair in many of these communities is preclusive to moving to where the jobs are (Graham & Pinto, 2021).

Yet despite the tragic statistics, there are remarkable pockets of hope we can look to and learn from. In contrast to low-income Whites, minorities, who had unequal access to good jobs and worse objective conditions to begin with, developed coping skills and supportive community ties in the absence of coherent public safety nets. Belief in education and strong communities has served them well in overcoming much adversity. African Americans remain more likely to believe in the value of a college education than are low-income Whites (Kerpelman, Eryigit, & Stephens, 2008). Minorities have built strong communities based on having empathy for their peers who fall behind and from jointly battling persistent discrimination, among other factors.

Low-income Whites remain sceptical of higher education, in part because it was not necessary to attain a stable, blue-collar lifestyle in the past. In contrast, low-income Blacks continue to believe in it as an upward path and have been narrowing education gaps with Whites over the past decades (see chapter 4 in Graham [2017] for a summary of trends across races). In keeping with that trend, our ongoing surveys of the hopes and aspirations of young adolescents in low-income neighbourhoods in Missouri are showing that, conditional on graduating high school, low-income minorities are more likely to pursue college than are their White counterparts.

Johns Hopkins sociologist Andrew Cherlin recently studied the children of former Bethlehem Steel workers in Baltimore (Cherlin, 2019). The mills, long since shuttered, were an anchor of the city's blue-collar jobs. The Black workers were recruited from the South in the 1950s, lived in segregated housing, and faced constant discrimination in the workplace. Yet most of their children attended college and left Dundalk, the neighbourhood surrounding the mills, for better parts of town. Yet, in keeping with the role of communities of empathy, many come back weekly to the local church to give back. The children of the White workers largely remained in Dundalk, did not attend college, and work in the gig economy. This example is a microcosm of the broader patterns of minority optimism for the future and related investments compared to the relative decline—and lack of intergenerational or geographic mobility—of low-income Whites.

Pain is a gateway into opioid addiction, meanwhile, and the lower likelihood that minorities are prescribed opioids ironically may have played a protective role. The vast increase of opioid prescriptions in the 2000s created a perfect storm. At the time that the medical community began to prioritise pain, opioid manufacturers such as Purdue Pharma began targeting the same declining blue-collar communities (where manual labour and pain often coincide), and adequate regulation lagged for decades. The so-called pill-mill towns in West Virginia and Kentucky are noteworthy, and those two states have amongst the highest levels of deaths of despair today.

The COVID-19 Shock

The entrance of COVID-19 pushed this crisis to an entirely new level. While initially COVID-19 hit low-income minorities in big cities the most, this changed with the nationwide spread of the virus by September 2020 and its reach to rural areas in the heartland which already had high levels of deaths of despair, poor underlying health conditions, and years of decline in the availability of accessible hospitals and health care. While population density is lower in these places, the COVID-19 mortality rate is very high in many of them (see our interactive tracker, cited above). The pre-existing low levels of health increased the vulnerability of these populations.

The stress and anxiety surrounding COVID-19 and the isolation caused by necessary lockdown policies has exacerbated vulnerabilities everywhere and surely in these hard-hit isolated places. While the economic shocks from the virus may be felt less in places where there are fewer industries left to fail, the other uncertainties caused by the virus also affect mental health. Concerns about eviction and job loss and the loss of existing community support—no matter how minimal—contribute to more isolation and despair among already vulnerable people and add new ones to the ranks.

Finally, an unintended outcome of the CARES Act—the relief package designed to boost the incomes of the vulnerable during COVID—is an increase in opioid and other overdose rates as a result of people with substance use disorders using their cash to purchase drugs (Maryland HIDTA, 2020). At the same time, lockdowns and the virus make it much more difficult for the Emergency Medical System (EMS) and other responders to get at-risk patients into treatment and makes it much harder time to follow their progress over time. The spillover effects of these trends will be long term. One of these is the increase in anxiety, depression, and suicide among the young, who are hit particularly hard by the lack of social contact and face an abysmal job market. Lack of hope and uncertainty about the future is a driving issue.

The results that we have to date are stark. First-responder data from the National EMS Information System (NEMSIS) shows significant increases

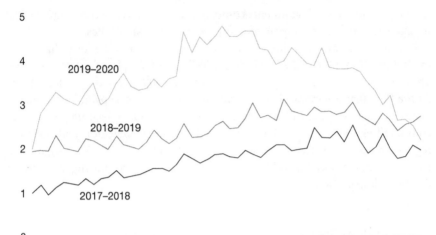

Figure 15.1 Opioid overdose: 2020 versus 2018–2019. Count of 911-initiated EMS activations with opiate-related overdose (thousands).
Figure by Carol Graham, The Brookings Institution. Source: Mann, C. (2020). "EMS by the Numbers: COVID-19 Update, December 10", NEMSIS Technical Assistance Center, https://nemsis.org/. For Figures 15.1–15.3, the numbers under the horizontal axis wrap around, with weeks 50–52 of the previous year starting at the origin, and then week 1 of the next year at the #1 spot and proceeding to week 49 at the end of the horizontal line.

in mental distress, overdose rates, and suicides. Mental health and overdose calls to first responders have doubled in 2020 compared to both 2018 and 2019 (Figures 15.1 and 15.2). Suicides have also increased, but at a lower rate (Figure 15.3).

Our wellbeing data from surveys conducted during COVID-19, in collaboration with the Social Policy School at Washington University in St. Louis, also show overall declines in mental health, drops in hope, and increases in anxiety. Remarkably, though, low income Blacks remain the most optimistic low-income race cohort, even though they are the most at risk from COVID-19. They have experienced increases in anxiety, but their levels remain lower than those of other cohorts, and they report the lowest levels of loneliness and hopelessness. They also report feeling more worthwhile than any other cohort, especially Whites (Figures 15.4 and 15.5). It seems that the same optimism and resilience that has helped African Americans cope with a history of adversity is also protective of mental health during the pandemic (Graham, Chun, Grinstein-Weiss, & Roll, 2020).

LIMITS OF HISTORIC AND EXISTING POLICIES

Past policies have focused largely on interdicting the supply of illegal drugs, which is a worthy cause but will not solve the demand problem. And even in

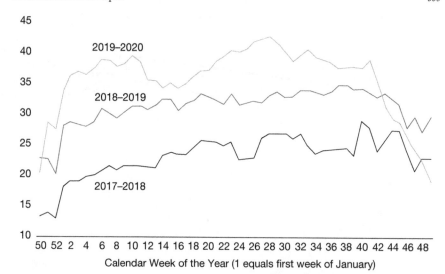

Figure 15.2 Mental and behavioral calls: 2020 versus 2018–2019. Count of 911-initiated
EMS activations related to mental and behavioral (thousands).
Figure by Carol Graham, The Brookings Institution. Source: Mann (2020).

the interdiction and tracking process, there is a lack of coordination between the
many efforts and a lack of connection to those concerned with the health effects
of the opioid crisis. The Office of National Drug Control Policy (ONDCP), for
example, coordinates several important tracking efforts, such as NEMSIS and
ODMAP (Overdose Map—the drug overdose tracking agency). The Substance

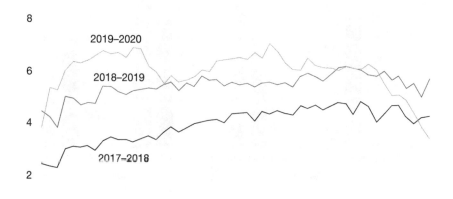

Figure 15.3 Suicides 2020 versus 2018–2019. Count of 911-initiated EMS activations
with suicide-related causes (thousands).
Figure by Carol Graham, The Brookings Institution. Source: Mann (2020).

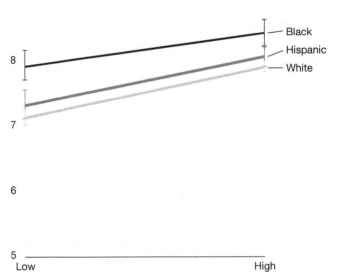

9

8

7

6

5

Low   High

INCOME

— Black
— Hispanic
— White

Figure 15.4 Differential optimism across race and income groups. Cantril ladder (0–10), 5 years after.
Figure by Carol Graham, The Brookings Institution, and Yung Chun, Washington University in St. Louis. Source: Graham et al. (2020) based on Wash U COVID Survey. Optimism is based on a question about expected life satisfaction in the future.

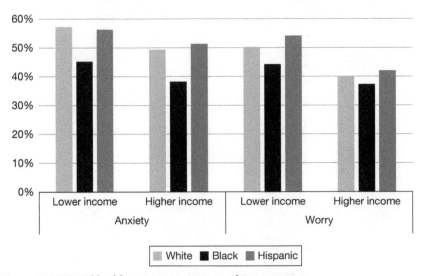

Figure 15.5 Mental health reports across race and income groups.
Figure by Carol Graham, The Brookings Institution, and Yung Chun, Washington University in St. Louis. Source: Chun and Graham, Social Policy Institute COVID Survey, Washington University in St. Louis (2020).

Abuse and Mental Health Services Agency (SAMHSA) does important work supporting research and tracking of suicides and other mental health illnesses, but this is not connected with the interdiction efforts. There is no shortage of committed people and agencies, but there is no coordinating body that connects drug supply-and-demand problems with trends in the causes of despair and especially economic decline. We need a coordinating body that connects those dealing directly with deaths of despair with those who are trying to deal with some of the root causes of the despair, including the decline of blue-collar jobs and the communities that used to support them. The intertwined problems of working-class decline and the increase in despair and death among these same cohorts should be treated as a conjoined national priority, not in separate silos.

Progress has been made on curtailing opioid prescribing practices, introducing new regulations, and prosecuting those companies that aggressively marketed these drugs in declining manufacturing and mining communities. Still, as noted above, that will not prevent already addicted people from switching from opioids to fentanyl, methadone, or any other drug that they can access.

None of these approaches has addressed the root causes of despair, which have been exacerbated in recent years by economic trends and COVID-19. There are many local-level efforts, some of which are creative and effective and could be generalised to other deprived communities. Yet they lack the capacity to go to scale and have little or no connection with or support from the federal government. First-responder efforts, which are critical and often entail efforts to get people experiencing addiction into treatment, suffer from the same problem. There have been some efforts to enhance federal and local coordination. ONDCP set up the High Intensity Drug Trafficking Areas (HIDTA) programme to coordinate the work of federal, state, and local policing bodies, for example. Yet there is still a lack of understanding of the connection between interdiction efforts and the needs of deprived communities, as well as of which activities should be scaled versus those that are successful only in their immediate geography.

More generally, there has also been a historical lack of attention to rural communities, which suffer from poor-quality education and healthcare, little access to broadband internet, and low civic participation among youth (Kawashima-Ginsberg & Sullivan, 2017). They often also lack the institutions and capacity to take advantage of existing state or federal resources. These trends have helped drive the decline in civic trust and belief in education and science, along with other trends that hamper any effective response to COVID-19 and to a recovery of the nation's economic productivity, health, and wellbeing.

THE PATH FORWARD

Reducing despair and its impact on society's health, longevity, wellbeing, and productivity is a complex, multifaceted problem that one policy alone cannot solve. It will require many approaches—some we know about and others that still need to be developed. Incorporating wellbeing metrics into data-gathering, policy design, and evaluation efforts going forward will make nations such as the United States more prepared for the next crisis of despair. At this juncture, though, immediate efforts to help reverse the crisis of despair are necessary.

As a first step in the United States, a federal coordinating body or interagency task force is needed that can provide logistical assistance and modest financial support to ongoing local efforts in deprived communities, as well as to better coordinate federal programmes, as in drug interdiction, that can bolster and scale local responses. Another role for the task force would be to marshal the use of tools such as our vulnerability indicator (discussed above) that provide information on where high levels of despair and economic decline intersect and reflect in the highest rates of mortality. Federal agencies, like Health and Human Services, Education, Labor, and Commerce/Economic Development, and place-based agencies like Housing and Urban Development and the Department of Agriculture, would be natural members of this coordinated effort.

This body or agency, with the full backing of the administration, could ensure that COVID-19 revitalisation programmes make combating deaths of despair a central theme of their work. We have efforts to promote economic development, and we have other efforts to connect people to teletherapy. Yet none of these explicitly puts deaths of despair at the centre, so we are likely not understanding the problem fully or responding to it adequately.

We have many examples of successful efforts from which to build—both within and outside the United States—including specific interventions that enhance the wellbeing of the isolated and desperate. Like wellbeing interventions, economic efforts to help revive deprived communities must be local and tailored to specific communities. Yet they also stand to gain a lot from the logistical support that could come from an agency or task force that serves as an information clearinghouse for local practitioners trying to learn from their counterparts in other counites, states, and nations.

SUCCESS STORIES TO BUILD FROM

Addressing societal despair is not a usual policy challenge, nor are there magic bullet solutions. Yet there are successful initiatives that we can learn and build from and that could serve as a benchmark for a coordinating agency to use to launch the process. Many countries around the world—such as the United Kingdom and New Zealand—have already made wellbeing a central policy priority, including using metrics of wellbeing in their official statistics as tools to assess budget priorities and the effects of policies to improve quality of life at the workplace or in health practices (including mental health), thereby enhancing productivity, the effects of changes in environmental policies, and more.

Key to the success of these efforts has been one or more high-level government officials making a strong commitment to the effort. In the United Kingdom, Lord Gus O'Donnell, former chief of cabinet under Prime Minsters Brown, Blair, and Cameron, championed the cause of wellbeing, from getting the metrics into the official statistics to making it a national government priority. Lord Richard Layard, meanwhile, a leading member of the Robbins Committee on higher education, an expert on unemployment and on the economics of happiness, led the charge to make mental health a priority via the creation of a Ministry of Loneliness and an initiative for the broader use of cognitive and behavioural therapy (CBT) to help combat depression. In New Zealand, Prime Minister Jacinda Arden has been a major driver of wellbeing as a national priority, and the Ministry of the Treasury has been the primary implementing organisation, placing wellbeing in a critical government agency and signaling that it is part of mainstream policy.

The British government also uses wellbeing metrics to design and evaluate policy interventions to enhance wellbeing in deprived or isolated populations or communities via the What Works Centre for Wellbeing (https://whatworkswellbe ing.org/), which receives both government and nongovernmental support to op- erate. The Centre supports academic scholars to design and implement the inter- ventions and then has them independently evaluated for cost-effectiveness (in both income and wellbeing terms).[1] The interventions are, for the most part, in- expensive and intuitive but yield important improvements in wellbeing. These in- clude increasing public participation in the arts, volunteering, and/or community environmental improvement programmes (especially for isolated individuals), interventions that seek to improve quality of life in the workplace, and training programmes for underprivileged youth.

There are also examples of successful efforts in the United States, although they tend to be local. The city of Santa Monica, for example, with initial support from a grant from Bloomberg and based on advice from an expert panel of scholars in the field, implemented the first annual wellbeing survey in the United States and for several years used the outcomes to frame municipal policy priorities. These included reducing the isolation and loneliness of low-income minorities via community-sponsored activities, such as group walks, involving local youth in art projects designed to enhance community wellbeing, and the provision of seed grants for small entrepreneurs who include a wellbeing focus in their projects. Again, many of the policies were simple and relatively inexpensive but improved the community's wellbeing, as assessed by the annual surveys (https://santamoni cawellbeing.org/about/wellbeing-index).

The Center for Creative Healing at the School of Public Health at the University of Louisville is designing and evaluating initiatives that encourage relevant industries such as healthcare providers and the makers of athletic equipment— to include and evaluate policies that enhance worker wellbeing. The Center is also active in solutions to address the opioid epidemic and racial division in the city. Importantly, they have the interest and logistical support of key local government officials there.

There are also examples in the arena of mental health. The Maryland Behavioral Health Administration (MBHA) has a wide range of programmes to address

1. For full disclosure, Graham is on the advisory panel of the What Works Centre for Wellbeing.

mental health issues of vulnerable populations in the state, including a pro-gramme to support the children of opioid patients and teach them resilience and coping skills based on age-appropriate messaging. In Wicomico County in Southern Maryland, first responders collaborate with mental healthcare providers when they respond to overdose calls to encourage people with addictions to get into treatment and then follow their progress overtime, when possible (COVID-19 has hampered these efforts for obvious reasons). The Center for Healthy Places at Salisbury University, Maryland, meanwhile, supports these efforts by providing logistical support from students in the social work programme.

There are also examples of economically oriented solutions for deprived com-munities. In a 2020 report on community revitalisation, Tim Bartik (2020) of the Upjohn Institute proposed a federal programme to provide block grants (at a cost of $12 billion per year) to communities with a high percent of people who are out of the labour force. The grants would cover economic development and em-ployment and training services, information services, and job retention support, among other things.

For two reasons, these programmes likely have more potential than grants to support individuals moving to communities where there are more jobs. The first is that, as our work has shown, these populations tend not to move, either due to health problems or to lack of skills and motivation to do so. The second is that, the more willing and able workers move out of these communities, the lower the chances of revitalisation in their labour markets. The provision of new jobs can also have spillover effects and encourage additional labour market partici-pation (it should be noted that these efforts could complement but are distinct from Opportunity Zones, which are aimed at labour markets rather than at more general community renovation). Additional efforts are needed to reach the most deprived and vulnerable communities.

Bill Galston and Mark Muro of Brookings, meanwhile, propose strategies to bridge the gap between regional growth poles and left-behind deprived com-munities. These include narrowing the gap in digital skills and in access to broadband internet, providing capital to businesses in falling-behind places, and identifying linkages to regional growth polls (Hendrickson, Muro, & Galston, 2018).

Efforts such as these also often require training for new kinds of jobs for the low-skilled as traditional jobs fade. These include training in medium-skill tech support, soft skills, and other less-traditional education offerings, particularly for the youth in these communities. Another policy that could complement these is the creation of a national service programme for high school gradu-ates, as Isabel Sawhill and Richard Reeves have proposed. They suggest that those who participate in a year of national service receive a grant for 2 years of tuition at a public college or university (Reeves & Sawhill, 2020). The service programme could also serve as a gateway into networks and experiences that youth living in deprived areas lack and be an equalising force and form of civic education.

WHAT IS MISSING

All these programmes can make a positive difference. But they will be much more effective if they are part of a coordinated effort and do not operate in silos. Individuals with very low levels of wellbeing are unlikely to take up opportunities such as job training programme unless their mental health issues are addressed. Those with substance use problems, for example, cannot recover in a vacuum and need access to treatment and follow up support.

Yet, in the United States today, insurance for and access to mental health-care is extraordinarily weak compared to other wealthy countries. According to SAMHSA, one in five US adults experienced mental illness in 2018, and one in 14 people aged 12 or older had a substance use disorder; yet, in 2017, despite the rising rates of overdoses and suicides, only $1 out of every $100 spent on health-care was for addiction treatment, and only $1 out of every $25 was for mental health and substance use disorders combined (Wellbeing Trust, 2020).

Youth in deprived communities will not participate in job training pro-grammes if they have no hope for the future or awareness of what kinds of opportunities that participation will lead to. First responders will not be very effective at getting those with addiction into treatment if they are not well-connected with local treatment providers or aware of what efforts have suc-ceeded and failed elsewhere.

SUMMARY

Despite the high levels of human suffering that preceded and were significantly exacerbated by COVID-19, there are also some surprisingly positive trends to build on as societies seek to recover from the COVID shock. Surveys find that, on average, humans are remarkably resilient and can face a wide range of challenges—from poverty to crime to health problems—and return to their initial high levels of wellbeing. As such, it is no surprise that in the countries for which we do have data, such as the United States, the United Kingdom, Ireland, and Sweden, average levels of wellbeing trended back upward to near pre-COVID-19 trends as soon as the lockdowns and the uncertainty surrounding them subsided (McCarthy, 2020; Office for National Statistics, 2020). Within the United States, groups that are traditionally resilient in wellbeing terms, such as poor Blacks and Hispanics, displayed this resiliency during the pandemic. While these same groups are much more likely to contract and/or die from COVID-19 (Graham et al., 2020), they also report better mental health and more optimism for the future than Whites during the pandemic. Low-income Blacks have higher levels of optimism than other low-income groups, and they also experienced less of a decline during COVID-19. The communities of empathy that they have built over time to combat disadvantage and discrimination play a fundamental role in sup-porting this resilience.

Still, the pandemic has highlighted how economic growth alone is not enough to sustain economies and societies. In the absence of a more comprehensive approach which supports societies' health and wellbeing in addition to growth, we will remain very vulnerable to the next societal shock, as well as to future waves of the COVID-19 pandemic. It has also emphasised how infectious diseases cross borders within and across countries and that ignoring the wellbeing of the poor and the vulnerable has broad costs within and beyond national borders.

Wellbeing metrics give policy-makers a tool to attach relative values to things such as lost jobs, lack of health insurance, and insecurity. As mentioned, many countries have adopted a wellbeing approach in their policies, most notably New Zealand, which, at the time of writing, has had success in controlling COVID-19. And, as we have written earlier (Graham & Pinto, 2021), New Zealand also has exceptionally high levels of public trust compared to those countries that have fared poorly in controlling the pandemic—such as the United States and India. Incorporating wellbeing into economic models and policy priorities would surely leave many other countries better prepared to handle crises in which the solutions hinge on public health systems and norms of public trust and cooperation.

In the United States, unless society's wellbeing becomes a national priority, a complete recovery from the COVID-19 shock is unlikely. The many local initiatives that exist are essentially operating in silos, with little ability to scale up or coordinate with other relevant actors elsewhere. And without a federal level commitment to wellbeing and mental health, the issue is likely to remained side-lined.

One positive sign is that many federal level agencies, such as the Federal Reserve, the Consumer Finance Protection Board, the CDC and Health, Human Services, and the Census Pulse survey, among others, have begun to include wellbeing questions in their official surveys. Tracking wellbeing and ill-being is a first step to mainstreaming the issue, as the experience of many other countries has shown.

More important though, is the signal that the creation of a federal entity dedicated to reducing despair would send about societal wellbeing as a national priority. That, in turn, would create a momentum of its own. The main objective is not to provide funds on a large scale or to create a new bureaucracy, but rather to provide logistical support and shared information and to prioritise the issue in the public dialogue. This will not be completely free of cost, but the costs of not addressing the problem will be significantly higher, in terms of both lost productivity and lost lives.

In the longer term, this may lead to the US government's following the UK and New Zealand examples to support new statistics collection efforts and learn from and support burgeoning local efforts. If one of the wealthiest countries in the world cannot combat premature mortality due to despair in a significant part of its population, its future health, civic cohesion, and economic potential will certainly decline. The many lessons from wellbeing research and policies are critical tools for the moment and for the future—in both the United States and in countries around the world.[2]

2. I thank Sarmed Rashid, formerly of the White House Task Force on opioids, and Amy Liu and Elaine Kamarck of Brookings for very helpful comments on an earlier version of this chapter, as well as the editors of this volume for additional insights.

REFERENCES

Bartik, T. (2020). *Helping America's distressed communities recover from the COVID-19 recession and achieve long-term prosperity*. Metropolitan Policy Program at Brookings. https://www.brookings.edu/research/helping-americas-distressed-communities-recover-from-the-covid-19-recession-and-achieve-long-term-prosperity/

Blanchflower, D., & Oswald, A. (2019). Unhappiness and pain in modern America: A review essay and further evidence for Carol Graham's *Happiness for All? Journal of Economic Literature, 57*, 385–402.

Cherlin, A. (2019). *In the shadow of Sparrows Point: Racialized labor in the white and black working classes*. Russell Sage Foundation Working Paper. https://www.russellsage.org/sites/default/files/In%20the%20Shadow%20of%20Sparrows%20Point.pdf

Funke, M., Shularick, M., & Trebesch, C. (2016). Going to extremes: Politics after financial crises, 1870–2014. *European Economic Review, 88*, 227–260.

Graham, C. (2017). *Happiness for all? Unequal hopes and lives in pursuit of the American dream*. Princeton University Press.

Graham, C., Chun, Y., Grinstein-Weiss, M., & Roll, S. (2020). *Well-being and mental health amid COVID-19: Differences in resilience across minorities and whites*. Brookings Institution. https://www.brookings.edu/research/well-being-and-mental-health-amid-covid-19-differences-in-resilience-across-minorities-and-whites/

Graham, C., & McLennon, S. (2021). Policy insights from the new science of well-being. *Behavioral Science and Policy, 6*, 1–20.

Graham, C., & Pinto, S. (2019). Unequal hopes and lives in the USA: Optimism, race, place, and premature mortality. *Journal of Population Economics, 32*, 665–733. https://doi.org/10.1007/s00148-018-0687-y

Graham, C., & Pinto, S. (2021). The geography of desperation in America: Labor force participation, mobility, place, and well-being. *Social Science and Medicine*. https://doi.org/10.1016/j.socscimed.2020.113612

Hendrickson, C., Muro, M., & Galston, W. A. (2018). *Countering the geography of discontent: Strategies for left-behind places*. Brookings Institution. https://www.brookings.edu/research/countering-the-geography-of-discontent-strategies-for-left-behind-places/

Herrin, J., Witters, D., Roy, B., Riley, C., Liu, D., & Krumholz, H. M. (2018). Population well-being and electoral shifts. *PLOS One, 13*, e0193401.

Kawashima-Ginsberg, K., & Sullivan, F. (2017). Sixty percent of rural millennials lack access to a political life. *The Conversation*, March 27. https://theconversation.com/study-60-percent-of-rural-millennials-lack-access-to-a-political-life-74513

Kerpelman, J., Eryigit, S., & Stephens, C. (2008). African American adolescents' future education orientation: Associations with self-efficacy, ethnic identity, and perceived parental support. *Journal of Youth & Adolescence, 378*, 997–1008.

Maryland HIDTA. (2020). *Maryland operational opioid command center, 2020 second quarter report*. https://beforeitstoolate.maryland.gov/wp-content/uploads/sites/34/2020/09/Second-Quarter-OOCC-Report-2020-Master-Copy-9-21-20-Update.pdf

McCarthy, J. (2020). U.S. emotions mixed after a tense month of COVID-19 response. *Gallup*. https://news.gallup.com/poll/306026/emotions-mixed-tense-month-covid-response.aspx

O'Connor, K., & Graham, C. (2019). Longer, more optimistic lives: Historic optimism and life expectancy in the United States. *Journal of Economic Behavior and Organization, 168*, 374–392.

Office for National Statistics (2020). *Coronavirus (COVID-19): Latest data and analysis on coronavirus (COVID-19) in the UK and its effect on the economy and society.* https://www.ons.gov.uk/peoplepopulationandcommunity/healthandsocialcare/conditionsanddiseases

Opportunity America, the American Enterprise Institute for Public Policy Research, and the Brookings Institution. (2018). *Work, skills, community: Restoring opportunity for the working class.* https://www.aei.org/research-products/report/work-skills-and-community-restoring-opportunity-for-the-working-class/

Pinto, S., Bencsik, P., Chuluun, C., & Graham, C. (2020). Presidential elections, divided politics, and happiness in the U.S.A. *Economica*, doi:10.1111/ecca.12349

Reeves, R., & Sawhill, I. (2020). *A new contract for the middle class.* The Brookings Institution Press.

Satel, S. (2019). The truth about painkiller addiction. *The Atlantic.* https://www.theatlantic.com/ideas/archive/2019/08/what-america-got-wrong-about-opioid-crisis/595090/

Sawhill, I. (2018). *The forgotten Americans: An economic agenda for a divided nation.* Yale University Press.

Wellbeing Trust. (2020). *Healing the nation: Advancing mental health and addiction policy.* https://healingthenation.wellbeingtrust.org

16

Inequality and the Transition from GDP to Wellbeing

RICHARD WILKINSON AND KATE PICKETT ∎

INTRODUCTION

As societies reach toward sustainability, there is a growing understanding that governments will have to replace their central aim of expanding gross domestic product (GDP) with policies devoted instead to increasing human wellbeing. However, in this chapter, we argue that dropping economic growth as a government objective may do little in itself to weaken the powerful drivers of growth which lie beyond government policy. To effect real change, we must focus attention on deeper structural reforms. And while the development of new measures of wellbeing will sharpen our focus, improvements in the quality of life will continue to depend on overcoming the powerful *political* forces which currently prevent reductions in things such as poverty, homelessness, unemployment, and food insecurity that dramatically depress wellbeing.

We go on to discuss the contrast between the co-existing high standards of material wellbeing in rich societies and the very high levels of stress, anxiety, and mental illness. As well as arguing that it is necessary to look at both the positive and negative sides of wellbeing, we go on to suggest the use of surveys that would help identify the *causes* of deficits in wellbeing and so facilitate policy responses. But, as we have shown in our previous work, material inequality between rich and poor is perhaps the single most important obstacle both to improving wellbeing and to realistic responses to the climate crisis. Until inequality is substantially

This chapter incorporates parts of a chapter originally entitled 'For Better or Worse' published in: Chris Deeming (Ed.) (2021). *The struggle for social sustainability: Moral conflicts in global social policy.* This revised version is published with permission of Policy Press (an imprint of Bristol University Press, UK).

reduced, our societies and political systems will remain highly dysfunctional, and progress in tackling the climate crisis and moving toward sustainable wellbeing will continue to be dangerously slow.

MOVING TO A FOCUS ON SUSTAINABILITY: TIGHTENING BELTS OR IMPROVING WELLBEING?

A crucial reason that governments everywhere drag their feet about the transition to environmental sustainability is that it is widely thought to depend primarily on a reduction in living standards. The popular view is that reducing carbon emissions not only involves tightening our belts and consuming less, but also doing without some of the pleasures in life such as giving up eating meat, stopping flying, using less plastic, and replacing private cars with public transport. In the public mind, that view inevitably makes facing the climate emergency a pretty dismal prospect, one to be avoided for as long as possible. That, in turn, means politicians are likely to regard action on the climate crisis and environmental degradation as an electoral liability.

To counter that view, many environmentalists have argued that it is possible to transition to sustainability while at the same time producing higher standards of human wellbeing (Costanza et al., 2018). This perspective is based primarily on three considerations. First, that in high-income countries, continued increases in happiness and life satisfaction are no longer closely linked to average material living standards and would not be damaged if levels of consumption were curtailed. Second, that sustainable societies could satisfy fundamental human social needs much better than high-income societies have been doing—for instance, by strengthening community life and reducing status competition. And third, that societies using renewable sources of power and electric public transport systems will be cleaner, safer, and quieter and so enable higher health standards. This perspective suggests that a transition to environmental sustainability involving large-scale socioeconomic restructuring can achieve major improvements in the real quality of our lives. Proposals involve everything from replacing increasing GDP per head as the central objective of government policy with the aim of maximising human wellbeing (see also Chapter 14, this volume) to much more radical demands for the abolition of capitalism itself.

WHAT FACTORS PROPEL A FOCUS ON ECONOMIC GROWTH?

The demand to replace GDP with wellbeing as the main objective of government policy has led—as this book shows—to a small academic industry devoted to understanding wellbeing and developing better ways to measure it. But it would be wrong to think that a mere substitution of aims would mean that wellbeing will increase or that the drivers of economic growth will lose their force. Both economic growth and standards of wellbeing are almost certainly propelled by more fundamental and poorly understood forces than government policy in itself.

That governments have little control of economic growth rates is shown by the many examples around the world where they have failed, despite constant attention from politicians and policy=makers, to achieve desired increases in these growth rates. Japan, for example, has had little or no growth for close to three decades—since the early 1990s—and successive governments in Britain have not only failed to achieve more than very slow growth but have also failed to halt the periodic economic booms and recessions.

Nor is this a superficial issue of getting policy right. It is often said that a minimum requirement for economic growth is a functional government, sufficiently in control to be able to provide stability and enforce the rule of law. Without these basics and in the absence of effective administrative institutions, governments would be ineffective, and so it might make little difference what policy they intended to implement—whether it is pro-growth or not. Although there is evidence that economic growth is *cross-sectionally* associated with measures of overall government effectiveness, it is less clear which way round that relationship works. Indeed, a study that looked at changes over time found that government effectiveness is unrelated to *subsequent* rates of economic growth. It concluded that the relationship probably goes from better economic performance to more effective government as increased prosperity improves administrative systems, strengthens the rule of law, and reduces corruption (Kurtz & Schrank, 2007).

There is still fundamental disagreement between governments of different political persuasions even on whether larger or smaller government is conducive to faster economic growth (Afonso & Furceri, 2010), and, when growth happens, there are usually many contending theories as to what made it possible. Rather than being primarily dependent on policy, we suspect that economic growth is likely to be an expression primarily of the simple fact that most people want to maximise their incomes and consumption, and most businesses want to maximise sales and profits. As Adam Smith famously pointed out, 'It is not from the benevolence of the butcher, the brewer, or the baker that we expect our dinner, but from their regard to their own self-interest' (Smith, 1937). And similarly, it is no doubt from their self-interest that the drive to expand their businesses comes.

For these and other reasons, many, including Karl Marx, have regarded growth as inherent to capitalism itself, rather than being dependent on government policy. Like these money making pressures, economic growth long preceded explicit government desire to foster GDP growth (probably by at least two centuries) and is likely to continue even when governments have shifted their focus. Rather than economic growth being dependent on government policy, we believe it will be difficult to discover how to stop it. Indeed, in present circumstances, it can easily be seen as if it were a natural expression of human avarice. Unless we find ways of addressing the income and profit maximising pressures at the roots of economic growth, they will continue to intensify the environmental crisis even after expanding GDP has ceased to be a government objective.

CURRENT LIMITATIONS IN MEASURING WELLBEING

With the strategic objective of making a sustainable society more attractive, people (ourselves included) have tried to present the transition to sustainability as a transition to a society which serves human wellbeing more broadly than the narrow concept of economic prosperity does now. This objective has often been supported by proposals to establish official systems for monitoring changes in population wellbeing based, for instance, on surveys of happiness and life satisfaction or on measures of what has been called 'economic wellbeing'. We suggest instead that measures of wellbeing should be developed which are designed to identify the preventable causes of low levels of wellbeing and so guide policy on what needs to be done to improve wellbeing. At the moment, many proposed measures of wellbeing do little to take us closer to understanding either the determinants of wellbeing or the policies that will, in any given circumstances, help us improve it. In a nutshell, measures of happiness may not tell us much about how to reduce unhappiness. In contrast, part of the influence of GDP in the past came from the assumption that it was a measure of good and valuable things produced in the economy. It was therefore regarded as both a measure *and* a determinant of wellbeing. Although we now know how very misleading these assumptions are when applied to the rich countries (Kubiszewski et al., 2013), it is a viewpoint which is likely to be less misleading in low-income countries today where many people continue to lack basic necessities.

A merit of health as a measure of wellbeing is that it is both a preeminent 'good' in itself and an indicator of a number of the most important components of wellbeing. Even when measured by death rates, it provides powerful indications of what is wrong with people's lives and living conditions—both material and psychosocial, including diet, housing, working conditions, air quality, and so on. That health is not widely recognised as a good indicator of wellbeing probably reflects a lack of understanding of its powerful social, economic, and psychological determinants. People still imagine health is determined overwhelmingly by medical care and health-related behaviour—like diet, smoking, and exercise. But what makes health a powerful indicator of wellbeing is that, as well as being influenced by material conditions, it is also highly sensitive to psychosocial factors that are particularly hard to measure objectively—including stress, friendship, conflict, insecurity and the quality of social relationships more widely. The happier people are, the less stressed; and the better their social and material circumstances, the longer they live (Steptoe, 2019). Indeed, there are good reasons for thinking that health is responsive to every step on Maslow's hierarchy of needs for attaining optimal human functioning. The so-called deaths of despair from drugs, alcohol, and suicide which, for the past 25 years, have pushed down life expectancy in the United States, particularly among middle-aged Whites, are an example of the importance of psychosocial factors (Case & Deaton, 2020; De Vogli, 2019; see also Chapter 15, this volume). Another example is the evidence of the impact of social relations on health. A meta-analysis of studies of the health effects of friendship and social integration found that they have as strong a protective effect on survival during a follow-up period gauging whether or not people smoke

(Holt-Lunstad, Smith, & Layton, 2010; House, Landis, & Umberson, 1988). More generally, chronic stress causes more rapid aging, making people vulnerable earlier to a wide range of diseases of later life. For example, there are strong links between depression (which is almost always accompanied by high levels of stress) and ischaemic heart disease mortality (Surtees et al., 2008).

In contrast to health, most of the so-called measures of economic wellbeing leave out psychosocial wellbeing entirely. That even societies which have reached almost unprecedented levels of physical comfort are, nevertheless, often marred by very high rates of misery, anxiety, and depression suggests the need for more appropriate measures of wellbeing. Survey data suggest that levels of stress are very high in most rich countries. A survey sponsored by the American Psychiatric Association reported that approximately 60% of American adults reported experiencing significant stress regarding a range of issues (American Psychiatric Association, 2017). A British survey found that 74% of the population often felt overcome by stress and unable to cope, 32% had had suicidal thoughts because of stress, and 16% had self-harmed as a result of stress (Mental Health Foundation, 2018). In France, 89% of the population said they were stressed some or all of the time and 83% thought their stress was bad enough to affect their health. Surveys that used diagnostic psychiatric interviews with random samples of the population in high-income countries found that, in any year, between 8% and 26% of the population suffer from mental illnesses (including substance use problems) of clinical severity (Demyttenaere et al., 2004; Wilkinson & Pickett, 2010). Nor are these problems diminishing. Over the past generation or so, the evidence suggests that rates of mental illness in rich countries have actually been rising (not simply recognised and reported more frequently).

While measures of economic wellbeing fail to index psychosocial stress and distress, subjective measures also have limitations. Many subjective measures are too superficial to be sensitive to how stress, anxiety, drug and alcohol problems, depression, and other mental illnesses reduce subjective wellbeing. For example, when, in January 2020 (before the COVID-19 pandemic), a Gallup survey in the United States asked people, 'In general are you satisfied or dissatisfied with the way things are going in your personal life at this time?', 90% replied that they were satisfied (McCarthy, 2020). This was despite roughly contemporaneous survey evidence of stress, anxiety, depression, and the problems of substance misuse that seem to underly the 'deaths of despair'. Similarly, the 2019 Ipsos Global Happiness Study reported that when Americans were asked, 'Taking all things together, would you say you are: Very happy, rather happy, not very happy, not happy at all?', 79% of them replied they were very happy or rather happy. In this situation it is clear that there are worse measures of wellbeing than health. The question is whether better ones can be devised.

IMPROVING MEASURES OF WELLBEING

Because questions about positive aspects of subjective wellbeing, such as levels of satisfaction and happiness, fail to reflect high rates of stress, anxiety, and mental illness, a solution might be to ask questions which also probe the negative side of wellbeing. Not only are rates of mental illness too high to be ignored in assessments of wellbeing, but there also is a growing body of theory and evidence to suggest that a large part of the burden of mental illness reflects forms of unhappiness attributable to aspects of social organisation and people's circumstances which we urgently need to address (Johnstone et al., 2018; Tibber, Walji, Kirkbride, & Huddy, 2021). Fortunately, there is a great deal of experience of how to ask questions about mental health and various forms of unhappiness in different areas of life—in relationships, money, work, or among schoolchildren. An example of the latter is a survey we conducted of schoolchildren in Bradford, United Kingdom, designed to identify those children whose wellbeing was particularly vulnerable during the COVID-19 pandemic (Pickett et al., 2021).

Rather than combining the different domains of wellbeing into one composite score, information on the separate domains is important because it can be used to identify causes of low wellbeing. If surveys of this kind were also to include information on aspects of people's objective situation, such as income, employment status, single-parent families, housing tenure, and housing conditions, it would be possible to build up data on the societal and environmental causes of low wellbeing. Estimates could be made of the damage to wellbeing caused by different aspects of people's circumstances. Decisions on what supplementary information to collect should be made to explore hypotheses about the determinants of wellbeing among the population. The value of compiling and collecting measures of wellbeing would clearly be greatly increased if measures of its possible determinants were collected at the same time. In short, a single government department or national statistical agency should be charged with measuring wellbeing, identifying the causes of deficits, and devising policies to increase wellbeing. This would operationalise the substitution of wellbeing for GDP and increase the likelihood of it making a real difference.

IS IT TOO LATE TO MAKE SUBSTANTIAL IMPROVEMENTS IN WELLBEING?

This approach to measuring wellbeing and identifying its determinants presupposes a level of social and economic stability that would provide a secure foundation on which improvements in quality of life could be made. However, the slow progress toward reducing world carbon emissions may mean that it is now misleading to suggest that we still have the possibility of creating a better world with rising standards of wellbeing. It looks increasingly likely that the future will be punctuated by a series of environmental emergencies—floods, storms, fires, droughts, crop failures, food, and water shortages, as well as increasing numbers of armed conflicts and refugees fleeing these threats. Government attention will increasingly be taken up with responding to these crises. As David Attenborough said when addressing the United Nations in 2021, it may be too late to make things better: perhaps all we can do is to try to make them get worse more slowly. A recent warning, signed by 11,000 scientists in 153 different countries, pointed to the continuing increases in world population, world GDP, meat consumption per head, deforestation, and air travel—all contributing to a continuing rise in greenhouse gas emission, global temperatures, and sea levels (Ripple, Wolf, Newsome, Barnard, & Moomaw, 2019). Their paper warned of 'potential irreversible climate tipping points . . . that could lead to a catastrophic "hothouse Earth", well beyond the control of humans' (p. 9) and emphasised that if we are to 'avoid untold suffering' we need 'an immense increase of scale in endeavours to conserve our biosphere' (p. 8). Failing that, temperatures are predicted, on current policies, to rise by close to 3° Celsius (some estimates are considerably higher) by the end of this century, with catastrophic consequences. Another report, from Future Earth, based on questionnaires sent to 222 scientists in 52 countries, found that more than one-third of them thought there was a real danger that interlinked emergencies 'might cascade to create global systemic crises' and 'ecosystem collapse' (Future Earth, 2020, p. 15).

Under such circumstances, what happens to human wellbeing would have little to do with current attempts to devise new measures of it. Inevitably, what policies best serve improvements in wellbeing will depend on the varying circumstances that populations are having to contend with. Wellbeing might turn out to be a question of ensuring adequate emergency supplies of food and shelter, the creation of standing emergency relief teams, and systems for evacuating people from danger and providing relief. For example, events such as the COVID-19 pandemic not only changed the determinants of wellbeing but also changed people's views of what constituted wellbeing, including raising the priority given to health and, during lockdown, the importance of positive social contact.

Though we may try to formulate theoretical scales of wellbeing based, like Maslow's hierarchy of needs, on concepts of human nature, the likelihood of increasing disruption means that the practical policy problem will shift dramatically toward reducing the limitations and threats to wellbeing in particular circumstances. Achieving high levels of sustainable wellbeing would then depend less on research and sound measures of wellbeing than on our ability to identify and respond to the coming threats to wellbeing.

Recent political trends suggest that the effective functioning of democratic systems has been influenced for the worse by popular reactions to increasing flows of refugees resulting from environmental and other disasters. Although the scale of migration seen in recent years is small in comparison with what might be expected to result from the advancing climate crisis, the public reaction has already contributed to the rise of populism, racism, and nationalism, effectively diverting political attention even further from the urgency of policies needed to counter the climate crisis or, for that matter, to increase wellbeing.

COHESIVE AND ADAPTABLE SOCIETIES

Nevertheless, the future is unpredictable. While always inherently unknowable, there are possibilities which might make the picture we have outlined a lot better or worse. The possibility that the outcomes could be even worse is suggested by the fact that the forecast temperature rises do not include the effects of some highly plausible major changes in natural feedback effects (e.g., deforestation, the loss of the albedo effect as ice melts, and increasing methane emissions as permafrost and ice—particularly over shallow areas of the Arctic Ocean—melt) (Wadhams, 2017), which are exacerbating climate change and could lead to runaway global warming. Moreover, the raised level of carbon dioxide already in the atmosphere means that climate disruption will undoubtedly get worse even if we were to make dramatic reductions in emissions immediately.

On the positive side, there are also possibilities of major technical developments which would make it much easier to reduce global carbon emissions. For example, as some—including the campaigning journalist George Monbiot—suggest, current developments of laboratory grown alternatives to meat may enable massive reductions in numbers of cattle and their methane production (Monbiot, 2020). Others hope that large-scale carbon capture will become a reality. There might also be major breakthroughs in battery technology that make it easier and cheaper to store electricity thus hastening the conversion to renewable power and electric transport. Nor do we know the longer-term effects on material consumption of the digital and information economy, which may be as profound—as economic and social theorist Jeremy Rifkin describes in his important book *The Zero Marginal Cost Society* (Rifkin, 2014). Essentially, by making it technically easy to copy all digitised materials accurately and in infinite numbers without cost, digitisation makes nonsense of copyright. And the expansion of the knowledge economy makes this possibility increasingly important.

We cannot, however, rely on these or any other possibilities rescuing us from the disastrous implications of the climate emergency. There can be little doubt that the most predictable part of the picture is that continuing increases in greenhouse gas concentrations in the atmosphere will lead to further environmental destruction.

When thinking about how we can be best prepared to deal with the extraordinarily difficult future we face, there are perhaps three key criteria. First, our societies need to be highly cohesive and adaptable. They must be willing to make the almost continuous changes in the way we live that are necessary to minimise our impact on the environment—changing our diets, reducing our need for transport, and developing renewable power sources, as well as converting the market economy from the production and consumption maximising economic leviathan it has become into a waste minimising system that would enable the long transition to sustainability. Second, achieving the necessary flexibility will require a high degree of solidarity, trust, and mutual support, backed by government policy. Only when people feel there is a social milieu and institutional structure which gives them a sense of security will they accept and participate in the necessary changes rather than opposing them as threats to their livelihood. This will require major modifications to how the market and institutions of wage labour work, including strong public services and reliable safety nets. To achieve this, we need to establish systems of mutual support and aid to areas hit by increasingly frequent threats, crises, and environmental disasters. These will need to include not only rescue teams and emergency supplies but also compensation for damage. And third, even if we can no longer feel confident that our societies will achieve new heights of wellbeing, we can at least remove some of the things which most obviously reduce the wellbeing of large sections of the population—things such as poverty, lack of education, and lack of political voice.

THE IMPORTANCE OF LOW INEQUALITY

A crucial determinant of how (and perhaps whether) populations come through the crises and disruptions of climate change and other immense challenges is likely to be the extent to which people respond with mutual support rather than simply fending for themselves. As we face the climate crisis, the danger is that the rich, and anyone who can afford to, will use their resources to establish themselves in protected safe havens while abandoning others to their fate.

Inequality is a strongly divergent social force. It leads people to be less likely to look out for each other and more likely to focus narrowly on their own safety and wellbeing (Wilkinson & Pickett, 2010, 2018). For example, research has shown that the societies that suffered worst during the COVID-19 pandemic were those with high economic inequality, such as the United States, Brazil, and the United Kingdom (Elgar, Stefaniak, & Wohl, 2020; Oronce, Scannell, Kawachi, & Tsugawa, 2020). They suffered higher rates of infection and higher death rates. In contrast, societies with lower inequalities of income and higher levels of social capital fared much better.

There is now little doubt that the extent of inequalities in income and wealth is likely to be the most powerful determinant of which societies will survive these tests and which will succumb to processes of social breakdown. In this section, we show that more equal societies—those with smaller income differences between rich and poor—are more cohesive, more adaptable, and perform better in almost all areas of social functioning.

Many studies show that the larger the income differences in a society, the weaker is local community life. The greater the inequality, the less likely people are to belong to local organisations and voluntary groups, the less likely they are to take part in community activities, and the less likely they are to know their neighbours. Research also shows that inequality makes people less likely to feel they can trust each other, their government, or other authorities—including scientists. In addition, violence (as measured by homicide rates) becomes very much more common in more unequal societies. Together, the studies confirm what many people have recognised intuitively over the centuries: that inequality increases social divisions and weakens social cohesion (Elgar et al., 2015; Ichida et al., 2009; Layte, 2012). And, as inequality increases, the social bonds of reciprocity and sense of community which, in more egalitarian societies, knit neighbourhoods together instead give way to self-interest, status competition, and a drive for self-advancement.

The causal process seems to be that bigger income differences make the divisions of class and status more powerful, increasing the idea that some people are 'worth' much more than others. As a result, we come to judge each other's personal worth even more by status while, at the same time, worrying more about how others judge us. Insecurities about our own self-worth increase, so we become more anxious about social comparisons and less at ease with other people (see also Chapter 4, this volume). In short, social relationships become increasingly marred by the social awkwardness and fears which accompany considerations of superiority and inferiority. As George Bernard Shaw said, 'Inequality of income takes the broad, safe, and fertile plain of human society and stands it on its edge so that everyone has to cling desperately to her foothold' (Shaw, 1928).

This in turn has serious implications for people's willingness to take action to solve common problems—including environmental ones. It makes people much less able or willing either to act together or even discuss shared problems. Social relations that have descended to this level are clearly described in Edward Banfield's book, *The Moral Basis of a Backward Society* (Banfield, 1967). Banfield describes the effects of a lack of social capital on life in a village in southern Italy. He explains how despite the village having obvious needs—such as to repair the road—there was no concept of people coming together to work on projects for the common good. Apart from a nepotistic loyalty to their own families, people regarded themselves and each other as motivated only by self-interest. The lack of trust and the suspicion directed toward anyone who did try to do anything in the public interest made cooperative activity almost impossible and placed severe limitations on practical progress in the village.

The antisocial effects of inequality can be seen at every level in society. For example, overseas development aid given by governments of more unequal countries falls further below the United Nations recommended standard of 0.7% of national income than it does in more equal societies. Even among children, research shows that bullying becomes much more common. Data from several different sources covering children between 8 and 14 years old show a powerful tendency for bullying to be more common in more unequal countries (Elgar, Craig, Boyce, Morgan, & Vella-Zarb, 2009). Instead of finding their peers 'kind and helpful', conflict becomes much increasingly common (Wilkinson & Pickett, 2010). Part of the explanation is likely to be that parents pass on their experience of adversity and conflict to their children—partly through parenting styles and probably partly through epigenetics processes through which gene expression changes in response to the behavioural and social environment.

The evidence that inequality has such widespread antisocial effects is too well established to doubt either the basic pattern or the causal processes (Pickett & Wilkinson, 2015). The first peer-reviewed research showing that health and violence were worse in more unequal countries, came out in the 1970s, and there are now hundreds of papers looking at these relationships in different ways and using different methods and controlling for possible 'confounders'. Indeed, as well as meta-analyses of multilevel models looking at the effects of changes in inequality over time, there are also studies which show the lag periods between changes in inequality and its effects.

Because inequality leads to the decline of community life, self-advancement takes over from concern for the common good. People's willingness to take action on the environment is greatly affected by how public-spirited they are; hence more unequal societies tend to do less for the environment (Wilkinson & Pickett, 2018). An international survey of business leaders found that those from more unequal countries attached a much lower priority to international environmental agreements. The same tendency can also be seen at the household level: the data show that people in more unequal countries recycle a smaller proportion of waste materials. They also use bicycles less, have higher carbon dioxide emissions per $100 of GDP per capita, and get less of their power from renewables. For the same reason, in more unequal countries there is likely to be both less pressure from public opinion to get governments to take decisive action on carbon emissions as well as more public opposition to any such action.

Inequality is particularly relevant to how we deal with environmental problems because it also increases consumerism—a major obstacle to sustainability. The more that money is seen as a measure of a person's worth and the goods we buy are used to enhance our appearance of status and success, the more desirous of accruing material wealth we become. As a result, studies show that people living in more unequal places spend more on status goods than do people in more equal societies (Bricker, Ramcharan, & Krimmel, 2014; Walasek & Brown, 2015a, 2015b). Indeed, the pressure to keep up appearances through consumption is so great that borrowing and bankruptcies go up in periods when inequality is high (Adkisson & Saucedo, 2012; Iacoviello, 2008). This means that if we are serious about the transition to sustainability, we must reduce the inequality which ramps up status competition and consumerism. This approach may also be helpful when thinking about how to overcome the forces behind economic growth and bring it to a halt.

Given the current very high levels of inequality and the lack of sufficiently far-reaching action to combat climate change, it is hard not to fear that the level of public-spiritedness and concern for the common good among the general population has become too weak to support the action necessary to combat the climate emergency. This situation has similarities to one faced by Britain during World War II, when priorities had to be changed to serve the war effort. In his essay *War and Social Policy*, Richard Titmuss described the thinking that went into the government's strategy. He said, 'If the cooperation of the masses was thought to be essential [to the war effort], then inequalities had to be reduced and the pyramid of social stratification had to be flattened' (Titmuss, 1958). As a result, the war was marked by far-reaching policies designed to make people feel the burden of war was equally shared. Income differences were rapidly reduced by progressive taxation, essential goods were subsidised, luxuries were taxed, and rationing was introduced for food, fuel, and clothing. Action on the climate emergency now needs a similar raft of egalitarian policies: without them, governments everywhere may face political opposition analogous to the Gilets Jaunes' (Yellow

Vest Movement) resistance to the French government's plan to raise fuel taxes (Chrisafis, 2018).

MUTUAL AID

Recovery from the recurring crises (floods, fires, storms, droughts, emergent infections, and increases in large-scale population displacement) that climate change is already bringing will be much more rapid if we not only have robust and well-prepared systems of support, but also a strong ethos of mutual aid. Rising inequality in so many countries over the past 40 years or so has, however, taken us in the opposite direction: weakening community life, strengthening the pursuit of self-advancement, reducing trust, and increasing violence. The increased number of homeless people on the streets in more unequal societies is another indication of the decline of mutual aid. This decline in the willingness of people in more unequal societies to help each other is underscored by findings from international survey data (Paskov & Dewilde, 2012).

The causal links between inequality and its effects are not difficult to understand. They start with our sensitivity to social relations—to friendship on the one hand and social hierarchy on the other. Because individual members of the same species have the same basic needs, there is almost always the possibility for repeated conflict between them—for food, shelter, territories, sexual partners, and so on. One way of avoiding endless conflict over access to each thing is simply for members to know who is strongest—who would win a fight for access. If you know who is strongest, you can predict the outcome, so the weaker can give way to the stronger without the need for actual conflict. Essentially, that is the basis of animal dominance hierarchies, including among non-human primates: the stronger are recognised as dominant and the weaker as subordinate, and the ranking system tends to be a hierarchy graded by strength (sometimes moderated by support from trusted allies). Everyone has to know his or her position in the ranking system and how to behave in relation to superiors and inferiors, when to give way and when not to. In effect, might is right and subordinates eat last. Getting this wrong is likely to result in injuries which may be life-threatening. Being as far up the hierarchy as possible is a huge advantage, not only in terms of access to food and other necessities, but also for reproductive opportunities and better survival chances for offspring. Hence powerful selective pressures have shaped our concern for social status. This is the prehuman origin—among our hominid ancestors—of our evolved sensitivity to social status. The dominance hierarchy was essentially a bullying hierarchy, ordered by fear and consequently highly stressful (see also Chapter 4, this volume).

That, however, is only half the story. The other half, in sharp contrast with our desire for dominance, is made up of our highly developed ability to be each other's best source of help, cooperation, love, learning, and assistance of every kind. In essence, we have the potential not only to be each other's worst rivals and greatest threats, but also to be each other's best source of cooperation, support, help, and security.

How is it, then, that we can contain the potential for two such opposite social characteristics? There is widespread agreement among anthropologists that the hunting and gathering societies of our human prehistory were, with few exceptions, highly egalitarian. They were marked by cooperation, food sharing, and reciprocity, with no sign of the pattern, common among animals, for the weakest to eat last or be excluded when food was scarce. Within these egalitarian societies, people with more prosocial characteristics, who were less selfish, better at sharing and reciprocity, were more likely to get selected as sexual partners and as collaborators for cooperative activities—processes which, through gradually selection, led to a more prosocial gene pool (Boehm, 2012). These societies have been described as not only consciously egalitarian, but sometimes as 'assertively' egalitarian. Indeed, the evidence suggests that people who were implacably antisocial were excluded and cast out of the sharing group—a treatment that amounted almost to a death sentence. And the best way of ensuring that you remained a secure member of the cooperative group was to have skills and perform tasks which others valued. That propensity has become enshrined as part of our evolved psychology, both in our capacity to get pleasure from doing things which others appreciate and in our desire to be valued by others.

In a nutshell, then, while the egalitarian social environment of our hunting and gathering human prehistory selected people for prosocial characteristics, the dominance hierarchies of our *pre*-human existence selected for the more antisocial strategies of self-advancement most consistent with self-preservation in dominance hierarchies. And it is not difficult to imagine how the advantages of cooperation could have become crucial.

We are left then with a psychological legacy containing both of these very different tendencies, and we, of course, use social strategies rooted in both all the time. With friends—usually chosen from among our near equals—we use egalitarian social strategies of sharing and reciprocity; we treat them as equals and we are careful not to put them down or give the impression we think we are better than they. But in settings where social status is important, we also know how to act snobbishly, stand on our dignity, name drop, and attempt to set ourselves apart and above those we regard as our social inferiors. Indeed, snobbishness has been described as driven by the desire for what divides people rather than for what unites them (Epstein, 2002).

Crucially important, however, is that our choice of social strategy is strongly influenced by our experience of the social environment. The bigger the differences in income and wealth, the more visible the differences in class and status become, and the more external wealth is seen as if it were a measure of individual worth.

Essentially these are the two opposite ways people can come together. At one extreme, scarce resources are allocated according to power differences used to serve self-interest, while, at the other, the allocation reflects the mutual recognition of each other's needs, sharing, and cooperation. Humans have, of course, lived in every kind of society from the most hierarchical and tyrannical to the most egalitarian, but the difference in the nature of social relationships makes more unequal societies much more stressful.

Because these contrasting systems of relationships require such different behavioural strategies, it seems likely that future research will reveal that there are epigenetic switches, controlling gene expression, to prepare our cognitive and emotional development for the world we find ourselves growing up in. Do we need the emotional and cognitive ability to fight for what we can get and learn not to trust others because we are all rivals, or should we be prepared for a world where empathy and reciprocity are important and we depend instead on gaining each other's trust and cooperation?

This interpretation of the effects of inequality fits well with what we know about the extraordinary sensitivity of human beings to the nature of social relationships. It explains why both low social status and bigger status differentials are such powerful stressors damaging health and why friendship is so highly protective of health.

INEQUALITY AND WELLBEING

As we have seen, the effects of inequality have very major implications for the health and wellbeing of populations. They are all the more important because they are key to redressing the contrast in rich countries between the unprecedentedly high material living standards on the one hand and their psychosocial failings and threadbare social fabric on the other.

This contrast has been shown many times. Although rising material standards are still needed in low-income countries where many do not yet have access to necessities, in middle- and high-income countries there are sharply diminishing increases to wellbeing associated with economic growth—so much so that, among high-income countries, further increases in material standards seem unrelated to wellbeing or improvements in health (Cutler, Deaton, & Lleras-Muney, 2006). The predictable implication is that having more and more of everything makes less and less difference. Whether you look at measures of happiness, life satisfaction, or life expectancy, the picture is the same. Wellbeing rises rapidly among poorer countries in the early stages of economic growth, but then levels out among the richer countries. The same basic story is told in analyses that use measures simply of economic wellbeing. Despite the failure to tackle serious relative poverty in high-income countries, those societies have reached material standards that should be regarded as a saturation point in terms of their material development. This contrasts with the evidence of huge deficits in emotional and psychological wellbeing we mentioned earlier among the populations of high-income countries.

FURTHER IMPROVEMENTS IN QUALITY OF LIFE

It is clear that further improvements in quality of life in high-income countries depend on switching attention from the material to the social environment. As we showed in our book, *The Inner Level* (Wilkinson & Pickett, 2018), reductions in inequality are key to improvements in psychosocial wellbeing across whole populations. At their core, the causal processes involve the effect of inequality on our worries about how we are seen and judged by others—status anxiety, social comparisons, and insecurities about self-worth.

A number of other ways of improving population wellbeing are also readily identified and need not await further research. The scale of relative poverty is a very major force that dramatically lowers wellbeing. Usually defined as living on less than 60% of the median income, relative poverty would—almost inevitably—be reduced by greater equality. Relative poverty has particularly serious consequences for children, affecting their education, health, and development: it blights their future. The Resolution Foundation has forecast that 37% of British children will, by 2023–2024, be growing up in relative poverty.

It is also clear that, since 2010, wellbeing in many countries has been seriously reduced by cuts in public services resulting from government austerity policies, so much so that death rates in some British population groups have risen and life expectancy for the population as a whole has ceased its long historical rise. Worst affected are women older than 85 years—the section of the population most in need of public services. But in Britain during the period 2011–2016, death rates among the whole population younger than 50 ceased to decline, and, among those in their late 40s, they have risen. It should not be imagined that these adverse trends are a sign that we have reached the limits of human longevity: not only does life expectancy continue to increase in some countries—even though it is already several years longer than in the United Kingdom or United States—but the adverse trends in the United Kingdom and United States also are most marked among the least well off, where life expectancy is lowest.

Overcoming problems such as homelessness, unemployment, or the injustice of the huge differences in life expectancy between rich and poor must all come high on the agenda for improving quality of life. Depending partly on the scale of socioeconomic inequalities in a country, healthy life expectancy in the most privileged areas may be 10, or sometimes even 20, years longer than in the most deprived areas of the same rich country.

We must not forget, however, that like many other factors that depress standards of wellbeing, it is largely politics and vested interests—rather than lack of knowledge—which have stopped these problems being addressed. Although the past decade has seen impressive progress in *recognising* the importance of reducing economic inequality, much less progress has been made in taking action to reduce it. Despite the facts that many international organisations (including the International Monetary Fund, the World Bank, the World Economic Forum, the Organisation for Economic Co-operation and Development, and Oxfam) have all emphasised the need for greater equality and that it is now enshrined as the 10th of the 17 United Nations Sustainable Development Goals, effective government action has rarely been forthcoming. There are parallels here with the huge rise in awareness of the climate crisis and the lack of adequate action. And though there are clear signs that opinion is beginning to switch from thinking that wellbeing rather than economic growth is the proper focus of government policy, only a tiny group of governments (including Finland, Iceland, New Zealand, and the devolved governments of Scotland and Wales) have actually made that switch (Coscieme et al., 2019; see also Chapter 13, this volume). Too often, the real political reasons for the failure to tackling things which depress wellbeing—such as deprivation, relative poverty, housing shortages, and unemployment—are ignored, and academics and policymakers act as if progress depended on better measurements or further research.

Whether or not it would take the end of capitalism to dethrone economic growth as the overriding aim of government, substituting wellbeing for growth as a measure of national performance might begin to change capitalism. It could provide a powerful public statement that in future we have to look elsewhere for improvements in the real quality of life. If that was accompanied by policies to decrease inequality, it would also help reduce consumerism, ease the transition to environmental sustainability, and improve psychosocial wellbeing.

SUMMARY

We have argued that replacing economic growth with wellbeing as the central objective of government policy may be much more difficult than has been recognised. It is unlikely that economic growth can be switched off simply by changing government policy. That is true because its most important drivers lie in the Gordian Knot that ties people's desire to maximise income into the desire of businesses to maximise sales and profits. In effect, no one knows how to stop destructive economic growth. However, we think a clue may lie in the way inequality increases status competition and consumerism; in a much more equal society, these forces become considerably weaker. Perhaps an additional clue lies in the experience of prehistoric hunter-gather societies. Because they had few needs and were almost always highly egalitarian, they were free of wasteful status competition, and so, despite being described as the 'original affluent societies' (Sahlins, 1998), they managed to avoid overexploiting their environment in terms of overhunting and overgathering for at least 200,000 years (Wilkinson, 1973).

We have also argued that maximising human wellbeing depends more on politics and less on the development of definitions and measures which, in themselves, tell us little about the determinants of wellbeing. There are a great many ways of increasing wellbeing which are already obvious to all: they include the reduction of poverty, unemployment, homelessness, lack of access to medical care, and many others. The reasons why they are ignored, despite the constant demands of pressure groups, are surely vested interests and politics.

It is likely that what people regard as wellbeing varies with circumstances, from culture to culture, and with ideology. Wellbeing may evade definition because it has no essential, unchanging core nature. The philosopher of science, Professor Sir Karl Popper, argued against what he called the 'essentialism' involved in trying to define every term, saying instead that we should simply seek to clarify our use of a word or a term when it proves problematic (Popper, 2014).

We discussed the radically different impressions that might be gained of the wellbeing of a society from measures of life-satisfaction, wellbeing, or happiness, on the one hand, and of stress, anxiety, and mental illness on the other. This is part of the mismatch between the levels of material comfort in rich societies today and their serious psychosocial failings. An important key to bridging this divide is, as a large body of evidence suggests, the scale of material inequality within societies. Inequality is divisive and socially corrosive. It exerts a powerful negative impact on wellbeing—including mental health—because it changes the nature of human relationships, which are one of the most powerful determinants of wellbeing. It places us in a hierarchy, one above the other, turning us into each other's superiors and inferiors. It increases the power of status and class, strengthens the idea that some people are worth much more than others, and so increases our feelings of insecurity about our own self-worth.

When considering the future of wellbeing, however, we should not forget that the intensifying climate crisis will not only increase insecurity, disruption, and loss of life almost everywhere, but it will also lead to political upheavals which could make improvements in wellbeing seem a distant luxury.

THE HAPPINESS-INEQUALITY PARADOX

People's reports of satisfaction with their own objective or subjective state are strongly influenced by culture. What makes that particularly important is that there seem to be national differences in reporting that vary systematically with inequality. This can make the international associations between inequality and differences in self-reported subjective wellbeing measures highly misleading. Evidence comes from two sources. First, although self-reported health—usually assessed with a question such as 'in general, would you say that your health is excellent, very good, good, fair, or poor?'—is quite a good predictor of mortality and morbidity *within* a country, it breaks down when you make comparisons *between* countries. Objectively, a country's death rate may be high or low, but that seems to bear no relation to whether or not people say their health is good. Among a group of rich developed countries, the country which had the *highest* life expectancy also had the *lowest* proportion of people who rated their health as good. Overall, there was a weak inverse tendency for countries with the best self-rated health to have *lower* life expectancy (Dorling & Barford, 2009). So, although life expectancy (based on objective death rates) was better in those countries with smaller income differences, self-reported health was not. The second example comes from a study of what its authors called 'self-enhancement bias' or 'illusory superiority'—a tendency of people to exaggerate their desirable qualities compared to others (Loughnan et al., 2011). The study showed that there was a much stronger tendency for people in more unequal societies to show a kind of narcissistic self-aggrandisement, with large majorities of the population claiming to be better than average.

The reason that people in more unequal societies have a greater tendency to exaggerate their positive characteristics is that inequality—as the research shows—increases people's status anxiety. In more unequal societies, there is a systematic tendency for people at every income level—from the poorest to the richest tenth—to worry more about what others think of them than do people in more equal societies (Layte & Whelan, 2014). As a result, they try harder to make a positive impression on others. If you live in a society where some people seem to be regarded as supremely important and others are treated as almost worthless, we end up using status as a measure of worth and worrying more about how others judge us. That has been shown to lead people living in more unequal societies to spend more on status goods—on flashy cars and clothes with expensive labels as a form or self-enhancement. In effect, inequality makes people more narcissistic, and indeed measures using the Narcissistic Personality Inventory have shown that narcissism has risen in the United States while income inequality increased.

We call this the 'happiness-inequality paradox'. Greater inequality makes people feel they have to hide signs of weakness or vulnerability and project instead an image of success, strength, and self-reliance. We suspect that for an American to answer a survey question on happiness by saying he or she is unhappy may feel like lowering their guard and an admission of failure, while for someone in a much more equal country to say they are happy might feel like complacency or bragging.

If researchers and policy-makers are not to lose sight of the benefits that greater equality brings to wellbeing, they need to understand the happiness-inequality paradox. Otherwise they could find themselves imagining that reducing inequality had no impact on subjective measures of wellbeing even though it reduces violence, improves objective measures of physical and mental health, strengthens trust and community life, reduces bullying, improves objective measures of child wellbeing, and more (Wilkinson & Pickett, 2010). While there are an increasing number of papers showing that more unequal societies have lower states of wellbeing and happiness, these effects are presumably smaller than they would be if it were not for the happiness-inequality paradox (Lous & Graafland, 2021; Oshio & Kobayashi, 2010; Verme, 2011).

REFERENCES

Adkisson, R. V., & Saucedo, E. (2012). Emulation and state-by-state variations in bankruptcy rates. *Journal of Socio-Economics, 41*(4), 400–407. doi:10.1016/j.socec.2012.04.008

Afonso, A., & Furceri, D. (2010). Government size, composition, volatility and economic growth. *European Journal of Political Economy, 26*(4), 517–532.

American Psychiatric Association. (2017). *Stress in America: The state of our nation*. https://www.apa.org/news/press/releases/stress/2017/state-nation.pdf

Banfield, E. C. (1967). *The moral basis of a backward society*. Free Press.

Boehm, C. (2012). *Moral origins: The evolution of virtue, altruism, and shame*. Basic Books.

Bricker, J., Ramcharan, R., & Krimmel, J. (2014). Signaling status: The impact of relative income on household consumption and financial decisions. Finance and Economics Discussion Series, Divisions of Research & Statistics and Monetary Affairs, Federal Reserve Board. https://static1.squarespace.com/static/5f75531c54380e4fb4b0f839/t/5faea51b54d01722c1951280/1605281052619/BrickerKrimmelRamcharan+%282 020%2C+MS%29+-+Signaling+Status.pdf

Case, A., & Deaton, A. (2020). *Deaths of despair and the future of capitalism*. Princeton University Press.

Chrisafis, A. (2018). Who are the gilets jaunes and what do they want? *The Guardian*.

Coscieme, L., Sutton, P., Mortensen, L. F., Kubiszewski, I., Costanza, R., Trebeck, K., . . . Fioramonti, L. (2019). Overcoming the myths of mainstream economics to enable a new wellbeing economy. *Sustainability, 11*(16), 4374.

Costanza, R., Caniglia, E., Fioramonti, L., Kubiszewski, I., Lewis, H., Lovins, H., . . . Pickett, K. (2018). Towards a sustainable wellbeing economy. *The Solutions Journal*. https://thesolutionsjournal.com/2018/04/17/toward-sustainable-wellbeing-economy/

Cutler, D., Deaton, A., & Lleras-Muney, A. (2006). The determinants of mortality. *Journal of Economic Perspectives, 20*(3), 97–120. doi:10.1257/jep.20.3.97

Demyttenaere, K., Bruffaerts, R., Posada-Villa, J., Gasquet, I., Kovess, V., Lepine, J. P., . . . Chatterji, S. (2004). Prevalence, severity, and unmet need for treatment of mental disorders in the World Health Organization World Mental Health Surveys. *JAMA, 291*(21), 2581–2590.

De Vogli, R. (2019). Mortality crises in high-income countries: Evidence from the United States, the United Kingdom, Italy, and Greece. https://www.researchgate.net/publication/342510723_MORTALITY_CRISES_IN_HIGH-INCOME_COUNTRIES_EVIDENCE_FROM_THE_UNITED_STATES_THE_UNITED_KINGDOM_ITALY_AND_GREECE

Dorling, D., & Barford, A. (2009). The inequality hypothesis: Thesis, antithesis, and a synthesis? *Health Place, 15*(4), 1166–1169.

Elgar, F. J., Craig, W., Boyce, W., Morgan, A., & Vella-Zarb, R. (2009). Income inequality and school bullying: Multilevel study of adolescents in 37 countries. *Journal of Adolescent Health, 45*(4), 351–359.

Elgar, F. J., Pförtner, T.-K., Moor, I., De Clercq, B., Stevens, G. W., & Currie, C. (2015). Socioeconomic inequalities in adolescent health 2002–2010: A time-series analysis of 34 countries participating in the Health Behaviour in School-Aged Children study. *The Lancet, 385*, 2088–2095. doi:10.1016/S0140-6736(14)61460-4.

Elgar, F. J., Stefaniak, A., & Wohl, M. J. (2020). The trouble with trust: Time-series analysis of social capital, income inequality, and COVID-19 deaths in 84 countries. *Social Science & Medicine*, 113365.

Epstein, J. (2002). *Snobbery: The American version*. Houghton Mifflin Company.

Future Earth. (2020). *Our Future on Earth 2020*. www.futureearth.org/publications/our-future-on-earth

Holt-Lunstad, J., Smith, T. B., & Layton, J. B. (2010). Social relationships and mortality risk: A meta-analytic review. *PLoS Med, 7*(7), e1000316. doi:10.1371/journal.pmed.1000316

House, J., Landis, K., & Umberson, D. (1988). Social relationships and health. *Science*, *241*, 540–545.

Iacoviello, M. (2008). Household debt and income inequality, 1963–2003. *Journal of Money, Credit and Banking*, *40*(5), 929–965. doi:10.1111/j.1538-4616.2008.00142.x

Ichida, Y., Kondo, K., Hirai, H., Hanibuchi, T., Yoshikawa, G., & Murata, C. (2009). Social capital, income inequality and self-rated health in Chita peninsula, Japan: A multilevel analysis of older people in 25 communities. *Social Science & Medicine*, *69*(4), 489–499.

Ipsos Global Advisor. (2019). Global happiness study: What makes people happy around the world. https://www.ipsos.com/sites/default/files/ct/news/documents/2019-08/Happiness-Study-report-August-2019.pdf.

Johnstone, L., Boyle, M., Cromby, J., Dillon, J., Harper, D., Kinderman, P., & Read, J. (2018). The power threat meaning framework. Paper presented at the British Psychological Society.

Kubiszewski, I., Costanza, R., Franco, C., Lawn, P., Talberth, J., Jackson, T., & Aylmer, C. (2013). *Beyond GDP: Measuring and Achieving Global Genuine Progress*, *93*, 57–68.

Kurtz, M. J., & Schrank, A. (2007). Growth and governance: Models, measures, and mechanisms. *Journal of Politics*, *69*(2), 538–554.

Layte, R. (2012). The association between income inequality and mental health: Testing status anxiety, social capital, and neo-materialist explanations. *European Sociological Review*, *28*(4), 498–511. doi:10.2307/23272534

Layte, R., & Whelan, C. T. (2014). Who feels inferior? A test of the status anxiety hypothesis of social inequalities in health. *European Sociological Review*, *30*, 525–535.

Loughnan, S., Kuppens, P., Allik, J., Balazs, K., de Lemus, S., Dumont, K., . . . Haslam, N. (2011). Economic inequality is linked to biased self-perception. *Psychological Science*, *22*(10), 1254–1258. doi:10.1177/0956797611417003

Lous, B., & Graafland, J. (2021). Who becomes unhappy when income inequality increases? *Applied Research in Quality of Life*, 1–18.

McCarthy, J. (2020). New high of 90% of Americans satisfied with personal life. *Gallup*. https://news.gallup.com/poll/284285/new-high-americans-satisfied-personal-life.aspx

Mental Health Foundation. (2018). *Stress: Are we coping?* https://www.mentalhealth.org.uk/publications/stress-are-we-coping

Monbiot, G. (2020). Lab-grown food will soon destroy farming—and save the planet. *The Guardian*.

Oronce, C. I. A., Scannell, C. A., Kawachi, I., & Tsugawa, Y. (2020). Association between state-level income inequality and COVID-19 cases and mortality in the USA. *Journal of General Internal Medicine*, 1–3.

Oshio, T., & Kobayashi, M. (2010). Income inequality, perceived happiness, and self-rated health: Evidence from nationwide surveys in Japan. *Social Science & Medicine*, *70*(9), 1358–1366.

Paskov, M., & Dewilde, C. (2012). Income inequality and solidarity in Europe. *Research in Social Stratification and Mobility*, *30*(4), 415–432.

Pickett, K., Ajebon, M., Hou, B., Kelly, B., Bird, P., Dickerson, J., . . . Lawlor, D. (2021). Vulnerabilities in child wellbeing among primary school children: A cross-sectional study in Bradford, UK. *medRxiv*. doi:10.1101/2021.01.10.21249538

Pickett, K. E., & Wilkinson, R. G. (2015). Income inequality and health: A causal review. *Social Science & Medicine, 128C*, 316–326. doi:10.1016/j.socscimed.2014.12.031

Popper, K. (2014). *Conjectures and refutations: The growth of scientific knowledge*. Routledge.

Rifkin, J. (2014). *The zero marginal cost society: The internet of things, the collaborative commons, and the eclipse of capitalism*. St. Martin's Press.

Ripple, W. J., Wolf, C., Newsome, T. M., Barnard, P., & Moomaw, W. R. (2019). World scientists' warning of a climate emergency. *BioScience*. doi:10.1093/biosci/biz088

Sahlins, M. (1998). The original affluent society. In J. Gowdy (Ed.), *Limited wants, unlimited means: A reader on hunter-gatherer economics and the environment* (pp. 5–41). Kluwer Academic Publishers.

Shaw, G. B. (1928). *The intelligent woman's guide to socialism and capitalism*. Transaction Publishers.

Smith, A. (1937). *The wealth of nations*. Modern Library.

Steptoe, A. (2019). Happiness and health. *Annual Review of Public Health, 40*, 339–359.

Surtees, P. G., Wainwright, N. W., Luben, R. N., Wareham, N. J., Bingham, S. A., & Khaw, K.-T. (2008). Depression and ischemic heart disease mortality: Evidence from the EPIC-Norfolk United Kingdom prospective cohort study. *American Journal of Psychiatry, 165*(4), 515–523.

Tibber, M. S., Walji, F., Kirkbride, J. B., & Huddy, V. (2021). The association between income inequality and adult mental health at the subnational level: A systematic review. *Soc Psychiatry and Epidemiology*, 1–24.

Titmuss, R. M. (1958). *Essays on the welfare state*. Unwin.

Verme, P. (2011). *Life satisfaction and income inequality*. World Bank Policy Research Working Paper No. 5574. https://papers.ssrn.com/sol3/papers.cfm?abstract_id=1774421

Wadhams, P. (2017). *A farewell to ice: A report from the Arctic*. Oxford University Press.

Walasek, L., & Brown, G. D. (2015a). Inequality and status seeking: Searching for positional goods in unequal US states. *Psychological Science, 26*, 527–533.

Walasek, L., & Brown, G. D. A. (2015b). Income inequality, income, and internet searches for status goods: A cross-national study of the association between inequality and well-being. *Social Indicators Research*, 1–14. doi:10.1007/s11205-015-1158-4

Wilkinson, R. (1973). *Poverty and progress: An ecological model of economic development*. Methuen & Co.

Wilkinson, R., & Pickett, K. (2010). *The spirit level: Why equality is better for everyone*. Penguin.

Wilkinson, R., & Pickett, K. (2018). The inner level: How more equal societies reduce stress, restore sanity and improve everyone's wellbeing. Penguin Random House.

17

An Economy Centred on Human and Ecological Wellbeing

LORENZO FIORAMONTI AND LUCA COSCIEME ■

INTRODUCTION

The concept of a 'wellbeing economy' (WE), an economy that puts the wellbeing of people and the planet first, is penetrating high-level policy-making, presenting an alternative to the mainstream 'growth' discourse centred on increasing a country's gross domestic product (GDP). The growing network of Wellbeing Economy Governments (WEGo) aims to be the 'wellbeing equivalent' of what the G7 or G20 are for economic growth (Boyce, Coscieme, Sommer, & Wallace, 2020; Coscieme et al., 2019; Fioramonti, 2017a; Hough-Stewart, Trebeck, Sommer, & Wallace, 2019). Members of WEGo, as well as other advocates of a WE, agree that human and ecological wellbeing is what we should care about collectively, not only in and of itself, but also as a (pre)condition to strengthen social cohesion and enhance environmental sustainability. The notion of a WE shifts away from material production and consumption as the main purpose of economic development to embrace a wide variety of social and environmental dynamics that are viewed as fundamental contributors to human and ecological wellbeing (Figure 17.1). Moreover, the WE tells a story of opportunities for human creativity that inspires collective action.

If we want to exert radical policy transformation within the next few years and, reasonably, before 2030, then we need a new paradigm that not only brings together citizens, entrepreneurs, professionals, scholars, and intellectuals, but also that offers to policy-makers a solutions-oriented view. In this chapter, we describe the tenets of the WE paradigm and analyse how the WE approach and language can be effective at triggering practical change at the institutional level and in society at large. We begin by describing what the WE is and the key differences between the growth-based approach and the wellbeing-based approach. We then

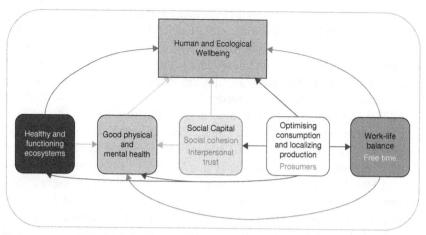

Figure 17.1 A wellbeing economy recognises that human and ecological wellbeing results from multiple contributors, going beyond the narrow view of progress as gross domestic product (GDP) growth.

discuss how the WE can become mainstream in policy design to drive a societal transformation. Ultimately, we explore practical solutions, discuss practices and tools for enabling a WE, and conclude with a vision for the future.

WHAT IS A WELLBEING ECONOMY?

The understanding of societal progress as economic growth is based on the conviction that material production and consumption is the main way to improve living standards and that both GDP and living standards can have limitless growth. Although some material growth is a necessity in most developing countries, studies have shown that very little correlation exists between further growth and wellbeing, especially in developed countries (Easterlin, 1995; Inglehart, Foa, Peterson, & Welzel, 2008; Kahneman & Krueger, 2006; Myers, 2000). Furthermore, research shows that only between 10% and 25% of the improvement in life expectancy over time is attributable to increases in income, given that living standards are impacted by factors like the quality of democracy, equality before the law, the development of welfare states, and legislation to protect people from unfair dismissal from work and eviction from housing, rather than income per se (Wilkinson, 2007).

From a wellbeing perspective, continuous material growth is not only unsustainable in so far as it takes a heavy toll on natural resources and ecosystems, but also because it has detrimental impacts on social cohesion as well as psychological and physical wellbeing (Wilkinson & Pickett, 2009). Furthermore, while over the past few years production and consumption may have become marginally more sustainable, several studies have demonstrated that total decoupling of GDP growth from greenhouse gas emissions and other forms of ecological degradation has not happened and probably cannot happen (Bastianoni, Coscieme, Caro, Marchettini, & Pulselli, 2019; Coscieme et al., 2019; Ward et al., 2016). With growth in GDP, inequalities have also grown, as well as psychological distress and the prevalence of noncommunicable diseases (Piketty, 2014; Stiglitz, 2012; Wilkinson & Pickett 2018; Alvaredo, Chancel, Piketty, Saez, & Zucman, 2018; see also Chapter 16, this volume). Increasing inequalities impact on many aspects of individual and societal wellbeing, including health, trust, happiness, and social and civic participation as well as crime rates, education, and social mobility (Wilkinson & Pickett, 2009, 2018). Since the 1980s, psychological disorders and distress such as anxiety and substance misuse have been increasing worldwide (World Health Organization, 2021; Yang et al., 2021) as has the prevalence of noncommunicable diseases, including obesity and diabetes (Di Cesare, 2019; see Chapter 9, this volume). This increase in inequality and the impacts on psychological and physical wellbeing point to the fact that the mainstream growth model has been falling short in delivering better health and living standards and equal opportunities for all.

The WE model is based on sustainable human and ecological wellbeing as the ultimate goal of economic activity and focuses on what we want to grow and what we want to contract in order to improve wellbeing. From the WE perspective, economic progress only occurs when in the service of human and ecological wellbeing and when progress brings about reduced inequalities. The WE places an overall vision at the centre of its discourse, making room for creativity, innovation, and definition of policy options that should be malleable enough to adapt to different contexts.

In Table 17.1, we report the key conceptual differences between the growth approach and the WE, focusing on key dimensions such as profitability, work, technology, and what indicators to use for measuring progress. In the following section, we elaborate on each of these dimensions in turn.

From a GDP growth perspective, any activity is profitable as long as the economic value of its output exceeds the market costs of its production, measured only in terms of capital invested and labour, with no regard for environmental/ social costs and gains. The WE, instead, completely redefines the concept of profitability in terms of contributions to wellbeing and the potential to deliver higher-order goals of social justice and planetary health. For example, a better work–life balance contributes to more profitability insofar as this frees up time for family care and improves noneconomic aspects of personal wellbeing. Any activity that positively contributes to social cohesion, children's wellbeing, healthy lifestyles, and ecological regeneration is profitable from a WE perspective (see Figure 17.1) (Kossek, Valcour, & Lirio, 2014; Lunau, Bambra, Eikemo, van der Wel, & Dragano, 2014).

The GDP growth approach only recognises formal market-based work and ignores voluntary work and unpaid housework and family care. From this standpoint, such unpaid activities do not generate any value insofar as they do not increase GDP and, to the contrary, keep workers away from performing 'productive' activities. In principle, the GDP growth economy welcomes any shift in

Table 17.1 KEY DIFFERENCES BETWEEN THE GROWTH APPROACH AND THE WELLBEING
ECONOMY (WE)

	Growth economy	Wellbeing economy
Development	Increase in GDP.	Increase in multidimensional wellbeing.
Profitability	Any activity generating market-based profit is considered profitable (regardless of its impact on society and the environment). It is encouraged as a driver of growth.	Profitability is viewed in multidimensional terms, according to social and environmental drivers of wellbeing. It is encouraged as it is viewed as a way to reduce negative effects and increase positive contributions.
Work	Only formal market-based work is recognised. Any unpaid activity should be replaced by its market-based alternative.	Any type of contribution to wellbeing should be valued as work, including receiving a remuneration. Quality work that delivers fundamental human needs is sought.
Technology	A fundamental driver of growth, especially if large-scale and proprietary.	A potential driver of wellbeing creation insofar as it is distributed, non-proprietary and optimising of production processes at the local level.
Indicators	GDP	Wellbeing dashboard (social, environmental, health, and economic indicators) and total cost accounting.

social production and reproduction that replaces informal care-based activities with their formal market-based alternatives: from schooling to care of the elderly, from food preparation to volunteering. In contrast, from a WE perspective, work equals any formal or informal, paid or unpaid contribution to collective human and ecological wellbeing. As a consequence, it must always be incentivised and guaranteed in economic policy and planning and also financially supported by the state through dedicated welfare programmes.

Technology is a fundamental driver of the GDP growth economy, with an esti-mated one-third to two-thirds of GDP growth directly coming from technological innovation (Bakker, Crafts, & Woltier, 2017). Large-scale and proprietary tech-nologies in particular, as well as highly sophisticated production processes, are the kind of innovations that stimulate GDP growth. A growing GDP economy is in turn a fertile ground for developing technologies that allow for the production of larger quantities of goods and services, further increasing consumption and GDP (and often funnelling enormous amounts of wealth into the hands of a few individuals). The WE represents technological breakthroughs as an opportunity but only insofar as technology is purposefully utilised to increase accessibility and nonproprietary distribution and when it helps to eliminate some harmful, degrading forms of work (Trebeck & Williams, 2019). Innovations based on peer-to-peer software and hardware, 3D printing, decentralised renewable energy systems (microgrids), and precision and regenerative agriculture have the potential to emancipate consumers from their dependency on mass production. Examples include peer-to-peer applications that allow people to produce energy on their rooftops and share their energy surplus within their own region (energy communities) thus bypassing the intermediation of large utility companies, or innovations that allow us to gather and use satellite and field data to make irrigation more effective, save water, and optimise the use of soil (precision agriculture). By localising and customising production and consumption, these innovations promote shorter value chains with less intermediaries, lower costs, and fewer environmental impacts. They also promote local empowerment, providing economic opportunities for every type of producer (including home-based production) while reducing the waste of resources (Fioramonti, 2017b). Moreover, these innovations are redefining the very meaning of producers and consumers, blurring the boundaries between the two, and enabling the emergence of *prosumer* models (European Environment Agency, 2019). These models, where consumers play an active role in the design and manufacture of products and services, can be an essential new ingredient in meeting basic needs in low-income countries and emancipate communities from global markets ranging from energy to food production (World Resources Institute, 2016).

Overall, the WE approach fundamentally alters our understanding of what creates value and when, thus requiring the adoption of multiple indicators and a system of total cost and benefit accounting. For instance, the costs society is paying for climate change caused by extraction and burning of fossil fuels are estimated on the scale of trillions of dollars annually (Nuccitelli, 2019). The indicators used for measuring progress in a WE include environmental quality and biodiversity indicators, as well as human health indicators (including mental health), social and natural capital indicators (such as measures of interpersonal trust, the proportion of the population involved in voluntary work, inequality measures, and the value of ecosystem services), and measures of innovation and circularity (including recycling and reuse rates). Furthermore, the adaptability of the WE concept allows for designing specific sets of indicators accounting for context-specific aspects influencing the wellbeing of local communities instead of imposing one single standard measure of progress across different realities (as is the case with GDP in the growth economy).

The WE overlaps, in part, with other alternatives to growth models. The *circular economy*, which replaces the concept of end of life with reducing, reusing, recycling, and recovering materials in production and consumption processes (Kirchherr, Reike, & Hekkert, 2017), overlaps with the WE as both aim at reducing waste and other environmental impacts of production and consumption. However, the circular economy does not include social aspects nor does it expressly redefine the goal of the economy away from growth (Giannetti et al., 2020). Other alternative models, such as the *care economy* or the *regenerative economy*, overlap with the WE but are focused on specific aspects, such as, respectively, recognising the importance of family care and voluntary work (Power, 2020) or exploring nature-based solutions to regenerate the social and ecological assets needed for wellbeing. These approaches are included in the WE, which is thus very much aligned with these models. Even broader overlaps exist between the WE and models based on the concept of fair consumption spaces (Akenji et al., 2021), such as the *doughnut economy* (Raworth, 2017). These models aim at ensuring necessary social foundations are met while respecting planetary boundaries (defined as the safe operating space for humanity within the Earth's biophysical system; Rockström et al., 2009) thus reorienting the goals of the economy toward improving ecological and social wellbeing.

CAN WELLBEING BECOME THE ECONOMIC MAINSTREAM?

The growing consensus around the concept of the WE is demonstrated by the expanding global network of the Wellbeing Economy Alliance (WEAll), which brings together more than 200 organisations and thousands of citizens. WEAll links and coordinates activities at all levels of the WE toward a common vision for the future where policies are framed in terms of human and ecological wellbeing, businesses exist to meet social needs and contribute to the regeneration of nature, and the rules of the economy are shaped by collaboration between government, business, and civil society (www.weall.org). In order for this to happen, WEAll is providing spaces to convene and connect stakeholders and is working to disseminate the existing knowledge and evidence base on wellbeing approaches in a coherent, solutions-oriented, and accessible format.

The positive and forward-looking language which characterises the WE approach is reflected in the WEAll's reference to five crucial elements of dignity, nature, connection, fairness, and participation (Sommer, 2019). This makes the WE approach more effective in aligning with like-minded efforts and initiatives for redesigning the economy, and it provides practical tools for citizens interested in shifting their lifestyles toward improving personal health and mitigating environmental impacts.

The implementation of the WE approach has been explored in a series of policy and action-oriented documents and initiatives promoted by WEALL. Notably, the Wellbeing Economy Policy Design Guide (Wellbeing Economy Alliance, 2021) describes principles and actions to design economic policies for ecological and people's wellbeing. The Guide includes recommendations and examples for co-creating a WE by engaging with governments, business, citizens, and other stakeholders, as well as indications on how to measure and assess wellbeing over time to support effective policy development. As a testament to the malleability of the WE approach, the principles and actions in the WE Policy Design Guide have been adapted to different contexts, as in developing post-COVID economic recovery pathways for Brazil (Girão et al., 2021) and the United States (Janoo, Fackenthal, Schwartz, Nuesse, & Sommer, 2021), as well as in the design of policies which focus on the associations between the environment and health (Laurent et al., 2021; see also Chapter 19, this volume).

The capacity of the WE approach to penetrate policy-making is evidenced by the Wellbeing Economy Governments network (WEGo). Within 2 two years from its launch, the network has come to include five national governments (Scotland, New Zealand, Iceland, Wales, and Finland), and it is expected to grow at a fast phase, with a number of other governments showing interest in being part of the group. The WEGo members are implementing concrete policies which replace GDP growth as the main goal of their national economies in favour of a more holistic approach to delivering wellbeing by taking care of the environment, people's health (including mental health), and social relations.

Scotland, for example, developed and implemented in 2018 a multidimensional National Performance Framework which considers the fundamental role of health, education, environmental quality, innovation, and inclusiveness for development (https://nationalperformance.gov.scot/). A public consultation led to cross-party consensus on a set of 81 national indicators of progress toward achieving 11 national outcomes including children, communities, culture, economy, entrepreneurial activity, education, environment, fair work and business, health, human rights, international, and poverty (Fisher, 2019).

In 2019, New Zealand launched its 'Wellbeing Budget', a set of development policies and accounting tools to advance what the 'GDP growth' approach neglects: that is, the quality of economic activities, real social benefits, and consequences such as inequality and damage to natural ecosystems (New Zealand Government, 2019). In order to do so, budget allocations are made according to their impacts on different components of wellbeing, beyond just considering the fiscal and economic implications, with a focus on collaboration across government and including long-term impacts on future generations (Dalziel & Saunders, 2020).

Following Scotland and New Zealand, other WEGo governments are rapidly moving in the same direction. For instance, Iceland has adopted a dashboard of 39 wellbeing indicators to guide national economic policies, which include education attainment, mental health, and the environmental costs of economic activities (BBC, 2019; Government of Iceland, 2019). The indicators are linked to the UN Sustainable Development Goals (SDGs), which further demonstrates the potential of the WE approach to be aligned with existing initiatives and frameworks and to enhance their focus on wellbeing (see also Chapter 21, this volume).

On December 2020, the Welsh Government published the report 'Wellbeing of Wales: 2020', with a list of indicators for assessing progress against seven national wellbeing goals on prosperity in terms of employment and education, resilience to climate change and other emergencies (including pandemics), physical and mental health, equality, community cohesion, culture and heritage, and global responsibility to carbon emissions. The report, required under the Wellbeing of Future Generations (Wales) Act 2015, makes no reference to 'economic growth', and GDP is left out of the 46 indicators for progress, which include measures of the status of ecosystems and biodiversity; the percentage of people who volunteer, as well as the gender pay difference; and the capacity of renewable energy equipment installed (Welsh Government, 2017, 2020). Similar to the wellbeing indicators adopted by Iceland, Wales wellbeing indicators are also connected with the SDGs.

These examples point to the potential of a WE for triggering system change, empowering citizens who are willing to adopt more sustainable lifestyles but find themselves in a space of constrained options for alternative consumption modes. Providing actionable solutions to policy-makers, the WE approach allows for policies for enabling behaviour change toward more sustainable lifestyles. These lifestyles might include vegan or vegetarian diets, a reduction in sugar and alcohol consumption, food waste reduction, renewable-based heating and electricity, electric mobility, car-free commuting, reduction of flights, and ride sharing, amongst many others (Akenji, Lettenmeier, Toivo, Koide, & Amellina, 2019), which can all be implemented and scaled-up within a WE framework where competition is replaced by collaboration and collective wellbeing is the main societal and policy goal.

Thanks to its ability to connect an overall and timely vision to a number of practical tools, the WE lends itself to several policy proposals that are becoming increasingly popular in today's world. Examples of these proposals include the following:

1. A shift to purpose-driven businesses with social and environmental aims in their DNA, using true cost accounting and leveraging supply chains and innovation for collective wellbeing. Requiring full corporate disclosure and reporting against clear benchmarks and increased accountability can move businesses away from a focus on short-term profit maximisation toward wider societal goals in business decision-making (Barth et al., 2020). For example, businesses can be required to include wellbeing objectives in their stated purpose and accounting or to implement total cost accounting systems for environmental and social externalities. Extended producer responsibility, sustainable design requirements, and regulations on planned obsolescence, together with government investments and actions that incentivise businesses with positive or lower environmental and social impacts and disincentivise businesses with negative ones, are all tools that can be used to redirect business behaviour.

2. Policies to encourage a circular and regenerative economy by incentivising new business models, as well as technical and social innovation for maximising wellbeing. These policies include the implementation of minimum recycled content targets, incentives for recycled materials, eco-design solutions, quality labels, repair and reuse, sustainability standards for public procurement, and separate waste collection, as well as a wellbeing-based fiscal reform by taxing more heavily all production and consumption that damages human and

ecological wellbeing while reducing tax on goods and services that, by contrast, produce positive wellbeing outcomes.

3. More appropriate systems of economic accounting, shifting from the System of National Accounts (SNA) to a dashboard of wellbeing indicators. The case of Scotland, New Zealand, Wales, and other governments of WEGo show how it is possible to build consensus on and implement frameworks of indicators for assessing budgets and national performance on the basis of impacts to wellbeing. Other examples include Bhutan's Gross National Happiness Index (see also Chapter 14, this volume) and the use of beyond-GDP indicators such as the Genuine Progress Indicator (GPI) in Canada (Anielski, 2018) and in some parts of the United States (e.g., Maryland and Vermont; see McGuire, Posner, & Haake, 2016; Zencey, 2018).

4. Shifting taxes from 'flows' (income) to 'harms' (pollution, waste) and 'stocks' (wealth, land). Taxes on wealth should be increased while taxes on income could be gradually reduced, with a view to encouraging people to perform useful professional activities rather than use 'rents' to earn profit. Moreover, value-added tax should be increased on harmful production and consumption (e.g., on unhealthy food and polluting energy), including an environmental border tax for adjusting prices on imports with significant ecological footprints. Land-value taxes of some form are already being implemented in more than 61 countries (Hughes, McCluskey, Sayce, Shepherd, & Wyatt, 2018) and have the potential to help correct wealth inequalities, deter speculative acquisitions, help economic development in areas where land values are low, increase the efficiency of land use, and boost government tax receipts (Barth et al., 2020).

5. New financing vehicles and incentives for directing private and public finance to regenerative activities/jobs. There is a need for assessing the environmental and social impacts of financial investments and implement science-based decisions into financial decision-making. Standards and labels could be developed to certify the contribution of financial investments for achieving wellbeing goals and international targets, for example on climate change. Long-term impacts and environmental risk assessment could be made mandatory for all financial institutions. This could stimulate investments and the design of incentives toward activities and jobs with positive contributions to wellbeing and the regeneration of nature.

6. Policies to support both predistribution and redistribution of income, wealth, and power. While redistribution of wealth (through taxation and benefits) is important, there is a need to create systems that entail a more equal distribution of access and wealth in the first place (Sennholz-Weinhardt, Meynen, & Wiese, 2021). More equal access to resources, technology, knowledge, and services could be achieved through more widely dispersed rights to access and through redefining ownership

toward less exclusive and more collective forms of managing wealth. By recognising the positive role of technology and innovation when distributed and nonproprietary, and by focusing on goals of collective wellbeing, reduced inequalities, and increasing levels of social cohesion and trust, the WE approach constitutes the right framework for predistribution and redistribution policies across income levels, gender, and other levels.

7. Appropriate policy instruments for enabling widespread access to consumption alternatives, including in the areas of nutrition, housing, and mobility, with benefits in terms of health, increasing social capital, poverty reduction, reduced socioeconomic marginalisation, and reduced environmental impacts. Policies and tools for enabling consumption options above societal needs and below ecological thresholds include investments in sustainable mobility and food market infrastructures, investments in renewable energy sources, taxes on high-sugar beverages, public land use designation for urban agriculture, and other supporting measures for enabling consumption alternatives with reduced environmental impacts (Akenji et al., 2021). In this context, engaging with consumers in a participatory approach for discussing viable lifestyle options, barriers to their adoption, and for co-developing future scenarios is essential (Hot or Cool Institute and Institute for Global Environmental Strategies, in press) and could be achieved by designing physical and virtual spaces for engagement.

8. A sustainable and humane work reform built upon serious and open dialogues on aspects such as a short working week, decent pay, control and autonomy at work, home office options, and a better work–life balance, as well as the redefinition of producers and consumers and the transactional, profit-driven activities that seek to separate them. In Iceland, a short working week trial revealed not only benefits in terms of employees' wellbeing (including stress reduction), but also benefits for companies, with productivity staying the same or even improving (Villegas & Knowles, 2021). Similar outcomes have been highlighted in Australia and Japan (Paul, 2019; Ziffer, 2020). The COVID-19 pandemic has triggered a global wave of new home-office opportunities across the globe, which has resulted in a massive reduction of carbon dioxide emissions and a significant improvement in work–life balance. Government subsides could be directed to workers who reduce their work time for taking care of their families or for expanding access to paid family leave and paid sick leave (Power, 2020). Globally, obligations could be implemented for companies to ensure living wages to all workers and compliance with the Global Framework Arrangements (GFAs), committing to upholding the core labour standards of the International Labour Organization (ILO), including the right to freedom of association in their own operations and in their supply chains (Hot or Cool Institute, 2021).

Together, these policy proposals and societal transformations (and many more) can be scaled-up to multiply the environmental and social benefits we are observing in their various manifestations today.

SUMMARY

The GDP growth economy brings about negative impacts to wellbeing that exceed its positive impacts. Redefining development in terms of wellbeing is essential to limit the risk of future pandemics as well as to build economies where health, environmental quality, and the promotion of thriving communities based on trust and solidarity are core priorities.

A wellbeing-based system of accounting should replace GDP as the main measure of progress. This accounting system will help us to identify the costs associated with highly centralised, polluting, and wasteful productions. Such a system would also highlight the economic contributions and external benefits of forms of production that GDP either downplays or ignores. If the unpaid activity of households and the social benefits to be derived from small, distributed businesses are fully accounted for, nonconventional economic actors will gain a much stronger voice in society. The beneficiaries that result from a shift from growth to wellbeing include families, communities, cooperatives, informal and small businesses, organic farmers, fair trade networks, and many more. This shift represents our most important goal if we want to move away from a world of degraded environment, recurring pandemics, impoverished social relations, compromised physical and psychological wellbeing, and an uncertain economic future and instead design an economy at the service of collective wellbeing.

REFERENCES

Akenji, L., Bengtsson, M., Toivo, V., Lettenmeier, M., Fawcett, T., Parag, Y., Saheb, Y., Coote, A., Spengenberg, J. H., Capstick, S., Gore, T., Coscieme, L., Wackernagel, M., & Kenner, D. (2021). 1.5-Degree lifestyles: Towards a fair consumption space for all. Hot or Cool Institute. https://hotorcool.org/wp-content/uploads/2021/10/Hot_or_Cool_1_5_lifestyles_FULL_REPORT_AND_ANNEX_B.pdf

Akenji, L., Lettenmeier, M., Toivo, V., Koide, R., & Amellina, A. (2019). 1.5-Degree lifestyles: Targets and options for reducing lifestyle carbon footprints. Technical Report. Institute for Global Environmental Strategies. https://www.iges.or.jp/en/publication_documents/pub/technicalreport/en/6719/15_Degree_Lifestyles_MainReport.pdf

Alvaredo, F., Chancel, L., Piketty, T., Saez, E., & Zucman, G. (2018). World inequality report 2018. World Inequality Lab. https://wid.world/document/world-inequality-report-2018-english/

Anielski, M. (2018). *An economy of well-being.* New Society Publishers.

Bakker, G., Crafts, N., & Woltjer, P. (2017). The sources of growth in a technologically progressive economy: The United States, 1899–1941. Economic History Working Papers, No: 269/2017. The London School of Economics and Political Science.

Barth, J., Abrar, R., Coscieme, L., Dimmelmeier, A., Hafele, J., Kumar, C., Mewes, S., Nuesse, I., Pendleton, A., & Trebeck, K. (2020). *Building a resilient economy. Analysing options for systemic change to transform the world's economic and financial systems after the pandemic.* ZOE-Institute for Future-Fit Economies.

Bastianoni, S., Coscieme, L., Caro, D., Marchettini, N., & Pulselli, F. M. (2019). The needs of sustainability: The overarching contribution of systems approach. *Ecological Indicators, 100,* 69–73.

BBC. (2019). Iceland puts well-being ahead of GDP in budget. https://www.bbc.com/news/world-europe-50650155

Boyce, C., Coscieme, L., Sommer, C., & Wallace, J. (2020). *Understanding wellbeing.* WEAll briefing papers: Little summaries of big issues. Wellbeing Economy Alliance.

Coscieme, L., Sutton, P., Mortensen, L. F., Kubiszewski, I., Costanza, R., Trebeck, K., Pulselli, F. M., Giannetti, B. F., & Fioramonti, L. (2019). Overcoming the myths of mainstream economics to enable a new wellbeing economy. *Sustainability, 11,* 4374.

Dalziel, P., & Saunders, C. (2020). *Wellbeing and economic policy: Lessons from New Zealand.* Squarespace. https://static1.squarespace.com/static/5a9f5444cef372803fb33678/t/5f51624dee9c5051818e4154/1599169140970/Wellbeing+Economy+Lessons+from+New+Zealand.pdf

Di Cesare, M., Soric, M., Bovet, P., Miranda, J. J., Bhutta, Z., Stevens, G. A., Laxmaiah, A., Kengne, A.-P., & Bentham, J. (2019). The epidemiological burden of obesity in childhood: A worldwide epidemic requiring urgent action. *BMC Med, 17*(1), 212. doi:10.1186/s12916-019-1449-8.

Easterlin, R. A. (1995). Will raising the incomes of all increase the happiness of all? *Journal of Economic Behavior Organization, 27*(1), 35–47.

Manshoven, S., Christis, M., Vercalsteren, A., Arnold, M., Nicolau, M., Lafond, E., Mortensen, L. F., & Coscieme. (2019). *Textiles and the environment in a circular economy.* Report of the European Environment Agency – European Topic Centre on Waste and Materials in a Green Economy. https://www.eea.europa.eu/publications/textiles-in-europes-circular-economy/textiles-in-europe-s-circular-economy

Fioramonti, L. (2017a). *Wellbeing economy: Success in a world without growth.* Pan Macmillan.

Fioramonti, L. (2017b). Well-being economy: A scenario for a post-growth horizontal governance system. Gross National Happiness USA. https://gnhusa.org/gnh/well-economy-scenario-post-growth-horizontal-governance-system/

Fisher, D. (2019). Wellbeing worldbeaters: New Zealand, Scotland, and Iceland. https://www.iwa.wales/agenda/2019/10/wellbeing-worldbeaters-new-zealand-and-scotland/

Giannetti, B. F., Almeida, C. M. V. B., Agostinho, F., Sulis, F., Coscieme, L., Pulselli, F. M., Bastianoni, S., & Marchettini, N. (2020). Enzo Tiezzi, turning pioneering into modern ideas: Tempos, ecodynamics, and sustainable economy. *Ecological Modelling, 431,* 109162. https://doi.org/10.1016/j.ecolmodel.2020.109162

Girão, A., Albuquerque, B., Hirszman, B., Casali, J. B., de Carvalho, J. D., & Bernardes Eloi, S. (2021). Brazil build back better: Principles for a Brazilian economic recovery. Wellbeing Economy Alliance & IONICA.

Government of Iceland. Indicators for measuring well-being. (2019). https://www.government.is/lisalib/getfile.aspx?itemid=fc981010-da09-11e9-944d-005056bc4d74

Hot or Cool Institute. (2021). Targets for slowing down fast fashion: Submission to the public consultation for the EU Strategy for Sustainable Textiles. Hot or Cool Institute.

Hot or Cool Institute & Institute for Global Environmental Strategies. (in press). Envisioning decarbonised urban lifestyles: Policies for 1.5-degree lifestyles cities in 2030. Hot or Cool Institute and Institute for Global Environmental Strategies.

Hough-Stewart, L., Trebeck, K., Sommer, C., & Wallis, S. (2019). What is a wellbeing economy? WEAll ideas: Little summaries of big issues. Wellbeing Economy Alliance.

Hughes, C., McCluskey, W., Sayce, S., Shepherd, E., & Wyatt, P. (2018). Investigation of potential land value tax policy options for Scotland. Report to the Scottish Land Commission. University of Reading.

Inglehart, R., Foa, R., Peterson, C., & Welzel, C. (2008). Development, freedom, and rising happiness: A global perspective (1981–2007). *Perspectives on Psychological Science, 3*(4), 264–285.

Janoo, A., Fackenthal, J., Schwartz, A., Nuesse, I., & Sommer, C. (2021). Rebuilding to a US wellbeing economy: 5 Principles for guiding economic recovery and policy action. Wellbeing Economy Alliance.

Kahneman, D., & Krueger, A. B. (2006). Developments in the measurement of subjective wellbeing. *Journal of Economic Perspectives, 20*, 3–24.

Kirchherr, J., Reike, D., & Hekkert, M. (2017). Conceptualizing the circular economy: Analysis of 114 definitions. *Reduce, Conserve, Recycle, 127*, 221–232.

Kossek, E. E., Valcour, M., & Lirio, P. (2014). The sustainable workforce: Organizational strategies for promoting work-life balance and wellbeing. In P. Y. Chen & C. L. Cooper (Eds.), *Work and wellbeing* (pp. 295–318). Wiley Blackwell. https://doi.org/10.1002/9781118539415.wbwell030

Laurent, E., Battaglia, F., Janoo, A., Galli, A., Dalla Libera Marchiori, G., Munteanu, R., & Sommer, C. (2021). Five pathways toward health-environment policy in a wellbeing economy. Wellbeing Economy Alliance.

Lunau, T., Bambra, C., Eikemo, T. A., van der Wel, K. A., & Dragano, N. (2014). A balancing act? Work-life balance, health and well-being in European welfare states. *European Journal of Public Health, 24*(3), 422–427.

McGuire, S., Posner, S., & Haake, H. (2016). Measuring prosperity: Maryland's genuine progress indicator. *Solutions, 3*(2), 50–58.

Myers, D. G. (2000). The funds, friends, and faith of happy people. *American Psychologist, 55*, 56.

New Zealand Government. (2019). The wellbeing budget. https://www.treasury.govt.nz/sites/default/files/2019-05/b19-wellbeing-budget.pdf

Nuccitelli, D. (2019). New report finds costs of climate change impacts often underestimated. *Yale Climate Connections.* November 18, 2019. https://yaleclimateconnections.org/2019/11/new-report-finds-costs-of-climate-change-impacts-often-underestimated/

Paul, K. (2019). Microsoft Japan tested a four-day work week and productivity jumped by 40%. *The Guardian.* 4 November, 2019. https://www.theguardian.com/technology/2019/nov/04/microsoft-japan-four-day-work-week-productivity

Piketty, T. (2014). *Capital in the twenty-first century.* Belknap Press of Harvard University Press.

Power, K. (2020). The COVID-19 pandemic has increased the care burden of women and families. *Sustainability: Science, Practice and Policy, 16*(1), 67–73.

Raworth, K. (2017). *Doughnut economics: Seven ways to think like a 21st-century economist.* Random House.

Rockström, J., Steffen, W., Noone, K., Persson, A., Chapin, F. S., Lambin, E. F., . . . Foley, J. A. (2009). A safe operating space for humanity. *Nature, 461*, 472–475.

Sennholz-Weinhardt, B., Meynen, N., & Wiese, K. (2021). Towards a wellbeing economy that serves people and nature. Oxfam and European Environmental Bureau.

Sommer, C. (2019). Telling the story of what we all need. https://weall.org/telling-the-story-of-what-we-all-need-blog-by-claire-sommer

Stiglitz, J. E. (2012). *The price of inequality: How today's divided society endangers our future.* W. W. Norton & Company.

Trebeck, K., & Williams, J. (2019). *The economics of arrival: Ideas for a grown up economy.* Policy Press.

Villegas, P., & Knowles, H. (2021). Iceland tested a 4-day workweek. Employees were productive – and happier, researchers say. *Washington Post.* https://www.washingtonpost.com/business/2021/07/06/iceland-four-day-work-week/

Ward, J. D., Sutton, P. C., Werner, A. D., Costanza, R., Mohr, S. H., & Simmons, C. T. (2016). Is decoupling GDP growth from environmental impact possible? *PLoS One, 11*(10), e01664733. doi:10.1371/journal.pone.0164733

Wellbeing Economy Alliance. (2021). Wellbeing economy policy design guide. Wellbeing Economy Alliance.

Welsh Government. (2017). National wellbeing indicators. https://gov.wales/national-wellbeing-indicators

Welsh Government. (2020). Wellbeing of Wales: 2020. https://gov.wales/wellbeing-wales-2020

Wilkinson, R., & Pickett, K. (2018). *The inner level.* Penguin Books.

Wilkinson, R., & Pickett, K. (2009). *The spirit level.* Penguin Books.

Wilkinson, R. G. (2007). Commentary: The changing relation between mortality and income. *International Journal of Epidemiology, 36*(3), 492–494.

World Health Organization. (2021). Mental health: Burden. https://www.who.int/health-topics/mental-health#tab=tab_2

World Resources Institute. (2016). The rise of the urban energy "prosumer". https://www.wri.org/insights/rise-urban-energy-prosumer

Yang, X., Fang, Y., Chen, H., Zhang, T., Yin, X., Man, J., Yang, L., & Lu, M. (2021). Global, regional and national burden of anxiety disorders from 1990 to 2019: Results from the Global Burden of Disease Study 2019. *Epidemiology and Psychiatric Sciences, 30,* e36. doi:10.1017/S2045796021000275

Zencey, E. (2018). *The Vermont genuine progress indicator project.* University of Vermont.

Ziffer, D. (2020). *Aussie firm's 'no-work Wednesday' concept goes global. ABC News,* January 7.

AND the Wellbeing of the Built and Natural Environments

18

Natural Capital, Ecosystem Services, and Subjective Wellbeing

A Systematic Review

DIANE JARVIS, PHIL LIGNIER, IDA KUBISZEWSKI, AND
ROBERT COSTANZA ■

INTRODUCTION

It has long been recognised that natural environments make important contributions to human wellbeing. However, the multiple pathways by which ecosystem benefits flow toward physical and mental wellbeing are less well understood. This makes it difficult to quantify or value the benefits we enjoy from experiencing nature or benefiting from hard to perceive ecosystem services, either *in situ* or remotely.

This chapter begins with an overview of the conceptual frameworks that have emerged over the past two decades seeking to describe the interlinked system of humans and the rest of nature. It then considers the growing body of empirical literature that has sought to measure the relationships between the natural environment and human wellbeing. In this chapter, we focus on a subjective wellbeing approach, also known as self-reported life satisfaction, while acknowledging the limitations of this approach in assessing overall wellbeing. We consider the various proxies for the environment that have been used when trying to empirically measure and quantify relationships with subjective wellbeing. Finally, we consider the lessons learned from this body of empirical research, seeking to both guide further research and to make recommendations for public policy approaches that can contribute to improved human wellbeing in the future.

THE COMPLEX SYSTEM OF HUMANS AND THE REST OF NATURE

The body of literature investigating the relationship between the wellbeing of humans and the natural environments they inhabit has grown significantly over recent years. It reflects a range of conceptual frameworks and methodological approaches emerging within separate academic disciplines and from multi- and transdisciplinary work. These frameworks seek to increase understanding of how human wellbeing depends on the natural environment.

The mechanisms by which the rest of nature contributes to human wellbeing are complex and operate as part of an interlinked and interdependent social-economic-environmental system. The physical extent and condition of the world's ecosystems and natural assets are frequently described using the term 'natural capital', representing the stock of environmental assets, while the flow of benefits that result from using natural capital are frequently described as 'ecosystem services'. In simplistic terms, ecosystem services are the benefits to humans provided as a result of the contributions of natural capital.

In some early conceptualisations of ecosystem services frameworks, the different types of services enjoyed from nature were considered in isolation and portrayed as a flow of benefits from nature toward humans; that is, a fairly simple, one-directional flow. Such frameworks generally recognised a number of different categorisations of ecosystem services, such as the regulating, provisioning, and cultural services model, underpinned by support services. A particularly well-known framework of this type is that presented within the Millennium Ecosystem Assessment (2005). *Regulating services* refer to the natural processes by which organisms mediate or moderate the environment in ways that affect humans, such as waste assimilation, water purification, storm protection, and carbon sequestration. *Provisioning services* refer to the provision of nutritional and non-nutritional outputs such as food, drinking water, and timber. Finally, *cultural services* refer to the nonmaterial outputs that affect the physical and mental states of people, whether *in situ* or remotely, and include providing aesthetic, intellectual, and spiritual benefits, such as ocean swimming, bush walking, scientific investigation and educational uses, and spiritual and religious interactions with the natural environment (Haines-Young & Potschin, 2018).

Early conceptualisations of the flow of benefits provided by ecosystems to wellbeing, in the form of ecosystem services, focused on the nature–human system alone, implying that the benefits to human wellbeing flowed directly from nature. Indeed, early definitions of sustainability focused on the substitutability of natural with physical capital as underpinning Hartwick's Law for (weak) sustainability (Hartwick, 1977). However, Costanza, de Groot, et al. (2014) highlighted that the benefits from natural capital flow when ecosystem services are created in interaction with social, human, and built capital (as depicted in Figure 18.1). This shows the inherent complementarity of the relationship between natural and other forms of capital. Understanding this system is further complicated by the overlapping and inseparable characteristics of

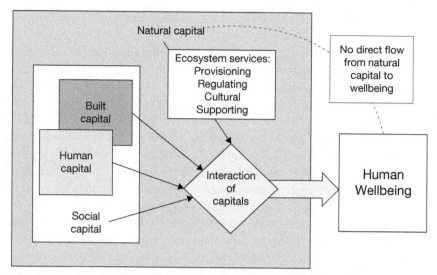

Figure 18.1 Human wellbeing depends on interactions among all four types of capitals. The benefits flow, in the form of ecosystem services that humans enjoy from natural capital, is therefore indirect, reflecting that nature is used together with complementary capitals, rather than a direct flow independent of other forms of capital. Adapted from Costanza, de Groot, et al. (2014).

many of the benefit flows (Stoeckl et al., 2014). Furthermore, in addition to private benefits flowing to individuals, many of the benefits from nature are inherently social. These benefits that are experienced at a community level are often greater than the sum of the benefits experienced separately by individuals (Stoeckl et al., 2018).

More recent developments in conceptualising the relationship between humans and the rest of nature recognise that, in addition to the flow of benefits from nature to people, there is also a reciprocal flow from people to nature. People have long recognised the need to maintain built capital; there is now a growing recognition that the sustainable use of nature requires the same logic be applied to natural capital. Thus, conceptualising a reverse flow of benefits recognises the important role that people play in providing stewardship services in protecting and caring for ecosystems and supporting their ability to provide a sustainable flow of ecosystem services (Costanza et al., 2017; De Groot et al., 2010; Díaz et al., 2015; Pascua, McMillen, Ticktin, Vaughan, & Winter, 2017).

Historically, studies of the nature–human relationship adopted a Western science lens, considering humans and nature to be two separate entities (Haines-Young & Potschin, 2018). This approach is opposed to those that consider humans and the rest of nature as interconnected and inseparable entities (Kenter, 2018; Pascua et al., 2017). Transdisciplinary work with First Nations Peoples recognises that the world views of many indigenous peoples takes a more holistic approach (see Chapter 7, this volume), whereby the benefits from the rest of nature to humans are inseparable from the actions taken by humans to protect and care for the rest of nature—their stewardship functions (Weir, Stacey, & Youngetob, 2011).

Recent transdisciplinary work extends the conceptual frameworks of the human–rest of nature system to incorporate the additional flows of benefits from human stewardship activities to human wellbeing (see Figure 18.2), irrespective of whether such stewardship activities contribute to increased environmental health or greater flow of benefits from ecosystem services (Stoeckl et al., 2021). This reflects that being involved in nature, and participating in activities on and for the environment, known as 'caring for Country' by the Australian Indigenous peoples, directly improves the wellbeing of those involved (Larson et al., 2020; Stoeckl et al., 2021). Providing environmental stewardship (Molsher & Townsend, 2016) has shown to have similar benefits to those gained from giving and volunteering (Black & Living, 2004; Choi & Kim, 2011). Recognising that people have stewardship obligations over the natural environment implies that they emotionally care, in addition to physically taking care of nature, and both aspects are likely to contribute to life satisfaction directly and also by indirect means, such as by contributing to people feeling that they have free choice and control over the direction of their lives (Sen, 1999), which has demonstrated links to happiness (Johnson & Krueger, 2006). Thus, human–nature links contribute to human wellbeing in many diverse ways beyond the direct flows of ecosystem services from nature that are more commonly considered to comprise nature's contribution to human wellbeing.

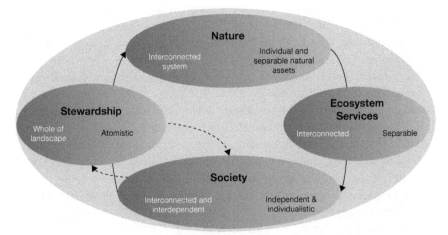

Figure 18.2 Nature and society form a cyclical and integrated system with reciprocal benefit flows from nature to people and from people to nature, plus the flow of benefits to human wellbeing from stewardship activities irrespective of benefits to nature resulting from those stewardship activities. Text on the right (within each oval) reflects that Nature, Society, Ecosystem Services, and Stewardship activities and can be conceptualised as simple and individualistic, while text on the left presents an alternate holistic interconnected worldview.
Adapted from Stoeckl et al. (2021). Figure reproduced under a Creative Commons CC-BY-NC-ND license.

MEASURING THE CONTRIBUTION OF THE REST OF NATURE TO HUMAN WELLBEING: THE LIFE SATISFACTION APPROACH

A wide range of research methodologies have attempted to measure the strength of the relationships among natural capital, ecosystem services, and human wellbeing. Such work recognises that understanding and quantifying the potential impacts of natural capital and ecosystem services on wellbeing and estimating the value of the benefits provided (either in monetary or relative terms) contributes to resource allocation decisions and improved public policy. Various proxy measures have been used to represent wellbeing (Costanza, Kubiszewski et al., 2014; Dolan, Peasgood, & White, 2008), including

1. subjective measures (discussed further below);
2. objective measures, including those based upon adjusted economic indicators such as the Genuine Progress Indicator (GPI) (Kubiszewski et al., 2013); and
3. composite measures that combine both types of measure.

Self-reported measures of overall life satisfaction or subjective wellbeing (SWB) assume that people are able to evaluate their own level of wellbeing and the quality of their lives (Diener, Suh, Lucas, & Smith, 1999). SWB can serve as a proxy for the economist's concept of utility (Kristoffersen, 2010). In this chapter, we focus on empirical studies seeking to understand the factors influencing subjectively measured wellbeing using one specific methodology: the life satisfaction (LS) approach. Simplistically, LS researchers ask questions such as 'How satisfied are you with your life as a whole?', and responses are then regressed against a variety of other factors. The coefficients of the equations provide information about the marginal contribution that these factors make to overall LS (or utility). The terms 'LS', 'happiness', and 'SWB' tend to be used interchangeably in the literature (Easterlin, 2003), along with the term 'quality of life', however each of these terms is conceptually distinct. Traditionally, the psychology literature distinguishes between the hedonic component (affect) of wellbeing and the eudaimonic component (cognitive evaluations of one's functioning in life) (Deci & Ryan, 2008) (see also Chapters 1, 2, and 3, this volume). While happiness is generally associated with hedonic wellbeing (short-lived emotions), LS is more closely related to cognitive judgements and intrinsic goals (in the Aristotelian tradition) (Engelbrecht, 2009) and has been found to correlate better with other national wellbeing predictors (Helliwell, 2003; Vemuri & Costanza, 2006). However, it has been argued that a composite SWB Index based on both happiness and LS was more reliable than either of its components (Inglehart, Foa, Peterson, & Welzel, 2008). Whilst there is some evidence of a reasonably strong relationship between the different concepts (psychological wellbeing and LS, and psychological wellbeing and positive and negative affect [Diener et al., 1999]), little correlation has been found between individual levels of LS and positive and negative affect (Organisation for Economic Co-operation and Development [OECD], 2013). Within the field of economics, LS has emerged as the preferred measure although the terms 'happiness' and 'SWB' are also used, and comparisons across the different measures are common in the literature (Engelbrecht, 2009). Other research has explored factors relating to satisfaction with specific domains of life (such as health, community, emotional wellbeing, etc.) and the relationship between these different domains (Cummins, 1996) but without a focus on how these different domains interrelate with the natural environment. Accordingly, while the focus here is on the evidence of links between LS and nature, further research exploring the association between the environment and different domains of wellbeing would also be helpful in improving our understanding of this complex relationship.

It is also important to recognise that the LS approach develops models that test whether there is a statistically significant relationship between LS and the different variables included within the model, and therefore the same caution should be applied when interpreting results of LS analysis as with any other research based on statistical models. That is, the research indicates when correlations are present, but this does not necessarily imply a causal relationship flowing from the variable to LS: it is possible that any identified association could alternatively indicate bidirectional causation or from LS to the other variable, or the apparent correlation could be spurious (e.g., when issues of endogeneity, omitted variables, or confounding variables are present).

The key challenge when using the LS approach for measuring the potential impact of the environment on wellbeing (as proxied by LS) is determining an appropriate proxy variable or variables to represent the role of the rest of nature within the LS model. A key component of this challenge is that humans do not necessarily perceive all the benefits that the rest of nature provides to them. Furthermore, the impacts on LS from the rest of nature are not always positive. Negative impacts can result from environmental degradation such as pollution, where the root cause is human activities, or from natural events such as earthquakes, volcanic eruptions, and extreme weather events, which themselves can be exacerbated (or potentially mitigated) by human intervention.

In summary, it is clear that natural capital is a multifaceted concept that contributes to wellbeing via a range of pathways: benefits can flow directly or via indirect routes, and the full range of benefits are derived through use and nonuse mechanisms, some of which are enjoyed *in situ* while other benefits can be enjoyed remotely. The environment has both stock and flow effects and is a complement to other (built, human, social, and cultural) capitals. The rest of nature can be considered both a 'stock' (a natural asset such as the Great Barrier Reef) and a 'flow' (the range of cultural, provisioning, and regulating ecosystem services that are provided by the Reef). Both stocks and flows contribute to LS separately, and their impacts can either reinforce each other or include trade-offs. It is this complexity of benefit flows combined with the social and interrelated nature of the benefits that generates the challenge in determining an appropriate indicator or proxy to represent the rest of nature: with a simple individual benefit being far easier to measure than complex social benefit flows (Stoeckl et al., 2018).

A number of reviews have looked at the use of LS in general (Ferrer-i-Carbonell, 2012; MacKerron, 2012) and the idea of using it to estimate environmental valuations (Ferreira & Moro, 2010; Welsch & Kühling, 2009). However, to our knowledge, no previous work has evaluated the relative performance of different proxy measures of nature in studies seeking to explore and explain how they contribute to wellbeing. In the next section, we seek to address this gap and thus provide an evidence base for both policy recommendations and future research opportunities.

METHODOLOGY ADOPTED FOR SEARCHING, CLASSIFYING, AND SYNTHESISING THE CONTRIBUTIONS OF THE REST OF NATURE TO LS

The Search and Screening Process

The target literature was identified via a process that involved systematically searching and screening relevant papers prior to synthesising the results. The Web of Science database was searched at the end of May 2019. The search was restricted to articles published from 1 January 2000 (reflecting that the LS approach is a fairly recent innovation, the use of which has grown substantially over the past two decades) to May 2019 and to articles published in English. Literature was selected based on the following search terms:

- Life Satisfaction OR Subjective Wellbeing OR Subjective Well-being
- Natural Capital OR Ecosystem* (where the * is a wild card implying any suffix).

The publications were initially screened based on Web of Science categories (excluding medical publications clearly focused on the physical and mental health aspects of wellbeing), then screened based on title, then subsequently screened based on abstract, and finally screened based on the full text. At each stage of the screening process papers clearly outside the scope of this study were excluded.

Following screening, 79 publications remained. These identified publications were supplemented by 8 additional publications identified by the authors from prior research, providing 87 eligible publications for critical appraisal and synthesis within this review.

Critical Appraisal and Synthesis

The publications were critically appraised and classified into a number of different themes representing analysis based on different types of environmental/natural capital indicators. Four clear indicator themes emerged from the analysis.

1. *Degree of human intervention* (28 papers): Indicators within this theme captured whether the local environment (neighbourhood, region etc.) reflected a state that had been heavily modified by human intervention

or was in a more 'natural', unmodified condition (e.g., urban/rural, or low population density/high density). Such indicators are simplistic but offer the advantage of being easy to quantify, and the data are easy to find. Measures of transport networks and connectivity were also included in this theme, recognising that the impact of transport networks may be nuanced; they are both an indicator themselves of increased development (hence reducing the 'naturalness; of the environment) but also provide opportunities for urban dwellers to visit more natural environments.

2. *Specific environmental goods and services* (36 papers): Indicators (subjective and objective) within this theme related to specific environmental 'goods' such as coverage of, proximity to, or satisfaction with pleasant places or features (e.g., green space, beach, national park).

3. *Adverse impacts* (40 papers): Indicators within this theme related to specific environmental 'ills', such as objective measures or subjective perceptions of pollution (e.g., air or water pollution) or proximity to somewhere unpleasant (e.g., a hazardous waste facility or polluted river).

4. *Overarching indicators* (24 papers): Indicators within this theme sought to represent the value of or satisfaction with natural capital or ecosystem services more broadly conceived (e.g., natural capital, ecosystem services, and environmental health).

During the appraisal process it was noted that some publications included indicators relating to one theme only whereas others included indicators relating to two or three. Furthermore, a number of the papers included more than one indicator relating to a specific theme. It was also notable that both subjective (based on perceptions) and objective (based on physical measures) indicators were included within a number of these themes, with some publications focusing on objective, others on subjective, and a further set including both subjective and objective indicators. The full list of publications included within this review, analysed by theme, are set out in the Appendix.

RESULTS AND DISCUSSION BY THEME

Summary of the Papers Reviewed

The publications included 65 studies relating to 18 individual countries, with the most highly represented countries being China and Australia. Additionally, 22 studies were based on cross-country comparisons for multiple different countries. Analysis by country is shown in Table 18.1.

The frequency of relevant publications across the years included within the reviewed period increased exponentially. During the first 5 years, only one relevant

Table 18.1 ANALYSIS OF PUBLICATIONS INCLUDED WITHIN THE REVIEW
BY CASE STUDY COUNTRY

Country	Number of papers	% of papers
Australia	13	15
Canada	1	1
Chile	1	1
China	15	17
Ecuador	2	2
Germany	5	6
India	1	1
Iran	1	1
Ireland	4	5
Italy	1	1
Japan	4	5
New Zealand	2	2
Spain	1	1
Switzerland	1	1
Taiwan	1	1
Turkey	2	2
UK	6	7
USA	4	5
Total single-country studies	65	75
Cross multiple countries studies	22	25
Total number of studies	87	100

paper was selected, rising to 13 papers (15% of total) for the second 5-year period, while the third and fourth 5-year periods contained 24 (28%) and 49 papers (56%), respectively (noting that the final period is potentially understated as it only contains 4 years and 5 months of publications) (Figure 18.3). This dramatic growth over time indicates both the increasing use and increasing acceptability of this approach as researchers recognise that it provides a powerful analysis tool.

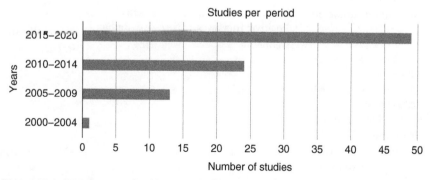

Figure 18.3 Distribution of publications over each 5-year period.

Theme 1: Degree of Human Intervention

Almost one-third of the papers selected for the study, 28 in total, included variables that could be classified as proxies of urbanisation or a degree of human intervention. These variables were further analysed between three subthemes: (1) population density (e.g., people per square kilometre; (2) indication of rural, remote, or far from city centre locations (e.g., distance to city centre; dichotomous variable indicating rural or urban; indicator of residence in either city, town, village or remote area; percentage urban/industrial/commercial coverage of region); and (3) proximity to transport networks (e.g., distance to railway station; indicators of being within a specified distance [say <5 km] from specified facility [say airport, station, main road, etc.]). The relationship between each variable and LS was then ascertained. Some papers included variables from more than one subtheme, and some included a number of different variables from within the transport subtheme, separately testing the impact of different types of transport networks (road, rail, etc). Some papers also include more than one model, with different results depending on the specific functional form of the model; hence one paper may be included in more than one of the groupings. Overall, the impact of 48 different variables from the subthemes is summarised in Table 18.2.

Whilst these types of variables are simple to define and easy to obtain, and consequently are fairly widely included within LS models, they are often found not to have a significant correlation with the respondent's LS. Such measures are too broad and imprecise to enable the effect of living in a natural environment to be determined. Indeed, such measures could be acting as proxies for many factors beyond living in or being connected to the natural world. These variables could also reflect the impacts of some or all elements of physical, social, and financial capital, rendering these variables unsuitable proxies for the benefits we gain from the environment.

Table 18.2 THE NUMBER OF VARIABLES DEMONSTRATING POSITIVE, NEGATIVE, OR NO IMPACT ON LIFE SATISFACTION (LS) OF DIFFERENT VARIABLES INDEXING DEGREE OF HUMAN INTERVENTION.

Degree of human intervention subtheme	Impact of variable on life satisfaction as a proxy for wellbeing		
	Positive: Increases wellbeing	Negative: Reduces wellbeing	No significant impact
Population density	2	3	12
Rural, remote, far from city centre	6	5	10
Proximity to transport networks	2	2	6
Total number of variables having this impact on wellbeing	10	10	28

The impact of population density was variable, suggesting that this may be a more important variable at a country scale rather than a regional scale. From the 13 single-country studies, population density had a positive impact on wellbeing in two of those studies (Ambrey & Shahni, 2017; Brereton, Clinch, & Ferreira, 2008) and a negative impact in one (Cuñado & de Gracia, 2012); no significant impact was found in the other 10 studies. For four cross-country studies, population density had no significant impact in two and was found to have a significant negative impact in two others (Maddison & Rehdanz, 2011; Menz & Welsch, 2010).

Measures indicating urbanised or city living compared to more regional or remote lifestyles were also found to have a mixed and frequently insignificant association with LS. Five studies found living in rural/remote locations contributed positively to LS (Ambrey & Fleming, 2012; Kopmann & Rehdanz, 2013; Sasaki, 2018; E. Wang, Kang, & Yu, 2017; Zhang & Wang, 2019) while five found a negative impact (Asadullah, Xiao, & Yeoh, 2018; MacKerron & Mourato, 2009; Requena, 2016; Winters & Li, 2017; Zorondo-Rodríguez et al., 2016). The remaining relevant studies found no significant impact. One study in particular found that the impact of rural residence was highly sensitive to the model specification, as positive, negative, and insignificant impacts were found depending on the form of the model (whether the model included variables indicating respondents' economic position relative to others, whether the model focused on full sample or subsamples selected by income groups), suggesting that the impact of rural or urban location could be mediated by the influences of absolute and relative incomes (Asadullah et al., 2018). Another study used rural/urban indicators (which were all insignificant) but also included dummy variables specifying whether respondents resided in one of the major metropolitan cities (Ambrey & Fleming, 2013). This study found that, compared to living in Sydney (the largest city in Australia), residing in one of the smaller metropolitan areas (Brisbane, Adelaide, Perth, Hobart, Darwin or Canberra) contributed positively to LS, while living in the second largest city, Melbourne, made no significant difference, suggesting that residing in smaller (less urban) rather than larger cities may be beneficial for LS.

The variables representing proximity to transport networks were also found to have highly mixed impacts, potentially due to the clear opportunities for both benefits (in the form of increased connectivity) and costs (noise, congestion, air pollution, etc.) to arise from being in the close vicinity of major roads, airports, etc. Thus, a study investigating regions of European countries found a positive impact from good coverage of roads, rail, and air for northern European countries but not those of central or southern Europe (Kopmann & Rehdanz, 2013). A study in Ireland found benefits from being fairly close to regional (<30 km) and international (30–60 km) airports (Brereton et al., 2008), while an Australian study found being within 5 kilometres of an airport negatively impacted LS (Ambrey & Fleming, 2013) as did being very close to a major road in Ireland (Brereton et al., 2008).

Thus, the relationship between LS and residing in a heavily built environment such as a large city, or a rural location, is unclear, likely due to the many confounding factors that could be having an impact. Some such possibilities are revealed by research focusing specifically on factors correlating with increased happiness or LS for city residents: for example, indicators of higher human capital have been shown to relate to higher levels of happiness within cities (Florida, Mellander, & Rentfrow, 2013) while larger cities are likely to contribute to longer commute times, which has been shown to reduce LS (Stutzer & Frey, 2008). Furthermore, complex links have been demonstrated between creativity (which itself can be fostered by interactions with nature), human capital, incomes, economic growth, and the aesthetic quality of a location (including natural scenery, parks, and green spaces) within cities, all factors that can impact on LS and which may contribute to the unclear relationship between urban or rural living and LS (Florida, 2014).

The findings from this theme broadly support the conceptual framework developed by Costanza, de Groot, et al. (2014), which proposes that for natural capital to provide human wellbeing benefits such capital needs to be in conjunction with the complementary human, built, and social capitals. High population density and city centre locations with good transport networks provide built capital but are unlikely to have sufficient quantities of natural capital to optimise wellbeing. In contrast, remote areas with low population density are unlikely to have sufficient built capital to enable the more abundant natural capital to be fully enjoyed. This effect may exacerbate differences seen when conducting cross-country comparisons of LS (and contributing factors), particularly between developed and developing countries (which are likely to have lower quality and quantity of built capital per capita). Hence, such variables are shown to have mixed or insignificant impacts on wellbeing and appear to be not overly robust to the precise specification of the model used. Accordingly, these variables appear to be too broad and unfocused to be able to clearly indicate the subtleties involved in the complex benefits flow from natural capital and the services provided by ecosystems.

Theme 2: Enjoyment of Specific Environmental Goods and Services

More than 40% of the papers selected for review, 36 in total, included variables that could be classified as proxies for the enjoyment of specific environmental goods and services. These variables were further analysed between a number of subthemes (Table 18.3) identifying the specific environmental services enjoyed (such as greenspace and urban parks, which were the most widely studied) and whether the variable provided an objective or subjective measure. The significance and direction of the relationship between each variable and LS is summarised in Table 18.3. Some papers included variables from more than one subtheme; thus the impact of 74 different variables across the papers and subthemes have been identified.

The most widely used variables (almost 50% of this theme) related to greenspaces, with a variety of measures used to indicate that natural greenspaces were accessible to those responding to the survey (Table 18.3). Studies that used a form of greenspace measure to indicate an environmental good found that (proximity to, extent of coverage in local region, use of, or quality of) greenspaces were generally (in 71% of the studies) positively related to LS. However, the relationship is somewhat ambiguous as a number of papers found no significant correlation. Furthermore, three papers found nonlinear or inverted-U shape relationships. A need exists for further research regarding the appropriate functional form of the relationship between greenspaces and wellbeing (linear or otherwise). These findings suggest greenspaces are an example of natural capital contributing to wellbeing as a complement to other capitals, as discussed earlier. That is, accessing greenspace may enhance wellbeing, but are individuals willing and able to access them alone and by foot, or do other factors, such as a need for a car or public transport to access the greenspace play a role as well? And, once there, is their enjoyment enhanced by footpaths, boardwalks, seating areas, etc.? And is their enjoyment enhanced by accessing the greenspace with others (friends, family, etc.)? The complementarity of this example of natural capital and the other capitals (built, social) adds complexity to the task of attempting to separately value the different contributors to overall LS and may have contributed to those studies with nonsignificant findings.

A similar pattern is seen when other proxy variables are considered. Approximately half have a positive relationship to LS, with no significant relationship being found in the rest. Similar nonlinear or complementary factors may apply to these other variables as to those discussed regarding greenspace.

Ambrey and Fleming (2011a) incorporated a number of variables representing a range of different coastal and inland water-based 'goods' in combination within their study, reflecting proximity to coasts, lakes, rivers, and creeks, and found a mix of relationships with wellbeing. Specifically, the relationship of proximity to rivers was negative, proximity to lakes was not significant, and proximity to coastal areas and creeks was found to be significantly positive. This study does not provide insights into potential reasons for these different associations, and there is not a large enough body of research into the impact of water-based environmental goods to be able to draw conclusions here. Potentially, the mixed findings could reflect trade-offs between benefits from proximity to water (such as attractive views, opportunities for leisure and fishing) and adverse outcomes such as risks of flooding or the presence of mosquitos. There is a growing interest in the use of water environments, or 'blue space', to promote human health and wellbeing (Britton, Kindermann, Domegan, & Carlin, 2020; Garrett et al., 2019; Wheaton, Waiti, Cosgriff, & Burrows, 2020). However, further research is recommended to understand the apparent mix of effects on wellbeing resulting from blue spaces.

The list in Table 18.3 includes a number of subjective variables measuring respondents' perceptions rather than objective measures: perceived amount of greenspace and urban parks, subjective quality or satisfaction with greenspace, and perceived increase in native forest cover. Generally, these subjective variables were positively correlated with LS (e.g., Ambrey & Fleming, 2013), which is consistent with other research, such as that which has shown self-reported attributes of greenspaces are associated more clearly with neighbourhood satisfaction than

Table 18.3 THE NUMBER OF VARIABLES DEMONSTRATING POSITIVE, NEGATIVE, OR NO IMPACT ON LIFE SATISFACTION OF DIFFERENT VARIABLES INDEXING DEGREE OF OPPORTUNITIES FOR ENJOYMENT OF ENVIRONMENTAL GOODS AND SERVICES

Enjoyment of environmental goods and services subtheme	Impact of variable on life satisfaction as a proxy for wellbeing		
	Positive: Increases wellbeing	Negative: Reduces wellbeing	No significant impact
Proximity to greenspace and urban parks	6[a]	0	3
Coverage of greenspace and urban parks	14[a]	1[b]	3
Use of greenspace and urban parks	1	0	2
Perceived amount of greenspace and urban parks	1	0	0
Subjective quality of, or satisfaction with, greenspace and urban parks	3	0	1
Proximity to coast or beach	10	0	4
Proximity to lake, river, water, brook, creek	2	1	6
Coverage of wetlands	0	0	3
Proximity to national park	1	0	2
Coverage of national park, reserve, protected area, forest etc	3	0	3
Perceived increase in native forest cover	1	0	0
Subjective scenic amenity or landscape quality	2	0	1
Total number of variables having this impact on wellbeing	44	2	28

[a]Some studies have found a significant nonlinear (inverted U-shape) relationship, with greenspace area (one study) and distance from greenspace (two studies) having a positive impact on wellbeing to a certain point, beyond which further increases in greenspace area/distance from greenspace having a negative impact (Ambrey & Fleming, 2011a; Bertram & Rehdanz, 2015).

[b]One study found the relationship to be negative and significant in the nonlinear model, but nonsignificant in the linear model (Kopmann & Rehdanz, 2013).

is physical reality (Hur, Nasar, & Chun, 2010). Subjective measures generally (not just in relation to the environment) have been found to correspond more strongly with self-reported subjective wellbeing or LS than objective measures (Cummins, 2000), and there can be discrepancies between subjective and objective measures, for example, between respondents' satisfaction with urban green areas and open space (Ma, Dong, Chen, & Zhang, 2018) and objective environmental indicators such as hectares of greenspace per capital within respondents' local region (Ambrey & Cartlidge, 2017), as has been noted in the literature (Kothencz & Blaschke, 2017). Moreover, respondents' perception of same size green spaces differ depending on their types: biodiversity, presence of old trees, density of trees, and the presence of recreational areas (Aoshima, Uchida, Ushimaru, & Sato, 2018).

Overall, the findings from this theme again broadly support the conceptualisations from Costanza, de Groot, et al. (2014). Environmental 'goods' contribute to wellbeing, particularly from the provision of cultural ecosystem services, such as leisure and recreation services, and the more spiritual services enjoyed from being 'close' to nature whether enjoyed directly *in situ* or more remotely. However, such benefits reduce as the distance from nature increases, implying reduced ease of access and increased need for the complementary built and human capital to facilitate the enjoyment of the natural benefit.

Theme 3: Adverse Impacts Arising from Specific Environmental 'Ills'

Approximately half (47%) of the papers selected, 40 in total, included variables that could be classified as proxies for the adverse consequences that result from environmental problems such as pollution and degradation of the environment. These variables were further analysed between the different types of pollution or other problems, including air pollution, water pollution, and proximity to landfill sites, amongst others (Table 18.4). Two papers included variables that, while pollution-related, in fact measured efforts to reduce pollution levels (i.e., indicators of efforts to reverse the impact of the environmental 'ill'); as these measures view pollution via a different lens, they have been shown separately (Table 18.5). Consideration was also given on whether each variable provided an objective or subjective measure of the issue, with these two types of measures shown separately within the table. As for other themes, the significance and direction of the relationship between each variable and LS was identified and summarised. Some papers included variables from more than one subtheme; thus the impact of 78 different variables across the papers and subthemes has been summarised in Table 18.4, plus two variables measuring reduced pollution are shown separately in Table 18.5 (i.e., 80 different variables in total related to this theme).

As can be seen from the analysis within Table 18.4, the topic of air pollution has received far more attention than other topics, with 74% of the variables relating to objective or subjective air pollution. The next most studied topic was water pollution (9%), with the remaining studies covering a variety of different

Table 18.4 THE NUMBER OF VARIABLES DEMONSTRATING POSITIVE, NEGATIVE, OR
NO IMPACT ON LIFE SATISFACTION OF DIFFERENT VARIABLES INDEXING DEGREE
OF IMPACTS FROM ENVIRONMENTAL 'ILLS'

Impact of environmental 'ills' subtheme	Impact of variable on life satisfaction as a proxy for wellbeing		
	Positive: Increases wellbeing	Negative: Reduces wellbeing	No significant impact
Proximity to landfill or hazardous waste	0	2	3
Objectively measured poor air quality: particulates pollution, and/or emissions of one or more gases	2	33	14
Subjectively measured perceived air pollution	0	7	2
Proximity to polluted river	0	0	2
Objectively measured water pollution	0	1	2
Subjectively measured perceived water pollution	0	1	1
Proximity to invasive species impacted location	0	1	0
Subjectively measured perceived noise pollution	0	1	2
Subjectively measured perceptions of impact of pollution in general	0	1	1
Reported having concerns about ozone layer	0	1	0
Reported having concerns about animal extinctions	1	0	0
Total number of variables having this impact on wellbeing	3	48	27

problems. Overall, the analysis reveals the unsurprising result that, in the majority of circumstances (62%), the presence of pollution or other environmental ills whether objectively or subjectively measured reduces wellbeing. However, this finding does vary if we consider the different types of pollution in more detail. In 69% of the instances where air pollution was the focus, a negative impact

Table 18.5 The number of variables demonstrating positive, negative, or
no impact on life satisfaction of different variables indexing degree
of impacts from indicators that environmental 'ills' are being reversed

Impact of reversed indicators within environmental 'ills' subtheme	Impact of variable on life satisfaction as a proxy for wellbeing		
	Positive: Increases wellbeing	Negative: Reduces wellbeing	No significant impact
% of industrial air emissions that have been treated	1	0	0
% of water discharges that have been treated	0	0	1
Total number of variables having this impact on wellbeing	**1**	**0**	**1**

on wellbeing was found, with most of the balance having no significant impact; however, in two papers, positive impacts were found. Beja (2012), in a multiple-country study, found context in the form of the development state of the country to be important. That is, emissions in developed countries generally reduce well-being but can have a positive impact in developing countries, presumably due to links between industrial activity (hence emissions) and income/jobs, which are generally found to benefit wellbeing. Goetzke and Rave (2015), in a single-country study drawing survey participants from across Germany, explained (and supported with econometric analysis) that the positive relationship they found between objectively measured air pollution and wellbeing was due to the air pollution being fully capitalised within the housing market (i.e., air pollution is factored into house prices, with housing in high-pollution areas being cheaper than housing in less-polluted areas, with the consequence that the negative impact of pollution on LS is counterbalanced by the positive effect on LS resulting from cheaper housing). Interestingly, alternate research has found that subjectively measured air pollution (as opposed to objectively measured pollution) is not fully capitalised within the housing market (Rehdanz & Maddison, 2008).

In comparison to the air pollution findings, the non–air pollution variables were found to have an insignificant impact in the majority of cases (55%), and, for those instances where the focus was water pollution, a negative impact on wellbeing was found in only 29% of cases (the remaining 71% showing no significant impact).

Considering the objective (proximity or actual measured pollution) variables compared to the subjective variables revealed little difference, with 62% and 61%, respectively, showing a negative impact on wellbeing.

The variables representing efforts to reduce the various forms of pollution supported the findings from the variables indicating the impact of the pollutions/ills themselves. Increasing the proportion of air emissions that are treated, thus reducing air pollution, had a positive impact on wellbeing, whereas for water emissions, increasing the proportion treated was not found to have a significant impact. Thus, again, air pollution problems appear to have a greater impact on wellbeing than problems with water quality.

The relationship between perception/awareness of environmental 'ills' and objective indicators, and between perception/awareness and LS, can be summarised as follows:

- Perceived air pollution (e.g., particulates such as PM10 or gases such as nitrogen dioxide [NO_2]) has been found to be strongly negatively related to LS (MacKerron & Mourato, 2009; Rehdanz & Maddison, 2008), as has noise pollution (van Praag & Baarsma, 2005).
- In some cases, the perception of pollution relates strongly with LS while objective measures of pollution do not (e.g., van Praag & Baarsma, 2005).
- Similar strongly negative relationships have been found between environmental awareness (ozone layer depletion, concerns about biodiversity) and LS (Ferrer-i-Carbonell & Gowdy, 2007).
- There is good evidence of a strong correlation between perceptions of air pollution and actual levels of air pollution (Li, Stoeckl, King, & Gyuris, 2017; MacKerron & Mourato, 2009).
- People with personal experience of air pollution (e.g., people with asthma and older people) display a higher sensitivity to the levels of air pollution (Day, 2007).

Overall, this theme clearly indicates that pollution, and environmental 'ills' more generally, have a negative impact on human wellbeing. These findings, in conjunction with the findings from theme 2, suggest a possible adaptation of the framework showing the indirect flows of ecosystem services from nature and involving the complementarity on other types of capitals (Costanza, de Groot et al., 2014). Instead, it appears that while enjoyment of the benefits of nature (ecosystem services) are indeed generally indirect, the reduction in wellbeing from a degraded or polluted environment (itself caused by human activities) may in fact have a direct and adverse impact on human health and wellbeing.

Theme 4: Overarching Measures of Ecosystems and Other Descriptors of Natural Capital

Around one-quarter (28%) of the papers selected for review, 24 in total, included variables that provide a more general or overarching measure of the impact of the environment on wellbeing rather than a specific element of the environment or the type of impact. These variables were further analysed between objective or subjective measures, with subjective indicators being more common within this

Table 18.6 The number of variables demonstrating positive, negative, or no impact on life satisfaction of different variables indexing degree of impacts from overarching indicators of the environment and natural capital

Impact of overarching environmental indicators subtheme	Impact of variable on life satisfaction as a proxy for wellbeing		
	Positive: Increases wellbeing	Negative: Reduces wellbeing	No significant impact
Objective measures of natural or less developed environments[a]	14	1	2
Subjective measures of contribution of nature/ ecosystems[a]	5	0	4
Subjective measures indication positive attitude toward conservation or environmental protection[a]	5	0	3
Total number of variables having this impact on wellbeing	24	1	9

[a]In all examples where a variable was measuring a degraded environment or concern about degradation or other problems, then measure reversed for consistency and comparability with other measures.

theme than elsewhere. Some papers included variables from more than one subtheme; the impact of 34 different variables (17 objective and 17 subjective) across the papers and subthemes is summarised in Table 18.6. As can be seen, these variables were found to be significantly and positively associated with wellbeing in a clear majority of cases (70%).

A diverse range of objective measures indicating a more natural environment were included and could be broadly categorised into a number of types including (1) values attributed to natural capital using World Bank wealth accounts; (2) values based on different indices (Normalised Difference Vegetation Index [NDVI]; diversity index; biocapacity index; environmental sustainability index; and ecosystem services production index); (3) counts of plant species, animal species, or crop species in a particular region; and (4) footprint measures (carbon footprint, ecological footprint, and impact of land use). Whichever type of measure was used, these objective variables were virtually always positively linked to wellbeing (in 82% of cases).

The subjective measures have been subdivided into two distinct categories. First were those measuring perceived benefits from or satisfaction with the environment, which were generally measured on a 1–5, 0–5, or best to worst type scale. Specific examples include 'perceived contribution of nature to wellbeing', 'perceived value of ecosystem services', a variety of satisfaction/dissatisfaction measures such as 'perceived satisfaction with the environment/nature', and 'perceived severity of environmental issues/worries'. Such measures were fairly evenly split between having a positive impact or no significant impact on LS, with a slight majority (56%) finding positive impacts. Studies using wider response scales (0–10) gave more positive impacts than those with narrower response scales (1–3) and intermediate response scales (0–5, 1–5) indicating a mix of significant and insignificant findings, perhaps indicating that fairly wide scales should be used to ensure that different attitudes can be differentiated. The second category described as subjective measures related to positive attitudes toward the environment, conservation, and environmental activism, which were found to be positively related to wellbeing 63% of the time. Of the variables found to have a positive relationship, three indicated that higher satisfaction with conservation activities was associated with improved wellbeing, while a fourth variable—namely, being concerned about the environment—was associated with lower wellbeing. The fifth variable is more complex, being a measure of activism. The question posed was 'Have you ever reported a situation that caused pollution?', with an affirmative 'yes' answer to the question being related to increased wellbeing; this indicates that the respondent must have encountered pollution (otherwise there would be nothing to report), but the act of taking action against the problem (reporting it) was sufficient to enhance wellbeing, rather than the pollution itself suppressing wellbeing, thus affirming the importance of people feeling they have the freedom to exercise control over their life and situation, as found in studies in many different contexts (e.g., Inglehart et al., 2008; Sen, 1999). This accords with findings from recent research, which found that those whose response to climate change was described as 'eco-anger' were prompted to take individual action which itself was related to improved mental health and wellbeing (reduced depression, anxiety, and stress), while alternate emotional responses to climate change classified as 'eco-depression' or 'eco-anxiety' were found to reduce the likelihood of the person taking individual action and were related to poor mental health outcomes (Stanley, Hogg, Leviston, & Walker, 2021).

The various indicators of environmental quality and its contribution to human wellbeing support the frameworks proposed by Costanza, de Groot, et al. (2014) and also that of Stoeckl et al. (2021). Not only does the environment itself contribute to wellbeing, but being actively involved in conservation/stewardship activities also contributes to wellbeing. Similarly, protests against environmental degradation or activities promoting conservation also contribute to human wellbeing even if such activities result in no direct benefits to nature itself (supporting the feedback loop from stewardship activities directly to societal wellbeing).

SUMMARY

This review sought to assess the relative abilities of variables based on different proxy measures of nature to explain variations in human wellbeing. The results revealed that simple and easy-to-obtain measures such as population density (theme 1) are too broad and unfocused to provide meaningful information regarding the complex relationship between humans and the rest of nature. Hence, more specific variables are required, with variables relating to access to specific environmental goods/services (theme 2) and to more overarching measures of natural capital (theme 4) generally related to improved human wellbeing, while exposure to environmental ills (theme 3) were generally found to directly reduce human wellbeing, perhaps through a combination of health and aesthetic impacts.

The insights from this review lead to a number of policy recommendations, the adoption of which could contribute to improved human wellbeing as follows:

- *Increase access to green space.* However, important questions remain regarding by how much and how close this access needs to be (linking to further research requirements below). It seems likely that a nonlinear, 'limiting factor' formulation is needed: that is, developing indicators and models that reflect that the impact of increasing green space on wellbeing will vary depending on the green space originally available and may also need to incorporate 'tipping points' at which level further increases in green space may have little impact on wellbeing or even change the direction of impact (see Chapter 21, this volume).
- *When developing policies to promote the use and enjoyment of nature, it is important to consider the complementary built, human, and social capital requirements* in addition to (but not as a replacement for) the extent and quality of the natural capital itself.
- *Reduce pollution!* It is very clear that environmental degradation and pollution in general, and air pollution in particular, whether perceived or measured objectively, have a very clear adverse effect on human health and wellbeing.
- *Increase opportunities for people to be involved in conserving and managing the natural environment,* as these types of stewardship activities provide multiple benefits including benefitting nature, benefitting humans by improving the flow of benefits back to humans from nature, and benefitting human wellbeing directly from their stewardship activities.

Future research recommendations generated from this work include the following:

- Further exploration of the nonlinearity of relationships between the correlating factors and wellbeing—particularly of environmental goods and services—is required to improve our understanding of how improvements to the environment may enhance wellbeing. Specific questions include gaining a better understanding of how much and what quality of environmental services are sufficient to optimise wellbeing benefits
- Further exploration of methods by which the complementarity of use of natural capital with other capitals can be reflected within the LS model
- Additional research to incorporate spatial and temporal scales and variations within the models
- Give consideration to additional moderators or potentially confounding factors that could usefully be built into future research models
- Further exploration of the reciprocity between stewardship/looking after nature, improved flow of ecosystem services, and improved human wellbeing, seeking to create a sustainable human–rest of nature system encapsulated by the Australian Indigenous motto 'healthy people, healthy country'.

Extending this review to also recognise the important impacts of climate and the effects of climate change on wellbeing would also be a valuable contribution to knowledge. There has been limited research on the climate–wellbeing relationship at this stage, which has mainly focused on inter-country comparisons (such as Maddison & Rehdanz, 2011), with one study of local-level influences in Ireland (Brereton et al., 2008). In addition to the impact of climate in isolation, such research would need to recognise that the impact of climate on wellbeing can relate to enjoyment of environmental goods (theme 2); that is, climate appears to influence the way we enjoy greenspaces and natural capital assets (Brereton et al., 2008). Furthermore, climate may also have an adverse impact on wellbeing: research has already indicated the adverse consequences of extreme weather events on LS such as drought (Carroll, Frijters, & Shields, 2009), floods (Fernandez, Stoeckl, & Welters, 2019), and extreme temperatures (Frijters & Praag, 1998). Climate change is the most prominent illustration of a 'reverse ill'; that is, human action negatively impacting on natural capital. Thus further research is needed into how climate interacts with natural and other forms of capital to impact wellbeing.

APPENDIX

Table 18.A1 SUMMARY OF PUBLICATIONS INCLUDED WITHIN THE REVIEW

Publication details	Theme 1: Degree of human intervention	Theme 2: Specific environmental goods or services	Theme 3: Adverse impacts	Theme 4: Overarching measures
Aguado, González, Bellott, López-Santiago, & Montes (2018)	✔			✔
Alfonso, Zorondo-Rodríguez, & Simonetti (2017)		✔		
Ambrey & Fleming (2013)	✔	✔		
Ambrey (2016a)	✔	✔		
Ambrey (2016b)		✔		
Ambrey & Cartlidge (2017)		✔		
Ambrey & Daniels (2017)				✔
Ambrey & Fleming (2014)	✔			✔
Ambrey & Fleming (2011a)		✔		
Ambrey & Fleming (2012)	✔	✔		
Ambrey & Fleming (2011b)	✔	✔		
Ambrey, Fleming, & Chan (2014)	✔	✔	✔	
Ambrey, Fleming, & Manning (2016)				✔
Ambrey & Shahni (2017)	✔	✔		
Aoshima et al. (2018)		✔		
Apergis (2018)			✔	
Asadullah et al. (2018)	✔			
Barrington-Leigh & Behzadnejad (2017)			✔	
Beja (2012)			✔	

(continued)

Table 18.A1 CONTINUED

Publication details	Theme 1: Degree of human intervention	Theme 2: Specific environmental goods or services	Theme 3: Adverse impacts	Theme 4: Overarching measures
Bertram & Rehdanz (2015)		✔		
Bonini (2008)				✔
Bravi & Sichera (2016)				✔
Brereton et al. (2008)	✔	✔	✔	
Cuñado & de Gracia (2012)	✔	✔	✔	
Diener & Tay (2015)			✔	✔
Dolan & Laffan (2016)	✔		✔	
Dong, Nakaya, & Brunsdon (2018)			✔	
Du, Shin, & Managi (2018)			✔	
Engelbrecht (2009)				✔
Engelbrecht (2012)				✔
Ferrer-i-Carbonell & Gowdy (2007)		✔	✔	
Ferreira et al. (2013)			✔	
Ferreira & Moro (2013)	✔	✔	✔	
Ferreira & Moro (2010)	✔	✔	✔	
Fleming, Manning, & Ambrey (2016)		✔		
Gao, Weaver Scott, Fu, Jia, & Li (2017)		✔		
Giovanis & Ozdamar (2016)			✔	
Goetzke & Rave (2015)			✔	✔
Guardiola & García-Quero (2014)				✔
Inoguchi & Fujii (2009)				✔
Jarvis, Stoeckl, & Liu (2017)				✔
Jones (2017)			✔	
Knight & Rosa (2011)				✔
Kopmann & Rehdanz (2013)	✔	✔		

Table 18.A1 CONTINUED

Publication details	Theme 1: Degree of human intervention	Theme 2: Specific environmental goods or services	Theme 3: Adverse impacts	Theme 4: Overarching measures
Krekel, Kolbe, & Wüstemann (2016)		✔		
Kubiszewski, Zakariyya, & Jarvis (2019)				✔
Kubiszewski, Jarvis, & Zakariyya (2019)				✔
Larson, Jennings, & Cloutier (2016)		✔		
Levinson (2012)			✔	
Liao, Shaw, & Lin (2015)			✔	✔
Liu, Liu, Huang, & Chen (2018)			✔	
Luechinger (2009)			✔	
Ma et al. (2018)	✔	✔		
MacKerron & Mourato (2009)	✔		✔	
MacKerron & Mourato (2013)		✔		
Maddison & Rehdanz (2011)	✔	✔		
Menz (2011)	✔		✔	
Menz & Welsch (2010)	✔		✔	
Moro, Brereton, Ferreira, & Clinch (2008)	✔	✔	✔	
Morrison (2011)		✔		
Orru, Orru, Maasikmets, Hendrikson, & Ainsaar (2016)			✔	
Ozdamar (2016)			✔	
Rajani, Skianis, & Filippidis (2019)				✔
Rehdanz & Maddison (2008)			✔	

(continued)

Table 18.A1 CONTINUED

Publication details	Theme 1: Degree of human intervention	Theme 2: Specific environmental goods or services	Theme 3: Adverse impacts	Theme 4: Overarching measures
Requena (2016)	✔			
Sasaki (2018)	✔			
Smyth, Mishra, & Qian (2008)		✔	✔	✔
Smyth et al. (2011)		✔	✔	
Tandoc Jr & Takahashi (2013)				✔
Taskaya (2018)		✔	✔	
Tsurumi & Managi (2015)	✔	✔		
Vemuri & Costanza (2006)				✔
Wang & Cheng (2017)			✔	✔
Welsch (2007)			✔	
Welsch (2006)			✔	
Welsch (2002)			✔	
White, Alcock, Wheeler, & Depledge (2013)		✔		
White, Pahl, Wheeler, Depledge, & Fleming (2017)		✔		
Winters & Li (2017)	✔	✔		
Yuan, Shin, & Managi (2018)		✔	✔	
Zhang & Wang (2019)	✔		✔	
Zhang, Liu, Zhu, & Cheng (2018)			✔	
Zhang, Shi, & Cheng (2017)				✔
Zhang, Zhang, & Chen (2017a)			✔	
Zhang, Zhang, & Chen (2017b)			✔	
Zorondo-Rodríguez et al. (2016)	✔			✔

REFERENCES

Aguado, M., González, J. A., Bellott, K. S., López-Santiago, C., & Montes, C. (2018). Exploring subjective well-being and ecosystem services perception along a rural–urban gradient in the high Andes of Ecuador. *Ecosystem Services, 34*, 1–10. doi:10.1016/j.ecoser.2018.09.002

Alfonso, A., Zorondo-Rodríguez, F., & Simonetti, J. A. (2017). Perceived changes in environmental degradation and loss of ecosystem services, and their implications in human well-being. *International Journal of Sustainable Development and World Ecology, 24*(6), 561–574. doi:10.1080/13504509.2016.1255674

Ambrey, C. L. (2016a). An investigation into the synergistic wellbeing benefits of greenspace and physical activity: Moving beyond the mean. *Urban Forestry & Urban Greening, 19*, 7–12. doi:10.1016/j.ufug.2016.06.020

Ambrey, C. L. (2016b). Urban greenspace, physical activity and wellbeing: The moderating role of perceptions of neighbourhood affability and incivility. *Land Use Policy, 57*, 638–644. doi:10.1016/j.landusepol.2016.06.034

Ambrey, C. L., & Cartlidge, N. (2017). Do the psychological benefits of greenspace depend on one's personality? *Personality and Individual Differences, 116*, 233–239. doi:10.1016/j.paid.2017.05.001

Ambrey, C. L., & Daniels, P. (2017). Happiness and footprints: Assessing the relationship between individual well-being and carbon footprints. *Environment, Development and Sustainability, 19*(3), 895–920. doi:10.1007/s10668-016-9771-1

Ambrey, C. L., & Fleming, C. M. (2011a). *The influence of the natural environment and climate on life satisfaction in Australia.* https://research-repository.griffith.edu.au/bitstream/handle/10072/390463/2011-01-the-influence-of-the-natural-environment-and-climate-on-life-satisfaction-in-Australia.pdf

Ambrey, C. L., & Fleming, C. M. (2011b). Valuing scenic amenity using life satisfaction data. *Ecological Economics, 72*, 106–115. doi:10.1016/j.ecolecon.2011.09.011

Ambrey, C. L., & Fleming, C. M. (2012). Valuing Australia's protected areas: A life satisfaction approach. *New Zealand Economic Papers, 46*(3), 191–209. doi:10.1080/00779954.2012.697354

Ambrey, C. L., & Fleming, C. (2013). Public greenspace and life satisfaction in urban Australia. *Urban Studies, 51*(6), 1290–1321. doi:10.1177/0042098013494417

Ambrey, C. L., & Fleming, C. M. (2014). Valuing ecosystem diversity in South East Queensland: A life satisfaction approach. *Social Indicators Research, 115*(1), 45–65. doi:10.1007/s11205-012-0208-4

Ambrey, C. L., Fleming, C. M., & Chan, A. Y.-C. (2014). Estimating the cost of air pollution in South East Queensland: An application of the life satisfaction non-market valuation approach. *Ecological Economics, 97*, 172–181. doi:10.1016/j.ecolecon.2013.11.007

Ambrey, C. L., Fleming, C. M., & Manning, M. (2016). The role of natural capital in supporting national income and social welfare. *Applied Economics Letters, 23*(10), 723–727. doi:10.1080/13504851.2015.1102839

Ambrey, C. L., & Shahni, T. J. (2017). Greenspace and wellbeing in Tehran: A relationship conditional on a neighbourhood's crime rate? *Urban Forestry & Urban Greening, 27*, 155–161. doi:10.1016/j.ufug.2017.08.003

Aoshima, I., Uchida, K., Ushimaru, A., & Sato, M. (2018). The influence of subjective perceptions on the valuation of green spaces in Japanese urban areas. *Urban Forestry & Urban Greening, 34,* 166–174. doi:10.1016/j.ufug.2018.06.018

Apergis, N. (2018). The impact of greenhouse gas emissions on personal well-being: Evidence from a panel of 58 countries and aggregate and regional country samples. *Journal of Happiness Studies, 19*(1), 69–80. doi:10.1007/s10902-016-9809-y

Asadullah, M. N., Xiao, S., & Yeoh, E. (2018). Subjective well-being in China, 2005–2010: The role of relative income, gender, and location. *China Economic Review, 48,* 83–101. doi:10.1016/j.chieco.2015.12.010

Barrington-Leigh, C., & Behzadnejad, F. (2017). Evaluating the short-term cost of low-level local air pollution: A life satisfaction approach. *Environmental Economics and Policy Studies, 19*(2), 269–298. doi:10.1007/s10018-016-0152-7

Beja, E. L. (2012). Subjective well-being approach to environmental valuation: Evidence for greenhouse gas emissions. *Social Indicators Research, 109*(2), 243–266. doi:10.1007/s11205-011-9899-1

Bertram, C., & Rehdanz, K. (2015). The role of urban green space for human well-being. *Ecological Economics, 120,* 139–152. doi:10.1016/j.ecolecon.2015.10.013

Black, W., & Living, R. (2004). Volunteerism as an occupation and its relationship to health and wellbeing. *British Journal of Occupational Therapy, 67*(12), 526–532. doi:10.1177/030802260406701202

Bonini, A. N. (2008). Cross-national variation in individual life satisfaction: Effects of national wealth, human development, and environmental conditions. *Social Indicators Research, 87*(2), 223–236. doi:10.1007/s11205-007-9167-6

Bravi, M., & Sichera, M. (2016). Valuing environmental and social quality impacts on subjective well-being. *Aestimum, 68,* 5. doi:10.13128/Aestimum-18722

Brereton, F., Clinch, J. P., & Ferreira, S. (2008). Happiness, geography, and the environment. *Ecological Economics, 65*(2), 386–396. doi:10.1016/j.ecolecon.2007.07.008

Britton, E., Kindermann, G., Domegan, C., & Carlin, C. (2020). Blue care: A systematic review of blue space interventions for health and wellbeing. *Health Promotion International, 35*(1), 50–69. doi:10.1093/heapro/day103

Carroll, N., Frijters, P., & Shields, M. A. (2009). Quantifying the costs of drought: New evidence from life satisfaction data. *Journal of Population Economics, 22*(2), 445–461. doi:10.1007/s00148-007-0174-3

Choi, N. G., & Kim, J. (2011). The effect of time volunteering and charitable donations in later life on psychological wellbeing. *Ageing and Society, 31*(4), 590–610. doi:10.1017/S0144686X10001224

Costanza, R., de Groot, R., Braat, L., Kubiszewski, I., Fioramonti, L., Sutton, P., . . . Grasso, M. (2017). Twenty years of ecosystem services: How far have we come and how far do we still need to go? *Ecosystem Services, 28,* 1–16. doi:10.1016/j.ecoser.2017.09.008

Costanza, R., de Groot, R., Sutton, P., van der Ploeg, S., Anderson, S. J., Kubiszewski, I., . . . Turner, R. K. (2014). Changes in the global value of ecosystem services. *Global Environmental Change, 26,* 152–158. doi:10.1016/j.gloenvcha.2014.04.002

Costanza, R., Kubiszewski, I., Giovannini, E., Lovins, H., McGlade, J., Pickett, K. E., . . . Wilkinson, R. (2014). Time to leave GDP behind. *Nature, 505*(7483), 283–285.

Cummins, R. A. (1996). The domains of life satisfaction: An attempt to order chaos. *Social Indicators Research, 38*(3), 303–328. doi:10.1007/BF00292050

Cummins, R. A. (2000). Objective and subjective quality of life: An interactive model. *Social Indicators Research, 52*(1), 55–72.

Cuñado, J., & de Gracia, F. P. (2012). Environment and happiness: New evidence for Spain. *Social Indicators Research, 112*(3), 549–567. doi:10.1007/s11205-012-0038-4

Day, R. (2007). Place and the experience of air quality. *Health & Place, 13*(1), 249–260. doi:10.1016/j.healthplace.2006.01.002

Deci, E. L., & Ryan, R. M. (2008). Hedonia, eudaimonia, and well-being: An introduction. *Journal of Happiness Studies, 9*(1), 1–11. doi:10.1007/s10902-006-9018-1

De Groot, R., Fisher, B., Christie, M., Aronson, J., Braat, L., Haines-Young, R., . . . Ring, I. (2010). Integrating the ecological and economic dimensions in biodiversity and ecosystem service valuation. In P. Kumar (Ed.), *The economics of ecosystems and biodiversity (TEEB): Ecological and economic foundations* (pp. 9–40). Routledge.

Díaz, S., Demissew, S., Carabias, J., Joly, C., Lonsdale, M., Ash, N., . . . Zlatanova, D. (2015). The IPBES conceptual framework: Connecting nature and people. *Current Opinion in Environmental Sustainability, 14*, 1–16. doi:10.1016/j.cosust.2014.11.002

Diener, E., Suh, E. M., Lucas, R. E., & Smith, H. L. (1999). Subjective well-being: Three decades of progress. *Psychological Bulletin, 125*(2), 276–302. doi:10.1037/0033-2909.125.2.276

Diener, E., & Tay, L. (2015). Subjective well-being and human welfare around the world as reflected in the Gallup World Poll. *International Journal of Psychology, 50*(2), 135–149. doi:10.1002/ijop.12136

Dolan, P., & Laffan, K. (2016). Bad air days: The effects of air quality on different measures of subjective well-being. *Journal of Benefit-Cost Analysis, 7*(1), 147–195. doi:10.1017/bca.2016.7

Dolan, P., Peasgood, T., & White, M. (2008). Do we really know what makes us happy? A review of the economic literature on the factors associated with subjective well-being. *Journal of Economic Psychology, 29*(1), 94–122. doi:10.1016/j.joep.2007.09.001

Dong, G., Nakaya, T., & Brunsdon, C. (2018). Geographically weighted regression models for ordinal categorical response variables: An application to geo-referenced life satisfaction data. *Computers, Environment and Urban Systems, 70*, 35–42. doi:10.1016/j.compenvurbsys.2018.01.012

Du, G., Shin, K. J., & Managi, S. (2018). Variability in impact of air pollution on subjective well-being. *Atmospheric Environment, 183*, 175–208. doi:10.1016/j.atmosenv.2018.04.018

Easterlin, R. A. (2003). Explaining happiness. *Proceedings of the National Academy of Sciences of the United States of America, 100*(19), 11176–11183. doi:10.1073/pnas.1633144100

Engelbrecht, H. J. (2009). Natural capital, subjective well-being, and the new welfare economics of sustainability: Some evidence from cross-country regressions. *Ecological Economics, 69*(2), 380–388. doi:10.1016/j.ecolecon.2009.08.011

Engelbrecht, H.-J. (2012). Some empirics of the bivariate relationship between average subjective well-being and the sustainable wealth of nations. *Applied Economics, 44*(5), 537–554. doi:10.1080/00036846.2010.510464

Fernandez, C. J., Stoeckl, N., & Welters, R. (2019). The cost of doing nothing in the face of climate change: A case study, using the life satisfaction approach to value the tangible and intangible costs of flooding in the Philippines. *Climate and Development, 11*(9), 825–838. doi:10.1080/17565529.2019.1579697

Ferreira, S., Akay, A., Brereton, F., Cuñado, J., Martinsson, P., Moro, M., & Ningal, T. F. (2013). Life satisfaction and air quality in Europe. *Ecological Economics, 88*, 1–10.

Ferreira, S., & Moro, M. (2010). On the use of subjective well-being data for environmental valuation. *Environmental and Resource Economics, 46*(3), 249–273. doi:10.1007/s10640-009-9339-8

Ferreira, S., & Moro, M. (2013). Income and preferences for the environment: Evidence from subjective well-being data. *Environment and Planning A: Economy and Space, 45*(3), 650–667. doi:10.1068/a4540

Ferrer-i-Carbonell, A. (2012). Happiness economics. *SERIEs, 4*(1), 35–60. doi:10.1007/s13209-012-0086-7

Ferrer-i-Carbonell, A., & Gowdy, J. M. (2007). Environmental degradation and happiness. *Ecological Economics, 60*(3), 509–516. doi:10.1016/j.ecolecon.2005.12.005

Fleming, C. M., Manning, M., & Ambrey, C. L. (2016). Crime, greenspace and life satisfaction: An evaluation of the New Zealand experience. *Landscape and Urban Planning, 149*, 1–10. doi:10.1016/j.landurbplan.2015.12.014

Florida, R. (2014). The creative class and economic development. *Economic Development Quarterly.* doi:10.1177/0891242414541693

Florida, R., Mellander, C., & Rentfrow, P. J. (2013). The happiness of cities. *Regional Studies, 47*(4), 613–627. doi:10.1080/00343404.2011.589830

Frijters, P., & von Praag, B. M. S. (1998). The effects of climate on welfare and well-being in Russia. *Climatic Change, 39*(1), 61–81. doi:10.1023/A:1005347721963

Gao, J., Weaver Scott, R., Fu, H., Jia, Y., & Li, J. (2017). Relationships between neighborhood attributes and subjective well-being among the Chinese elderly: Data from Shanghai. *BioScience Trends, 11*(5), 516–523.

Garrett, J. K., White, M. P., Huang, J., Ng, S., Hui, Z., Leung, C., . . . Wong, M. C. S. (2019). Urban blue space and health and wellbeing in Hong Kong: Results from a survey of older adults. *Health Place, 55*, 100–110. doi:10.1016/j.healthplace.2018.11.003

Giovanis, E., & Ozdamar, O. (2016). Structural equation modelling and the causal effect of permanent income on life satisfaction: The case of air pollution valuation in Switzerland. *Journal of Economic Surveys, 30*(3), 430–459. doi:10.1111/joes.12163

Goetzke, F., & Rave, T. (2015). Regional air quality and happiness in Germany. *International Regional Science Review, 38*(4), 437–451. doi:10.1177/0160017615589008

Guardiola, J., & García-Quero, F. (2014). Buen vivir (living well) in Ecuador: Community and environmental satisfaction without household material prosperity? *Ecological Economics, 107*, 177–184. doi:10.1016/j.ecolecon.2014.07.032

Haines-Young, R., & Potschin, M. (2018). *Common International Classification of Ecosystem Services (CICES) V5.1 and Guidance on the application of the revised structure.* https://cices.eu/content/uploads/sites/8/2018/01/Guidance-V51-01012 018.pdf

Hartwick, J. M. (1977). Intergenerational equity and the investing of rents from exhaustible resources. *American Economic Review, 67*(5), 972–974.

Helliwell, J. F. (2003). How's life? Combining individual and national variables to explain subjective well-being. *Economic Modelling, 20*(2), 331–360. doi:10.1016/s0264-9993(02)00057-3

Hur, M., Nasar, J. L., & Chun, B. (2010). Neighborhood satisfaction, physical and perceived naturalness and openness. *Journal of Environmental Psychology, 30*(1), 52–59. doi:10.1016/j.jenvp.2009.05.005

Inglehart, R., Foa, R., Peterson, C., & Welzel, C. (2008). Development, freedom, and rising happiness: A global perspective (1981–2007). *Perspectives on Psychological Science, 3*(4), 264–285. doi:10.1111/j.1745-6924.2008.00078.x

Inoguchi, T., & Fujii, S. (2009). The quality of life in Japan: The quality of life in Confucian Asia: From physical welfare to subjective well-being. *Social Indicators Research, 92*(2), 227–262.

Jarvis, D., Stoeckl, N., & Liu, H.-B. (2017). New methods for valuing, and for identifying spatial variations, in cultural services: A case study of the Great Barrier Reef. *Ecosystem Services, 24*, 58–67. doi:10.1016/j.ecoser.2017.02.012

Johnson, W., & Krueger, R. F. (2006). How money buys happiness: Genetic and environmental processes linking finances and life satisfaction. *Journal of Personality and Social Psychology, 90*(4), 680–691. doi:10.1037/0022-3514.90.4.680

Jones, B. A. (2017). Invasive species impacts on human well-being using the Life Satisfaction Index. *Ecological Economics, 134*, 250–257. doi:10.1016/j.ecolecon.2017.01.002

Kenter, J. O. (2018). IPBES: Don't throw out the baby whilst keeping the bathwater: Put people's values central, not nature's contributions. *Ecosystem Services, 33*, 40–43. doi:10.1016/j.ecoser.2018.08.002

Knight, K. W., & Rosa, E. A. (2011). The environmental efficiency of well-being: A cross-national analysis. *Soc Sci Res, 40*(3), 931–949. doi:10.1016/j.ssresearch.2010.11.002

Kopmann, A., & Rehdanz, K. (2013). A human well-being approach for assessing the value of natural land areas. *Ecological Economics, 93*, 20–33. doi:10.1016/j.ecolecon.2013.04.014

Kothencz, G., & Blaschke, T. (2017). Urban parks: Visitors' perceptions versus spatial indicators. *Land Use Policy, 64*, 233–244. doi:10.1016/j.landusepol.2017.02.012

Krekel, C., Kolbe, J., & Wüstemann, H. (2016). The greener, the happier? The effect of urban land use on residential well-being. *Ecological Economics, 121*, 117–127. doi:10.1016/j.ecolecon.2015.11.005

Kristoffersen, I. (2010). The metrics of subjective wellbeing: Cardinality, neutrality, and additivity. *Economic Record, 86*(272), 98–123. doi:10.1111/j.1475-4932.2009.00598.x

Kubiszewski, I., Costanza, R., Franco, C., Lawn, P., Talberth, J., Jackson, T., & Aylmer, C. (2013). Beyond GDP: Measuring and achieving global genuine progress. *Ecological Economics, 93*, 57–68.

Kubiszewski, I., Jarvis, D., & Zakariyya, N. (2019). Spatial variations in contributors to life satisfaction: An Australian case study. *Ecological Economics, 164*, 106345.

Kubiszewski, I., Zakariyya, N., & Jarvis, D. (2019). Subjective wellbeing at different spatial scales for individuals satisfied and dissatisfied with life. *PeerJ, 7*, e6502–e6502. doi:10.7717/peerj.6502

Larson, L. R., Jennings, V., & Cloutier, S. A. (2016). Public parks and wellbeing in urban areas of the United States. *PLoS One, 11*(4), e0153211–e0153211. doi:10.1371/journal.pone.0153211

Larson, S., Stoeckl, N., Jarvis, D., Addison, J., Grainger, D., Watkin Lui, F., . . . Yanunijarra Aboriginal Corporation RNTBC. (2020). Indigenous land and sea management programs (ILSMPs) enhance the wellbeing of indigenous Australians. *International Journal of Environmental Research and Public Health, 17*(1), 125. doi:10.3390/ijerph17010125

Levinson, A. (2012). Valuing public goods using happiness data: The case of air quality. *Journal of Public Economics*, *96*(9–10), 869–880. doi:10.1016/j.jpubeco.2012. 06.007

Li, Q., Stoeckl, N., King, D., & Gyuris, E. (2017). Exploring the impacts of coal mining on host communities in Shanxi, China – Using subjective data. *Resources Policy*, *53*, 125–134. doi:10.1016/j.resourpol.2017.03.012

Liao, P.-S., Shaw, D., & Lin, Y.-M. (2015). Environmental quality and life satisfaction: Subjective versus objective measures of air quality. *Social Indicators Research*, *124*(2), 599–616. doi:10.1007/s11205-014-0799-z

Liu, N., Liu, R., Huang, J., & Chen, L. (2018). Pollution, happiness, and willingness to pay taxes: The value effect of public environmental policies. *Problemy Ekorozwoju*, *13*(1), 75–86.

Luechinger, S. (2009). Valuing air quality using the life satisfaction approach. *The Economic Journal*, *119*(536), 482–515. doi:10.1111/j.1468-0297.2008.02241.x

Ma, J., Dong, G., Chen, Y., & Zhang, W. (2018). Does satisfactory neighbourhood environment lead to a satisfying life? An investigation of the association between neighbourhood environment and life satisfaction in Beijing. *Cities*, *74*, 229–239.

MacKerron, G. (2012). Happiness economics from 35,000 Feet. *Journal of Economic Surveys*, *26*(4), 705–735. doi:10.1111/j.1467-6419.2010.00672.x

MacKerron, G., & Mourato, S. (2009). Life satisfaction and air quality in London. *Ecological Economics*, *68*(5), 1441–1453. doi:10.1016/j.ecolecon.2008.10.004

MacKerron, G., & Mourato, S. (2013). Happiness is greater in natural environments. *Global Environmental Change*, *23*(5), 992–1000. doi:10.1016/j.gloenvcha.2013.03.010

Maddison, D., & Rehdanz, K. (2011). The impact of climate on life satisfaction. *Ecological Economics*, *70*(12), 2437–2445. doi:10.1016/j.ecolecon.2011.07.027

Menz, T. (2011). Do people habituate to air pollution? Evidence from international life satisfaction data. *Ecological Economics*, *71*, 211–219. doi:10.1016/ j.ecolecon.2011.09.012

Menz, T., & Welsch, H. (2010). Population aging and environmental preferences in OECD countries: The case of air pollution. *Ecological Economics*, *69*(12), 2582–2589. doi:10.1016/j.ecolecon.2010.08.002

Millennium Ecosystem Assessment. (2005). *Ecosystems and human well-being: General synthesis*. Island Press.

Molsher, R., & Townsend, M. (2016). Improving wellbeing and environmental stewardship through volunteering in nature. *EcoHealth*, *13*(1), 151–155. doi:10.1007/ s10393-015-1089-1

Moro, M., Brereton, F., Ferreira, S., & Clinch, J. P. (2008). Ranking quality of life using subjective well-being data. *Ecological Economics*, *65*(3), 448–460. doi:10.1016/ j.ecolecon.2008.01.003

Morrison, P. S. (2011). Local expressions of subjective well-being: The New Zealand experience. *Regional Studies*, *45*(8), 1039–1058. doi:10.1080/00343401003792476

Organisation for Economic Co-operation and Development (OECD). (2013). *OECD guidelines on measuring subjective well-being*. https://www.oecd-ilibrary.org/docserver/9789264191655-en.pdf?expires=1636333796&id=id&accname=ocid53019 574&checksum=E4CBCE0C47519DDD1614C0BAD38705AF

Orru, K., Orru, H., Maasikmets, M., Hendrikson, R., & Ainsaar, M. (2016). Well-being and environmental quality: Does pollution affect life satisfaction? *Quality of Life Research*, *25*(3), 699–705. doi:10.1007/s11136-015-1104-6

Ozdamar, O. (2016). Exposure to air pollution and crime in the neighbourhood: Evidence from life satisfaction data in Turkey. *International Journal of Social Economics, 43*(12), 1233–1253. doi:10.1108/IJSE-01-2015-0018

Pascua, P. A., McMillen, H., Ticktin, T., Vaughan, M., & Winter, K. B. (2017). Beyond services: A process and framework to incorporate cultural, genealogical, place-based, and indigenous relationships in ecosystem service assessments. *Ecosystem Services, 26*, 465–475. doi:10.106/j.ecoser.2017.03.012

Rajani, N. B., Skianis, V., & Filippidis, F. T. (2019). Association of environmental and sociodemographic factors with life satisfaction in 27 European countries. *BMC Public Health, 19*(1), 534–538. doi:10.1186/s12889-019-6886-y

Rehdanz, K., & Maddison, D. (2008). Local environmental quality and life-satisfaction in Germany. *Ecological Economics, 64*(4), 787–797. doi:10.1016/j.ecolecon.2007.04.016

Requena, F. (2016). Rural–urban living and level of economic development as factors in subjective well-being. *Social Indicators Research, 128*(2), 693–708. doi:10.1007/s11205-015-1051-1

Sasaki, H. (2018). Do Japanese citizens move to rural areas seeking a slower life? Differences between rural and urban areas in subjective well-being. *Bio-based and Applied Economics, 7*(1), 1. doi:10.13128/BAE-24045

Sen, A. (1999). *Development as freedom.* Oxford University Press.

Smyth, R., Mishra, V., & Qian, X. (2008). The environment and well-being in urban China. *Ecological Economics, 68*(1), 547–555. doi:10.1016/j.ecolecon.2008.05.017

Smyth, R., Nielsen, I., Zhai, Q., Liu, T., Liu, Y., Tang, C., . . . Zhang, J. (2011). A study of the impact of environmental surroundings on personal well-being in urban China using a multi-item well-being indicator. *Population and Environment, 32*(4), 353–375. doi:10.1007/s11111-010-0123-z

Stanley, S. K., Hogg, T. L., Leviston, Z., & Walker, I. (2021). From anger to action: Differential impacts of eco-anxiety, eco-depression, and eco-anger on climate action and wellbeing. *Journal of Climate Change and Health, 1*, 100003.

Stoeckl, N., Farr, M., Larson, S., Adams, V. M., Kubiszewski, I., Esparon, M., & Costanza, R. (2014). A new approach to the problem of overlapping values: A case study in Australia's Great Barrier Reef. *Ecosystem Services, 10*, 61–78. Doi:10.1016/j.ecoser.2014.09.005

Stoeckl, N., Hicks, C., Farr, M., Grainger, D., Esparon, M., Thomas, J., & Larson, S. (2018). The crowding out of complex social goods. *Ecological Economics, 144*, 65–72. doi:10.1016/j.ecolecon.2017.07.021

Stoeckl, N., Jarvis, D., Larson, S., Larson, A., Grainger, D., & Ewamian Aboriginal Corporation. (2021). Australian Indigenous insights into ecosystem services: Beyond services towards connectedness: People, place and time. *Ecosystem Services, 50*, 101341. doi:10.1016/j.ecoser.2021.101341

Stutzer, A., & Frey, B. S. (2008). Stress that doesn't pay: The commuting paradox. *Scandinavian Journal of Economics, 110*(2), 339–366. doi:10.1111/j.1467-9442.2008.00542.x

Tandoc Jr, E. C., & Takahashi, B. (2013). The complex road to happiness: The influence of human development, a healthy environment and a free press. *Social Indicators Research, 113*(1), 537–550. doi:10.1007/s11205-012-0109-6

Taskaya, S. (2018). Environmental quality and well-being level in Turkey. *Environmental Science and Pollution Research International, 25*(28), 27935–27944. doi:10.1007/s11356-018-2806-4

Tsurumi, T., & Managi, S. (2015). Environmental value of green spaces in Japan: An application of the life satisfaction approach. *Ecological Economics, 120,* 1–12. doi:10.1016/j.ecolecon.2015.09.023

van Praag, B. M. S., & Baarsma, B. E. (2005). Using happiness surveys to value intangibles: The case of airport noise. *The Economic Journal, 115*(500), 224–246.

Vemuri, A. W., & Costanza, R. (2006). The role of human, social, built, and natural capital in explaining life satisfaction at the country level: Toward a National Well-Being Index (NWI). *Ecological Economics, 58*(1), 119–133.

Wang, B. Z., & Cheng, Z. (2017). Environmental perceptions, happiness and pro-environmental actions in China. *Social Indicators Research, 132*(1), 357–375. doi:10.1007/s11205-015-1218-9

Wang, E., Kang, N., & Yu, Y. (2017). Valuing urban landscape using subjective well-being data: Empirical evidence from Dalian, China. *Sustainability, 10*(2), 36. doi:10.3390/su10010036

Weir, J., Stacey, C., & Youngetob, K. (2011). *The benefits of caring for country.* Australian Institute of Aboriginal and Torres Strait Islander Studies (AIATSIS).

Welsch, H. (2002). Preferences over prosperity and pollution: Environmental valuation based on happiness surveys. *Kyklos, 55*(4), 473–494. doi:10.1111/1467-6435.00198

Welsch, H. (2006). Environment and happiness: Valuation of air pollution using life satisfaction data. *Ecological Economics, 58*(4), 801–813. doi:10.1016/j.ecolecon.2005.09.006

Welsch, H. (2007). Environmental welfare analysis: A life satisfaction approach. *Ecological Economics, 62*(3-4), 544–551. doi:10.1016/j.ecolecon.2006.07.017

Welsch, H., & Kühling, J. (2009). Using happiness data for environmental valuation: Issues and applications. *Journal of Economic Surveys, 23*(2), 385–406. doi:10.1111/j.1467-6419.2008.00566.x

Wheaton, B., Waiti, J., Cosgriff, M., & Burrows, L. (2020). Coastal blue space and wellbeing research: Looking beyond western tides. *Leisure Studies, 39*(1), 83–95. doi:10.1080/02614367.2019.1640774

White, M. P., Alcock, I., Wheeler, B. W., & Depledge, M. H. (2013). Would you be happier living in a greener urban area? A fixed-effects analysis of panel data. *Psychological Science, 24*(6), 920–928. doi:10.1177/0956797612464659

White, M. P., Pahl, S., Wheeler, B. W., Depledge, M. H., & Fleming, L. E. (2017). Natural environments and subjective wellbeing: Different types of exposure are associated with different aspects of wellbeing. *Health & Place, 45,* 77–84. doi:10.1016/j.healthplace.2017.03.008

Winters, J. V., & Li, Y. (2017). Urbanisation, natural amenities and subjective well-being: Evidence from US counties. *Urban Studies, 54*(8), 1956–1973. doi:10.1177/0042098016631918

Yuan, L., Shin, K., & Managi, S. (2018). Subjective well-being and environmental quality: The impact of air pollution and green coverage in China. *Ecological Economics, 153,* 124–138. doi:10.1016/j.ecolecon.2018.04.033

Zhang, P., & Wang, Z. (2019). PM2.5 concentrations and subjective well-being: Longitudinal evidence from aggregated panel data from Chinese provinces. *International Journal of Environmental Research and Public Health, 16*(7), 1129. doi:10.3390/ijerph16071129

Zhang, S., Liu, B., Zhu, D., & Cheng, M. (2018). Explaining individual subjective well-being of urban China based on the four-capital model. *Sustainability, 10*(10), 3480. doi:10.3390/su10103480

Zhang, S., Shi, Q., & Cheng, M. (2017). Renewable natural capital, the biocapacity, and subjective well-being. *Journal of Cleaner Production, 150,* 277–286. doi:10.1016/j.jclepro.2017.03.021

Zhang, X., Zhang, X., & Chen, X. (2017a). Happiness in the air: How does a dirty sky affect mental health and subjective well-being? *Journal of Environmental Economics and Management, 85,* 81–94. doi:10.1016/j.jeem.2017.04.001

Zhang, X., Zhang, X., & Chen, X. (2017b). Valuing air quality using happiness data: The case of China. *Ecological Economics, 137,* 29–36. doi:10.1016/j.ecolecon.2017.02.020

Zorondo-Rodríguez, F., Grau-Satorras, M., Kalla, J., Demps, K., Gómez-Baggethun, E., García, C., & Reyes-García, V. (2016). Contribution of natural and economic capital to subjective well-being: Empirical evidence from a small-scale society in Kodagu (Karnataka), India. *Social Indicators Research, 127*(2), 919–937. doi:10.1007/s11205-015-0975-9

An Integrated Approach to Health and Wellbeing in Response to Climate Change

SOTIRIS VARDOULAKIS AND HILARY BAMBRICK ■

INTRODUCTION

Climate change—from intensified and more frequent extreme weather to long-term geographic and seasonal shifts in temperature and rainfall—caused by the emission of greenhouse gasses from the burning of fossil fuels and other sources is detrimental to our health and wellbeing. We begin this chapter by describing the range of primary, secondary, and tertiary adverse health effects of climate change, as well as highlighting how these impacts are unevenly distributed, with poorer nations and people disproportionately affected. We go on to present a series of cases studies from around the world to illustrate these diverse and substantial deleterious consequences. Because some level of climate change is already occurring and will continue for some decades even with urgent action to reduce fossil fuel use, adaptation to protect health from its worst effects is now essential. In our final section, we therefore offer suggestions for protecting and improving health and wellbeing in a climate-changing world. We demonstrate how reducing greenhouse gas emissions and adapting to climate change can bring multiple benefits to health and wellbeing from improved air quality in cities, healthier diets, and more sustainable healthcare, transport, and housing conditions.

IMPACTS OF CLIMATE CHANGE ON WELLBEING

'Climate change' encompasses all the consequences of planetary warming, the rise in mean global temperatures caused primarily by the emission of greenhouse gasses from our burning of fossil fuels (coal, oil, and gas) and the loss of forests. The Earth has warmed, on average, by 1.10°C so far above pre-industrial levels (Intergovernmental Panel on Climate Change [IPCC], 2021); parts of the world are warming at a more rapid rate than others. The oceans are absorbing a lot of the excess heat and carbon dioxide (the primary greenhouse gas), and large landmasses, such as Australia, have warmed more than the global average, having reached a 1.44°C increase in average temperatures since Australian weather records began in 1910 (Commonwealth Scientific and Industrial Research Organisation [CSIRO] and the Australian Government Bureau of Meteorology, 2020). The increase in average temperatures means a shift in the distribution of weather and a pushing out of extremes. The Arctic, for example, also warming twice as fast as the global average, has just had two consecutive summers where temperatures reached more than 30°C above average (https://arcticwwf.org/work/climate/).

Not just temperatures are becoming more extreme, but also other weather events such as heavy rainfall and severe storms. There is now more energy in the Earth system, and a warmer atmosphere can hold more water, so the weather has become extreme across a number of fronts (IPCC, 2021).

'Health' in this chapter invokes the definition from the World Health Organization (WHO, 2020): that is, a state of 'complete physical, mental and social wellbeing and not merely the absence of disease or infirmity' and that good health is a right of all people. The WHO also note that the distribution of good health may be inequitable between countries, but that good health is an underlying requirement of peace and security, is something that requires work and cooperation, and is of benefit to everyone. The healthy development of children is seen as fundamental, as is the provision of health education to all.

Climate change is detrimental to human health and wellbeing in multiple ways, including challenging the principles of equity and healthy child development, relating to both the changes in averages and the increasing extremes. The impacts of climate change on human health and wellbeing can be described as falling into three types: primary, or the most direct impacts, as when a heatwave causes people to become sick; secondary, which are less direct and mediated by their impact on environmental factors, as when a drought causes crops to fail and consequently a food shortage; and tertiary impacts on health, which are more complex and more diffuse, such as trauma and population displacement resulting from a conflict over resources made scarce by the changing climate (Butler & Harley, 2010).

Primary (Direct) Impacts

Extreme weather events, such as heatwaves, floods, droughts, storms, and wildfires, directly affect our wellbeing, and their effects can be short and/or long term. Short-term impacts may be as catastrophic as the direct loss of life, onset or exacerbation of serious illness, or loss property and livelihood (IPCC, 2012).

Heatwaves (i.e., periods of hot weather that last several days) are detrimental to our health and wellbeing. From 1998 to 2017, more than 166,000 people died due to heatwaves worldwide, including more than 70,000 who died during the 2003 heatwave in Europe (WHO, 2021a). These health effects are exacerbated by the *urban heat island effect* in cities, which are hotter than surrounding less built-up areas (Heaviside, Macintyre, & Vardoulakis, 2017). Extreme heat damages physical and mental health and wellbeing in many ways. It increases respiratory and cardiovascular problems and diminishes quality of sleep and emotional wellbeing. Droughts, which often coincide with periods of hot weather, have been shown to substantially increase the incidence of suicide in rural populations, particularly among male farmers and their families (Hanigan, Butler, Kokic, & Hutchinson, 2012). The risk of wildfires increases in extremely dry and hot conditions, weather that is becoming more frequent and prolonged with climate change. Wildfires and volcanic activities directly affected 6.2 million people between 1998 and 2017, with 2,400 additional deaths worldwide from suffocation, injuries, and burns (WHO, 2021b), and with many more deaths attributed to poor air quality over larger areas affected by these events (Vardoulakis, Marks, & Abramson, 2020). Wildfires affect animals and crops and disrupt transportation, communications, power and gas services, and water supply. Wildfires also have a significant effect on mental health and psychosocial wellbeing in the communities affected (Rodney et al., 2021).

Floods are common extreme events, affecting more than 2 billion people worldwide between 1998 and 2017 (WHO, 2021c). They are caused by rivers exceeding capacity due to heavy rain or snow melt, overflowing dams, or by storm surges, tropical cyclones/hurricanes, and tsunamis affecting coastal areas. In many parts of the world, the frequency and severity of floods is increasing due to climate change and other factors (Tabari, 2020). Floods can cause direct injury and loss of life due to drowning as well as due to electrocution and carbon monoxide poisoning during drying up operations. Floods have also been linked to diarrheal and vector-borne diseases, such as malaria, particularly in low-income countries (Ahern et al., 2005). Although more difficult to quantify, it is believed that the longer-term effects of floods on mental health and wellbeing are substantial, including common mental health symptoms (anxiety, depression, irritability, and sleeplessness) and posttraumatic stress disorder (Fernandez et al., 2015). The longer-term mental health effects of extreme events—and their broader consequences for social and workplace participation and productivity—are likely to be severely underestimated.

Secondary (Environmentally Mediated) Impacts

Climate change interacts with environmental pollutants and allergens in the air in multiple ways. Increasing temperatures can alter atmospheric circulation patterns, emissions, and reaction rates of chemicals, which in turn affect the distribution of certain harmful air pollutants such as ground-level ozone (i.e., ozone close to the Earth's surface), fine particles, and a range of volatile organic compounds (Kinney, 2018). Wildfires generate huge quantities of smoke that can travel long distances and affect air quality in major population centres. As mentioned previously, wildfires are becoming more frequent and intense in most part of the world (Xu et al., 2020). Air pollutants, such as fine particles and ozone, can exacerbate a range of health conditions, including respiratory and cardiovascular problems. Exposure over many years to high levels of wood smoke or certain volatile organic compounds such as benzene and formaldehyde increases the risk of cancer. Air pollutants and aeroallergens can also trigger asthma attacks and allergic rhinitis (i.e., hay fever), affecting the wellbeing and quality of life of a large proportion of the global population (Baldacci et al., 2015).

Changes in the climate affect vegetation in many complex ways. Higher temperatures and carbon dioxide levels in the atmosphere may promote certain invasive vegetation species, like ragweed in Europe, which release large quantities of pollen (Rasmussen, Thyrring, Muscarella, & Borchsenius, 2017). It has been suggested that climate change may result in earlier and more prolonged pollen seasons, which would in turn deteriorate respiratory health and wellbeing, especially in asthma and allergy sufferers (Beggs & Bambrick, 2005).

Climate change is also likely to increase the occurrence of weather conditions (i.e., wet winters, warmer springs, and hot summers) in temperate regions that cause thunderstorms, which can put people with pollen allergies at risk of 'thunderstorm asthma' (Shamji & Boyle, 2021). Thunderstorm asthma can happen when there is a lot of pollen in the air and the weather is hot, dry, windy, and stormy. In November 2016, Melbourne, Australia experienced the world's largest epidemic thunderstorm asthma event, which resulted in 3,365 additional respiratory-related presentations to emergency departments, 476 excess asthma-related admissions to hospital, and 10 fatalities (Thien et al., 2018).

Climate change is affecting the safety and supply of food and water in many parts of the world, through both increases in temperatures and changes in rainfall patterns (IPCC, 2020). Too little or too much rain, or rain at the wrong time, can damage crops and reduce yields, while warmer temperatures mean that some crops are no longer viable where they previously flourished. Pome fruits (e.g., apples and pears), for example, require a period of cool minimum temperatures in order to produce fruit (Thomson, McCaskill, Goodwin, Kearney, & Lolicato, 2014). It is not just the overall amount of rain, but the intensity that matters as well. Cyclones and severe storms cause damage to staple and cash crops, such as Cyclone Winston destroying half of Tonga's food crops in 2016, or Cyclone Debbie destroying winter vegetable crops in Australia in 2017. The intensity of such events is increasing with climate change. Globally, regions that are already marginal for growing food, for example, are likely to become increasingly at risk of crop failure. Kummu, Heino, Taka, Varis, and Viviroli (2021) estimate that unchecked greenhouse gas emissions will render nearly a third of productive land 'unsafe' for crop and livestock production.

Both drought and flooding risk water supplies. Drought reduces both overall supply and quality by increasing the concentration of pathogens. Too much rain can wash contaminants into the catchment, and floods can damage supply infrastructure. Changes to rainfall patterns with climate change are less certain than trends in warming, but increases in extremes are likely. Even in areas with an overall drying trend, such as eastern Australia, the intensity of rainfall when it does occur will be increased. The trend toward increasing intensity of rainfall events associated with warmer global temperatures has been apparent for a number of years (Lehman, Coumou, & Frieler, 2015).

Climate change is one of many factors affecting the global distribution of infectious diseases, in addition to causing changes in agriculture and farming practices, urbanisation, deforestation, and loss of biodiversity. Many infectious diseases, including vector-, water-, and food-borne diseases, are sensitive to weather and climatic changes (Wu, Lu, Zhou, Chen, & Xu, 2016). The effect on vector-borne diseases such as malaria and dengue fever is mainly due to the expansion of areas infested with mosquitoes and related changes in their number and feeding activity that increase the intensity of transmission. Mosquitos and other infectious disease vectors, such as ticks, operate within a range of optimal climatic conditions, including temperature and rainfall, which are affected by climate change (Rocklov & Dubrow, 2020). Malaria and dengue have a large impact on population health and wellbeing mainly in low- and middle-income countries. Lyme disease is the most common vector-borne disease affecting humans in high-income countries in the temperate Northern Hemisphere (Caminade, McIntyre, & Jones, 2019).

Temperature and rainfall also influence the survival and dissemination of water- and food-borne pathogens. Unsafe water used for drinking and for the cleaning and processing of food is a key risk factors contributing to water- and food-borne diseases (i.e., diarrheal diseases) mainly affecting young children in Africa and Asia (Cissé, 2019). In addition to infectious diseases, the transport of chemicals, such as heavy metals and organic compounds, in the environment is affected by floods and droughts. These extreme events are becoming more frequent and intense in many parts of the world because of climate change, thus increasing the risk of water, soil, and food contamination.

Sea level rise, with its associated coastal erosion, salination, and flooding, is one of the most pressing climate-related issues for coastal communities, particularly in small island developing states in the Pacific and elsewhere (McIver et al., 2016). The distress associated with recurrent flooding and related environmental impacts can significantly affect individual and community behaviour and wellbeing. The prospect of forced migration to other islands and countries due to climate change and sea level rise can raise fears of having to abandon land, culture, and customs, and this fear is a source of mental stress. Sea level rise also poses a risk to infrastructure, estuaries, wetlands, coral reefs, and beaches in larger, wealthy countries such as Australia and the United States, directly and indirectly affecting the physical and mental health and wellbeing of coastal communities.

Tertiary (Complex and Diffuse) Impacts

As climate change threatens resources such as land, water, and food, conflicts arising from increasing scarcity are likely, alongside population displacement and forced migration (Balsari, Dresser, & Leaning, 2020). Reduced productivity means a decline in incomes and loss of livelihoods, particularly in areas that are already marginal for agriculture; hence, climate change acts directly against the alleviation of poverty worldwide. It is these types of complex, diffuse, downstream effects of climate change that disrupt whole human systems that will conceivably bring the heaviest burden to human health and wellbeing (Bowles, Butler, & Friel, 2014). These are also the impacts that are least amenable to lending themselves to quantified projections for the future and also the least readily measured as they unfold in the present.

Climate change is also driving species loss. Geographic and seasonal boundaries are shifting, narrowing, or even abolishing the ecological niches in which certain species thrive (Bellard, Bertelsmeier, Leadley, Thuiller, & Courchamp, 2012). Mobile species may be able to keep up with the changing parameters, but other species on which they depend (i.e., plants) may not. Human health depends on a healthy, biodiverse environment, but climate change is threatening the existence of species. Aside from the ecosystem services that biodiverse environments provide, such as keeping water catchments healthy, mere exposure to a biodiverse environment and engagement with green space keeps people healthy through reduced cardiovascular risk factors and improved immune function (Rook, 2013; Roslund et al., 2020) and better mental health (Aerts, Honnay, & Van Nieuwenhuyse, 2018). Many medical therapies, such as the anti-inflammatory aspirin and antimalarial quinine, are also derived from nature. Humans have described perhaps less than 10% of the Earth's larger species (Chivian & Bernstein, 2004) and an even tinier proportion of microbial species, and so we are losing species that are still unknown, thus limiting our potential to discover new therapeutic compounds.

Extreme events associated with climate change, such as floods, droughts, heatwaves, and wildfires, have all been linked to deteriorating mental and emotional health and wellbeing in those affected. These effects, which encompass distress symptoms, suicide rates, and clinical disorders (depression, anxiety, sleep disturbances, and post-traumatic stress disorder), can be immediate or delayed and even affect proximal populations not directly exposed (Cianconi, Betrò, & Janiri, 2020). They affect people and communities in different ways depending on their geographic location, occupation, and access to resources, information, and protection. Certain communities and occupations are typically at higher risk, for example farmers, outdoor workers, and coastal communities, which may experience loss of income and displacement. Young children, the elderly, minority groups, those with existing illness or disability, and in general population groups with less ability to take protective action and adapt (e.g., because of their socioeconomic status) are at higher risk of experiencing psychological effects.

In addition to extreme events, a range of other consequences of environmental and climate change that occur more slowly (e.g., sea level rise, deforestation, desertification, and increasing average temperatures) can cause distress. Landscape modification in particular may cause a profound sense of detachment from a familiar 'home' environment, a sense of distress that has been termed 'solastalgia' (Albrecht et al., 2007). This tends to be more powerful for First Nations, such as the Maori communities of New Zealand and the Aboriginal and Torres Strait Islander communities of Australia, due to their strong connection with Country (Middleton, Cunsolo, Jones-Bitton, Wright, & Harper, 2020). There is generally a dearth of information about the health consequences of climate change and related mitigation policies for First Nations. Much of the evidence that currently exists is from Western perspectives, which has serious limitations in relation to Indigenous health (Jones, Macmillan, & Reid, 2020).

Inequities in Climate Risks to Health and Wellbeing

Climate change does not affect the health and wellbeing of people equally. Wealthy countries are able to provide more of a socioeconomic buffer to their populations than poorer countries (e.g., they have more buying power for importing food and reliable electricity supply for keeping buildings cool) and poorer countries often have less favourable climates for food production even without the added uncertainty and extremes arising from climate change. These inequities also play out within countries, with wealthier and more socially advantaged people having more resources available to deal with the challenges of climate change. For example, in an extreme event, those who have the means to avoid exposure to the event (e.g., easier access to transport and alternative places to stay) will be more likely to survive. For example, during hot conditions socially disadvantaged groups are less able to avoid extreme heat exposure by using air-conditioning or accessing cool spaces (Hansen et al., 2011). In Australia, people in remote Indigenous communities often rely on expensive and non-renewable electricity generation methods, such as diesel generators. Characteristics that contribute to relative disadvantage when it comes to avoiding the worst of climate change include being elderly, disabled, or with chronic illness; having a job that involves exposure to climate risks (e.g., being an outdoor or factory worker without air-conditioning); living in poor-quality housing or being homeless; being Indigenous or from a minority group; and, worldwide—given the weighted distribution of poverty and marginalisation—being female.

    Gender plays a part in susceptibility to climate risks due to differential poverty, social status, and activities affecting exposure, particularly in low-income countries. Women are overrepresented among the world's poor (poverty increases risk), have lower social status (reduced access to education and resources that might be protective, including, e.g., the ability to swim in a flood or access warning information), and have domestic and carer responsibilities that increase risks to health and wellbeing, such as collecting water and fuel wood or working in fields where disease-carrying mosquitoes may be present.

CASE STUDIES

Here we discuss contrasting examples of climate change–related health risks affecting countries or regions around the world and the implications for the wellbeing of their populations.

Pacific Islands

Climate change poses an existential risk to many low-lying small island developing states in the Pacific Ocean. Nearly all Pacific islanders are vulnerable to sea-level rise that can cause flooding that threatens life and destroys houses, crops, and infrastructure (McIver et al., 2016). Low-lying coral atolls and reef islands, such as Kiribati, Marshall Islands, and Tuvalu, with less than 2 metres average elevation above sea level, are among the most vulnerable nations in the world to climate change. For example, the Republic of Marshall Islands, with 24 inhabited, mostly remote atolls and islands, is exposed to a variety of climate-related risks, including recurrent coastal flooding, tropical storms, and droughts. Climate change impacts in the Marshall Islands are exacerbated by underlying vulnerabilities, including high levels of poverty, limited freshwater resources, and the majority of the population living in coastal areas (Nurse et al., 2014). In Kiribati, some villages already flood during 'king tides', and efforts are being made to protect freshwater wells (Cauchi, Moncada, Bambrick, & Correa-Velez, 2021).

In general, climate change–related risks are particularly serious for Pacific islanders because of their typically limited financial resources; geographic isolation and minimal diversity in local food sources; high incidence of vector-borne diseases, including dengue outbreaks in many islands; and high prevalence of chronic health conditions such as obesity and diabetes. Despite these limitations—or perhaps in recognition of them—Pacific Islands are at the global forefront of adaptation planning to protect the health and wellbeing of their populations.

Australian Bushfires

There is increasing consensus that climate change was the underlying cause of the prolonged dry and hot conditions that led to the unprecedented bushfires in eastern Australian during the 'Black Summer' of 2019–2020 (Vardoulakis et al., 2020). The fires burned 20 times more land than in an average summer, directly caused 33 deaths, destroyed around 3,000 homes, and killed or displaced an estimated 3 billion animals. Millions of Australians were exposed to hazardous bushfire smoke that blanketed Sydney, Brisbane, Canberra, and Melbourne, with more than 400 deaths attributed to the smoke (Borchers Arriagada et al., 2020). Ash and toxic runoff from fire-affected areas had an impact on aquatic life, drinking water quality, and agricultural industries (Robinne et al., 2021).

The Australian Black Summer fires were not a single or rare one-off event. Many other regions around the world, including California, Southern Europe, Southeast Asia, and the Amazon, have also been affected by catastrophic wildfires which have caused many deaths and massive destruction of infrastructure and ecosystems in recent years. We should be prepared for more frequent and intense wildfire events under climate change conditions. Land use planning and forest management are important for reducing fuel load and protecting populations (Bowman et al., 2013), but tackling climate change is essential for reducing the long-term risk of wildfires in Australia and around the world.

Torres Strait Islands, Australia

Torres Strait Islands at the tip of Australia's Cape York are especially vulnerable to climate change, having a tropical monsoon climate and rainfall variability that is set to increase. The remoteness of the communities in Torres Strait already contribute to challenges in health service delivery, and the islands have a high burden of chronic illness such as diabetes and cardiovascular disease. Underlying health conditions such as these increase vulnerability to heat-related illness, which will become more of a concern as the temperatures rise, especially because higher temperatures occur with high humidity. When humidity is high, our bodies accumulate heat more easily because there is no evaporative cooling occurring with sweating. This puts people in the islands at high risk of heat rash, heat exhaustion, stroke, and heart attacks. Other climate-associated health challenges in Torres Strait include increased potential for vector-borne disease, including dengue and malaria (endemic in nearby Papua New Guinea), a shortage of safe drinking water, reduced coastal and ocean productivity threatening seafood sources, psychological distress relating to sea level rise, loss of resources and cultural heritage, and population displacement (Hall, Barnes, Canuto, Nona, & Redmond, 2021; Halls & Crosby, 2020).

European Heatwaves

One of the most devastating manifestations of climate change was the European heatwave of the summer of 2003, which caused more than 70,000 additional deaths across Europe (Robine et al., 2008). Many of these deaths were in elderly people living in large cities of France and other European countries, where urban heat islands, overheating of residential apartments, and weak social support networks exacerbated the impact of the heatwave. This extremely high impact on mortality resulted in adaptation action, with several European countries developing operational heatwave plans aiming to minimise health risks associated with heat. However, it should be noted that most studies focusing on the health effects of heat and heatwaves come from Europe and North America, with far fewer studies conducted in other world regions (e.g., South and Southeast Asia), which are likely to be significantly affected (Campbell, Remenyi, White, & Johnston, 2018).

PROTECTING AND IMPROVING HEALTH AND WELLBEING IN A CLIMATE-CHANGING WORLD

There is clearly an urgent need for policy action to protect physical and mental health from climate change. Well-designed policies aimed at reducing greenhouse gas emissions from different sectors (e.g., power generation, industry, transport, agriculture, and buildings) and improving the climate resilience of our infrastructure and services will bring multiple health benefits (Gao et al., 2018). In this section we provide some examples.

Housing

Most of us spend the majority of our time indoors, mainly in our homes, workplaces, and schools. Therefore, the interaction between climate change and the built environment is particularly important for our health (see also Chapter 20, this volume). Building structures are primarily intended to provide shelter and enhance wellbeing, but they are also associated with a range of health hazards such as indoor air pollution, heat and cold, mould, and respiratory infectious diseases (e.g., tuberculosis and COVID-19). These are influenced by climatic conditions and the way we adapt to them, for example, through building ventilation, heating and cooling, and insulation.

Measures aimed at reducing greenhouse gas emissions in the built environment (e.g., by improving insulation) have the potential to reduce health impacts and improve wellbeing through improved thermal comfort and indoor air quality. Increased airtightness of dwellings reduces energy losses and infiltration of smoke from wildfires and other outdoor sources, but it can increase levels of indoor pollutants, such as tobacco smoke, radon, and carbon monoxide in certain cases, so that adequate ventilation needs to be provided (Vardoulakis et al., 2015).

Climate change typically has a disproportionate impact on poorer households, which may not have the means to adapt to higher temperatures or take protective action against wildfire smoke, for example, by installing cooling and filtration systems and better doors and windows.

Transport

In addition to buildings, another form of infrastructure that can be adversely affected by climate change is transport in cities, particularly in rural areas and in coastal areas prone to flooding (Younger, Morrow-Almeida, Vindigni, & Dannenberg, 2008). Extreme heat can also cause road and railway buckling, pavement cracking, and potholes.

Transport and access to services are essential to our health and wellbeing. Land use planning and urban form strongly influence transport accessibility and use and, consequently, our health and wellbeing. In most places around the world, motorised transport—including public transport—still depends heavily on fossil fuels and thus contributes substantially to greenhouse gas emissions. Active travel (i.e., walking and cycling) not only reduces emissions of greenhouse gasses and other air pollutants, but also provides substantial health benefits in relation to improved physical activity, community cohesion, and road safety (see also Chapter 9, this volume). These multiple benefits make active travel an attractive intervention for mitigating against climate change and improving health and wellbeing.

However, unintended negative effects are also possible, such as migration of polluting sources, road injuries, or exacerbation of health inequities if the measures are not well-designed or implemented (Vardoulakis & Kinney, 2019).

Green and Blue Spaces

Protection from increasing temperatures under climate change conditions requires a range of adaptation measures at the individual, community, and population levels. These might include relatively simple behavioural adaptation measures such as wearing light clothing, avoiding outdoor activities during peak temperatures, and using air conditioning at home or work. However, increased air conditioning use will also increase energy consumption, which exacerbates climate change unless renewable energy is used. Thus, infrastructure interventions are needed to adapt to increasing temperatures in the long run, particularly in cities where the urban heat island effect exacerbates overheating. Among them, the extended use of vegetation and water features has been very popular in high-income countries, but technologies aiming to increase the albedo (i.e., reflectivity) of cities are also gaining momentum (Santamouris, 2014). Green infrastructure, such as parks and street trees, can reduce the intensity of the urban heat island effect, although their effectiveness depends on many factors including the selection of vegetation species and canopy design (Salmond et al., 2016). Reflective (or 'cool') roofs increase the albedo of cities and thus reduce ambient temperatures as well as indoor building temperatures. The combinations of vegetation, water features, and albedo enhancement in buildings and other urban surfaces (e.g., streets and pavements) can help offset projected increases in temperature and related impacts on population health and wellbeing (Vardoulakis & Kinney, 2019).

Building Community Resilience

Regardless of mitigation strategies aimed at putting the brakes on climate change, temperatures will continue to increase for some decades to come even if rapid greenhouse gas reduction strategies were put in place globally today. This means that on top of the adverse impacts that humans are already experiencing, such as those relating to extreme events, surviving and perhaps thriving in our changing climate will require us to adapt where and how we live. Healthier populations will be more resilient to the effects of climate change (e.g., extreme heat), and having adequate economic resources to hand is also protective in managing crises. For example, governments in wealthy countries, such as the United States and Australia, provided significant increases in income support to ameliorate the employment crisis arising from the COVID-19 pandemic. In Australia, this provision of what was in effect a liveable, universal basic income served to nearly eliminate poverty overnight (Australian Council of Social Service [ACOSS], 2020). People who were previously struggling to pay for housing, food, and essential medicines were suddenly not having to make a choice among these necessities. If such a basic income programme were installed permanently, underlying population health and wellbeing would greatly improve.

The built environment shapes our interactions with others, as does the provision of means for creating social capital, such as through community sports and other activities. Improved social cohesion, where people know and care for others in the community, is protective against climate-associated ill health (e.g., as people look out for their neighbours in an extreme event). Perceptions of neighbourhood safety are also protective, with fewer people dying in heatwaves in neighbourhoods that are perceived as safe since windows are opened at night to let cooler air through the house (Gronlund, 2014).

Local production of food may also protect health and wellbeing in an increasingly challenging climate, with a diversification of crops and multiple sites protecting against weather damage, while reduced transportation distance improves freshness through reduced time to table and contributes to lower emissions. Shifting toward diets that are predominantly plant-based is also healthier for people and the planet (Macdiarmid & Whybrow, 2019; see also Chapter 9, this volume).

Health systems and services will need to become well-prepared for climate change, with infrastructure that is built to appropriately climate resistant standards (e.g., against heat, fire, storms, and floods), with better planning for public health prevention (e.g., early warning systems for heat or vector-borne disease) and for dealing with the aftermath of extreme events. Much of what we can expect as impacts on health systems and services is fairly predictable and merely a matter of intensity or scale, but the thunderstorm asthma events in Melbourne have shown us that unusual or unforeseen events associated with climate can be devastating.

SUMMARY

Climate change affects our physical and mental health and wellbeing in multiple ways. From extreme weather events, to wildfires, to food and water insecurity, the consequences of climate change can be dangerous, frightening, and paralysing. The lack of sufficient action on climate change mitigation from governments globally is causing significant mental health distress ('eco-anxiety'), particularly among young people who will be living in a future climate that is increasingly hostile. While policy and practice remain largely inadequate, climate change advocacy remains imperative. Taking part in climate advocacy instils hope for the future and is shown to be beneficial for mental health (Nairn, 2019).

However, there are also reasons to be optimistic as scientific evidence, technological advancement, and societal pressure are paving the way toward a zero-carbon future. Drastic reductions in greenhouse gas emissions and equity-oriented adaptation to climate change can deliver a range of health benefits. Reduced reliance on fossil fuels for energy generation, reduced dependency on polluting private vehicles, climate-sensitive housing design, greener and more liveable cities, and healthier and more sustainable diets are all actions that are good for our health and wellbeing. Accounting for all these health benefits strengthens the case for ambitious climate change mitigation targets and adaptation plans worldwide.

REFERENCES

Aerts, R., Honnay, O., & Van Nieuwenhuyse, A. (2018). Biodiversity and human health: Mechanisms and evidence of the positive health effects of diversity in nature and green spaces. *British Medical Bulletin, 127,* 5–22.

Ahern, M., Kovats, R. S., Wilkinson, P., Few, R., & Matthies, F. (2005). Global health impacts of floods: Epidemiologic evidence. *Epidemiologic Reviews, 27*(1), 36–46. https://doi.org/10.1093/epirev/mxi004

Albrecht, G., Sartore, G-M., Connor, L., Higginbotham, N., Freeman, S., Kelly, B., . . . Pollard, G. (2007). Solastalgia: The distress caused by environmental change. *Australasian Psychiatry, 15,* S95–S98.

Australian Council of Social Service (ACOSS). (2020). *Survey shows increased jobseeker payment allowing people to eat regularly, cover rent and pay bills.* https://www.acoss.org.au/media_release/survey-shows-increased-jobseeker-payment-allowing-people-to-eat-regularly-cover-rent-and-pay-bills-2/

Baldacci, S., Maio, S., Cerrai, S., Sarno, G., Baïz, N., Simoni, M., . . . HEALS Study. (2015). Allergy and asthma: Effects of the exposure to particulate matter and biological allergens. *Respiratory Medicine, 109,* 1089–1104.

Balsari, S., Dresser, C., & Leaning, J. (2020). Climate change, migration, and civil strife. *Current Environmental Health Reports, 7,* 404–414.

Beggs, P. J., & Bambrick, H. J. (2005). Is the global rise of asthma an early impact of anthropogenic climate change? *Environmental Health Perspectives, 113,* 915–919.

Bellard, C., Bertelsmeier, C., Leadley, P., Thuiller, W., & Courchamp, F. (2012). Impacts of climate change on the future of biodiversity. *Ecology Letters, 15,* 365–377.

Borchers Arriagada, N., Palmer, A. J., Bowman, D. M., Morgan, G. G., Jalaludin, B. B., & Johnston, F. H. (2020). Unprecedented smoke-related health burden associated with the 2019–20 bushfires in eastern Australia. *Medical Journal of Australia, 213,* 282–283.

Bowles, D. C., Butler, C. D., & Friel, S. (2014). Climate change and health in earth's future. *Earth's Future, 2,* 60–67.

Bowman, D. M., Murphy, B. P., Boer, M. M., Bradstock, R. A., Cary, G. J., Cochrane, M. A., . . . Williams, R. J. (2013). Forest fire management, climate change, and the risk of catastrophic carbon losses. *Frontiers in Ecology and the Environment, 11,* 66–67.

Butler, C. D., & Harley, D. (2010). Primary, secondary, and tertiary effects of eco-climatic change: The medical response. *Postgraduate Medical Journal, 86,* 230–234.

Caminade, C., McIntyre, K. M., & Jones, A. E. (2019). Impact of recent and future climate change on vector-borne diseases. *Annals of the New York Academy of Sciences, 1436,* 157–173.

Campbell, S., Remenyi, T. A., White, C. J., & Johnston, F. H. (2018). Heatwave and health impact research: A global review. *Health & Place, 53,* 210–218.

Cauchi, J. P., Moncada, S., Bambrick, H., & Correa-Velez, I. (2021). Coping with environmental hazards and shocks in kiribati: Experiences of climate change by atoll communities in the equatorial pacific. *Environmental Development*, *37*, 100549.

Chivian, E., & Bernstein, A. S. (2004). Embedded in nature: Human health and biodiversity. *Environmental Health Perspectives*, *112*, A12–13.

Cianconi, P., Betrò, S., & Janiri, L. (2020). The impact of climate change on mental health: A systematic descriptive review. *Frontiers in Psychiatry*, *11*. https://doi.org/10.3389/fpsyt.2020.00074

Cissé, G. (2019). Food-borne and water-borne diseases under climate change in low- and middle-income countries: Further efforts needed for reducing environmental health exposure risks. *Acta Tropica*, *194*, 181–188.

Commonwealth Scientific and Industrial Research Organisation (CSIRO) and the Australian Government Bureau of Meteorology. (2020). *State of the climate 2020*. https://www.csiro.au/en/research/environmental-impacts/climate-change/state-of-the-climate

Fernandez, A., Black, J., Jones, M., Wilson, L., Salvador-Carulla, L., Astell-Burt, T., & Black, D. (2015). Flooding and mental health: A systematic mapping review. *PLoS One*, *10*, e0119929.

Gao, J., Kovats, S., Vardoulakis, S., Woodward, A., Wilkinson, P., Gu, S., . . . Liu Q. (2018). Public health co-benefits of greenhouse gas emissions reduction: A systematic review. *Science of the Total Environment*, *627*, 388–402.

Gronlund, C. J. (2014). Racial and socioeconomic disparities in heat-related health effects and their mechanisms: A review. *Current Epidemiology Reports*, *1*, 165–173.

Hall, N. L., Barnes, S., Canuto, C., Nona, F., & Redmond, A. M. (2021). Climate change and infectious diseases in Australia's Torres Strait Islands. *Australian and New Zealand Journal of Public Health*, *45*, 122–128.

Hall, N. L., & Crosby, L. (2020). Climate change impacts on health in remote indigenous communities in Australia. *International Journal of Environmental Health Research*, 1–16.

Hanigan, I. C., Butler, C. D., Kokic, P. N., & Hutchinson, M. F. (2012). Suicide and drought in New South Wales, Australia, 1970–2007. *Proceedings of the National Academy of Sciences*, *109*, 13950–13955.

Hansen, A., Bi, P., Nitschke, M., Pisaniello, D., Newbury, J., & Kitson, A. (2011). Residential air-conditioning and climate change: Voices of the vulnerable. *Health Promotion Journal of Australia*, *22*, 13–15.

Heaviside, C., Macintyre, H., & Vardoulakis, S. (2017). The urban heat island: Implications for health in a changing environment. *Current Environmental Health Reports*, *4*, 296–305.

Intergovernmental Panel on Climate Change (IPCC) (2012). *Managing the risks of extreme events and disasters to advance climate change adaptation. A special report of Working Groups I and II of the Intergovernmental Panel on Climate Change*. Cambridge University Press.

Intergovernmental Panel on Climate Change (IPCC). (2020). *Climate change and land: An IPCC special report on climate change, desertification, land degradation, sustainable land management, food security, and greenhouse gas fluxes in terrestrial ecosystems. Summary for policymakers*. IPCC.

Intergovernmental Panel on Climate Change (IPCC). (2021). Summary for policymakers. In V. Masson-Delmotte, P. Zhai, A. Pirani, S. L. Connors, C. Péan, S. Berger, . . . B.

Zhou (Eds.), *AR6 climate change 2021: The physical science basis. Contribution of Working Group I to the Sixth Assessment Report of the Intergovernmental Panel on Climate Change.* Cambridge University Press. https://www.ipcc.ch/site/assets/uplo ads/2018/11/SR1.5_SPM_Low_Res.pdf

Jones, R., Macmillan, A., & Reid, P. (2020). Climate change mitigation policies and co-impacts on indigenous health: A scoping review. *International Journal of Environmental Research and Public Health, 17,* 9063.

Kinney, P. L. (2018). Interactions of climate change, air pollution, and human health. *Current Environmental Health Reports, 5,* 179–186.

Kummu, M., Heino, M., Taka, M., Varis, O., & Viviroli, D. (2021). Climate change risks pushing one-third of global food production outside the safe climatic space. *One Earth, 4,* 720–729.

Lehman, J., Coumou, D., & Frieler, K. (2015). Increased record-breaking precipitation events under global warming. *Climatic Change, 132,* 501–515.

Macdiarmid, J. I., & Whybrow, S. (2019). Nutrition from a climate change perspective. *Proceedings of the Nutrition Society, 78,* 380–387.

McIver, L., Kim, R., Woodward, A., Hales, S., Spickett, J., Katscherian, D., . . . Ebi, K. L. (2016). Health impacts of climate change in pacific island countries: A regional assessment of vulnerabilities and adaptation priorities. *Environmental Health Perspectives 124,* 1707–1714.

Middleton, J., Cunsolo, A., Jones-Bitton, A., Wright, C. J., & Harper, S. L. (2020). Indigenous mental health in a changing climate: A systematic scoping review of the global literature. *Environmental Research Letters, 15,* 053001.

Nairn, K. (2019). Learning from young people engaged in climate activism: The potential of collectivizing despair and hope. *YOUNG, 27,* 435–450.

Nurse, L. A., McLean, R. F., Agard, J., Briguglio, L. P., Duvat-Magnan, V., Pelesikoti, N., . . . Webb, A. (2014). Small islands. In V. R. Barros, C. B. Field, D. J. Dokken, M. D. Mastrandrea, K. J. Mach, T. E. Bilir, . . . L. L. White (Eds.), *Climate change 2014: Impacts, adaptation, and vulnerability. Part b: Regional aspects. Contribution of Working Group II to the Fifth Assessment Report of the Intergovernmental Panel on Climate Change* (pp. 1613–1654). Cambridge University Press.

Rasmussen, K., Thyrring, J., Muscarella, R., & Borchsenius, F. (2017). Climate-change-induced range shifts of three allergenic ragweeds (ambrosial.) in Europe and their potential impact on human health. *PeerJ – Life & Environment, 5,* e3104.

Robine, J-M., Cheung, S. L. K., Le Roy, S., Van Oyen, H., Griffiths, C., Michel, J-P., & Herrmann, F. H. (2008). Death toll exceeded 70,000 in Europe during the summer of 2003. *Comptes Rendus Biologies, 331,* 171–178.

Robinne, F. N., Hallema, D. W., Bladon, K. D., Flannigan, M. D., Boisramé, G., Bréthaut, C. M., . . . Wei, Y. (2021). Scientists' warning on extreme wildfire risks to water supply. *Hydrological Processes, 35,* e14086.

Rocklöv, J., & Dubrow, R. (2020). Climate change: An enduring challenge for vector-borne disease prevention and control. *Nature Immunology, 21,* 479–483.

Rodney, R. M., Swaminathan, A., Calear, A. L., Christensen, B. K., Lal A., Lane J., . . . Walker I. (2021). Physical and mental health effects of bushfire and smoke in the Australian Capital Territory 2019-20. *Frontiers in Public Health, 9,* 682402.

Rook, G. A. (2013). Regulation of the immune system by biodiversity from the natural environment: An ecosystem service essential to health. *Proceedings of the National Academy of Sciences, 110,* 18360–18367.

Roslund, M. I., Puhakka, R., Gronroos, M., Nurminen, N., Oikarinen, S., Gazali, A. M., . . . ADELE Research Group. (2020). Biodiversity intervention enhances immune regulation and health-associated commensal microbiota among daycare children. *Science Advances, 6*, eaba2578.

Salmond, J. A., Tadaki, M., Vardoulakis, S., Arbuthnott, K., Coutts, A., Demuzere, M., . . . Wheeler, B. W. (2016). Health and climate related ecosystem services provided by street trees in the urban environment. *Environmental Health, 15*, S36.

Santamouris, M. (2014). Cooling the cities – A review of reflective and green roof mitigation technologies to fight heat island and improve comfort in urban environments. *Solar Energy, 103*, 682–703.

Shamji, M. H., & Boyle, R. J. (2021). What does climate change mean for people with pollen allergy? *Clinical & Experimental Allergy, 51*, 202–205.

Tabari, H. (2020). Climate change impact on flood and extreme precipitation increases with water availability. *Scientific Reports, 10*(1), 13768. https://doi.org/10.1038/s41598-020-70816-2

Thien, F., Beggs, P. J., Csutoros, D., Darvall, J., Hew, M., Davies, J. M., . . . Guest. C. (2018). The Melbourne epidemic thunderstorm asthma event 2016: An investigation of environmental triggers, effect on health services, and patient risk factors. *The Lancet Planetary Health, 2*, e255–e263.

Thomson, G., McCaskill, M., Goodwin, I., Kearney, G., & Lolicato, S. (2014). Potential impacts of rising global temperatures on Australia's pome fruit industry and adaptation strategies. *New Zealand Journal of Crop and Horticultural Science, 42*, 21–30.

Vardoulakis, S., Dimitroulopoulou, C., Thornes, J., Lai, K-M., Taylor, J., Myers, I., . . . Wilkinson, P. (2015). Impact of climate change on the domestic indoor environment and associated health risks in the UK. *Environment International, 85*, 299–313.

Vardoulakis, S., & Kinney, P. (2019). Grand Challenges in Sustainable Cities and Health. Frontiers in Sustainable Cities 1. https://www.frontiersin.org/articles/10.3389/frsc.2019.00007

Vardoulakis, S., Marks, G., & Abramson, M. J. (2020). Lessons learned from the Australian bushfires. *JAMA Internal Medicine, 180*, 635.

World Health Organization (WHO). (2020). *Constitution of the World Health Organization, WHO Basic Documents* (49th ed.). https://apps.who.int/gb/bd/

World Health Organization (WHO). (2021a). *Heatwaves.* https://www.who.int/health-topics/heatwaves#tab=tab_1

World Health Organization (WHO). (2021b). *Wildfires.* https://www.who.int/health-topics/wildfires#tab=tab_1

World Health Organization (WHO). (2021c). *Floods,* https://www.who.int/health-topics/floods#tab=tab_1

Wu, X., Lu, Y., Zhou, S., Chen, L., & Xu, B. (2016). Impact of climate change on human infectious diseases: Empirical evidence and human adaptation. *Environment International, 86*, 14–23.

Xu, R., Yu, P., Abramson, M. J., Johnston, F. H., Samet, J. M., Bell, M. L., . . . Guo, Y. (2020). Wildfires, global climate change, and human health. *New England Journal of Medicine, 383*, 2173–2181.

Younger, M., Morrow-Almeida, H. R., Vindigni, S. M., & Dannenberg, A. L. (2008). The built environment, climate change, and health. *American Journal of Preventive Medicine, 35*, 517–526.

20

Wellbeing and the Built Environment

A Case Study in the Application of Broad-Based Participatory Design

**MARGARETTE LEITE, SERGIO PALLERONI, AND
BARBARA SESTAK ■**

INTRODUCTION

It may seem shocking today to think that until the past decade or so, human wellbeing was not the stated main goal of architecture or the built environment as a whole. Client-driven programming, cost, constructability, and energy and material efficiency were the terms most commonly used to guide the decision-making around buildings and public spaces. That is not to say that designers of the built environment did not aspire to create spaces that made people feel comfortable, safe, and healthful, but that, as a goal, the term 'wellbeing' was vague and uncommon in professional circles and the way to evaluate and achieve it was subject to opinion due to lack of empirical evidence and metrics. Attempts to move the field toward a more human-centred design of the built environment linking the psychological, physical, societal, and environmental imperatives of wellbeing have come from a variety of social movements like social justice work and the sustainability movement, as well as from the realm of public health. These movements, while arising from their own specific perspectives have, over time, come to overlap in many of their basic principles and in some of their strategies. This is a positive move to be sure and one that suggests that the goals of wellbeing, however broad and difficult to define, are nonetheless gaining in acceptance and importance within the industry.

There is one particular strategy for ensuring greater accountability and, arguably, greater success in accomplishing these shared goals which, in our opinion, holds the greatest hope for success in any project that seeks to serve particular communities or the public as a whole. It is one that has emerged from the social justice perspective and public interest design. It is the implementation of multivoice, multipartner processes that ensure participation from all community members and stakeholders including, and most importantly, those typically excluded, that holds the greatest promise for achieving the goal of wellbeing in its broadest sense.

This chapter looks at the connection between goals of human wellbeing and current practices in the design of the built environment. We begin by describing the emergence of the greater use of community participatory design in the development of built environments. We then use the Oregon-based Smart Academic Green Environment (SAGE) green modular classroom as a case study project that was predicated on goals of public interest design, including an evaluation of its merits based on more recent industry-defined definitions of wellbeing as they relate to built environments.

COMMUNITY PARTICIPATORY DESIGN AND THE BUILT ENVIRONMENT

In the United States, architecture in particular and urban planning to some degree have long been driven by fee-based interactions initiated by clients of means through a serialised and intimidating process of design and construction. These processes are carried out by highly trained professionals in specialised and separated fields. In addition, they have proceeded largely outside the public eye and in ways that are not transparent to the communities they are meant to serve. The result is that 90% of humanity is not served by architects or designers.

This reality was the catalyst that spurred a series of social justice movements beginning in the 1960s to offer services to that 90% in an effort to create a more human-centred, relevant, and socially just response to communities in need. The movement created community design centres (CDCs) and design build programmes in universities around the country, like the Basic Initiative, Design Corps, and Rural Studio. These programmes leveraged student talent and labour to work with low-income communities to build housing and community service centres. The movement spurred other organisations like the nonprofit Social Economic Environmental Design (SEED) network, which encourages through award programmes and other outreach efforts design professionals, architects, planners, and builders to address the 'triple bottom line' of social, environmental, and economic goals for all built works. In addition, numerous publications by the SEED network, like *Expanding Architecture*, promote the works of architects and educators who use design as a tool to empower physically, socially, and politically underserved communities (see Gámez and Rogers [2008] for a fuller discussion of this social justice history of public interest design). These efforts have given rise to the term *public interest design* (PID), and, in the past decade, a number of universities throughout the United States have begun to offer PID certificate or degree programmes.[1]

This type of work seeks to achieve community-initiated design and construction through a participatory process that includes a multiplicity of voices. Often this process is framed as a social contract between the designers, client community, and other associated stakeholders to empower the community to act as co-producer of the built project.[2] This type of work, by necessity, must address the economic and environmental disparities suffered by marginalised communities that are most affected by environmental hazards of air and water pollution, limited infrastructure access, and a host of other maladies.

The lessons of these more inclusive design processes have begun to impact the design of public buildings in many jurisdictions across the country which are now mandating community participatory design processes as a requirement for all building approvals. This is clearly an important step in recognising the value that users of these built spaces, and other often forgotten stakeholders, bring to the table, one that is generally filled with professionals far removed from the eventual use and impact of the proposed work. These kinds of engagement follow various processes and modes of participation, and many are truly genuine and successful. Many others, however, see the requirement as a hindrance to timeliness and efficiency and as a box they simply need to check. It is our opinion that by highlighting the advances in multivoice processes and co-authored buildings and urban designs, the advantages and obvious benefits of these endeavours can begin to redefine the industry as a whole.

SUSTAINABILITY AND THE BUILT ENVIRONMENT

In recent decades, concern regarding the impact that the construction and maintenance of our built environments has unleashed on the climate and other natural systems of our planet has bolstered a worldwide conversation around sustainability. These conversations have led to the development of metrics for evaluating the impacts buildings have, resulting in an ever-increasing number of rating systems that encourage, and, in some cases, depending on building type and jurisdiction, require specific action in this realm.

In their nascence, rating systems such as Leadership in Energy and Environmental Design (LEED) were focused on the environmental aspects

1. The authors' own professional programme in architecture offers a graduate certificate in PID through its Center for Public Interest Design (www.centerforpublicinterestdesign.org). Although the first such degree was offered in 2016, the growth in the field has meant that now more than 40 universities offer a similar degree programme in the United States.

2. See the SEED Evaluator, which supports architects, developers, client communities, and stakeholders to establish social contracts to support the key needs and asks of communities to ensure that they remain central and are addressed by the final built solution (https://seednetw ork.org/seed-evaluator/).

of building practices, namely energy, material, and infrastructure efficiencies. Others, like the Living Building Challenge (LBC), focused initially on net zero energy usage. As these rating systems have evolved, the goals associated with responsible building development and construction have expanded to include psychological factors such as natural daylighting and safe space, health factors related to air quality and material composition, and social responsibility to communities impacted by buildings. In fact, recent changes have included the integration of SEED and other social metrics into the LEED certification process. These systems and strategies for greater accountability are laudable and long-overdue, and they represent one way to simplify the process. However, these systems, in their attempts to streamline requirements, reduce the answers to important questions to a limited set of responses that can be checked off a list as a way to apply points to a sought-after score. In addition, rating systems are mostly voluntary and generally expensive. These are some of the criticisms that have been aimed at rating systems in the United States.

PUBLIC HEALTH AND THE BUILT ENVIRONMENT

As sustainability and then resiliency gained traction in the built environment, obesity became a parallel focus in public health (see Chapter 9, this volume). Obesity and its impact on chronic diseases such as heart disease, cancer, and stroke have overtaken infectious diseases as leading causes of death. In the past half century, we have designed physical activity out of our daily lives and become basically an indoor species, spending more than 93% of our lives indoors with very little physical work and recreation in our lives.[3]

In an attempt to address this and other unhealthy trends, the American Institute of Architects' (AIA) design and health initiative was launched in 2014 promoting Six Approaches to Achieving Health through Built Environment, Design and Policy. This initiative centred on environmental quality, natural systems, physical activity, safety, sensory environments, and social connectedness and was tied closely to another initiative for evidence-based design, the AIA Design and Health Research Consortium, intended to promote university-led research in design and health.[4] This shift away from focusing only on building performance to including how building environments (e.g., air quality, ventilation, and daylight access) impact users in terms of health, absenteeism, productivity, and so on has been dramatic.

---

3. The change has been particularly dramatic in the United States, where the average citizen has gone from spending 48% of their lives outdoors after World War II to more than 93% indoors today. See EPA research on this phenomenon and its impact on health and disease in https://www.epa.gov/report-environment/indoor-air-quality.

4. For information on the Design and Health Research Consortium, see http://architectsfoundation.org/health/aia-design-health-research- consortium/.

This data-driven emergence of the importance of health and wellness in built environments has helped to expand the definition of 'client' to include building users. It also spurred both LEED and LBC to include the verification of building performance over a specified period of time (1–2 years generally), a move toward post-occupancy evaluation of buildings that includes user satisfaction. In addition, the WELL Standard introduced the requirement that an organisation's culture and business operations should be centred around health and wellness.

It is also heartening that the US General Services Administration (GSA) is now piloting Fitwell for all federal building projects. Fitwell is a building certification programme that supports healthier workplace environments to help improve occupant health and productivity. Involvement in Fitwell is voluntary and is led by individual GSA regions, but the effort to create regional standards is allowing the GSA to address regional priorities and differences in use and culture.

FROM INDIVIDUAL BUILDINGS TO WHOLE NEIGHBOURHOODS

These changes to our understanding of the impacts of built environments on our health and wellness apply not only to individual homes and buildings but also to entire urban blocks and neighbourhoods. An individual's health is determined as much by their housing conditions, neighbourhood, urban planning decisions, transportation options, and energy usage as by the person's medical care. Intervention means looking upstream to how our food is produced, how we design our homes and buildings, and how we lay out our cities.

As a result, architects have started to turn their attention to the NYC Active Design Guidelines which were published in 2010 by the City of New York to provide architects and urban designers with a manual of strategies for creating neighbourhoods, streets, outdoor spaces, and buildings that encourage walking, bicycling, and active transportation and recreation. The LEED rating system has been expanded from individual buildings to now include ratings for neighbourhoods or groups of buildings. LEED ND (Neighbourhood Development) is for new land development projects or redevelopment projects containing residential uses, nonresidential uses, or a mix. It is designed to create better, more sustainable, well-connected neighbourhoods. At an even larger scale, LEED for Cities and Communities has metrics for entire cities and subsections of a city that measure and manage the city's water consumption, energy use, waste, transportation, and human experience. With a data-driven emphasis, it benchmarks social, economic, and environmental performance against national and global standards.

Likewise, public mental health is impacted in a similar way by the spaces we inhabit. Connection to nature can ease mental fatigue, restore a person's capacity to pay attention, and increase student learning. *Place attachment*, which refers to the psychological and social connections people feel with certain places (homes, neighbourhoods, and other settings in which they grew up) draw people together, influence the development of social ties, and enhance the development of community.

In turn, social connectedness helps communities and societies function more effectively and predicts higher levels of happiness and wellbeing and better health. Community resilience, the ability to bounce back after disaster, is also influenced by preparedness planning, community design, and social networks, as demonstrated by more recent natural disasters like those in Japan and Chile.

CASE STUDY: THE SAGE GREEN MODULAR CLASSROOM

As a vehicle for exploring the connection between built space and notions of wellness, the rest of this chapter describes the SAGE green modular classroom project, a modest building designed with the intent of creating a better learning environment that addresses the physical, mental, intellectual, and emotional health of its users and the larger community of which they are an important part. The description includes the actual process of design as well as the architectural design decisions and their implications to the health of a particular type of community: namely, a school. The project predated much of the more recent developments in both rating systems and incentive programmes that now pursue wellness in various forms. This description of the project is followed by an evaluation of its merits with respect to these current developments and draws conclusions that are consistent with our approach to best practices for achieving wellness goals in constructed environments.

The modular classroom, or 'portable', long a maligned but necessary answer to the underfunding of public schools, is heir to a long history of expediency and neglect. These spaces essentially house but fail to nurture the youngest members of our society for a significant amount of their lives and do so for increasingly larger numbers of children each year.

The SAGE green modular classroom project, initiated in 2010, and carried out by students and faculty at Portland State University, led to the design and implementation of an alternative to these ubiquitous classrooms. The project goal was to design a healthy, environmentally sustainable, and, most importantly, still affordable option for school modulars in the US Pacific Northwest (see Figure 20.1). The process by which it proceeded was unconventional as compared to standard practice for the commissioning of school buildings in the United States and was planned according to PID principles. These PID practices and protocols included strategies for the integration of many points of view and diverse disciplines to address a multiplicity of goals. They guided the process of engagement with the client, professionals, and communities involved because more recent guidelines regarding wellness and buildings were not yet available.

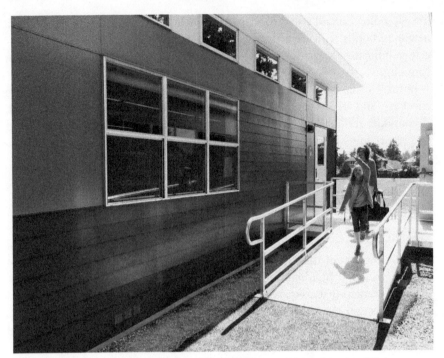

Figure 20.1 A SAGE classroom at Edmonds School District, Washington, US. Courtesy of Peter Simon.

The Problem for Schools

Modular classrooms are becoming the primary structures in which US children will be educated for the foreseeable future (see Figure 20.2). Today, more than 50% of new classroom space is provided by modular classrooms, often referred to as 'portables'. While these classrooms may provide a cheap solution for schools in need of additional space quickly, a growing body of evidence shows that choosing cost over quality may be creating significant health risks and performance-related deficiencies for many of our students as well as low-quality buildings with negative ecological impacts on our environments. This reliance on modular classrooms is an outgrowth of primarily economic factors that have led to a national crisis in school funding and, as a result, increased investment in these inexpensive and poorly made modular classrooms, investments that are often kept out of the public eye and policy discussions. This economic dilemma creates very real and long-term impacts for the host community and its children, making it clear that the design and commissioning of these classrooms should involve all impacted communities in collaboration with designers, school administrators, health experts, green building professionals, and modular industry partners. Because of the career PID focus of the authors, this kind of public, multidisciplinary approach was used to design the SAGE classroom.

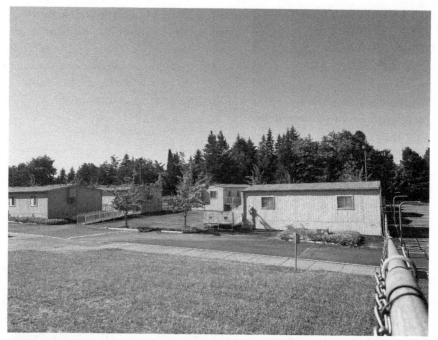

Figure 20.2 Entire schools are now often constructed of modulars, especially in California, where population growth and its mobility have led to modular classrooms becoming a norm.
Courtesy of Margarette Leite.

The vast majority of modular classrooms in the United States are unhealthy, uninspiring, and unsustainable. Nevertheless, they are the spaces in which a large percentage of our students are schooled (in the United States, that number is 6 million). In Portland, Oregon, alone, portable classrooms in use number in the thousands. Many of them are 60–80 years of age, making these 'temporary classrooms' quite permanent. With age, these poorly constructed classrooms degrade along with the environmental conditions experienced by the students and teachers who must occupy them. They are *de facto* permanent solutions to overcrowding created by fluctuations in enrolment and our collective failure to provide reliable and reasonable funding to our public schools. While these problems have their roots in earlier political and economic policy choices, given our present economic and social conditions, they are likely to continue into the future.

The Upsides and Downsides of Modulars

Despite the obvious problems associated with modular classrooms, they fulfil an important need in the United States and abroad, and there are some compelling and positive reasons for our continuing reliance on them. For one, fluctuating enrolments make investments in brick-and-mortar schools and additions to them questionable propositions. It may serve a school better to create a fleet of temporary, portable structures that can move as the need for them shifts. In addition, the very nature of their rapid construction, procurement, and installation serves the needs of the school system schedule. In addition, in Portland, Oregon, where new construction for schools must be paid through the passage of bonds, modular classrooms can be purchased from maintenance and operations budgets because they are considered emergency measures.

The greatest advantage to the use of modulars would seem to be the low cost of these structures. While the above-cited benefits are significant, the cost savings may not be as great as would be expected depending on the particular jurisdiction. In Portland, Oregon, for example, the average cost of a modular unit and its installation in 2009 was between $250,000 and $300,000. Today that cost has risen to close to $350,000, much of it driven by seismic codes that are considerable, particularly in the Portland area.[5] It could be argued that a brick-and-mortar addition would not be much more costly. In fact, the modular unit makes up barely half that cost. The rest is made up largely of site work costs, with management fees, permitting, furniture, and equipment added to make the classroom useful for teaching. Since site work and soft costs are unpredictable and largely unavoidable, manufacturers of modulars are pressed continually to provide a cheaper product in order to meet schools' ever-increasing funding shortages.

A considerable amount of research has been focused on modular classrooms in California. Of the 300,000 modular classrooms in use in American schools in 2011, 90,000 of those were in California. One in every three children in California was schooled in a modular classroom in 2011, and the numbers are considerably higher today.[6] With the growing number of students in modular classrooms have come post-occupancy impact studies which point to decreased performance and increased health-related issues among students and teachers and show a direct correlation to the poor environmental conditions of modular classroom environments (Shendell, Winer, Stock et al., 2004; Shendell, Winer, Weker, & Colome, 2004).

Underpinning much of the health-related complaints associated with modulars are their reliance on poorly designed and underperforming heating, ventilation, and air-conditioning (HVAC) systems that can lead to a host of respiratory illnesses in children as well as create challenging conditions for learning.[7] Other undesirable attributes include few window openings and poor building orientation. Both can lead to insufficient exposure to natural daylight, which research shows is critical to student wellbeing and educational performance. To make matters worse, a poorly built structure made of cheap materials will degrade quickly over

5. Data from 2009 obtained from Portland Public School District.

6. 2011 Annual Report on Relocatable Classrooms, Modular Building Institute.

7. http://www.insidescience.org/content/hidden-risks-modular-classrooms/1269.

time, exposing children to contaminants and pollutants that are particularly toxic to young bodies. Finally, their lack of design attention and architectural character as well as their apparent haphazard placement on school campuses leaves communities stigmatised and uninspired.

Community Participatory Processes

The SAGE classroom project was initiated through academic channels as a way to begin a community-wide discussion about the preponderance of modular classrooms and to look at what could be done to address some of the negative issues associated with them (see Figure 20.3). It was launched through the convening of a symposium and community design charrette (group brainstorming activity), which, for the first time, brought all of the stakeholders in the region together, from parents, teachers, and school officials to members of the modular construction industry. In addition to arriving at potential scenarios to address modular design problems, the symposium helped bridge what had been to that point one of the main roadblocks: distrust among the various stakeholders. However, the conference and charrette also revealed that behind the mistrust and historical lack of transparency, all stakeholders recognised the shortcomings of the current state of affairs and shared a commitment to changing the system. This alliance, created out of shared concern, helped advance the next steps in the process. Students of architecture and engineering acted as facilitators and were encouraged to continue their involvement in the project by further investigating the various solutions generated at the charrette in collaboration with the alliance of stakeholders from the conference. The public charrette and the follow-up research and coursework helped to create a network of community members that served as grassroots supporters for the plan to design an alternative classroom for Oregon students. In addition, it laid the groundwork for a collaborative relationship between design faculty and students and a modular building manufacturer, Blazer Industries (an Oregon-based company, recognised as a US leader in modular construction). This collaboration has proved crucial to the success of the project by bringing the expertise of the manufacturer into a human-centred discussion involving school administration, parents, and schoolchildren.

Public Advocacy as Community Engagement

In addition to symposia and charrette work, architecture students and faculty expanded the role typically associated with the architect to include community advocate, human subjects researcher, project manager, and curator of public processes. They took part in brainstorming activities with schoolchildren to appreciate their perspectives, met with parent groups and teachers to invite ideas and understand priorities, solicited design ideas at school events through innovative play with scale models and site games, and presented design ideas at public venues

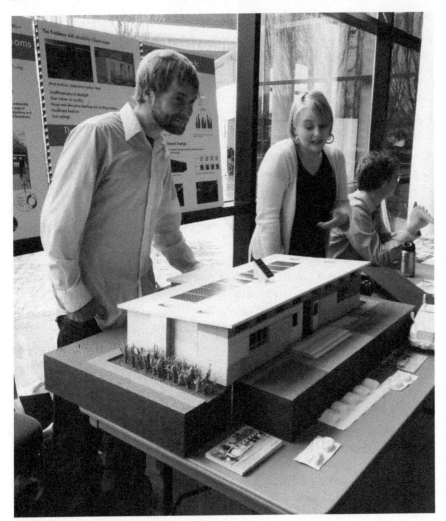

Figure 20.3 Students and faculty of the SAGE design team engaged the community through various forums to solicit their expert opinion as well as their buy-in and participation in the development of the SAGE classroom.
Courtesy of SAGE design team.

like the Oregon Museum of Science and Industry (a supporter of new ideas and forward thinking in the community). These public exchanges were curated to give each participant a voice, using activities designed to solicit thought rather than guide inquiry, to encourage participants to be co-authors of the design.

The processes of inquiry outlined above also tapped into other efforts nationally in school design, modular construction, manufacturing, and even pedagogy. The conference brought many national leaders in related fields together and opened a line of inquiry and exchange that informed many of the design efforts. Projects such as Eco-Mod, led by John Quale at the University of Virginia, and

Mark Anderson's (2007; UC Berkeley) efforts in prefabricated green buildings and classrooms, were among some of the projects that influenced the design team's work. Exchange also occurred through numerous conferences, published papers, and funded research exchanges which allowed the team to expand its expertise and collaborators to what eventually became a *de facto* regional effort with support both from parents, school districts, the industry, and even elected officials to create consensus and decision-making at the larger scale.

Expanding the Stakeholder Pool

The political support that helped mobilise the project came from a state-mandated focus on K-12 education and from a unique consensus process referred to as Oregon Solutions. The process was created by Governor Kitzhaber and provided the state with a mechanism to conduct an informed public process of discovery into issues and initiatives that could benefit the state as a whole. The Green Modular Classroom project was designated an official Oregon Solution in 2011, at a time when the state was struggling with public backlash against growing enrolments and funding gaps in its schools. This designation, while not financially supported, receives project management assistance from the state and helps to identify an issue as being of regional significance, with the political backing of the Governor's office to bring it greater awareness in the eyes of the citizenry. It gave the project regional momentum and a broader support that helped bring together a number of important stakeholders who took part in working through the design of a healthier, more energy efficient, and more aesthetically exciting classroom for Oregon students. This consortium was critical to addressing the multifaceted issues that included financial accessibility, building code interpretation, and energy-efficient engineering. It is unusual in a design and implementation process to be able to sit at a table that includes design and engineering teams as well as code officials, school administrators, and other stakeholders all involved in the production marketing of the subject of your efforts. It allows for spontaneous exchanges and decision-making, and for even unexpected insights to occur that uncover bottlenecks and problems in the system. In the traditional, linear method of practice, these innovations could not occur, and problems may become unsurmountable. It allows for each member in this process to step back and appreciate the larger picture and the importance of their role in the system. In retrospect, much of the success in getting the SAGE on the ground was due to the advances made within this industry and stakeholder roundtable.[8]

The Green Modular Classroom Task Force met on a regular basis for more than 1 year, with the stated mission of creating a prototype classroom. The close working relationship that was forged through the symposium and the Oregon

8. For more information on the Oregon Solutions process, see the website http://orsolutions. org/). Several projects covering a range of needs statewide are showcased.

Solutions process has allowed the design team to work closely with the manufacturers to identify opportunities for cost saving and innovation. The process began
with the identification of current efficiencies within the system that would be ad-
vantageous to retain.

Building on Existing Efficiencies

Current construction practices for modular structures are maximised for efficiency in terms of materials, time, and money. They are models of lean production, and finding savings in their construction costs was clearly a challenge for
the team. These structures are built to maximise transportable sizes and minimise
on-site construction finishing and detailing, which suits the quick installation
time required by school schedules. In the current market, the most commonly
ordered configuration is a two-classroom unit. This configuration is provided in
two long halves brought on two transport vehicles. Each half is approximately
14 × 64 feet (4 × 20 metres) in dimension, and the halves are connected on site
along a 'mate line' creating two classrooms of approximately 28 × 32 feet (8.5 × 10
metres). Despite its spatial limitations, this configuration accommodates a fairly
large number of students per classroom. In Oregon, most are ordered as 'dry'
units without toilets or water facilities. We chose to accept these basic dimen-
sional constraints and efficiencies.

Reducing Environmental and Material Waste by Increasing
Portability and Reducing Site Infrastructure

Thinking sustainably means thinking of modular classrooms as long-term investments rather than disposable structures. But that does not mean they need
to be permanent. Improving the structure and durability of the units can make
them both sturdier and easier to move. Increased portability can make them
more useful in increasingly unpredictable enrolment environments, thus allowing
school districts to move them around as needed. Most current modulars are not
sturdy enough to be moved more than once. In addition, Portland's seismic requirements are considerable, making continuous concrete stem wall foundations
that raise the unit 30 inches (76 cm) above grade the most expedient for modular
classrooms. This represents a considerable cost in terms of foundations and permanent ramps. The use of steel rather than wooden floor structures allows the
modular unit to last longer and to be located closer to the ground. This reduces
the need for the long, unsightly ramps associated with most modulars. Shorter
ramps can be made to be reused and can move with the unit. Steel floor structures
can also reduce the amount of concrete required in foundation structures, reducing not only infrastructure costs, but also site impact and eventual demolition
waste. The creation of more durable structures, the inclusion of reusable ramps,

and the reduction of site infrastructure contribute to the creation of a commodity of greater value for resale and reuse by school districts while also reducing the burden on the environment.

In terms of finish materials, the choice of low- to no-volatile organic compound (VOC) materials promotes improved air quality, more tactile surfaces, and the perception of a healthy and safe environment. The classrooms exclude the use of US Green Building Council (USGBC) red-list materials such as polyvinyl chlorides and formaldehydes. Instead, they promote the inclusion of cork on walls for pinup and noise reduction, bio-based sheet flooring, and cement-based siding for their VOC-free and durable makeup.

Rethinking HVAC for Health, Performance, and Energy Efficiency

Most modular classrooms are outfitted with HVAC systems that are oversized for heating and cooling and undersized for ventilation. Poorly ventilated spaces can contribute to the growth of molds and the accumulation of pollutants in the indoor air. The source of some of these pollutants is often the modular itself because many are built with cheap, low-quality materials that off-gas VOCs. Poor ventilation also contributes to higher levels of carbon dioxide in the classrooms, which is directly linked to reduced student performance and motivation. As shown in Figure 20.4, researchers at the Lawrence Berkeley Labs in California discovered that just 1,000 parts per million (ppm) of carbon dioxide in the air, a common amount found in our studies of Portland modulars, can impact cognitive performance by 25–45%, and, at 2,500 ppm, certain types of performance like initiative and basic strategy can drop to dysfunctional levels (Satish et al., 2012). As a comparison, outdoor concentrations of carbon dioxide are typically 380 ppm.

In addition to air quality concerns, the operation of these systems can create noise levels that reduce auditory clarity, preventing students from hearing their lessons and affecting the teacher's ability to engage students in conversation and exchanges. They can also produce inconsistent and uneven distribution of air, with concurrent discomfort to those in close proximity to air outlets.

The SAGE classroom uses a 'whole building design' approach to systems design by considering the students in the classroom as a primary thermal resource (see Figure 20.5). It does not take much time for numerous active bodies to generate enough heat to raise the temperature inside a classroom. As the needs of the classroom are driven primarily by fresh air provision, this can be provided simply by energy recovery ventilation (ERV). The bonus effect is that ERVs can provide considerably better air quality since the system conditioning is performed through outdoor air exchange rather than conditioning the indoor air, like conventional HVAC systems. The use of ERVs allowed the team to address a core goal of 100% fresh air in the classrooms, reducing carbon dioxide levels to natural outdoor air concentrations.

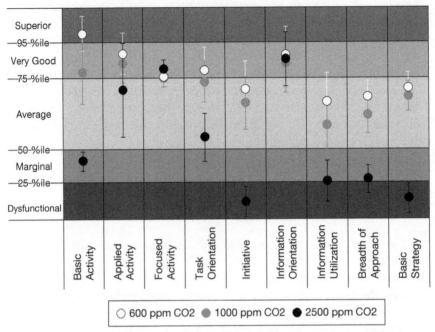

Figure 20.4 Results of the Department of Energy's Lawrence Berkeley National Laboratory's air quality studies found that high concentrations of carbon dioxide (CO_2) can significantly impair students' cognitive performance, as this chart from their study demonstrates. These results, released as the SAGE classroom was being designed and engineered, impacted the design team's approach to air quality.
Courtesy of Lawrence Berkeley Laboratories.

For cooling, natural ventilation is induced by the select placement of operable windows, ceiling fans, and the use of a phase-change material made of a wax-based substance that is placed within the stud wall cavity and that significantly reduces heat transfer through walls. This system serves as our base model. In cases where summer use is critical or where climatic conditions are different, high-efficiency heat pumps can boost cooling and reduce heating energy usage and noise disturbance. As an additional upgrade, ventilation can be boosted with roof-mounted, solar-powered ventilators. Each of these moves also reduces the need for the active systems that can produce noise and air flow disturbances.

Natural Light for Student Wellbeing and Energy Savings

In the Northwest region of the United States, where cloud cover is consistent during most of the year, natural light is an important asset that architects are challenged to understand and master in order to provide its benefits to building occupants.

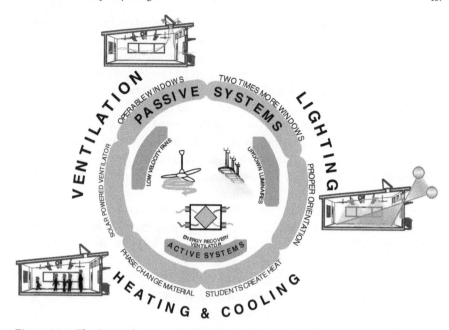

Figure 20.5 The SAGE classroom approach focuses on the whole building, balancing light, energy, and ventilation with a focus on student health, learning, and sense of connection.
Courtesy of SAGE design team.

Studies by Judith Heerwagen, and Susan Ubeholde at University of California (UC) at Berkeley, as well as Northwest regional power companies (Pacific Gas and Electric [PGE]), have compiled a strong body of evidence on the impact of natural light on children's health and cognitive performance (Heerwagen, 2011; Heschong Mahone Group, 1999). Judith Heerwagen, in particular, an internationally recognised figure in the field of learning environments for children and a member the SAGE classroom research team, has written and spoken extensively about the importance of natural daylight and views to nature and the outdoors to the wellbeing, work productivity, and educational performance of human beings in general and young minds and bodies in particular. She supports her findings with research done in hospitals and care settings (Heerwagen, 1998). Researchers found that patients in spaces with access to greater levels of natural light experienced less stress and anxiety, reduced needs for pain relief, and lower overall healthcare costs as a result. In addition, her work points to the importance of the variable qualities present only in natural light which can counteract boredom and passivity. Windows provide access to natural light, but they can also provide another important opportunity for impacting student performance. Teachers, in their efforts to focus student attention on their lessons, tend to keep shades down to reduce distraction from the outdoor environment. However, views to the outdoors and to natural elements in the environment can actually alleviate afternoon sleepiness and anxiety.

With this new appreciation and awareness of the impacts of light on human potential has come a range of methods and simulation tools that allow the architect
to determine how best to introduce natural light into the building and even create
light-neutral environments (i.e., those that do not require artificial light during
daylight hours). The research has, in turn, generated a body of design metrics, and
key research institutions such as UC Berkeley and Luma Laboratories in Portland
and Seattle, as well as numerous others in the United States and internationally,
are advancing this understanding and its application in building design. The evidence from the research by these institutions was largely in place when the SAGE
classroom was first designed and guided much of the development of the classroom since.

To achieve well-lit spaces in buildings, proper orientation to the sun's path
is also necessary. Most modular classrooms in the United States are designed
without a specific site in mind and are, therefore, orientation-neutral since they
must eventually accommodate themselves to preexisting school campuses. To
deal with this lack of predictable orientation, the traditional modular is built with
little consideration for natural light, resulting in few windows and depending entirely on artificial lighting.

Light-neutrality in the SAGE classroom is achieved by the creation of a row of
clerestory windows along the high side of the classroom, as well as view windows
below (see Figure 20.6). The clerestory windows can be oriented to achieve the
greatest access to sunlight, while lower windows bring in ambient light and views.
Additionally, the simple inclusion of additional framing to allow for doors on
either side of each classroom allows the portable the flexibility to be placed with
the clerestory in the ideal orientation to provide natural lighting while allowing
the entrance to be placed wherever it meets the needs of the school, even if it is
eventually moved to a new location. Proper orientation also reduces solar heat

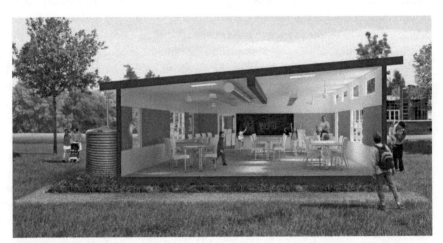

Figure 20.6 Section of a SAGE classroom with daylight penetration described by
computer modelling.
Courtesy of SAGE design team.

gain and loss, allowing the SAGE classroom to meet the traditional sustainability metrics of energy performance.

Aesthetics and Identity

One last sad fact related to the use of modular classrooms to solve our space and funding shortages is the legacy we leave for our children that can only be translated as a lack of concern, or at the very least, an inattention to the aesthetics of our educational structures. Today's hastily constructed and poorly performing boxes, with little consideration to their aesthetics, often appear to be parked on school campuses rather than thoughtfully sited. They can be stigmatising to many communities, and they signify a complete abdication of the respect and value we once placed on our institutions of education and, in effect, our children. School buildings constructed in the earlier part of the 20th century were monuments to the value we, as a society, placed on education, and they often grounded the identity of a community. Local schools continue to be hubs of shared experiences for their communities, and, through them, residents come to know and connect with neighbours and come to act on issues of mutual concern. The condition and quality of their school impacts a student's and a community's sense of self-worth. By the same token, current modular classrooms do not convey to children that they are valued and that their education is important to adult society. Adults do not accept these spaces for their own places of work. How, then, can we place our most vulnerable and future citizens in such uninspired spaces? The SAGE classroom, despite its low cost, strives to provide engaging, colourful, and well-designed units made of quality materials that help to shift that message and regain the pride and trust of children and communities.

At the end of the yearlong design process, the first prototype was constructed by modular distributor Pacific Mobile Structures and was exhibited at the 2012 USGBC international Greenbuild Conference in San Francisco. The project received an International Public Interest Design Award from the SEED network in 2013, and five awards to date from the Modular Building Institute, including first place for Green Building in 2020. As of the writing of this chapter, more than 120 classrooms have been built and placed, serving approximately 3,000 students in the Pacific Northwest.

Constructive Critical Overview of the SAGE Green Modular Classroom Project Through a Wellbeing Lens

In 2014, the Acting US Surgeon, General Rear Admiral Boris Lushniak, stated, 'Architects are public health workers. We have a partnership—public health professionals and architects and planners. Our minds have to talk because we have an influence on America's public health that we're only now beginning to grasp' (cited in Weeks, 2014). This quote is based on the premise that to change the health problems the country is experiencing, we need to 'go upstream' to prevent them from happening. Health is defined in the constitution of the World Health Organization (1946) as complete physical, mental, and social wellbeing; its definition thus extends beyond the absence of disease to include multiple dimensions of comfort and wellbeing. Design plays an important role in promoting or discouraging physical activity, the availability of healthy food to eat, the quality of the air we breathe and the water we drink, the risk of injuries throughout our environments, our mental health due to the quality and sensory conditions of the spaces we occupy, and the ways in which we form social bonds; all of which is compounded by the health disparities found in different communities. The interface and interactions among public health officials and the design professions is critical to understanding the complexity of the issues at hand. To do so, it is necessary to begin thinking across disciplines and across a variety of spatial scales—regional, city, neighbourhood, and building—and over a variety of time scales out to a fairly distant time horizon. The tools of evidence-based design, guided by health impact assessments and community engagement, are all critical to this effort.

The definition of wellbeing is broad. For architects, as outlined in the American Institute of Architects' (AIA) Six Approaches to Achieving Health Through Built Environment, Design, and Policy, it encompasses environmental quality, natural systems, physical activity, safety, sensory environments, and social connectedness. While not every project covers each of these approaches, some aspect of each can be incorporated into every design. Examples of each of these elements include the following:

- *Environmental quality*: Preventing, mitigating, or reversing quantifiable chemical and microbial, water, and air pollutants that directly or indirectly affect populations
- *Natural systems*: Natural forms, diverse species, and ecosystems that influence design
- *Physical activity*: Exercise, recreational activity, and activities that comprise everyday life, including labour, commuting, and chores
- *Safety*: Protection from physical or psychological harm caused by accidental injury or crime
- *Sensory environments*: Perceived olfactory, tactile, acoustic, and aesthetic qualities of space that contribute to the physical, mental, and emotional wellbeing of people
- *Social connectedness*: The networks of relationships that bind people together.

So how does the SAGE classroom address these more recently established metrics?

Consciously or not, the design of the SAGE classroom addresses some aspect of each of the above approaches, with a major focus in three primary areas: the quality of the air, the quality and types of lighting, and the social connectivity of both students and the larger community. Though anchored in these three primary metrics, the framing of each of these within the public forums that identified them was comprehensive enough to account for all six approaches identified by the AIA.

Schools are unique built environments because the high density of occupants is generally higher than the average workplace. Children spend long hours in the classroom, second only to the amount of time spent at home, and classrooms are also workplaces for teachers and staff. Children are especially vulnerable to environmental hazards that will have long-term health impacts, and school maintenance (or lack thereof) can be a contributing factor. The SAGE classroom contributes to the wellness of its users in three major ways.

First, the air quality is greatly improved over previous modular designs by the use of an ERV system providing 100% fresh air while also eliminating the need for a larger ducted HVAC system and eliminating noise. The use of nontoxic materials throughout the building as well as increased airflow eliminates the issue of mould that was prevalent in older module classrooms.

The second main contribution of the SAGE classroom to its users' wellbeing is in terms of lighting. Adequate, even, glare-free, balanced-spectrum lighting is an important environmental quality in schools. The SAGE classroom has 2–4 more square feet (.2 × .4 square metres) of windows than standard modular classrooms, large operable view windows, both clerestory windows and skylights, mini-blinds on all windows for manually controlled light, a higher and angled ceiling bringing light deeper into the classroom and increasing perceived room size, and automatic dimming luminaries that adjust to daylight levels to save energy but also provide an overall balanced lighting system.

Optimal lighting provides daylight and outdoor views. A series of studies on the performance of 21,000 second- through fifth-grade students in California, Washington, and Colorado, which analysed 2,000 classrooms, found that students with the most daylighting in their classrooms progressed 20% faster on math tests and 26% faster in reading compared to their counterparts in classrooms with the least daylight (Heschong Mahone Group, 1999). With some variations, these findings were very similar whether the daylight was from the roof area or on the walls. The amount of daylight in a classroom will vary depending on the orientation of the module. The SAGE classroom was designed with additional structural framing to allow for different door placements depending on the portable's location. This is critical for making the SAGE classroom adaptable to different sites and still maintain its health impacts.

These improved lighting elements stemming from the window design also improved access to natural settings. Stimuli and the tasks of everyday life can make relentless demands on our ability to pay attention and process information and can result in mental fatigue. The consequences of mental fatigue include becoming inattentive, withdrawn, irritable, distractible, impulsive, and accident-prone. There is growing experimental evidence that natural settings have the capacity to alleviate mental fatigue and restore a person's capacity to pay attention. This attention-restoring ability includes views through windows. The positioning of windows in the SAGE classroom allows for those outside views.

The third primary contribution of the SAGE classroom to its users' wellbeing relates to social connectivity. Some places draw people together and thus support the development of social ties and enhance the development of social capital and the resiliency of a community. There is no one way for designers to create the positive emotion of place attachment, but we can increase the likelihood that such ties develop by creating spaces that are attractive, support social interactions, and invite people to linger. This is a strong possibility for the students using the SAGE classroom due to its high level of physical and spatial qualities that make it a unique and positive space with which the students can identify. The process of creating the design also created connections to the larger community of all the individuals who were part of the design process, and the community charrettes involving parents and neighbours helped them to feel some ownership of the SAGE classroom as well. It is not just the space, but the process of creating the space that helped to create that social capital.

In summary, consciously or not, the designers created a more energy-efficient, longer-lasting building, but, more importantly, they also created a healthier building, with natural daylight and outdoor views that impact students' learning and a positive value of self, and a design process that included a variety of community voices. This process allowed the community's voices as well as those of design experts and environmental scientists, who rarely share the same forum, to essentially coproduce the SAGE classroom.

SUMMARY

The preceding evaluation describes the ways in which the SAGE classroom project has been able to meet the goals of wellness in the built environment as defined from the standpoint of public health. In doing so, it actually demonstrates the value of a multivoice, expanded stakeholder, participatory design process that is the hallmark of PID work. While the design team did not set out to consciously meet the metrics defined by either ratings programmes (too expensive a prospect for the tight budget of the classroom) or the specific guidelines from a public health standpoint listed above and post-dating the classroom's design, the classroom was able to address the full range of goals we now associate with a broader definition of wellbeing that includes social, economic, physical, psychological, and environmental dimensions. This stems from the fact that the inclusion of a greater number of voices, and particularly those typically excluded, will, by definition, promote the interests and therefore wellbeing of the broadest number of people. In short, it is the process that matters. Had the project been approached using primarily the tools of either ratings systems or public health guidelines, it might have failed to create the buy-in, ownership, and best interests of the users that inclusivity ensures.

Community participatory process, expanding the stakeholder pool, and co-authored building design represent the democratisation of a long-standing system of opacity and exclusion, and, while messy, time-consuming, and sometimes unpredictable, portend a movement whose time has come. The academy and profession are being challenged to respond to the overwhelming needs of the voiceless. These processes attempt to break down the walls that divide us as they address the right of all communities to be heard.

REFERENCES

Anderson, M. (2007). *Prefab prototypes: Site specific design for off-site construction.* Princeton Architectural Press.

Gámez, J. L. S., & Rogers, S. (2008). Introduction: An architecture of change. In B. Bell & K. Wakeford (Eds.), *Expanding architecture: Design as activism* (pp. 18–25). Metropolis Books.

Heerwagen, J. (1998). Design, productivity and wellbeing. What are the links? Paper presentation at AIA Conference on Highly Effective Facilities, Cincinnati, OH.

Heerwagen, J. (2011). The experience of daylight. *Daylight Architecture.* https://www.livi ngdaylights.nl/wp-content/uploads/2017/01/Heerwagen-2010.-The-experience-of-daylight.-Daylight-Architecture.pdf

Heschong Mahone Group. (1999). Daylighting in schools: An investigation into the relationship between daylighting and human performance. Pacific Gas and Electric Company.

Satish, U., Mendell, M., Shekhar, K., Hotchi, T., Sullivan, D., Streufert, S., & Frisk, W. (2012). Is CO_2 an indoor pollutant? Direct effects of low-to-moderate CO_2 concentrations on human decision-making performance. *Environmental Health Perspectives, 120,* 1671–1677. doi:10.1289/ehp.1104789

Shendell, D., Winer, A., Stock, T., Zhang, L., Zhang, J., Maberti, S., & Colome, S. (2004). Air concentrations of VOCs in portable and traditional classrooms: Results of a pilot study in Los Angeles County. *Journal of Exposure Science & Environmental Epidemiology, 14,* 44–59.

Shendell, D., Winer, A., Weker, R., & Colome, S. (2004). Inadequate ventilation in portable classrooms: Results of a pilot study in Los Angeles County. *Indoor Air, 14,* 154–158. doi:10.1111/j.1600-0668.2004.00235.x.

Weeks, K. (2014, April) Health is not a building typology. *Architect Magazine.* https://www.architectmagazine.com/design/health-is-not-a-building-typology_o

World Health Organization. (1946). *Constitution.* https://www.who.int/about/governa nce/constitution

FURTHER READING

Architecture for Humanity. (2009). Architecture for humanity, open architecture challenge: Classroom. https://www.archdaily.com/30098/finalists-announced-for-the-open-architecture-challenge-architecture-for-humanity

Bell, B., & Wakeford, K. (Eds.) (2008). *Expanding architecture: Design as activism.* Metropolis Books.

Coates, T. (2010). The littlest schoolhouse. *Atlantic Monthly.*

Dannenberg, A. L., Frumkin, H., & Jackson, R. (Eds.). (2011). *Making healthy places: Designing and building for health, well-being and sustainability.* Island Press.

Fischer, T. (2002). The once and future profession. *Archvoices*. AIA Online. https://usmo dernist.org/AIACH/AIACH-2002-08.pdf

Fulcher, M. (2010). Prefab schools debate heats up. *Architects Journal*, 1(1), 2–9.

Hawthorne, C. (2011). Prefab: The dream that refused to die. *Metropolis*.

Heerwagen, J. (2008). Psychosocial value of space. *Whole building design guide*. National Institute of Building Science.

Johnson, K. (2012). School district bets future on real estate. *New York Times*.

Modular Building Institute White Pages. https://www.modular.org/?gclid=CjwKCAiA zKqdBhAnEiwAePEjkpxYyFsMFcr-t4Ieq2gGQbtEna12zJXIcxmoChjgEQ10DTuq XtTuthoCjDoQAvD_BwE

Modular Building Institute. (2011). Annual report on permanent modular construction. Modular Building Institute.

Modular Building Institute. (2011). Annual report on relocatable buildings. Modular Building Institute.

Oregon Solutions website http://orsolutions.org/.

U.S. Environmental Protection Agency. (1989). Report to Congress on indoor air quality: Volume 2. EPA/400/1-89/001C. U.S. Environmental Protection Agency.

Wilson, E. O. (1984). *Biophilia*. Harvard University Press.

21

Sustainable Wellbeing and the United Nations Sustainable Development Goals

ROBERT COSTANZA, IDA KUBISZEWSKI, AND
LORENZO FIORAMONTI ■

INTRODUCTION

In this chapter, we investigate alternative methods to relate the United Nations Sustainable Development Goals (SDGs) to overall measures of sustainable wellbeing that can motivate and guide the process of global societal change. We first discuss the evolution and content of the SDGs. We then discuss alternative methods to relate the SDGs to sustainable wellbeing, including objective and subjective indicators of wellbeing, and an integrated approach. We then investigate what an aggregate Sustainable Wellbeing Index (SWI) that connects with the SDG dashboard might look like. Here, we first analyse several options for how to construct such an index and then propose a way forward that builds a hybrid approach. Finally, we propose linking the SDGs and our SWI to a comprehensive, nonlinear, systems dynamics model that can track both stocks and flows of built, human, social, and natural capital and make projections into the future under different policy scenarios.

This chapter draws heavily from work first published as: Costanza, R. et al. (2016). Modelling and measuring sustainable wellbeing in connection with the UN Sustainable Development Goals. *Ecological Economics, 130*, 350–355.

THE UN SUSTAINABLE DEVELOPMENT GOALS

The SDGs were agreed to at the UN 2030 Agenda for Sustainable Development (United Nations, 2015). They are an improvement and expansion on the previous UN Millennium Development Goals (MDGs). They address some of the systemic barriers to sustainable development and contain a more extensive coverage of and balance between the three dimensions of sustainable development—social, economic, and environmental—and their institutional/governance aspects. In addition, the SDGs apply to all countries, not just developing countries, as the MDGs did. The SDG process provides an opportunity to trigger systemic change to build a sustainable future in an increasingly interconnected world. However, with 17 goals supported by 169 targets and more than 200 indicators, the SDG process provides diluted guidance at best since the goals have limited capacity to be translated into concrete and measurable policies at the national or local level. This is to be expected, given the complex political negotiations that led to the SDGs.

The SDG measurement process is still at an early stage, with additional work needed to elaborate on (1) the complex interconnections between the goals, (2) the means–ends continuum toward achieving an overarching goal, and (3) a 'narrative of change' to describe the societal shifts needed to achieve the goals. Policy reforms to achieve the SDGs, and a better understanding of how this may happen within the existing socioeconomic and geopolitical circumstances, are required (Costanza, 2014; Ostrom, 2014).

At present, the SDGs are still a list of objectives. They lack an overarching goal with clear metrics of progress toward that goal and ways to integrate all the subgoals (Costanza, McGlade, Lovins, & Kubiszewski, 2014a). Table 21.1 shows the 17 proposed SDGs clustered according to the three subgoals originally proposed by Daly (1992) of sustainable scale, fair distribution, and efficient allocation. These are embedded in the 'means–ends' spectrum presented in Figure 21.1, which shows the relationship between the 'ultimate end' of sustainable, equitable, and prosperous wellbeing and the intermediate means of the economy, society, and the environment as opportunities to achieve it.

One important point of clarification is that sustainability is impossible to measure directly. It can only be assessed after the fact. Therefore, any measure of 'sustainability' is a prediction of which characteristics of the system might ultimately be sustainable (Costanza & Patten 1995; Garnåsjordet, Aslaksen, Giampietro, Funtowicz, & Ericson, 2012). The requirement for 'sustainable scale' is based on the idea that a sustainable system cannot deplete natural capital or damage ecosystem services beyond a certain 'safe operating space' (Rockström et al., 2009). We need a system that is both sustainable and desirable, including the contributions of natural, social, human, and built capital assets (Costanza et al., 2013). Ultimately, to properly assess sustainability and desirability will require both (1) a better, more integrated understanding of what contributes to individual, community, national, and global wellbeing (see other chapters in this volume); and (2) an integrated system-dynamics modelling approach to understand the complex interactions of these contributions and the possible futures of the system. The

Table 21.1 The 17 Sustainable Development Goals (SDGs) (UN 2015) clustered under the three elements of sustainable wellbeing shown in Figure 21.1.

Efficient allocation: Building a living economy

Goal 7.   Ensure access to affordable, reliable, sustainable, and modern energy for all

Goal 8.   Promote sustained, inclusive and sustainable economic growth, full and productive employment and decent work for all

Goal 9.   Build resilient infrastructure, promote inclusive and sustainable industrialization and foster innovation

Goal 11. Make cities and human settlements inclusive, safe, resilient and sustainable

Goal 12. Ensure sustainable consumption and production patterns

Fair distribution: Protecting capabilities for flourishing

Goal 1.   End poverty in all its forms everywhere

Goal 2.   End hunger, achieve food security and improved nutrition, and promote sustainable agriculture

Goal 3.   Ensure healthy lives and promote well-being for all at all ages

Goal 4.   Ensure inclusive and equitable quality education and promote life-long learning opportunities for all

Goal 5.   Achieve gender equality and empower all women and girls

Goal 10. Reduce inequality within and among countries

Goal 16. Promote peaceful and inclusive societies for sustainable development, provide access to justice for all and build effective, accountable and inclusive institutions at all levels

Goal 17. Strengthen the means of implementation and revitalize the global partnership for sustainable development

Sustainable scale: Staying within planetary boundaries

Goal 6.   Ensure availability and sustainable management of water and sanitation for all

Goal 13. Take urgent action to combat climate change and its impacts*

Goal 14. Conserve and sustainably use the oceans, seas and marine resources for sustainable development

Goal 15. Protect, restore and promote sustainable use of terrestrial ecosystems, sustainably manage forests, combat desertification, and halt and reverse land degradation and halt biodiversity loss

SDGs represent an important step in building global consensus on what kind of world is desirable. Sustainability, in the sense of longevity, is certainly one of the characteristics of a desirable world, but it can only be predicted, not measured directly.

ALTERNATIVE METHODS TO RELATE THE SDGS TO SUSTAINABLE WELLBEING

The SDGs provide a detailed dashboard or list of 17 goals and associated targets and the indicators to guide the transition to sustainable development. Some argue that

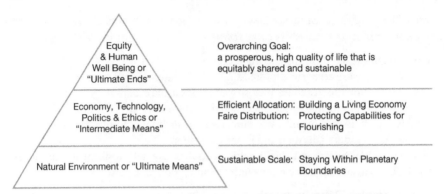

Figure 21.1 The 'means–ends' spectrum showing the three elements of sustainable wellbeing used to cluster the Sustainable Development Goals (SDGs) in Table 21.1. From Costanza et al. (2014a).

a dashboard approach is sufficient and the only feasible option. We disagree and contend that dashboards and aggregate indicators are *not* mutually exclusive—in fact, they are both essential. For example, having a well-instrumented dashboard in your car is essential, but so is knowing where you are going and whether you are making progress toward your destination. As baseball star Yogi Berra once quipped: 'If you don't know where you're going, you end up somewhere else'. We must first decide where we are going—that is, our overarching goal—in order to measure progress toward it. The 17 SDGs are best seen as subgoals, or means to this larger end (Table 21.1). We are certainly not recommending throwing out the dashboard, but merely recognising that the dashboard and an aggregated indicator of overall progress toward our shared goal are *both* necessary if we hope to achieve our goal. The SDGs acknowledge this need in Target 17.19, which states: 'By 2030, build on existing initiatives to develop measurements of progress on sustainable development that complement gross domestic product, and support statistical capacity-building in developing countries'.

Objective Versus Subjective Indicators

Examinations of wellbeing often fall under two headings, objective and subjective indicators. Objective indicators of wellbeing include, for example, indices of economic production, literacy rates, life expectancy, and other data that are gathered without a subjective evaluation by the individual being assessed. However, we must acknowledge that the subjective judgement of the researcher is involved in the process of defining and gathering objective indicators. Objective indicators may be used independently or in combination to form summary indexes, such as the UN's Human Development Index (HDI-UNDP, 1998) or the OECD Better Life Index (Durand, 2015). Objective indicators help us gather standardised data less affected by social comparison and local adaptation (e.g., minimising the degree to which wellbeing is largely a function of comparing one's life to others, which is vulnerable to adaptative preferences and cultural bias).

Subjective indicators typically rely on survey or interview tools to gather respondents' own assessments of their lived experiences in the form of self-reported overall life satisfaction, happiness, wellbeing, or some other near synonym. Rather than presume the importance of various life domains (e.g., life expectancy or material goods), subjective measures can tap the perceived significance of the domain (or 'need') to the respondent. Diener and Suh (1999) provide convincing evidence that subjective indicators are valid measures of what people *perceive to be* important to their happiness and wellbeing. Nevertheless, there are individuals who cannot provide subjective reports or whose subjective reports may not be as trustworthy in reflecting their true wellbeing because of the influence of transient mood, recent remembered events, cultural norms, personality, framing, priming, and a multitude of other factors that cannot be fully controlled for in a survey (Campbell, Converse, & Rodgers, 1976; Kahneman 2011; Schwarz & Strack, 1991; see also Chapter 15, this volume). Also, individuals may have limited information and cognitive capacity to understand what objectively contributes to their sustainable wellbeing. Many ecosystem services fit into this category since most people are unaware of the complex relationships involved (see later discussion).

An Integrated Approach to Wellbeing

What seems best, then, is to attempt an approach to wellbeing that combines objective and subjective indicators. An integrative definition of wellbeing would be as follows (Costanza et al., 2007a): wellbeing is the extent to which objective human needs are fulfilled in relation to personal or group perceptions of subjective wellbeing (Figure 21.2). Humans have basic needs for subsistence, reproduction, security, affection, etc. (see Table 21.1). Such wellbeing is assessed by individuals' or groups' responses to questions about happiness, life satisfaction, utility, or welfare. The relation between specific human needs and perceived satisfaction with each of them can be affected by mental capacity, cultural context, information, education, personality, inequality within society, and the like, often in quite complex ways. Moreover, the relation between the fulfilment of human needs and overall subjective wellbeing is affected by the (time-varying) weights individuals, groups, and cultures give to fulfilling each of the human needs relative to the others.

With this definition, the role of policy is to create opportunities for human needs to be met, understanding that there exists a diversity of ways to meet any particular need (Figure 21.2). Built, human, social, and natural capital (Costanza et al., 1997, 2014b, 2014c, 2014e; Costanza, Hart, Kubiszewski, & Talberth, 2014d) represent one way of categorising those opportunities. Time is also an independent constraint on the achievement of human needs. Social norms affect both the weights given to various human needs when aggregating them to overall

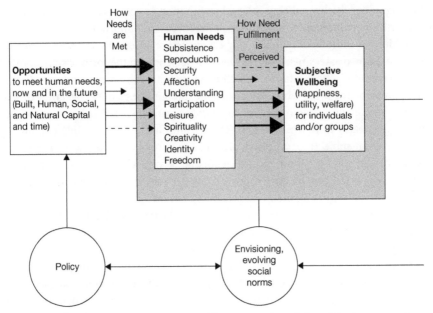

Figure 21.2 Wellbeing as the interaction of human needs and the subjective perception of their fulfilment, as mediated by the opportunities available to meet the needs.

individual or social assessments of subjective wellbeing and also policy decisions about social investments in improving opportunities. Social norms evolve over time due to collective population behaviour (Azar, 2004). The evolution of social norms can be affected by conscious shared envisioning of preferred states of the world (Costanza, 2000; Costanza et al., 2014e).

In this chapter, we investigate what an aggregate SWI that connects with the SDG dashboard might look like. We first analyse several options for how to construct such an index and then propose a way forward that builds a hybrid approach. Finally, we propose linking the SDGs and our SWI to a comprehensive, nonlinear, systems dynamics model that can track both stocks and flows of built, human, social, and natural capital and make projections into the future under different policy scenarios. This is an essential and often overlooked step in the process. The gross domestic product (GDP) has been so widely accepted partly because of its links to the System of National Accounts (SNA) and the underlying static, linear input–output model of the economy. We need a new, integrated, dynamic systems model to underlie and integrate the SDG goals and aggregate wellbeing indicators.

EXISTING GENERAL APPROACHES

Many alternative approaches to aggregate indicators of societal wellbeing and progress have been developed over the years. Three basic approaches have been used in developing these indicators. We first discuss these basic approaches and then discuss how these approaches might be applied to the SDGs.

Consumption, Production, and Wealth Indicators

Conventional measures of national progress, like GDP, are based on production and consumption of goods and services exchanged in markets (with the occasional imputed value). GDP was never designed as a measure of societal wellbeing. However, a popular assumption, derived from utilitarian philosophy, is that—all else being equal—more consumption leads to higher wellbeing and that therefore GDP per capita and its growth can be used as proxies for national wellbeing (Costanza et al., 2014d). This assumption has been challenged for decades, and the problems with using GDP as an indicator of national wellbeing are well known (Costanza et al. 2014b; Fioramonti, 2013, 2017; Fleurbaey & Blanchet, 2013; Stiglitz, Sen, & Fitoussi, 2009). For example, the United Nations Development Programme (1996) identified five types of GDP growth that are actually negative indicators: (1) jobless growth (the economy gets bigger with more buying and selling of goods and services, but without creating more jobs), (2) voiceless growth (an apparently successful economy rides on the back of the suppression of civil rights, union membership, and democracy), (3) ruthless growth (accompanying high or rising inequality), (4) rootless growth (culturally destructive effects of economic globalisation), and (5) futureless growth (that steals our collective future by depending on the unsustainable consumption of finite natural resources).

Several alternatives have been devised that attempt to correct some of the problems with GDP. These include Green GDP (Boyd, 2007; Li & Lang, 2010), Genuine Savings (Hamilton & Clemens, 1999; Pillarisetti, 2005), the Inclusive Wealth Index (UNU-IHDP and UNEP, 2014), and the Index of Sustainable Economic Welfare (ISEW; Daly & Cobb, 1989), also known as the Genuine Progress Indicator (GPI; Talberth, Cobb, & Slattery, 2007). For example, the GPI is calculated by starting with personal consumption expenditures, a measure of all spending by individuals and a major component of GDP, weighting it by income distribution to recognise the impacts of inequality on societal welfare (Wilkinson & Pickett, 2009; see also Chapter 16, this volume) and making more than 20 additions and subtractions to account for 'goods' and 'bads' which are not included in conventional measures of income. 'Goods' include volunteer work and work in the family, and 'bads' include the costs of divorce, crime, pollution, and the depletion of natural capital. The GPI has been estimated for several countries and has been formally adopted by the states of Maryland and Vermont in the United States. Results show that when growing inequality and environmental costs are incorporated, GPI has not been growing at all in many countries over the past several decades (Kubiszewski et al., 2013).

The SDGs include some costs and benefits not incorporated in the GPI (e.g., gender equality, urban resilience, and accountable institutions). One could create a 'GPI SDG' that incorporated these factors as well as other changes that have been suggested. One characteristic of GPI is that it is denominated in monetary units, making it directly comparable with GDP but also requiring that all the elements be assessed in monetary units. These valuations can be quite difficult and imprecise. But one should keep in mind that GDP itself is not as precise as often assumed, especially due to technological transformations in our economy (e.g., the digital revolution) and the partial and patchy data behind it (especially but not exclusively in developing countries) which therefore requires a growing number of imputations (Fioramonti, 2013, 2014, 2017).

Aggregation of all the SDG Indicators into a Unitless Index

One could build an aggregate, unitless indicator from the 232 SDG indicators (or more than 650 indicators, if all the subdivisions are included). The well-known problem with this approach is how to weight the different indicators. There are several examples of this approach (Costanza et al., 2014a). One example that builds on the 'ends–means' spectrum is the 'degrowth accounts' proposed by O'Neill (2015). Another example, the OECD Better Life index (http://www.oecd betterlifeindex.org/), is built from 11 elements, each with one or two indicators. These elements are housing, income, jobs, community, education, environment, civic engagement, health, life satisfaction, safety, and work–life balance. In the default mode, each element is ranked on a 1–10 scale. The scores are displayed as a flower diagram (i.e., with the strength of the different elements represented by petals of different sizes) so one can quickly see which elements are high and low for each country. To get an overall score, the elements are averaged together, initially weighted equally. However, one can change the weights on the website and observe the effects on the rankings. The OECD is collecting a survey of user weightings, and this could be used to construct a weighted index. But weighting all the SDG indicators via surveys seems too ambitious, while a simple unweighted average seems arbitrary and not in line with different national priorities. Furthermore, for many of the SDGs and associated goals and indicators, data will not be available for all countries in the short and medium term. Similar concerns can be raised with respect to new indices—such as the Social Progress Index (recently adopted in Massachusetts and Paraguay) and the Legatum Prosperity Index—which aggregate various dimensions of wellbeing, social capital, and prosperity.

Contributions to Subjective Wellbeing

Another approach to weighting is to construct a regression model with all indicators as the independent variables and some existing independent approximation of wellbeing—for example, subjective life satisfaction scores—as the dependent variable (Kubiszewski et al., 2022). This would provide statistically derived weights in terms of degree of correlation with the dependent variable. The main challenge here is what to choose as the dependent variable. Subjective wellbeing, from international/national public opinion surveys, has been suggested by some as the most appropriate dependent variable and the most appropriate national policy goal (Layard, 2005). There has been some research with statistical models that include subjective wellbeing as the dependent variable and built, human, natural, and social capital indicators as the independent variables (Abdallah et al., 2007; Kubiszewski, Zakariyya, & Costanza, 2018; Kubiszewski et al., 2022; Vemuri & Costanza, 2006). These approaches successfully predict more than 70% of the variation in subjective wellbeing across countries. As an example, the World Happiness Report (Helliwell et al., 2016) developed regressions of subjective wellbeing against a range of independent variables that explained 73% of the variation across countries. Even more impressively, a study showed that a mere 8 of the 232 SDG indicators for which sufficient data were available can explain 84% of the variation in subjective wellbeing across countries (Kubiszewski, Mulder, Jarvis, & Costanza, 2021).

However, it is also well known that individuals' perceptions are limited in that they may be influenced by cultural factors, thus making international comparisons difficult. For example, studies comparing levels of happiness and depression in China and the United States showed that, although the Chinese seem less happy (Spencer-Rodgers, Peng, Wang, & Hou, 2004) and optimistic (Lee & Seligman, 1997) than their American counterparts, people living in the United States are more depressed than the Chinese (Demyttenaere, 2004). This may show the greater operation of mental illness stigma in some cultures which results in the underreporting of symptoms such as depression. Measures of subjective wellbeing are also limited by the fact that people may be unaware of some of the factors that contribute to their wellbeing (Kahneman, 2011). For example, the contributions of natural capital and ecosystem services may not be well perceived by individuals and may not show up in life satisfaction surveys, even though studies indicate that these services contribute far more to sustainable wellbeing than does GDP (Costanza et al., 1997; 2014c). Individuals do not directly perceive the climate regulation benefits of forests or the storm protection benefits of coastal wetlands, although these may be critical contributors to their sustainable wellbeing.

A HYBRID APPROACH

All the approaches mentioned above have positive and negative aspects. So the question becomes: Can we construct a hybrid indicator that incorporates most of the positive aspects and minimises the negative aspects of these various measurement approaches? As Costanza et al. (2014b) conclude,

> The successor to GDP should be a new set of metrics that integrates current knowledge of how ecology, economics, psychology, and sociology collectively contribute to establishing and measuring sustainable wellbeing. The new metrics must garner broad support from stakeholders in the [UN SDG] conclaves. (p. 285)

Against this backdrop, one potential hybrid SWI could be a combination of three basic parts, each covering the contributions to sustainable wellbeing from the dimensions of the economy, nature, and society, respectively. In the following section, we elaborate on each of these in turn before integrating them as our proposed hybrid measure.

Net Economic Contribution: E

The GPI can be thought of as a measure of the *net* contribution of economic (production and consumption) elements to wellbeing. As we have seen, it weights personal consumption by income distribution, adds some positive economic elements left out of GDP, and subtracts a range of costs that should not be counted as benefits. Although some costs to natural and social capital are included in GPI, many others are missing (e.g., loss of community cohesion due to the social disruptions caused by economic growth), and we also need a way to measure and include the positive benefits to wellbeing from natural and social capital. We therefore need to supplement the current GPI with additional cost estimates (from the SDGs or elsewhere, including its targets and proposed indicators) as well as measurements of the positive contributions of natural and social capital.

Natural Capital/Ecosystem Services Contribution: N

The positive contributions of natural capital and the ecosystem services it provides have been estimated in spatially explicit form and can be valued in different units, including monetary units (Costanza et al., 1997, 2014c; Sutton & Costanza, 2002). These can be estimated at the country level as well as at subnational and regional scales. For example, the Wealth Accounting and Valuation of Ecosystem Services (WAVES) project of the World Bank (https://www.waves partnership.org/) is actively pursuing this agenda, as are several other initiatives, including the new Intergovernmental Science-Policy Platform on Biodiversity and Ecosystem Services (IPBES; http://www.ipbes.net/), the Economics of Ecosystems and Biodiversity (TEEB; http://www.teebweb.org/), the Economics of Land Degradation (ELD) initiative (http://eld-initiative.org/), and the Ecosystem Services Partnership (ESP; http://www.fsd.nl/esp).

Social Capital/Community Contribution: S

The positive contributions to wellbeing from social capital could be captured via surveys of the various components of life satisfaction and measures of community health as described in other chapters in this volume. For example, the World Values Survey as well as regional barometers (e.g., Eurobarometer and Afrobarometer) ask questions about trust and other aspects of social capital.

However, we will need to add additional survey questions that ask explicitly about the value of community and social capital in addition to individual life satisfaction. Objective measures of community physical and mental health like infant mortality, life expectancy, access to healthcare, and rates of depression could also be incorporated into this component.

Figure 21.3 shows the 17 SDGs and how they contribute to each of the three categories mentioned above. These categories correspond to the three basic goals outlined in the framework of *ecological economics* (Costanza, 1991; Costanza et al., 2013, 2014d; Daly, 1990) and the three basic components of sustainability. Note that many of the SDG subgoals contribute to more than one category.

Ultimately, a pluralistic approach that allows several options to be investigated will be required in the short term, and a consensus-building process will be needed to narrow down the possibilities to those that are most useful in assessing overall progress toward sustainable wellbeing. But, for a start, we propose the following:

$$SWI = f(E, N, S), \tag{1}$$

where:
SWI = Sustainable Wellbeing Index
E = Net economic contribution
N = Natural Capital/Ecosystem Services contribution
S = Social capital/Community contribution.

How these three elements combine to produce SWI is important. They are not linear combinations since the absence of any one of these factors would lead to zero SWI. At the same time, they are not purely multiplicative with the possibility for infinite SWI. For example, it is clear that increases in material standards make a very major difference to wellbeing in poorer countries where many people lack basic necessities. But as countries get richer, further increases in material standards make less and less difference to wellbeing. In richer countries, social capital and community may be the limiting factors. We therefore propose that a 'limiting factor' approach might be a better option. For example, an equation like the following might work:

$$SWI = L_{max} * (E / (k_e + E)) * (N / (k_n + N)) * (S / (k_s + S)), \tag{2}$$

where:
L_{max} = the maximum achievable SWI when all factors are simultaneously at their maximum.
k_e = the 'half-saturation constant' of E—the value of E where the result of this term achieves half its maximum value
k_n = the 'half-saturation constant' of N
k_s = the 'half-saturation constant' of S.

In this equation, each of the terms approaches 1 as the variable approaches infinity. As all the terms approach 1, SWI approaches L_{max}. The larger the half-saturation constant relative to the size of the variable, the slower is the approach

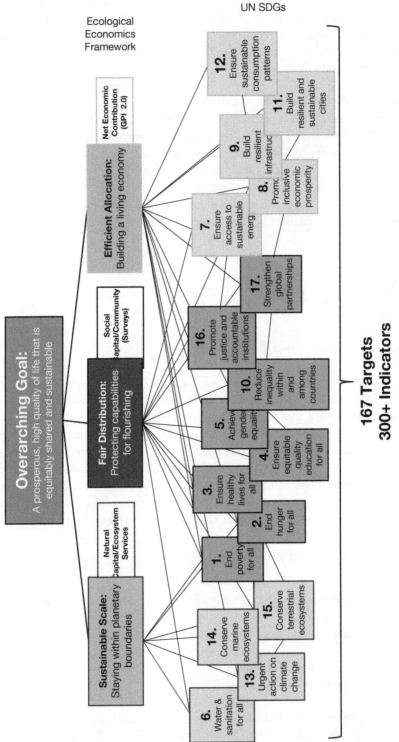

Figure 21.3 The relationship of the 17 UN Sustainable Development Goals (SDGs) to the framework of ecological economics and the overarching goal of a sustainable, equitable, and prosperous system.

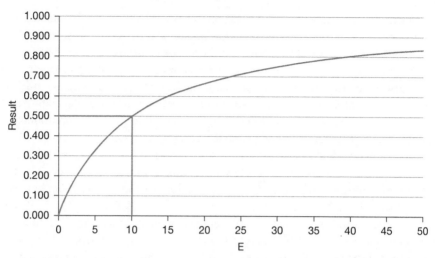

Figure 21.4 Example of limiting factor type curve, where: Result = E/(k_e + E) for a value of k_e =10. k_e is the 'half-saturation constant' or the value of E where Result reaches 50% of its maximum value.

to 1. Any one of the variables can be the 'limiting factor.' For example, if E is very large, its term in the equation will be close to 1. But if S is small, its term will be a small fraction that will reduce and limit SWI. Figure 21.4 is an example of the relationship for (E/((k_e +E)).

This approach is based on the idea that the best system is one that achieves the overarching goal of a *simultaneously* prosperous, high quality of life that is equitably shared and sustainable (Figure 21.1). The goal is not infinite growth but balanced sufficiency, equity, and sustainability.

Many countries have words that encapsulate this overarching goal as the essence of the 'good life'. For example, the Swedish term *lagom* means roughly 'just the right amount, equitably shared' (Costanza, 2015). In parts of Latin America, this concept is encapsulated in terms such as *buen vivir* and *pura vida*, while in Africa it connects with collective welfare traditions like *ubuntu*. We are searching for a way to quantify and guide progress toward the goals that many cultures implicitly share.

COMPREHENSIVE SYSTEMS DYNAMICS MODELLING

One of the reasons that GDP has achieved such dominance as an indicator of national progress is that it is integrated with an underlying model of the economic system. The model used is the basic linear input–output structure originally developed by Leontief (1941). It is a linear accounting model of monetary flows from sector to sector in the economy and to 'final demand'—the output to households, government, capital formation and net exports—which is GDP. In this accounting model, the inputs and outputs from each sector of the economy (such as agriculture, manufacturing, services, etc.) have to balance. It does not account for stocks of capital assets except as a flow of 'capital formation' that is part of final demand. It is the basis of the SNA that all countries currently use.

We need to replace the misuse of GDP as a measure of national success with not just an alternative indicator of wellbeing, but also with a dynamic, nonlinear, systems model of the entire system of the economy-in-society-in-nature that keeps track of both stocks and flows, and one that can deal with nonmonetary stocks and flows. Figure 21.5 is a simplified example. The input–output structure of the economy could be embedded in this model, but it would have to go far beyond that to account for the costs and benefits from natural and social capital and the dynamics of capital formation and decline. Versions of such models exist (Boumans et al., 2002; Costanza, Leemans, Boumans, & Gaddis, 2007b; Victor, 2018), and several are currently in further development. This approach could help to build better assessments of progress toward sustainable wellbeing. These models can also span several time scales, including past, present, and future scenarios, allowing us to make better predictions of what sets of policies are actually sustainable and desirable and overcome the short-termism that afflicts much of current policy.

SUMMARY

The agreed UN SDGs are a major achievement in the development of shared goals for all of humanity. The SDGs have been agreed to by all UN Member States, and they include economic, social, and environmental elements. However, they lack an overarching goal and an effective aggregate indicator of progress toward that goal. One could argue that such an aggregate indicator is not necessary (or possible) and that the pursuit of the individual goals will be sufficient to achieve sustainable development. That might be true if the goals were independent of each other and they all contributed to the overarching goal equally. This is obviously not the case, especially in the context of the widely different situations in each country. We need an aggregate indicator that can assess the relative contribution of each of the SDGs and their interactions with each other in order to assess overall progress. We have suggested three fundamental categories that could make up a hybrid indicator and how these categories could be combined, but we also propose the development of an underlying systems dynamics model to assess interactions and synergies over space and time, including both stocks and flows, causes and effects. It is also necessary to develop a framework of policy reforms and societal change that make the achievement of the SDGs possible at both national and global levels. In today's interconnected world, the SDGs cannot be achieved unless there is sustainable wellbeing globally. We hope that the SDG process will continue in the direction we have proposed in order to speed the approach to a sustainable and desirable future.

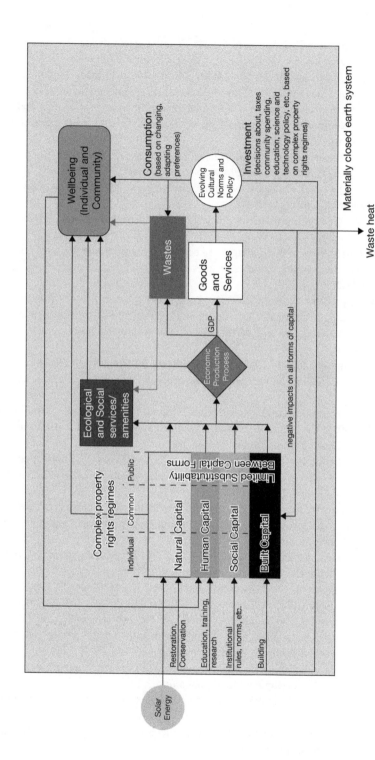

Figure 21.5 'Full world' model of the whole system.
From Costanza et al. (2014e).

490 TOWARD AN INTEGRATED SCIENCE OF WELLBEING

REFERENCES

Abdallah, S., Thompson, S., & Marks, N. (2008). Estimating worldwide life satisfaction. *Ecological Economics*, 65, 35–47. doi:10.1016/j.ecolecon.2007.11.009

Boumans, R., R. Costanza, J. Farley, M. A. Wilson, R. Portela, J. Rotmans, . . . Grasso, M. (2002). Modeling the dynamics of the integrated earth system and the value of global ecosystem services using the GUMBO model. *Ecological Economics*, 41, 529–560.

Boyd, J. (2007). Nonmarket benefits of nature: What should be counted in green GDP? *Ecological Economics*, 61, 716–723.

Campbell, A., Converse, P. E., & Rodgers, W. L. (1976). *The quality of American life: Perceptions, evaluations, and satisfactions.* Russell Sage Foundation.

Costanza, R. (Ed.). (1991). *Ecological economics: The science and management of sustainability.* Columbia University Press.

Costanza, R. (2014). A theory of socio-ecological system change. *Journal of BioEconomics.* 16, 39–44. doi:10.1007/s10818-013-9165-5

Costanza, R. (2015). How to build a 'lagomist' economy. *The Guardian* 4/6/2015. http://www.theguardian.com/sustainable-business/2015/apr/06/lagomist-economy-consumerism-quality-of-life

Costanza, R., Alperovitz, G., Daly, H., Farley J., Franco, C., Jackson, T., . . . P. Victor, P. (2013). Building a sustainable and desirable economy-in-society-in-nature. *ANU ePress.* http://epress.anu.edu.au/titles/building-a-sustainable-and-desirable-economy-in-society-in-nature

Costanza, R., Cumberland, J. C., Daly, H. E., Goodland, R., Norgaard, R., Kubiszewski, I., & Franco, C. (2014e). *An introduction to ecological economics* (2nd ed.). Taylor and Francis.

Costanza, R., d'Arge, R., de Groot, R., Farber, S., Grasso, M., Hannon, B., . . . van den Belt, M. (1997). The value of the world's ecosystem services and natural capital. *Nature*, 387, 253–260.

Costanza, R., de Groot, R., Sutton, P., van der Ploeg, S., Anderson, S., Kubiszewski, I., . . . Turner, R. K. (2014c). Changes in the global value of ecosystem services. *Global Environmental Change*, 26, 152–158.

Costanza, R., Fisher, B., Ali, S., Beer, C., Bond, L, Boumans, R., . . . Snapp R. (2007a). Quality of life: An approach integrating opportunities, human needs, and subjective well-being. *Ecological Economics*, 61, 267–276.

Costanza, R. Hart, M., Kubiszewski, I., & Talberth, J. (2014d). Moving beyond GDP to measure well-Being and happiness. *Solutions*, 5, 91–97.

Costanza, R., Kubiszewski, I., Giovannini, E., Lovins, H., McGlade, J., Pickett, K. E., . . . Wilkinson, R. (2014b). Time to leave GDP behind. *Nature*, 505, 283–285.

Costanza, R., Leemans, R., Boumans, R., & Gaddis, E. (2007b). Integrated global models. In R. Costanza, L. Graumlich, & W. Steffen (Eds.), *Sustainability or collapse? An integrated history and future of people on earth* (pp. 417–446). MIT Press.

Costanza, R., McGlade, J., Lovins, H., & Kubiszewski, I. (2014a). An overarching goal for the UN Sustainable Development Goals. *Solutions*, 5, 13–16.

Costanza, R., & Patten, B. C. (1995). Defining and predicting sustainability. *Ecological Economics*, 15, 193–196.

Daly, H. E. (1990). Toward some operational principles of sustainable development. *Ecological Economics*, 2, 1–6.

Daly, H. E. (1992). Allocation, distribution, and scale: Towards an economics that is efficient, just, and sustainable. *Ecological Economics*, 6, 185–193.

Daly, H. E., & Cobb Jr., J. B. (1989). *For the common good: Redirecting the economy toward community, the environment, and a sustainable future.* Beacon Press.

Demyttenaere. K. (2004). WHO World Mental Health Survey Consortium: Prevalence, severity and unmet need for treatment of mental disorders in the World Health Organization World Mental Health Surveys. *JAMA*, *291*, 2581–2590.

Durand, M. (2015). The OECD better life initiative: How's life? and the measurement of well-being. *Review of Income and Wealth*, *61*, 4–17.

Fioramonti, L. (2013). *Gross domestic problem: The politics behind the world's most powerful number.* Zed Books.

Fioramonti, L. (2014). *How numbers rule the world: The use and abuse of statistics in global politics.* Zed Books.

Fioramonti, L. (2017). *The world after GDP: Economics, politics and international relations in the post-growth era.* Polity Press.

Fleurbaey, M., & Blanchet, D. (2013). *Beyond GDP: Measuring welfare and assessing sustainability.* Oxford University Press.

Garnåsjordet, P. A., Aslaksen, I., Giampietro, M., Funtowicz, S., & Ericson, T. (2012). From statistics to policy: Sustainable development indicators. *Environmental Policy and Governance*, *22*, 322–336.

Hamilton, K., & Clemens, M. (1999). Genuine savings rates in developing countries. *The World Bank Economic Review*, *13*, 333–356.

Kahneman, D. (2011). *Thinking, fast and slow.* Macmillan.

Kubiszewski, I., Costanza, R., Franco, C., Lawn, P., Talberth, J., Jackson, T., & Aylmer, C. (2013). Beyond GDP: Measuring and achieving global genuine progress. *Ecological Economics*, *93*, 57–68.

Kubiszewski, I., Jarvis, D., & Zakariyya, N. (2019). Spatial variations in contributors to life satisfaction: An Australian case study. *Ecological Economics*, *164*, 106345.

Kubiszewski, I., Mulder, K., Jarvis, D., & Costanza, R. (2022). Toward better measurement of sustainable development and wellbeing: A small number of SDG indicators reliably predict life satisfaction. *Sustainable Development*, *30*, 139–148.

Kubiszewski, I., Zakariyya, N., & Costanza, R. (2018). Objective and subjective indicators of life satisfaction in Australia: How well do people perceive what supports a good life? *Ecological Economics*, *154*, 361–372.

Kubiszewski, I., Zakariyya, N., & Jarvis, D. (2019). Subjective wellbeing at different spatial scales for individuals satisfied and dissatisfied with life. *PeerJ* 7, e6502.

Layard, R. (2005). *Happiness: Lessons from a new science.* Penguin.

Lee, Y., & Seligmam, M. (1997). Are Americans more optimistic than the Chinese? *Personality and Social Psychology Bulletin*, *23*, 32–40.

Leontief, W. W. (1941). *The structure of the American economy, 1919–1929: An empirical application of equilibrium analysis.* Harvard University Press.

Li, V., & Lang, G. (2010). China's "Green GDP" experiment and the struggle for ecological modernisation. *Journal of Contemporary Asia*, *40*, 44–62.

O'Neill, D. W. (2015). The proximity of nations to a socially sustainable steady-state economy. *Journal of Cleaner Production*, *108*, 1213–1231.

Ostrom, E. (2014). Do institutions for collective action evolve? *Journal of BioEconomics*, *16*, 3–30. doi:10.1007/s10818-013-9154-8.

Pillarisetti, J. R. (2005). The World Bank's 'genuine savings' measure and sustainability. *Ecological Economics, 55,* 599–609.

Rockström, J., Steffen, W., Noone, K., Persson, Å., Chapin, III, F. S., Lambin, E. F., . . . Foley, J. (2009). A safe operating space for humanity. *Nature, 461,* 472–475.

Schwarz, N., & Strack, F. (1991). Evaluating one's life: A judgment model of subjective wellbeing. In F. Strack, M. Argyle, & N, Schwarz. (Eds.), *Subjective well-being: An interdisciplinary perspective* (pp. 27–47). Pergamon Press.

Spencer-Rodgers J., Peng, K., Wang, L., & Hou, Y. (2004). Dialectial self-esteem and East-West differences in psychological well-being. *Personality and Social Psychology Bulletin, 30,* 1416–1432.

Stiglitz, J., Sen, A., & Fitoussi, J.-P. (2009). *Report of the Commission on the Measurement of Economic Performance and Social Progress.* https://www.voced.edu.au/content/ngv%3A44133

Sutton, P. C., & Costanza, R. (2002). Global estimates of market and non-market values derived from nighttime satellite imagery, land use, and ecosystem service valuation. *Ecological Economics, 41,* 509–527.

Talberth, D. J., Cobb, C., & Slattery, N. (2007). *The Genuine Progress Indicator 2006: A tool for sustainable development.* https://sustainable-economy.org/wp-content/uploads/GPI-2006-Final.pdf

Vemuri, A. W., & Costanza, R. (2006). The role of human, social, built, and natural capital in explaining life satisfaction at the country level: Toward a National Well-Being Index (NWI). *Ecological Economics, 51,* 119–133.

Victor, P. A. (2018). *Managing without growth: Slower by design, not disaster.* Edward Elgar Publishing.

Wilkinson R. G., & Pickett, K. (2009). *The spirit level: Why greater equality makes societies stronger.* Bloomsbury Press.

United Nations Development Programme. (1996). *Human development report 1996.* Oxford University Press.

United Nations. (2015). *Transforming our world: The 2030 agenda for sustainable development.* https://sustainabledevelopment.un.org/post2015/transformingourworld/publication

UNU-IHDP and UNEP (2014). *Inclusive wealth report 2014. Measuring progress toward sustainability.* Cambridge University Press.

For the benefit of digital users, indexed terms that span two pages (e.g., 52–53) may, on occasion, appear on only one of those pages.

Tables, figures, and boxes are indicated by *t*, *f*, and *b* following the page number